1972

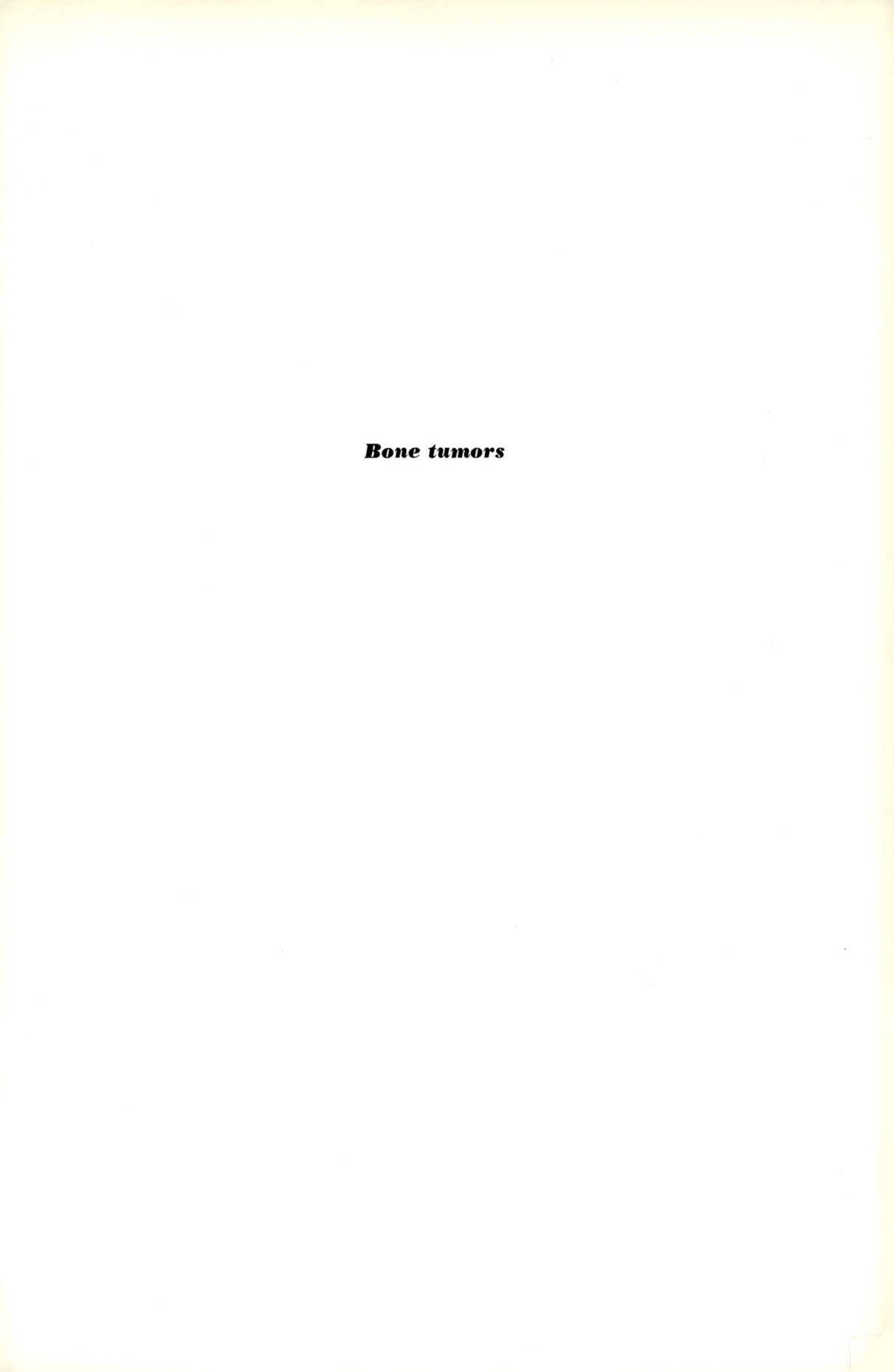

Bone tumors

FOURTH EDITION

BONE TUMORS

LOUIS LICHTENSTEIN, M.D.

Clinical Professor of Pathology, University of California, San Francisco
Professor Extraordinario, National University of Mexico
Honorary Member, Spanish Orthopedic Society (SECOT)
Honorary Member, Western Orthopedic Association
Fellow, New York Academy of Medicine
Consultant in Pathology, Orthopedic Department of St. Joseph's Hospital, San Francisco
Consultant in Pathology, Children's Hospital, San Francisco
Consultant in Pathology, U. S. Naval Hospital, Oakland
Consultant in Orthopedic Pathology, Mt. Zion Hospital and Medical Center, San Francisco

With 496 illustrations in 252 figures

THE C. V. MOSBY COMPANY
Saint Louis   1972

Fourth edition

Copyright © 1972 by The C. V. Mosby Company

All rights reserved. No part of this book may be reproduced in any manner without written permission of the publisher.

Previous editions copyrighted 1952, 1959, 1965

Printed in the United States of America

International Standard Book Number 0-8016-3004-5

Library of Congress Catalog Card Number 78-184330

Distributed in Great Britain by Henry Kimpton, London

To my son Bob
and
To my wife Stella

Preface to fourth edition

Six years pass quickly, and advances in the field make it desirable once again to revise *Bone Tumors*. In doing so, I wish to express my feeling of appreciation to my readers around the world, wherever they may be, who have kept the book in active circulation for two decades. The current literature even in this limited segment of oncology continues to expand like an accordion, but the efficient services of my medical librarian, Prudence H. Hamilton, have kept my assignment from becoming onerous.

The format of the book has been preserved, but scarcely a chapter has been left unchanged. A brief new chapter on certain rare primary tumors of bone not previously considered has been introduced, dealing notably with leiomyosarcoma and malignant mesenchymoma. A fresh concept of so-called adamantinoma of the tibia, and occasionally other bones, as dermal inclusion tumors has been presented. Also, recent observations on malignant change in occasional instances of chondroblastoma, chondromyxoid fibroma, and benign osteoblastoma have been duly noted. Although the size of the text has not been appreciably increased, some 40 new illustrations, mostly roentgenograms, have been added to graphically depict new or interesting facets of many subjects, with a view to enhancing the book's usefulness. These have all been selected from my consultation material.

As always, the book remains pragmatic, and the emphasis throughout is on accurate diagnosis as an essential basis for effective treatment and realistic prognosis.

Louis Lichtenstein
3903 Middlefield Road
Palo Alto, Calif. 94303

Preface to first edition

This book is the outgrowth of a long series of studies on primary tumors of bone pursued in collaboration with Dr. Henry L. Jaffe during the period 1938-1948, while working at the Hospital for Joint Diseases in New York. These investigations were based upon the accumulated material of the hospital, richly supplemented by case material from other sources, much of it referred for consultation. As a result, certain old ideas were of necessity revised and a number of new clinical, radiologic, and pathologic concepts were advanced, which found expression in individual papers dealing with many of the benign and malignant primary bone tumors and also with a number of non-neoplastic lesions of bone sometimes mistaken for tumors. To designate some of these distinctive lesions appropriately, new names had to be coined, such as benign chondroblastoma, chondromyxoid fibroma, non-osteogenic fibroma, fibrous dysplasia, eosinophilic granuloma, and aneurysmal bone cyst, which have since gained wide acceptance.

I have been repeatedly urged by my colleagues in pathology, radiology, and orthopedic surgery, particularly, to make the individually published papers dealing with bone tumors more readily available by incorporating their subject matter into a monograph. In the course of preparation of this book, the previously published articles have all been revised and brought up to date, while certain new sections dealing with subjects not previously covered; namely, osteogenic sarcoma; tumors of vascular, fat-cell, and nerve origin; so-called adamantinoma of limb bones; carcinoma metastatic to bone; and the skeletal manifestations of tumors of hematopoietic origin, have been added to enchance its usefulness and give more complete coverage of the field. Further, since as much mischief is done by overdiagnosis as by failure to recognize malignant tumors promptly, a section has been added as an appendix, dealing with certain non-neoplastic lesions of bone which are sometimes mistaken for tumors; e.g., fibrous dysplasia, eosinophilic granuloma, aneurysmal bone cyst, and myositis ossificans, among others. With this exception, no extraneous subjects have been introduced.

Emphasis has been placed throughout the book upon accurate diagnosis as a basis for appropriate treatment, through familiarity with the distinctive features of each of the neoplasms presented. The time is long since past when it might be said with some justification that the clinical history, the x-ray picture, or the response to treatment were more valuable than the pathologist's opinion. Inasmuch as the usefulness of some of the existing books in the field is seriously marred by pathologic inaccuracies, I have made it a special point to discuss or illustrate only cases in which I have had the opportunity personally to establish or verify the diagnosis by tissue examination. On the other hand, it is not intended to imply that the pertinent clinical data and the roentgenograms are not important in an analysis of the problem in diagnosis and therapy, although there are some pathologists naïve enough to believe that one can make sound recommendations in regard to treatment from a biopsy slide alone. In this book, illustrative roentgenograms have been freely utilized as a uniquely useful tool in determining the extent and topography of various skeletal lesions, and in judging their probable behavior on the basis of what they have done to the bone.

The relatively few blood chemical alterations that are of diagnostic importance have been considered in connection with each of the neoplasms concerned. It requires no lengthy dissertation to point out that in osteogenic sarcoma the serum alkaline phosphatase value is often elevated, that in approximately half the cases of multiple myeloma one observes hyperglobulinemia and/or hypercalcemia, that in carcinoma metastatic to the skeleton rapid demineralization may result in moderate hypercalcemia, and that in the case of prostatic carcinoma specifically, one commonly observes increased alkaline and acid phosphatase activity.

Problems in therapy have likewise been considered in relation to each of the neoplasms discussed. The emphasis throughout has been placed upon sound therapeutic indications, and beyond these, I do not feel that a competent surgeon needs to be told how to perform thorough curettement, resection, or amputation, any more than a skilled radiotherapist requires details of technique in most situations.

In the interest of clarity and conciseness, the regional treatment of bone tumors has been rejected as entailing unnecessary and confusing repetition. Further, no attempt has been made to employ considerations of embryologic development as window dressing, although a few specific allusions have been made when indicated. In the matter of bibliography, selected articles have been cited, and no attempt has been made to list all of the pertinent references. The literature pertaining to many of the bone tumors has become so voluminous, that it would be virtually impossible to catalogue it, even if it were desirable to do so.

I am indebted to Ruth Cordish and Lloyd Matlovsky for their painstaking illustrating in the matter of x-ray reproductions and photomicrographs; to Dr. Alex Griswold for his meticulous proofreading and general criticism of the text; and to my numerous colleagues and friends in pathology, radiology, and orthopedic surgery who have generously placed much of the interesting case material at my disposal. It would not have been possible to complete this book in its present form without their sustained interest and gracious cooperation.

Louis Lichtenstein

Los Angeles, California

Foreword to pathologists

It is my impression that standards in the reliable pathologic appraisal of tumors and tumorlike lesions of bone have risen perceptibly since the first edition of this book appeared. In correspondence with pathologists throughout the country seeking help with their problems in this field, I find fewer men who fail to display good insight and many more who are reasonably well informed but want moral support or encounter atypical tumors or mavericks, so to speak, for which they have no precedents in their own experience. With reference to these unusual cases, it has been my privilege to be of assistance in resolving some of the questions, and it is the accumulation and study of this valuable material that makes it possible in time to develop new concepts.

Although this is less complimentary, I feel obliged to stress once again that some pathologists still venture opinions having a bearing on treatment and prognosis (or expect me to do so) from slide interpretation alone, without fully realizing the collateral importance of the pertinent roentgenograms and of an adequate history, including the surgeon's findings. To function in this field simply as a slide reader without benefit of good clinical orientation can be disastrous at times, since the location of a lesion or what it has done to the bone (as a portent of its growth potential and probable behavior in the future) can conceivably be as significant as its cytologic picture. For example, the criteria outlined (Chapter 15) for the recognition of early chondrosarcomas apply strictly to central cartilage tumors of bone and not at all to the growing cartilage caps of osteochondromas in young patients, or to periosteal chondromas, or necessarily to extraskeletal cartilage tumors, which have a different natural history. To cite another instance in point, a lesion of myositis ossificans at the height of its activity may appear ominous enough cytologically to suggest osteogenic sarcoma, but only if one were uninformed as to the history and the location of the mass *outside* of the contiguous bone. One could go on in this vein, but suffice it to say that this is one branch of pathology in which effective medical communication is of prime importance.

Getting down to more mundane considerations, it may be in order to comment briefly on the problems of obtaining satisfactory bone sections. Altogether, I find that, while some laboratories turn out consistently good or excellent bone sections many more leave a great deal to be desired. By and large, a pathologist gets only as good a preparation from his tissue technician as he expects, and otherwise competent technicians can be taught to improve the quality of their bone preparations. Without going into details of procedure, a few practical suggestions may be helpful. Tissue blocks should be carefully trimmed, so as to be neither too large nor more than several millimeters in thickness, and here a band saw can often be used to advantage. Whenever possible, bits of soft tissue that do not require decalcification should be processed separately, since these afford the best cellular detail. Not infrequently one has to dig them out of the bone lesion with a knife point. Fixation in Zenker's solution often yields better results than conventional formalin fixation, but this is not essential. Also, irrespective of whether one uses nitric acid or formic acid (in adequate volume) for decalcification, perhaps speeded up by an electrode device, or whether one resorts to modern chelating agents, meticulous attention must be given to the determination of the earliest point of adequate decalcification. When a bone block can be readily pierced with a pin, it is usually ready for cutting. The time required obviously varies from specimen to specimen, so that assembly-line production methods will not do. Inadequate treatment causes shattering of cement lines when the block is cut, while overdecalcification (an equally common fault) tends to obscure cellular detail. In the matter of staining, my own preference is for a deep hematoxylin (Harris) and a relatively light eosin stain.

For the rapid diagnosis of bone tumors, the frozen section approach can often be used to advantage as a guide to the choice of appropriate surgical procedure, for a quick line on prognosis and, at times, to obviate delay in amputation when this is clearly indicated. It is essential to counterstain with eosin in addition to using a nuclear stain (hematoxylin is preferred), since otherwise it is possible to overlook patches of osteoid or new bone. However, one must be wary of jumping to serious conclusions from equivocal evidence, and sometimes it is prudent to wait for paraffin sections. Pathologists whose experience in this field is limited may be reluctant to accept responsibility for a frozen section diagnosis. I do not believe that they should be expected necessarily to do so.

The value of needle biopsy of bone lesions is a controversial subject that often engenders strong feelings. This approach to diagnosis has many strong adherents in Latin America (Argentina, especially) and some in this country, mainly in institutions with very large clinic populations and relatively few hospital beds, where they have made a virtue of necessity. My own impression is that the method has only limited usefulness when applied to bone tumors specifically, in lesions in vertebral bodies (provided the operator is skilled in localization), with foci of metastatic carcinoma (where the finding of even a few cell nests affords an unequivocal diagnosis), and in some few primary tumors of strikingly uniform cytology, such as myeloma or chordoma (in which one can often obtain a representative field of diagnostic value by random sampling). In most other situations, speaking quite candidly, I dislike needle biopsy and shy away from it (if there is any alternative) in the belief that the meager cytologic picture thus obtained is frequently not representative of the lesion as a whole, nor too informative, and may in fact be misleading as often as it is helpful. It's something like riding a bicycle with your hands tied behind your back: it's a good trick if you get away with it, but if you hit an obstacle, you're apt to fly over the handlebars and break your neck.

Louis Lichtenstein

Contents

1 General remarks on the clinical management of bone lesions that may be tumors, 1

2 General remarks on roentgenographic interpretation of skeletal lesions, 3

3 Classification of primary tumors of bone, 7

Tumors of cartilage-cell or cartilage-forming connective tissue derivation, 9
Tumors of osteoblastic connective tissue derivation, 11
Tumors of nonosteoblastic connective tissue derivation, 12
Tumors of mesenchymal connective tissue origin, 13
Tumors of hematopoietic origin, 13
Tumors of nerve origin, 13
Tumors of vascular origin, 14
Tumors of fat-cell origin, 14
Tumors of notochordal derivation, 14
Dermal inclusion tumors (so-called adamantinoma), 14
Tumors of smooth muscle origin, 14
Malignant mesenchymoma of bone, 15

4 Osteocartilaginous exostosis (osteochondroma), 17

Clinical features, 17
Pathologic observations, 19
Treatment and prognosis, 25
Summary, 28

5 Solitary enchondroma of bone; enchondromatosis, 29

Clinical features, 29
Roentgenographic picture, 32
Pathologic observations, 34
Treatment and prognosis, 36
Skeletal enchondromatosis, 38
Summary, 42

6 Benign chondroblastoma of bone, 45

Clinical features, 47
Pathology, 50
Treatment and prognosis, 53
Summary, 55

xv

xvi   Contents

7 Chondromyxoid fibroma of bone, 57

Clinical features, 58
Gross pathologic features and their roentgenographic reflection, 62
Microscopic appearance, 63
Treatment and prognosis, 67
Summary, 68

8 Unusual benign and malignant chondroid tumors of bone, 70

Poorly differentiated chondroid tumors, 74
Mesenchymal chondrosarcoma, 74
Chondroblastic sarcoma, 76
Multicentric chondroblastic sarcoma, 80
Atypical benign chondroblastoma, 82
Atypical chondromyxoid fibroma, 84
Summary, 88

9 Osteoid-osteoma, 89

Diagnosis, 90
Pathology, 94
Treatment and prognosis, 99
Summary, 100

10 Benign osteoblastoma, 103

Clinical features, 104
Pathologic features, 110
Differentiation from other lesions, 112
Treatment and prognosis, 117
Malignant change in osteoblastoma, 118
Summary, 119

11 Nonosteogenic fibroma of bone (nonossifying fibroma, metaphyseal fibrous defect, fibrous cortical defect), 121

Clinical features, 125
Roentgenographic findings, 128
Pathologic features, 128
Treatment, 132
Summary, 133

12 Giant-cell tumor of bone (osteoclastoma), 135

Clinical features, 138
Roentgenographic appearance, 143
Gross pathology, 144
Microscopic pathology, 147
Grading of giant-cell tumors, 150
Problems in therapy, 158
Summary, 163

13 Tumors of bone of vascular origin, 166

Hemangioma, 166
Malignant hemangioendothelioma, 173
Hemangiopericytoma (glomus), 177
Lymphangioma, 182

Contents   xvii

14 Tumors of nerve origin, 185

15 Chondrosarcoma of bone, 190

    Clinical features, 193
    Roentgenographic findings, 196
    Central chondrosarcoma, 196
    Peripheral chondrosarcoma, 198
    Extension and metastasis, 203
    Treatment, 208
    Summary, 212

16 Osteogenic sarcoma of bone, 215

    Clinical features, 217
    Roentgenographic appearance, 219
    Pathologic features, 220
    Sarcoma complicating Paget's disease, 228
    Osteogenic sarcoma developing in multicentric foci, 230
    Treatment and prognosis, 233
    Ossifying parosteal sarcoma (juxtacortical osteogenic sarcoma, parosteal osteogenic sarcoma, parosteal "osteoma"), 240

17 Fibrosarcoma of bone, 244

    Treatment and prognosis, 254
    Multicentric fibrosarcomas of bone, 254

18 Ewing's sarcoma, 256

    Clinical features, 259
    Roentgenographic findings, 261
    Pathologic features, 264
    Microscopic findings, 264
    Differentiation from neuroblastoma with skeletal metastases, 267
    Differentiation from carcinoma and other malignant tumors with skeletal involvement, 270
    Treatment and prognosis, 272

19 Plasma-cell myeloma (multiple myeloma), 277

    Clinical features, 280
    Problems of diagnosis, 284
    Skeletal alterations and their roentgenologic reflection, 285
    Hematologic observations of diagnostic importance, 287
    Significant biochemical changes in cases of multiple myeloma, 289
    Extraskeletal myelomatous infiltrations, 292
    Significant renal changes in cases of multiple myeloma, 294
    Amyloidosis in relation to multiple myeloma, 296
    Relationship of apparently solitary myeloma and multiple myeloma, 298
    Cytologic character of multiple myeloma, 301
    Treatment, 304
    Summary, 305

20 Skeletal manifestations of other tumors of hematopoietic origin, 311

    Chronic myeloid leukemia, 311
    Acute leukemias, 312
    "Lymphosarcoma," 315
    Primary reticulum-cell sarcoma of bone, 317
    Hodgkin's disease, 323

21 *Lipoma and liposarcoma of bone, 330*

22 *Chordoma, 335*

23 *Dermal inclusion tumors in bone (so-called adamantinoma of limb bones), 343*

24 *Other rare malignant tumors in bone, 349*

25 *Carcinoma metastatic to the skeleton, 352*

26 *Tumors of periosteal origin, 370*
Benign tumors, 371
Malignant tumors, 376

Appendixes

A *Some nonneoplastic lesions of bone that may be mistaken for tumors, 384*

B *Tumors of synovial joints, bursae, and tendon sheaths, 407*
Tumorlike lesions of debatable pathologic nature, 409
Benign tumors, 417
Malignant tumors, 420

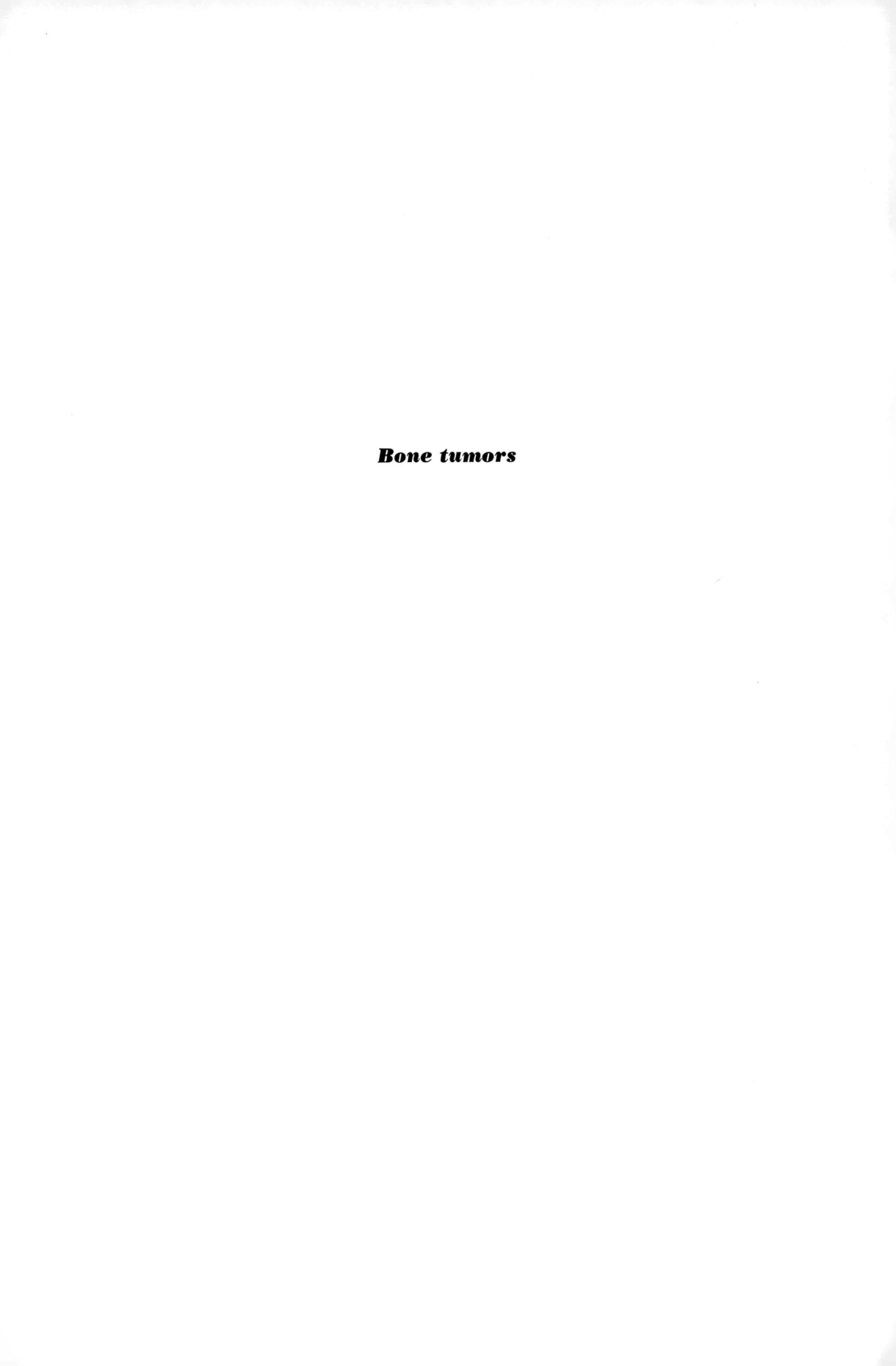

Bone tumors

Chapter 1

General remarks on the clinical management of bone lesions that may be tumors*

This brief introductory chapter seems to me to be as valid today as it was when it was first written almost twenty years ago, and it has therefore been retained without change in this fourth edition. The admonition is directed mainly toward physicians and surgeons who see bone tumors only occasionally or whose experience with them is still limited.

Before launching into specific details, it seems important at the outset for overall orientation to emphasize certain basic general principles entailed in the recognition and appropriate treatment of bone lesions that may be neoplasms. (If any of these views are restated in subsequent chapters, the repetition is intentional and deemed justified by the importance of the points stressed.)

1. If a patient complains of persistent pain, swelling, or limitation of motion in an extremity or some other skeletal part, obtain good roentgenograms promptly. If these disclose a significant skeletal lesion that may be neoplastic, do not guess at its interpretation but obtain a reliable opinion. Roentgenograms are essential in determining the extent and topography of various skeletal lesions and in judging their probable behavior on the basis of what they have done to the bone. It must be recognized, however, that radiologic interpretation has its inherent limitations and that, as a rule, biopsy is required for definitive diagnosis. Despite the impression that still prevails in some quarters, there are no pat formulas for the roentgen-ray diagnosis of bone tumors, and most of the allegedly pathognomonic signs, while sometimes helpful, are often fallacious (Chapter 2).

2. The problem in diagnosis should be analyzed before surgery is undertaken since the choice of procedure, whether it be conservative biopsy, curettement, resection, or amputation, varies with circumstances. Needle biopsy, incidentally, has only limited usefulness in the diagnosis of bone lesions. The planning of an advantageous approach often calls for good liaison between surgeon,

*Lichtenstein, L.: Primary malignant tumors of bone, CA, A Bulletin of Cancer Progress 4:12, 1954.

radiologist, and pathologist. While this principle appears self-evident and is generally recognized as sound, in actual practice some men pay only lip service to it and seek advice after the fat is already in the fire, so to speak. An important corollary is that the pathologist must be more than a slide reader, if he is to function efficiently in this field, and should have the benefit of good clinical orientation before venturing an opinion as to diagnosis and/or prognosis.

3. Definitive treatment, whether by surgery or irradiation, should be predicated upon accurate pathologic diagnosis. The time is long since past when it might be said with some justification that the clinical history, the roentgenogram, or the response to treatment was more valuable than the pathologist's opinion. I am unalterably opposed to blind irradiation of skeletal lesions believed to represent tumors, except perhaps for palliation of far-advanced malignant tumors in inaccessible sites. By the same token, I am categorically opposed to radical surgery undertaken on the strength of a roentgen-ray impression alone, however well founded it may seem. What appears to be an obvious osteogenic sarcoma, for example, justifying ablation of an extremity, may conceivably prove to be a lesion of sclerosing metastatic carcinoma.

4. If roentgen therapy is the treatment of choice for whatever reason, employ the smallest dose calculated to be effective, if only because of the potential hazard of postirradiation sarcoma (after a latent interval usually of five years or more).

5. In dealing with what appears to be a malignant bone tumor, before resorting to radical surgery, obtain expert opinion if there is any reasonable doubt in regard to the diagnosis of sarcoma. Apart from any medicolegal liability entailed, it is possible that the lesion is not so serious as you think. Thus, osteomyelitis may simulate Ewing's sarcoma on occasion, as may rapidly developing lesions of eosinophilic granuloma. Instances of aneurysmal bone cyst are occasionally mistaken for aggressive giant-cell tumors and sometimes for osteogenic sarcoma. With reference to lesions held to represent osteogenic sarcoma, one must be particularly careful to make certain that the condition does not represent some other less serious lesion exhibiting active new bone formation for whatever reason, e.g., periosteal ossification, myositis ossificans (in an active stage), ossifying hematoma, or exuberant callus. In the matter of recognizing and treating skeletal lesions in general, it is my impression that more mischief is done currently through overdiagnosis than through failure to recognize malignant tumors promptly.

6. If, on the other hand, the malignant nature of a bone lesion has been clearly established, treat it without undue delay and as aggressively as may be necessary. The result of compromise and temporizing (too little and too late) is usually complete therapeutic failure. In dealing with early chondrosarcoma, for example, delay many sometimes mean the difference between cure and ultimate fatality. This urgency may apply also to instances of central fibrosarcoma and primary reticulum-cell sarcoma, which can also be cured if they are appropriately treated before metastasis has developed.

Chapter 2

General remarks on roentgenographic interpretation of skeletal lesions

Radiologists today are much more sophisticated in regard to bone tumors and tumorlike lesions than they were some twenty years ago, and this introductory section therefore does not have quite the impact that it did when it was first written. The views expressed, however, seem to me to be still valid, and the chapter, therefore, has been retained in this fourth edition without significant change. It is directed mainly toward younger radiologists (and orthopedists) whose experience with skeletal lesions is still limited.

Despite the impression that once prevailed, there are no pat formulas for the roentgen diagnosis of bone tumors, and most of the allegedly pathognomonic signs, while sometimes helpful, are often fallacious. It is true, for example, that a sclerosing tumor in the lower end of a femur, which has obviously penetrated the cortex and provoked the formation of perpendicular radiopaque striations within the cuff of tumor tissue beneath the raised periosteum, will in all probability prove to be an osteogenic sarcoma. On the other hand, if a radiologist necessarily expects this distinctive appearance as a criterion for diagnosis, he is very likely to miss more than half of all the osteogenic sarcomas that he encounters, because the indications of new bone formation and of periosteal reaction to cortical perforation by tumor are often much more subtle. In fact, there are an appreciable number of osteogenic sarcomas, mainly of osteolytic type, whose roentgen appearance is so equivocal that it is hardly possible to venture any definitive diagnosis prior to biopsy, although one may perhaps suspect the presence of a malignant neoplasm. As for the particular sign commonly alluded to, not only is this not constant, as indicated, but it is also not actually specific. That is to say, the finding of perpendicular striae of periosteal new bone is not in itself an indication necessarily of osteogenic sarcoma, inasmuch as it may be observed on occasion as a reaction to the presence of metastatic carcinoma, Ewing's sarcoma, or even tuberculosis of the shaft of a long bone.

To cite another instance in point, while it is true that an occasional lesion of

Ewing's sarcoma may manifest reactive striations of periosteal new bone laid down parallel to the cortex (so-called "onionpeel" effect), most lesions will not present this appearance. Moreover, this pattern of periosteal new bone apposition, when present, is not in itself indicative necessarily of Ewing's sarcoma, for it may be observed at times with active osteomyelitis and even in an occasional instance of osteogenic sarcoma. Actually, the presenting lesion in a case of Ewing's sarcoma that is still in an early stage of its evolution is usually reflected roentgenographically by a vaguely mottled area of rarefaction without any clearly discernible periosteal reaction, so that it may not be readily distinguishable from a focus of osteomyelitis. In a more advanced stage, when the tumor has already broken through the cortex and produced an overlying soft tissue mass, its appearance will readily suggest a malignant neoplasm, although again this picture may not be at all distinctive and at times simulates that of osteogenic sarcoma.

Continuing in the same vein, the roentgenographic picture formerly held to characterize giant-cell tumor of bone, namely, that of an expanded lesion presenting a trabeculated pattern suggesting an agglomeration of "soap bubbles," is not the picture presented by most instances of (untreated) genuine giant-cell tumor. Actually, this allegedly pathognomonic sign is distinctly misleading. Most giant-cell tumors grow too rapidly to provoke the pattern indicated. The latter is much more likely to be encountered with other lesions (e.g., hemangioma, nonosteogenic fibroma, fibrous dysplasia, enchondroma, or chondromyxoid fibroma) that grow more slowly and therefore permit the development of reactive grooves and spurs on the endosteal surface of the attenuated cortex overlying the lesion. More significant insofar as a diagnosis of giant-cell tumor is concerned are the location of the area of rarefaction in the end of the affected limb bone (especially in a patient past the age of 15 years), thinning and expansion of the cortex particularly on one side, and the absence of periosteal new-bone formation over the thinned and expanded cortex. However, as indicated elsewhere, even these features are not infallible guides to the correct diagnosis, and it is important to recognize that on occasion a chondrosarcoma (which does not display telltale calcification), a central fibrosarcoma (which has not as yet broken through the cortex), or even a solitary focus of myeloma may produce a roentgen picture not readily distinguishable, with any degree of assurance at least, from that of giant-cell tumor. It follows as an obvious corollary that one must reserve judgment as to the diagnosis in such cases until an adequate biopsy has been examined. By the same token, the wisdom of the practice of instituting radiation therapy on the strength of a roentgen impression alone, unverified by biopsy, is open to serious criticism.

Still another instance in which an oft-repeated radiologic cliché may actually render a disservice relates to the emphasis placed upon the presence of multiple punched-out defects in many bones, and particularly the calvarium, as a distinguishing hallmark of multiple myeloma. While no one will deny that some cases of far-advanced myeloma present this picture, it is essential to bear in mind that others present merely vaguely defined rarefactions in a number of bones and that still others show widespread osteoporosis without any obvious localized defects (reflecting diffuse infiltration of the bone marrow by myeloma). Furthermore, as is now generally recognized, an appreciable number of cases of myeloma present a single sizable localized area of rarefaction (in the vertebral column, an innominate bone or a long bone, for example) as their initial manifestation, without any demonstrable roentgen evidence of involvement of the remainder of the skeleton. As for the calvarium in particular, this may fail to show outspoken involvement even in well-established cases of myeloma in which clear-cut defects are obvious in other bones. Moreover, the presence of multiple osteolytic defects in the skull is not in itself an indication necessarily of multiple myeloma, inasmuch as comparable defects may be observed occasionally with metastatic carcinoma.

The foregoing comment is not intended to detract from the great value of the roentgenographic findings as an indispensable clue to the diagnosis of tumors and tumorlike lesions of bone. On the contrary, it is intended to emphasize the necessity for objective interpretation rather than undue reliance upon outdated criteria that were not predicated upon sound pathologic correlation. As a basis for diagnosis, one must think in terms of the actual pathologic lesion at hand, its topography and location, its apparent rate of growth, and what it has done to the bone, and any attempt to operate in a world of shadows divorced from pathologic reality is fraught with hazard. It is of considerable value, incidentally, in sharpening one's diagnostic acumen to follow through by examining actual specimens obtained at surgery or autopsy and taking roentgenograms of these specimens and also of specimen slices as indicated for comparison with the clinical films.

In the interest also of an objective approach to problems in diagnosis, I wish to emphasize the importance of the use of precise language in describing the roentgen appearance of bone lesions in general as essential to clear thinking about them. For example, a circumscribed area of rarefaction is not necessarily a cyst, although it is often loosely designated as such. To be sure, such a lesion may actually contain fluid, but more often it is found on surgical exploration to be solidly filled with fibrous tissue, tumor cartilage, or some other type of tumor tissue. To cite another instance in point, certain lesions are often described as trabeculated, implying that they are traversed by osseous septa, when actually the effect observed reflects the projection on a flat plate of irregularities on the inner contour of the shell of bone delimiting the lesion peripherally.

It is essential also to bear in mind that roentgenographic interpretation has its inherent limitations, and that not infrequently even a skilled observer possessed of the essential clinical data must be content to record a tentative impression subject to verification by biopsy, or to suggest two or more plausible alternate possibilities. To cite a pertinent instance, an equivocal lesion in the upper shaft of a humerus of a child or a young adult may conceivably represent a focus of fibrous dysplasia, or an enchondroma (devoid of telltale calcific stippling), or a latent bone cyst that has moved away from the epiphyseal plate region. In such an instance it may be quite difficult prior to surgical exploration to forecast the precise nature of the lesion, and one does not lose face by admitting this.

Many advances have been made in the field of skeletal pathology in recent years and, specifically, many new lesions, both neoplastic and nonneoplastic, have been clearly delineated as clinical and pathologic entities. These new concepts must be gradually assimilated and, self-evident though this may seem, one must keep an open mind in regard to them. The dogmatism of a few radiologists saying, in effect, that if you disagree with me, you must be wrong, hardly seems justified or conducive to progress.

Finally, it is of the utmost importance to stress the basic principle that roentgen impressions of skeletal lesions should be verified by tissue examination before one proceeds with definitive treatment, whatever that may be. As indicated, I am strongly opposed to blind irradiation, except perhaps for palliation of an obviously advanced malignant neoplasm in an inaccessible site. If an open biopsy or surgical treatment is not contemplated for whatever reason, then at least one should resort to needle aspiration biopsy, whenever possible, in the hope (though not necessarily the expectation) that it may yield information of diagnostic value. As has already been noted, for example, a lesion in the lower end of a femur whose x-ray picture seems clearly to resemble that of a giant-cell tumor may on occasion prove to be a sarcoma requiring prompt ablation rather than irradiation. By the same token, I am categorically opposed to radical surgery undertaken on the strength of a roentgen diagnosis alone, however well founded it may seem. In this connection, I recall the pertinent instance of a tumor in the upper end of a humerus presenting all the roentgenographic features held to characterize osteogenic sarcoma, which proved on biopsy to represent a focus of metastatic carcinoma. It is a relatively simple matter in such cases to obtain a small bit of tumor tissue to confirm the clinical impression.

Chapter 3

Classification of primary tumors of bone

It appears logical to preface any treatise on tumors developing within bone with a classification, for, as Ewing has aptly stated, unless the surgeon or the pathologist is familiar with what *may* happen in bone, he is hardly able to recognize what *has* happened. It is true that a number of such classifications have already been advanced, but their usefulness is marred by pathologic inaccuracies, lack of completeness, or undue preoccupation with minor subdivisions of dubious significance and with theoretical considerations of histogenesis. I feel justified, therefore, in using my own listing of primary tumors appearing within bone as a structure and involving, at one time or another, not only the osseous tissue proper and the bone marrow, but also the supporting connective tissue along with its component nerves, blood vessels, and fat.

This classification (see table on page 8), reflecting current concepts, provides within its framework a place for all known primary neoplasms of bone including those recently delineated as pathologic entities, with the exception only of the odontogenic tumors and the comparatively uncommon tumors arising from the periosteum, whose biologic behavior sets them apart as a group unto themselves (Chapter 26). It includes the benign as well as the malignant primary tumors. When this classification was first drawn up (1951), a place was reserved for the malignant counterpart of each of the benign tumors, in the event that they might be observed subsequently. It has taken quite a few years, but some of these tumors that were postulated on theoretical grounds have now materialized, notably those resulting from malignant change in chondroblastoma, chondromyxoid fibroma, and benign osteoblastoma. The scheme has been made as streamlined as possible in the interest of clarity and conciseness and lists only neoplastic entities that have been described as such or that can be readily identified on pathologic examination, if one is familiar with them. To be sure, it reflects my personal views, and in some few debatable instances (e.g., Ewing's sarcoma of bone) necessarily entails arbitrary decisions as to histogenetic origin. Be that as it may, this classification is presented for consideration as a helpful working hypothesis, along with pertinent comment in support of the proposed

Classification of primary tumors of bone

	Benign tumors of bone		Malignant counterpart (if any)	Malignant tumors of bone (arising through malignant change or independently)
Of cartilage-cell or cartilage-forming connective tissue derivation	Peripheral	Osteocartilaginous exostosis (multiple exostosis)	Peripheral chondrosarcoma	Chondrosarcoma
	Central	Enchondroma (skeletal enchondromatosis)	Central chondrosarcoma	
		Benign chondroblastoma	Malignant (metastasizing) chondroblastoma	
		Chondromyxoid fibroma	Locally aggressive and frankly malignant tumors	
		Poorly differentiated chondroid tumors	Mesenchymal chondrosarcoma	
			Chondroblastic sarcoma	
Of osteoblastic derivation		Osteoma	(Not known)	Osteogenic sarcoma { Central, Parosteal }
		Osteoid-osteoma	(Not known)	
		Benign osteoblastoma	Osteogenic sarcoma	
Of nonosteoblastic connective tissue derivation		Desmoplastic fibroma	(Not known)	Fibrosarcoma
		Nonosteogenic fibroma	Fibrosarcoma	
		Least aggressive giant-cell tumors → More aggressive and malignant giant-cell tumors → Frankly malignant giant-cell tumors		
Of mesenchymal connective tissue origin		———		Ewing's sarcoma
Of hematopoietic origin		———		Multiple myeloma
				Chronic myeloid leukemia
				Acute leukemias { Reticulum-cell sarcoma, "Lymphosarcoma", Hodgkin's disease }
				Malignant lymphoma
Of nerve origin		Neurofibroma / Neurilemoma / Ganglioneuroma	Malignant schwannoma	
Of vascular origin		Hemangioma / Hemangiopericytoma (glomus)	Malignant hemangioendothelioma	Hemangioendothelioma
Of fat-cell origin		Lipoma		Liposarcoma
Of notochordal derivation		———		Chordoma
Of dermal derivation		———		Dermal inclusion tumors (so-called adamantinoma)
Of mixed mesenchymal origin		———		Malignant mesenchymoma

categories. In this book, it will serve as a framework of reference for the various benign and malignant primary neoplasms of bone which will be discussed in the chapters that follow.

Tumors of cartilage-cell or cartilage-forming connective tissue derivation

As indicated, the tumors that are composed of frank cartilage or that appear to be derived from cartilage-forming connective tissue are bracketed in this group. A significant distinction is maintained between those that develop peripherally as cartilage-capped exostoses (osteocartilaginous exostosis or osteochondroma) and those that develop centrally within the interior of the affected bone. The tendency manifested in the French and Italian literature, particularly, to lump together the osteocartilaginous exostoses and the enchondromas as related expressions of a vague category of so-called "osteogenic disease" is strongly to be deprecated as seeking to obliterate well-established and useful distinctions.

In regard to *osteocartilaginous exostoses,* which, as is well known, may be solitary or multiple (hereditary multiple exostosis[17]), one can maintain with some cogency that they actually represent an expression of a skeletal developmental anomaly. While that is true, they are undoubtedly tumors in a clinical sense and, moreover, in the case of multiple exostoses at least, they not infrequently give rise to chondrosarcoma through activated growth of their cartilage caps. Incidentally, such peripheral chondrosarcomas are sometimes mislabeled as instances of osteogenic sarcoma, owing to the fact that the older portion of the tumor, particularly, is likely to be rather heavily calcified and ossified.

The most frequently encountered benign central cartilage tumor is the common *enchondroma,*[23] which is composed of facets of mature hyaline cartilage. Occasionally, especially when it is situated within a long bone, it may undergo malignant change and insidious conversion to central chondrosarcoma.[31] As is well known also, enchondromas may be multiple (skeletal enchondromatosis) and at times exhibit a tendency to monomelic or predominantly unilateral distribution (Ollier's disease). In such cases, the tendency to malignant transformation is rather strong, and the development of chondrosarcoma in some one, or even two or more, cartilage foci simultaneously, is not unusual. On the other hand, one may of course encounter instances of fully evolved central chondrosarcoma in which there is no evidence to indicate that the neoplasm developed on the basis of a preexisting enchondroma.

Also included in this group is the tumor formerly regarded as the calcifying or chondromatous variant of giant-cell tumor, which Jaffe and I[19] have designated as *benign chondroblastoma of bone.* Its recognition is of some practical importance, inasmuch as instances of it are sometimes overdiagnosed as chondrosarcoma or even osteogenic sarcoma, with the attendant recommendation of ablation. The distinctive pathologic and clinical features that set it apart from genuine giant-cell tumors and justify its inclusion among the bone tumors derived from cartilage-forming connective tissue have been emphasized elsewhere.[34] For the reasons indicated, and also because the capital epiphysis of the humerus is one of its less common sites of origin, the eponym *Codman's tumor* is avoided. This peculiar neoplasm responds satisfactorily to thorough curettement, and I have not observed any instances of aggressiveness or spontaneous malignant change, although a few such instances have been recorded in recent literature.

Still another tumor that seems clearly to belong in this category, though not composed of full-fledged hyaline cartilage, is the distinctive benign tumor which Jaffe and I[20,29] christened *chondromyxoid fibroma of bone* in 1948. This tumor also is likely to be mistaken for chondrosarcoma or myxosarcoma if one is not familiar with it. Occasionally it may recur locally after curettement, especially in children. The malignant counterpart of this neoplasm is comparatively rare. As indicated elsewhere, the tumor is usually encountered in a bone of a lower limb, although instances of it have been observed in other sites. It has been interpreted as a peculiarly differentiated connective tissue tumor exhibiting, in the course of its evolution, certain chondroid and also myxoid traits that hallmark the lesion cytologically.

Apart from benign chondroblastoma and chondromyxoid fibroma, there is a gamut of peculiar tumors of bone designated as chondroid for convenient reference, which exhibit in common subtle or more obvious indications of cartilage-forming connective tissue derivation. These are discussed in Chapter 8. Some are poorly differentiated or mesenchymal and show only focal areas of cartilage and chondroid matrix microscopically. Another clinically important group has been interpreted as low-grade chondroblastic sarcoma. This category of benign and malignant chondroid tumors of bone is one that requires further exploration, and we still have much to learn about it.

It is pertinent at this point to comment briefly upon the question of the existence of primary tumors that may be appropriately designated as myxoma or myxosarcoma of bone and to indicate why no provision has been made for categorizing such tumors in the proposed classification. It is true that Bloodgood[2] reported a number of tumors under this head, but his pathologic data afford only the vaguest indication of what he may actually have been dealing with. One of his illustrated cases may conceivably have represented an instance of chondromyxoid fibroma of bone, while some others that had more serious consequences may well have been chondrosarcomas. It is well known that chondrosarcomas, especially the larger ones, may undergo degeneration and cystic softening in places, and that such areas may present a myxoid appearance histologically. This tendency apparently accounts for the listing in Ewing's classification of "myxosarcoma" as a subgroup in the "chondroma series." I see no valid reason to so dignify a minor secondary feature that does not alter the clinical behavior of the tumor, or its basic character, and, for the same reason, I abjure such confusing combination names as chondromyxosarcoma. In dealing with osteogenic sarcoma also, one may occasionally observe fields of malignant myxoid connective tissue, especially at the periphery, although not in the more representative, central portion of the neoplasm. The designation of "myxoma" has also been applied to certain tumorlike, myxoid connective tissue lesions in jaw bones particularly. It should be noted also that Stout in his A.F.I.P. fascicle on tumors of the soft tissues makes mention in passing (F5-79) of myxomas in bones "where curettage has sometimes resulted in lasting cures," but without further details it is difficult to surmise precisely what he was referring to. As for the tumor reported as "myxoma of bone" by Bauer and Harrell (1954), this seems clearly to represent an instance of chondromyxoid fibroma, as do also the tumors reported as such by Scaglietti and Stringa.

Tumors of osteoblastic connective tissue derivation

The name *osteoma* is a much abused one, which is often employed to characterize a miscellaneous group of lesions, some of which are not even neoplastic. Thus, it has been used loosely to denote burned-out osteochondromas in which the cartilage cap has involuted, bony spurs induced by trauma or inflammatory reaction, the condition of hyperostosis frontalis interna, as well as certain lesions of fibrous dysplasia developing in the facial and jaw bones particularly. Further, the eburnated, localized, single or multiple hyperostoses that one occasionally observes on the calvarium have also been called osteomas. These are generally fully evolved bony protuberances by the time one has occasion to examine them, and there is no way of telling at this stage whether they had their origin in neoplastic osteoblastic activity. In this classification, in keeping with current usage, the term *osteoma* is restricted specifically to the designation of certain bony growths of appreciable size, which arise particularly in the bones of the skull preformed in membrane, and are rather prone to extend into the orbit or into one or another of the paranasal sinuses. On rare occasions, one may observe comparable tumors in other bones as well. Cytologically, these growths are composed essentially of osteoblastic connective tissue, forming abundant osteoid and new bone, which may eventually become rather compact and mature.

Osteoid-osteoma

Osteoid-osteoma is now widely accepted as a distinct entity, although some observers apparently still are not certain that the lesion represents a genuine neoplasm. Jaffe and I[18,22] have already stated the reasons for interpreting this lesion as a peculiar benign tumor, rather than the result of infection or some other nonneoplastic reparative process, and nothing would be gained by reiterating them here. It is true that the incipient phase of the lesion requires further elucidation, and that in some early cortical lesions, particularly, one may still observe a residual focus of peculiarly condensed and reconstructed original bone undergoing invasion and resorption by osteoblastic connective tissue. When fully evolved, this nidus is composed essentially of a highly vascularized substratum of osteogenic connective tissue that is actively depositing osteoid matrix and trabeculae of atypical new bone. This can be plausibly interpreted as a neoformation despite its relatively small size, as a rule. Occasional osteoid-osteomas may attain substantial size and measure as much as 5 or 6 cm. in their long axis.

Benign osteoblastoma

Benign osteoblastoma is a category that includes certain osteoid- and bone-forming tumors, other than osteoma, so-called, and classical osteoid-osteoma. These benign osteoblastic tumors include the ones previously called osteogenic fibroma, as well as those referred to provisionally as "other osteoid tissue-forming tumors" in my earlier classification of primary tumors of bone. The designation of "giant osteoid osteoma" introduced by Dahlin and Johnson (Chapter 10) has reference to the same category. Their recognition is of practical importance in that they may be mistaken for giant-cell tumor, though without sound justification, or for osteogenic sarcoma and as such be treated more aggressively than their benign nature requires. Spontaneous malignant change in osteoblastoma to osteosarcoma has been noted, but this is rather unusual.

Tumors of nonosteoblastic connective tissue derivation

The rather common benign connective tissue growth designated as *nonosteogenic fibroma*[21] is one that was delineated in 1942. As the name implies, the lesion is interpreted as a benign neoplasm derived from mature marrow connective tissue that exhibits no tendency to bone formation. The extensive roentgenographic studies of Caffey would seem to indicate that "benign cortical defects" are a milder, evanescent expression of the same lesion. However one interprets the lesion, it represents a clear-cut clinical and pathologic entity, easily recognized roentgenographically in most instances and readily identified by tissue examination. Cytologically, it presents a distinctive pattern of whorled bundles of spindle-shaped connective tissue cells, interspersed among which there are occasional small, compressed multinuclear giant cells. In some pertinent lesions, though by no means all, areas containing foam-cell aggregates may make their appearance, apparently as a secondary feature.

The propriety of listing *giant-cell tumor of bone* among the tumors composed of connective tissue cells that are not bone-forming is now generally accepted, regardless of what special significance one attaches to the multinuclear cells that hallmark the lesion cytologically. I have no serious objection in principle to the name *osteoclastoma* preferred by British physicians, although the designation of giant-cell tumor is so firmly rooted in the American literature that one can never hope to displace it. Be that as it may, if one adheres to a strict definition[24,30] of what should be regarded as giant-cell tumor and strips away all of the alleged variants so-called, then what is left constitutes a formidable neoplasm. It has become increasingly evident that, while giant-cell tumors are not necessarily "sarcomas," neither are they all "benign," and that, with respect to potential seriousness, they may run the whole gamut from one extreme to the other. There appears to be substantial agreement, among pathologists at least, that, while many giant-cell tumors are successfully treated by thorough curettement or irradiation, some are undoubtedly aggressive and prone to recur, and occasional ones behave like frank sarcomas.[41] An occasional giant-cell tumor is found to be malignant on initial tissue examination, but more often one has to reckon with malignant change incidental to one or more local recurrences.

Tumors of mesenchymal connective tissue origin

By listing Ewing's sarcoma under this heading, I[32] take my stand with those who accept this malignant neoplasm as a tumor entity, distinct and apart from primary reticulum-cell sarcoma of bone marrow[36] (though freely conceding, as Willis maintains, that the diagnosis is often applied uncritically to instances of other tumors, especially carcinoma and neuroblastoma metastatic to the skeleton, and malignant lymphoma involving the bone marrow primarily). At the same time, like many pathologists, I no longer accept Ewing's contention that the tumor is of endothelial origin. I am more inclined to the belief that the tumor cells are probably derived from the undifferentiated mesenchymal connective tissue framework of the marrow, and that, in most instances, the neoplasm is of multicentric origin, thus accounting for its grave prognosis despite prompt radical surgery or effective irradiation of the presenting skeletal tumor focus.

Tumors of hematopoietic origin

Under this heading there are listed the various neoplasms that are derived from the blood-forming cells of the bone marrow. These tend to become more or less systematized and to involve the hematopoietic organs generally, although occasional ones (e.g., certain instances of myeloma[33] and malignant lymphoma[11]) may appear initially within a single bone and apparently remain localized there for some time. These tumors of hematopoietic origin include multiple myeloma, chronic myeloid leukemia, the acute leukemias, and the various expressions of malignant lymphoma, namely, reticulum-cell sarcoma,[36,38] lymphoblastic and lymphocytic lymphoma (lymphosarcoma[11]), and Hodgkin's disease.[10,39]

Tumors of nerve origin

This category provides a place for the very occasional neurofibromas[45] and neurilemomas (neurinoma, schwannoma[7,13,37]) that have been encountered within bone. These neoplasms are apparently derived from the connective tissue cells or the Schwann cells of nerves that accompany the nutrient blood vessels of bone. While there has been no comprehensive description to date of malignant schwannomas developing within bone (rather than invading it secondarily), there is no reason a priori why such neoplasms should not arise there occasionally, and, hence, a niche has been provided for them. I have refrained from using the designation *neurogenic sarcoma* in this connection, in keeping with the sharp contention of Stout[42] that there is no sound basis for the supposition that there is a special variety of nerve fibrosarcoma that can be designated a "neurogenic sarcoma." An apparently unique instance of mature ganglioneuromas in multiple bone sites has been recorded (Chapter 14). There are also observations indicating that neuroblastoma metastases in bone (and other sites) may mature as ganglioneuromas in children who survive long enough for this to happen.

Tumors of vascular origin

The simple plexiform and cavernous hemangiomas require no particular comment in this connection, except perhaps to point out that they occur rather infrequently in bone. Several instances of glomus tumor arising within bone are now on record,[26] as well as a few less differentiated hemangiopericytomas (Chapter 13). As for the malignant neoplasms, a limited number of more or less aggressive hemangioendotheliomas of bone have been recorded. Apparently none of these developed through malignant change in a previously benign hemangioma of bone in the course of its clinical observation, although I have seen this happen after irradiation. In the matter of nomenclature, the designation of malignant hemangioendothelioma is preferred to angiosarcoma or angioblastic sarcoma. Lymphangioma is seldom encountered in bone; more often, one sees multiple foci there as part of a congenital systemic disorder.

Tumors of fat-cell origin

Although the development of a lipoma within fatty bone marrow should occasion no great surprise, for some reason or other such tumors are comparatively rare. However, a number of convincing cases with illustrations have been recorded in recent years (Chapter 21). The existence of primary liposarcoma of bone has also been firmly established.

Tumors of notochordal derivation

It is generally accepted that chordoma develops by neoplastic proliferation of notochordal vestiges situated within the nucleus pulposus of intervertebral discs or, occasionally, within one or more vertebral bodies.

Dermal inclusion tumors (so-called adamantinoma)

The histogenesis of this category of so-called adamantinomas is a problem that requires a fresh point of view. There is general agreement that the resemblance of these tumors to adamantinoma of jaw bones is a superficial one. It is apparent also that over the years a variety of neoplasms have been dumped into this category mainly because they happened to arise in the tibia. If the hemangioendotheliomas and mesenchymal sarcomas (and possibly other tumors) that do not really belong there are stripped away, then one is left with a hard core of distinctive neoplasms that may be appropriately designated as dermal inclusion tumors. Many of them resemble basal-cell carcinoma; some of them contain squamous-cell nests; and occasional ones are reminiscent of adnexal skin tumors of sweat gland origin. It seems logical to postulate that they have their origin in misplaced embryonal rests (the old Cohnheim theory).

Tumors of smooth muscle origin

A few primary leiomyosarcomas in bone have been observed (Chapter 24), presumably arising from proliferating smooth muscle cells in the media of a blood vessel.

Malignant mesenchymoma of bone

This unusual category of malignant tumors in bone comprises those with two or more different mesenchymal components (Chapter 24). Liposarcoma and osteogenic sarcoma appear to be a favorite combination, but others have also been noted.

References

1. Bergstrand, H.: Ueber eine eigenartige, wahrscheinlich bisher nicht beschriebene osteoblastische Krankheit in den langen Knochen der Hand und des Fusses, Acta Radiol. 11:597, 1930.
2. Bloodgood, J. C.: Bone tumors, myxoma, Ann. Surg. 80:817, 1924.
3. Budd, J. W., and Macdonald, I.: A modified classification of bone tumors, Radiology 40:586, 1943.
4. Changus, G. W., and Stewart, F. W.: Malignant angioblastoma of bone. A reappraisal of adamantinoma of long bone, Cancer 10:540, 1957.
5. Coley, B. L.: Neoplasms of bone and related conditions: their etiology, pathogenesis, diagnosis, and treatment, New York, 1949, Paul B. Hoeber, Inc., pp. 14-15.
6. Dawson, E. K.: Liposarcoma of bone, J. Path. Bact. 70:513, 1955.
7. DeSanto, D. A., and Burgess, E.: Primary and secondary neurilemmoma of bone, Surg. Gynecol. Obstet. 71:454, 1940.
8. Ewing, J.: The classification and treatment of bone sarcoma. Report of the International Conference on Cancer, London, 1928, New York, 1928, William Wood & Co., pp. 365-376.
9. Ewing, J.: A review of the classification of bone tumors, Surg. Gynecol. Obstet. 68:971, 1939.
10. Falconer, E. H., and Leonard, M. E.: Skeletal lesions in Hodgkin's disease, Ann. Intern. Med. 29:1115, 1948.
11. Gall, E. A., and Mallory, T. B.: Malignant lymphoma; a clinicopathologic survey of 618 cases, Am. J. Pathol. 18:381, 1942.
12. Geschickter, C. F., and Copeland, M. M.: Tumors of bone, ed. 3, Philadelphia, 1949, J. B. Lippincott Co., p. 27.
13. Gross, P., Bailey, F. R., and Jacox, H. W.: Primary intramedullary neurofibroma of the humerus, Arch. Pathol. 28:716, 1939.
14. Haas, S. L.: In Dean Lewis' Practice of surgery, Hagerstown, Md., 1927, W. F. Prior Co., Inc., vol. 2, p. 15.
15. Hatcher, C. H.: The diagnosis of bone sarcoma, Rocky Mt. Med. J. 45:968, 1948.
16. Hicks, J. D.: Synovial sarcoma of tibia, J. Path. Bact. 67:151, 1954.
17. Jaffe, H. L.: Hereditary multiple exostosis, Arch. Pathol. 36:335, 1943.
18. Jaffe, H. L.: Osteoid-osteoma of bone, Radiology 45:319, 1945.
19. Jaffe, H. L., and Lichtenstein, L.: Benign chondroblastoma of bone. A re-interpretation of the so-called calcifying or chondromatous giant-cell tumor, Am. J. Pathol. 18:969, 1942.
20. Jaffe, H. L., and Lichtenstein, L.: Chondromyxoid fibroma of bone. A distinctive benign tumor likely to be mistaken especially for chondrosarcoma, Arch. Pathol. 45:541, 1948.
21. Jaffe, H. L., and Lichtenstein, L.: Non-osteogenic fibroma of bone, Am. J. Pathol. 18:205, 1942.
22. Jaffe, H. L., and Lichtenstein, L.: Osteoid-osteoma: further experience with this benign tumor of bone, with special reference to cases showing the lesion in relation to shaft cortices and commonly misclassified as instances of sclerosing nonsuppurative osteomyelitis or cortical-bone abscess, J. Bone Joint Surg. 22:645, 1940.
23. Jaffe, H. L., and Lichtenstein, L.: Solitary benign enchondroma of bone, Arch. Surg. 46:480, 1943.
24. Jaffe, H. L., Lichtenstein, L., and Portis, R. B.: Giant-cell tumor of bone. Its pathologic appearance, grading, supposed variants and treatments, Arch. Pathol. 30:993, 1940.
25. Jaffe, H. L., and Mayer, L.: An osteoblastic osteoid tissue-forming tumor of a metacarpal bone, Arch. Surg. 24:550, 1932.
26. Lattes, R., and Bull, D. C.: A case of glomus tumor with primary involvement of bone, Ann. Surg. 127:187, 1948.
27. Lederer, A., and Sinclair, A. J.: Malignant synovioma simulating "adamantinoma of tibia," J. Path. Bact. 67:163, 1954.
28. Lichtenstein, L.: Benign osteoblastoma. A category of osteoid and bone-forming tumors other than classical osteoid-osteoma, which may be mistaken for giant-cell tumor or osteogenic sarcoma, Cancer 9:1044, 1956.

29. Lichtenstein, L.: Chondromyxoid fibroma of bone, Am. J. Pathol. **24**:686 (Abstr.), 1948.
30. Lichtenstein, L.: Giant-cell tumor of bone. Current status of problems in diagnosis and treatment, J. Bone Joint Surg. **33-A**: 143, 1951.
31. Lichtenstein, L., and Jaffe, H. L.: Chondrosarcoma of bone, Am. J. Pathol. **19**: 553, 1943.
32. Lichtenstein, L., and Jaffe, H. L.: Ewing's sarcoma of bone, Am. J. Pathol. **23**:43, 1947.
33. Lichtenstein, L., and Jaffe, H. L.: Multiple myeloma. A survey based on thirty-five cases, eighteen of which came to autopsy, Arch. Pathol. **44**:207, 1947.
34. Lichtenstein, L., and Kaplan, L.: Benign chondroblastoma of bone. Unusual localization in femoral capital epiphysis, Cancer **2**:793, 1949.
35. Luck, J. V.: Bone and joint diseases. Pathology correlated with roentgenological and clinical features, Springfield, Ill. 1950, Charles C Thomas, Publisher, pp. 439-440, 484-485.
36. Parker, F., Jr., and Jackson, H., Jr.: Primary reticulum cell sarcoma of bone, Surg. Gynecol. Obstet. **68**:45, 1939.
37. Peers, J. H.: Primary intramedullary neurogenic sarcoma of ulna, Am. J. Pathol. **10**: 811, 1934.
38. Sherman, R. S., and Snyder, R. E.: The roentgen appearance of primary reticulum cell sarcoma of bone, Am. J. Roentgenol. **58**:291, 1947.
39. Steiner, P. E.: Hodgkin's disease; the incidence, distribution, nature and possible significance of the lymphogranulomatous lesions in the bone marrow, Arch. Pathol. **36**:627, 1943.
40. Stewart, F. W.: Primary liposarcoma of bone, Am. J. Pathol. **7**:87, 1931.
41. Stewart, F. W., Coley, B. L., and Farrow, J. H.: Malignant giant cell tumor of bone, Am. J. Pathol. **14**:515, 1938.
42. Stout, A. P.: Fibrosarcoma, the malignant tumor of fibroblasts, Cancer **1**:30, 1948.
43. Stout, A. P.: Hemangiopericytoma. A study of twenty-five new cases, Cancer **2**:1027, 1949.
44. Stout, A. P.: Tumor Seminar, J. Missouri M. A., pp. 259-291, April, 1949 (see p. 280).
45. Uhlmann, E., and Grossman, A.: von Recklinghausen's neurofibromatosis with bone manifestations, Ann. Intern. Med. **14**:225, 1940.
46. Wheelock, M. C.: The pathology of bone tumors, J. Iowa Med. Soc. **38**:522, 1948.
47. Willis, R. A.: Pathology of tumours, London, 1948, Butterworth & Co., Ltd., p. 670.

Chapter 4

Osteocartilaginous exostosis (osteochondroma)

It seems appropriate to begin a discussion of benign tumors of bone with osteocartilaginous exostosis or osteochondroma, as it is often designated, since the latter is by far the most common of the benign tumors. It may be encountered on practically any bone preformed in cartilage, but is observed most often on the long limb bones and, particularly, their metaphyseal regions. As is well known, the lesion may be solitary or multiple (hereditary multiple exostosis). Since solitary osteochondroma may be regarded as a limited expression or *forme fruste* of hereditary multiple exostosis[5] that represents a systematized anomaly of skeletal development, one may question the propriety of regarding the growth as a genuine neoplasm. However, since it is undoubtedly a tumor in the clinical sense and may on occasion give rise to peripheral chondrosarcoma through activated growth of its cartilage cap, it appears logical to so classify it.

Whether single or multiple, an osteocartilaginous exostosis represents, as its name implies, a cartilage-capped bony growth protruding from the surface of the affected bone. At the site of the exostosis the cortical bone is defective and the bony mass constituting the bulk of the exostosis merges with the underlying spongiosa. The lesion appears to have its basis essentially in perverted activity of the periosteum that tends to form anomalous foci of metaplastic cartilage. These cartilage foci by continued growth and endochondral ossification may give rise to manifest exostoses. It seems not unlikely, furthermore, as Keith[7] has expounded, that defective modeling of the bone (diaphyseal aclasis) contributes to the broadening and blunting of the affected metaphyseal region. This is a feature that one is more likely to observe in cases of multiple exostosis. The present discussion will be concerned mainly with the lesion in its solitary form. For detailed consideration of hereditary multiple exostosis the reader is referred to a comprehensive article by Jaffe[5] dealing with that subject. A more recent, heavily illustrated article of clinical and pathologic value is that of Bethge.[2]

Clinical features
Sex and age incidence

A series of over 200 hospital cases that I have analyzed indicates that there is apparently no significant difference in sex incidence and that, in regard to age incidence, the condition in the great majority of instances manifests itself clinically during adolescence or childhood and occasionally even in infancy. Approximately four fifths of the patients operated upon were under 21 years of age.

Clinical complaints

The slow growth of the tumor and the lack of serious disability induced by it are reflected in the comparatively long interval that usually elapses between the recognition of the bony protuberance by the patient and the time he seeks surgical treatment, for whatever reason. Occasionally, an osteochondroma may become painful as it enlarges, especially on motion of the affected part. Sometimes following trauma, one may observe a fracture through the stalk of an exostosis. In particular, osteochondromas springing from the ankle and foot bones may occasion difficulty on walking or wearing shoes. Not infrequently, patients become concerned for cosmetic reasons or because of fear of cancer.

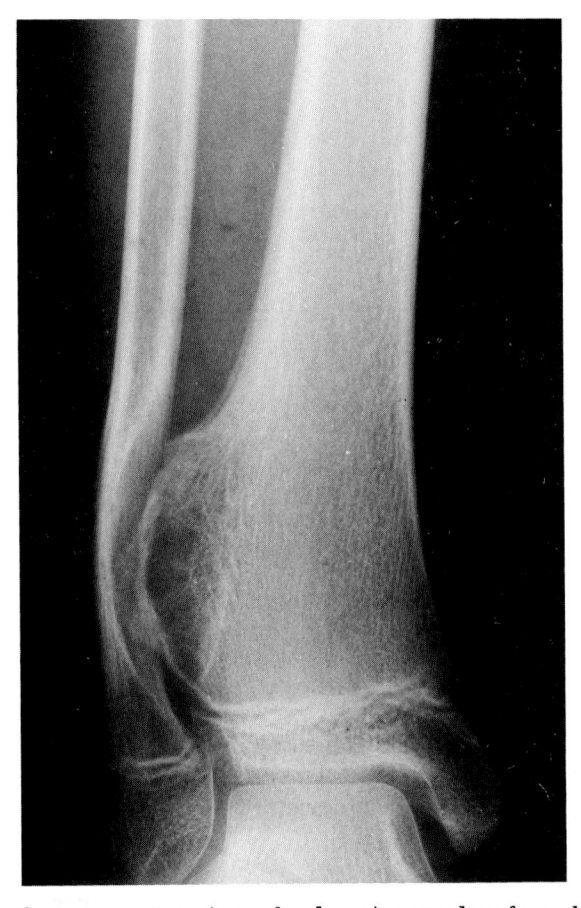

Fig. 4-1. Osteocartilaginous exostosis (osteochondroma) protruding from the lower end of a tibia and gouging out a defect in the contiguous fibula.

Finally, osteocartilaginous exostoses that have become quite large may cause difficulty through pressure on impinged nerves, as in the case illustrated in Fig. 4-5 and in the remarkable instance reported by Gokay and Bucey[4] in which a bulky osteochondroma of the lumbar vertebral column caused symptoms of compression of the cauda equina. In another unusual case reported recently by Chiurco,[3] fatal spinal cord compression ensued.

Localization

Although osteochondromas not infrequently spring from flat bones (rib, scapula, clavicle, iliac bone, or the spinous process of a vertebral body), they are most often encountered, as noted, on the long tubular bones. By far the commonest locations are the lower metaphysis of the femur and the upper metaphysis of the tibia.

Pathologic observations

An osteocartilaginous exostosis, as indicated, is a sessile or stalked bony protuberance of variable size and contour, jutting from the affected bone. The sessile exostoses may be plateaulike, or roughly hemispheric, or cauliflower-like with a rather knobby surface. The same variation in contour pattern also holds for many of the stalked exostoses with comparatively short stems. On the other hand, some of the more tubular or conical exostoses may present pronged or spiked ends.

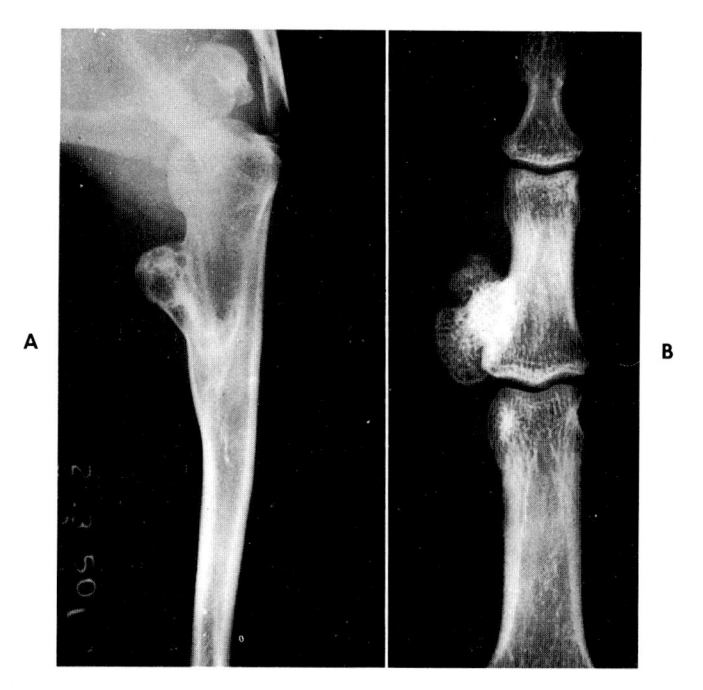

Fig. 4-2. A, Roentgenogram of another solitary exostosis springing from the upper end of a humerus. B, Roentgenogram of an unusual osteochondroma of a phalanx of a finger.

20 Bone tumors

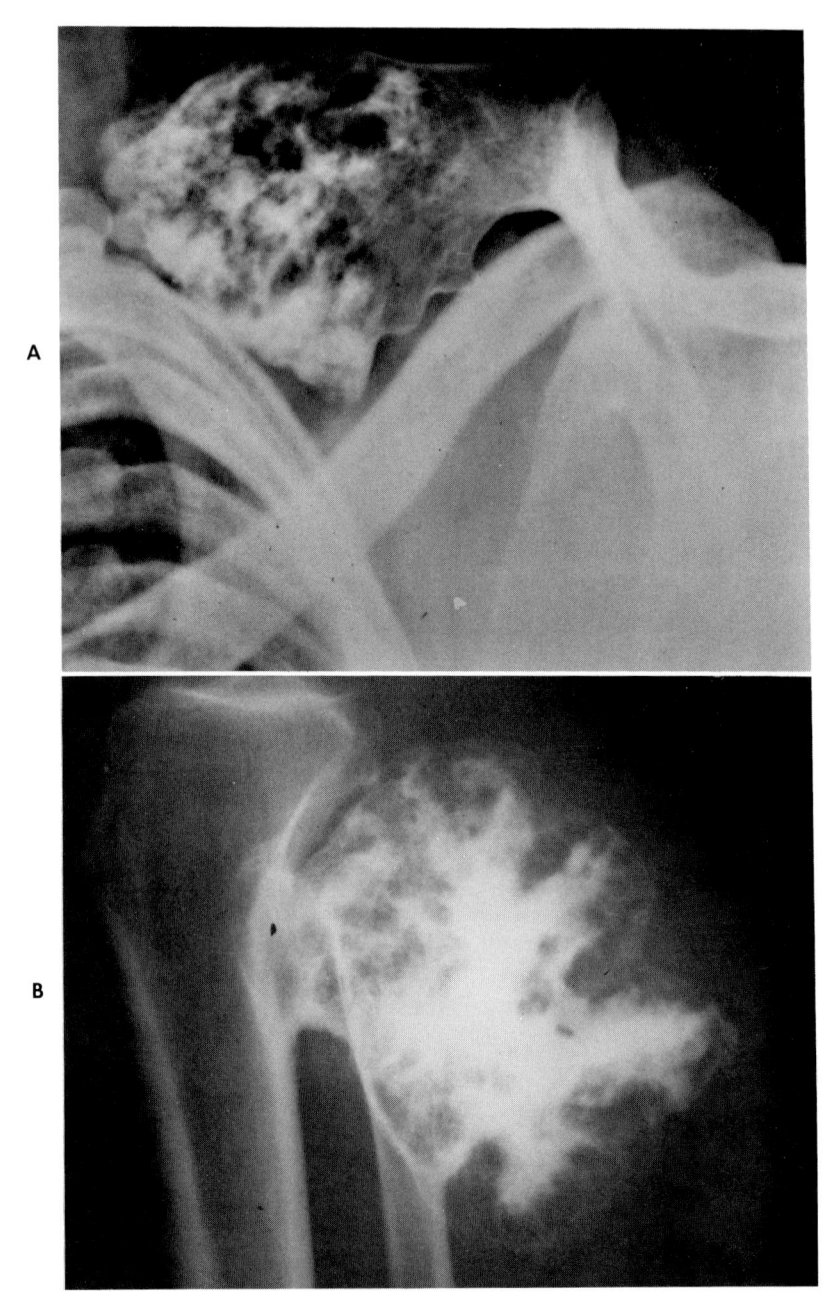

Fig. 4-3. A, Roentgenogram of a stalked osteochondroma springing from a scapula. The mottled radiopacity reflects faulty resorption and reconstruction of calcified and ossified cartilage beneath the cap. **B,** Roentgenogram of a comparable, large osteochondroma arising from the upper fibula. Its huge size and the heavy calcification and ossification should not be interpreted as portents of malignant change. Note that the periphery of the exostosis is well outlined and shows no indication of recent active growth.

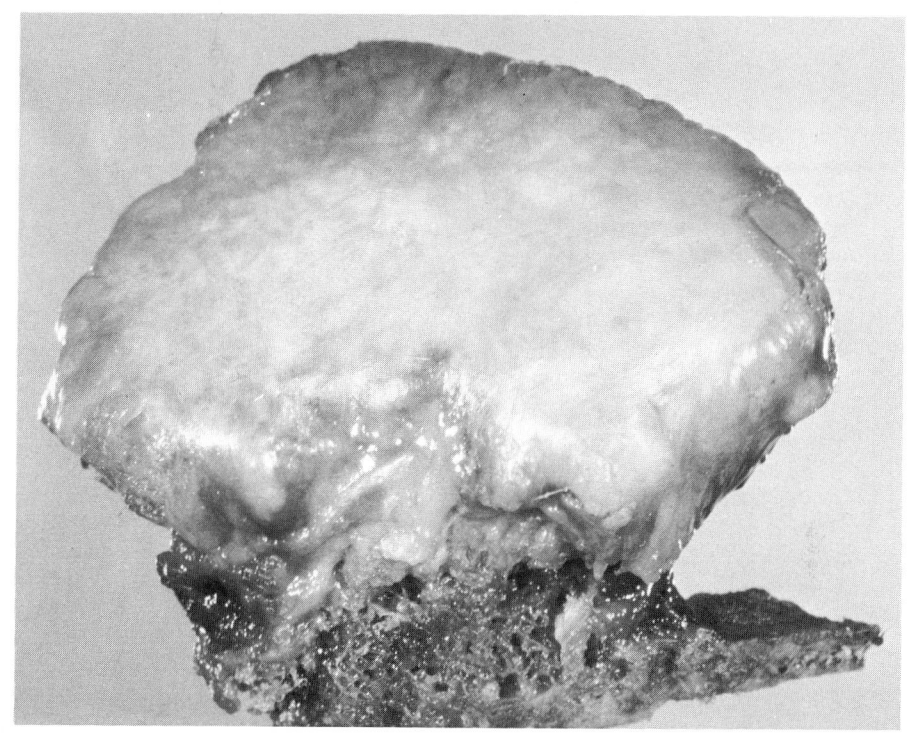

Fig. 4-4. Photograph (enlarged) of a sessile osteochondroma of a scapula, the entire surface of which was capped by cartilage that measured up to 4 mm. in thickness. (Courtesy Letterman General Hospital, San Francisco, Calif.)

Equally wide variation prevails as to size, so that one finds exostoses as small as 1 cm. and as large as 10 cm. or more in diameter. Whatever its size and shape may be, the exostosis is covered by periosteum that adheres closely to the irregular surface contour. The periosteal covering is continuous with that of the adjacent cortical bone. This rather avascular, collagenous connective tissue covering may be delicate, but more often it is comparatively thick, as periosteum goes, and attempts to peel it away from the exostosis show it to be composed usually of a number of layers. When this is accomplished, one observes, as a rule, that the surface of the exostosis is capped, in part or altogether, by a layer of blue-white hyaline cartilage. In general, the younger the patient presenting the exostosis, the more prominent will be its cartilage cap, since the latter tends eventually to involute. Section through a cartilage-capped exostosis perpendicular to its surface reveals further that the thickness of the peripheral cartilage zone usually varies from 1 to 3 mm., and occasionally its thickness may be as much as 5 to 6 mm. If the cartilage cap measures as much as 1.0 cm. or more in thickness, then one has cause for serious concern over the possibility of chondrosarcomatous change. On the undersurface of this cartilage cap, if endochondral ossification is still in progress, one observes a thin, yellowish growth zone or plate, and

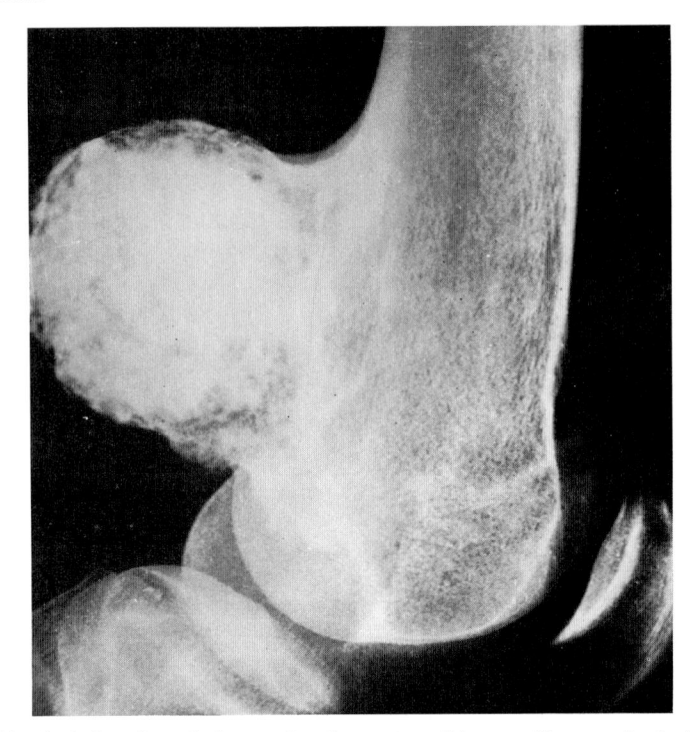

Fig. 4-5. Old calcified and ossified osteochondroma in a 54-year-old man who had been aware of its presence for more than twenty years. The growth caused increasing limitation of flexion and eventually paresthesia from stretching of the lateral popliteal nerve. Examination of the specimen showed a persistent cap of calcified cartilage that exhibited no evidence of recent growth.

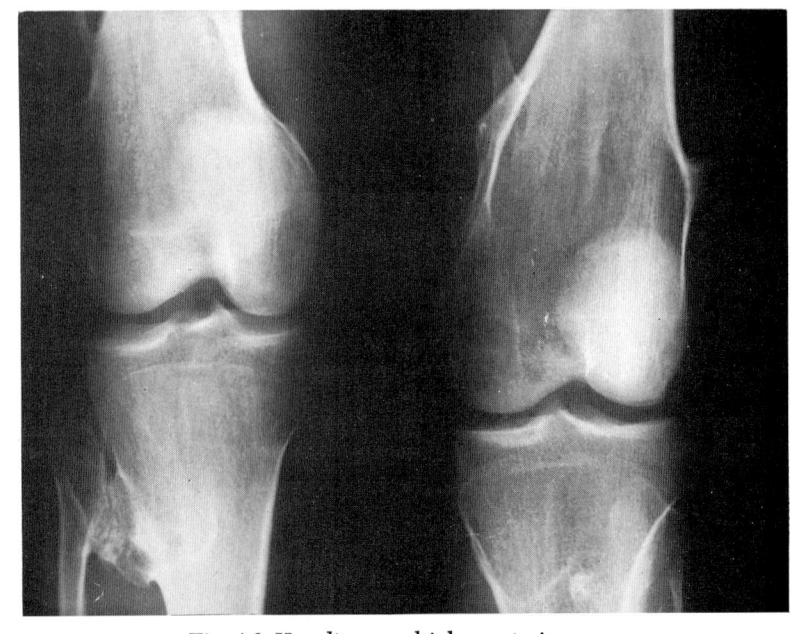

Fig. 4-6. Hereditary multiple exostosis.

beneath this, spongy bone comprising the bulk of the lesion. The marrow is usually fatty but may be myeloid in places (Fig. 4-8).

Microscopic examination of the cartilage cap of an exostosis that is still actively growing is likely to show foci of proliferating cartilage cells in its deeper layers, reminiscent of the proliferating zone of articular cartilage. As indicated, an osteocartilaginous exostosis grows by endochondral ossification of its proliferating cartilage, after the manner of growth at an epiphyseal cartilage plate. Similarly, its enlargement ceases when this growth zone becomes closed off by a thin plate of bone. There is also a tendency to gradual resorption of the cartilage cores within the subchondral trabeculae of bone adjacent to the growth zone. In some instances, however, these cartilage cores persist for a longe time, if not indefinitely. Occasionally, when the process of resorption and reconstruction in this subchondral zone has been particularly faulty, one observes fibrosed marrow im-

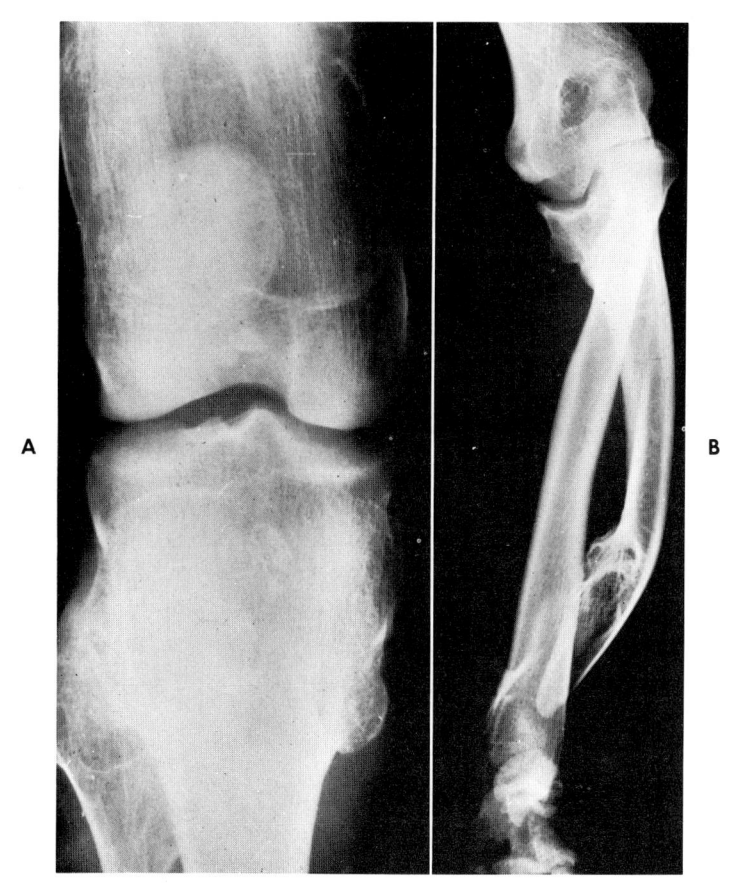

Fig. 4-7. A, Roentgenogram demonstrating the broadening and blunting of the affected bone ends frequently observed in multiple exostosis. B, Roentgenogram illustrating the characteristic deformity of the forearm bones in multiple exostosis.

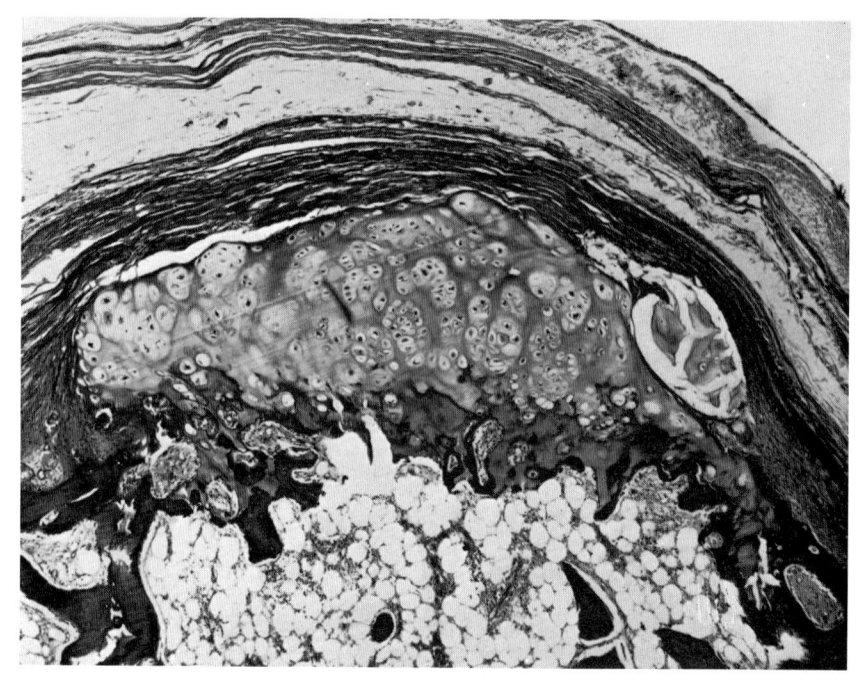

Fig. 4-8. Osteocartilaginous exostosis (osteochondroma). Photomicrograph showing a portion of its cartilage cap. (×40.)

pregnated by calcium detritus, as well as irregularly dispersed fields of heavily calcified cartilage intermingled with bone (Fig. 4-3, A).

The age at which growth of an exostosis ceases is distinctly variable. In general, however, it coincides roughly with the end of the growth period of the individual and often precedes it by several or many years. Thus, one not infrequently observes cessation of growth in specimens from adolescents or even children. In a young adult, the cap of an exostosis is likely to be composed of quiescent cartilage exhibiting calcification and other regressive changes. In older adults, the cartilage cap tends ultimately to involute and gradually disappear, although remnants of it may persist even into the fourth and fifth decades. These residual cartilage nests, although dormant, apparently retain a latent capacity for reactivated growth, affording an explanation for the occasional development of peripheral chondrosarcoma in later life.

Bursae developing over osteocartilaginous exostoses

The development of such bursae is not uncommon, particularly in the case of larger exostoses impinging upon muscles and tendons, and their occurrence has long been recognized (so-called "exostosis bursata"[9]). Such a bursal sac, when present, is likely to be attached around the base of the exostosis. As a rule, it contains mucinous fluid and its lining sometimes comes to resemble synovium. It is not uncommon also to find fibrin rice bodies attached to the lining or lying free

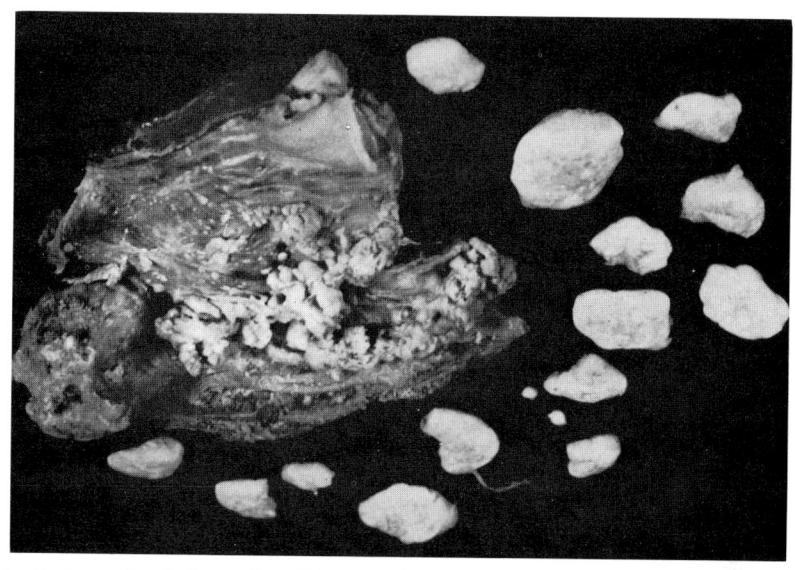

Fig. 4-9. Photograph of the wall and lining of a bursa that developed over an exostosis on the shaft of a femur and contained numerous calcified chondral bodies.

within the sac, and, occasionally, calcified chondral bodies resembling joint mice are encountered. I have observed a rather unusual specimen of a bursa developing around an exostosis of a femur, which contained fully 13 calcified, roentgenographically discernible bodies, ranging in size from 1 to 2.5 cm. in greatest dimension (Fig. 4-9).

Postirradiation exostoses

It is noteworthy that following irradiation of tumors in children, exostoses have been described as one of many postirradiation skeletal effects or complications. I have not had occasion to examine any of them, however, and there is some doubt in my mind whether such exostoses actually have cartilage caps or whether they are simply small bony protuberances.

Treatment and prognosis

When an osteocartilaginous exostosis is surgically extirpated, its periosteal covering should also be removed rather than stripped back, since, theoretically at least, it may contain or subsequently re-form the cartilage nidus of a recurrent lesion. In actual practice, however, I observed no local recurrences in a series of some 50 patients who had been operated upon, even though some of the exostoses, at least, had been removed subperiosteally.

Peripheral chondrosarcoma as a complication

As noted, the remnants of the cartilage cap of a solitary exostosis may occasionally, after a latent interval of many years, exhibit a spurt of renewed growth

26   Bone tumors

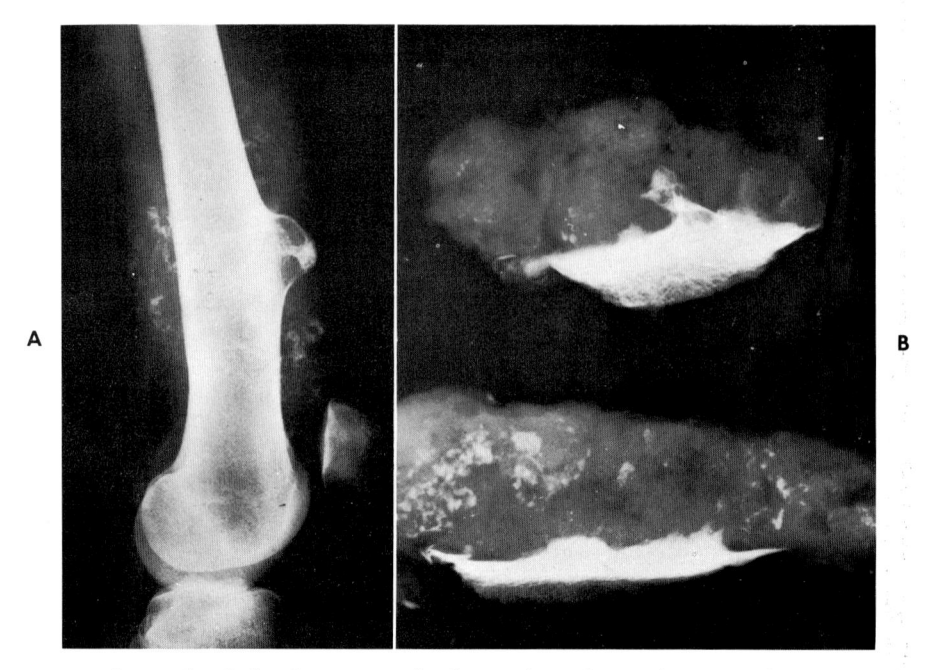

Fig. 4-10. **A,** Peripheral chondrosarcoma developing from the cartilage cap of an exostosis on the lower shaft of a femur. **B,** Roentgenograms of serial slices of the tumor specimen showing more clearly its relation to the exostosis and also focal calcification of the neoplastic cartilage.

and undergo malignant transformation to chondrosarcoma.[8] In some instances this may follow closely upon an injury to the affected site. The development of chondrosarcoma in such cases is usually a slow and insidious process requiring many months or even several years for its evolution, and such tumors may attain appreciable size before they are recognized clinically. Roentgenographically, they characteristically manifest rather heavy calcification and ossification especially in the older portion of the growth, which tends to mask their serious nature. By the same token, they may be underdiagnosed as calcifying and ossifying chondromas even by the pathologist on the basis of tissue examination, if proper significance is not attached to the finding of atypical cartilage-cell nuclei in the actively growing peripheral portion of the lesion as an indication of early chondrosarcomatous change.[8] It seems important to emphasize therefore that any osteocartilaginous exostosis in an adult, and occasionally even in a younger patient, which takes on a spurt of growth, should be regarded as already a chondrosarcoma, irrespective of how much calcification and ossification it exhibits. As such, it should be widely excised at the time of the initial surgical intervention in order to avoid local recurrence of the neoplasm in bulkier and more aggressive form (Figs. 4-10 and 4-11).

It is noteworthy that Anderson, Popowitz, and Li[1] recently reported an instance in which an unusual sarcoma, interpreted as fibrosarcoma, arose in a soli-

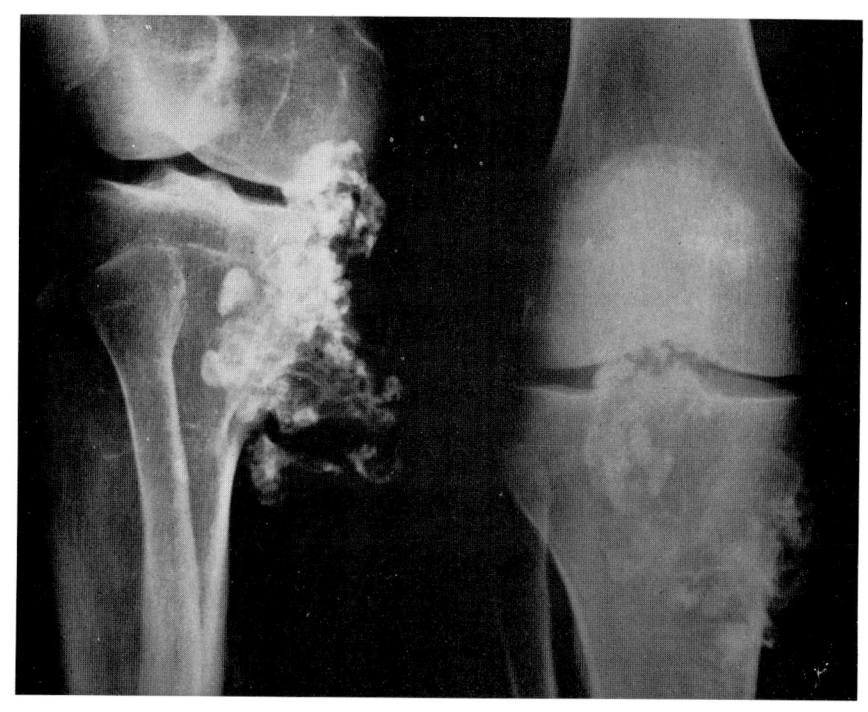

Fig. 4-11. Peripheral chondrosarcoma developing through activated growth of the cartilage cap of an exostosis (apparently solitary) of the upper tibia of a 48-year-old man. The patient had complained of discomfort and gradual enlargement of the affected area for three months. At exploration a fist-sized circumscribed cartilaginous tumor mass was encountered, surrounding a bony projection on the posterolateral surface of the tibia. Roentgenograms, lateral and anteroposterior views.

tary osteochondroma. This would seem to be a rarity. When one considers how common solitary osteochondromas are, the incidence of chondrosarcoma as a complication appears fortunately to be rather low and probably does not exceed 1% to 2%, judging by our experience. I have observed only a few such instances in recent years (two on a humerus and one in the ischial tuberosity), and they are distinctly unusual. One seems hardly justified on that basis alone in advocating the mandatory surgical removal of all exostoses as a routine preventive measure. On the other hand, one should recommend periodic roentgen examination of exostoses that are not removed, particularly in adults, to make certain that they have remained quiescent. It is important to note, however, that the comparable incidence of chondrosarcoma in cases of multiple exostosis is significantly higher. In this connection, Jaffe reported the development of chondrosarcoma in 3 of 28 cases of hereditary multiple exostosis (11%) and pointed out that the incidence of malignant change in this same group might ultimately be appreciably higher, since the majority of the patients were still young at the time the survey was made.

Summary

Osteocartilaginous exostosis or so-called osteochondroma is by far the most common of the benign tumors of bone. The present survey is based upon a study of more than 200 cases. Although osteochondromas not infrequently spring from flat bones, they are most often encountered on the long tubular bones. The commonest locations are the lower metaphysis of the femur and the upper metaphysis of the tibia. As its name implies, the lesion represents a cartilage-capped bony growth protruding from the surface of the affected bone. Like the comparable lesions in hereditary multiple exostosis, the solitary exostosis appears also to have its basis in perverted activity of the periosteum that tends to form anomalous foci of metaplastic cartilage. In fact, the weight of evidence lends support to the view that the condition represents a limited or abortive expression of multiple exostosis, the most common of the systematized anomalies of skeletal development. In keeping with this view is the fact that the condition manifests itself clinically in the great majority of instances in adolescence or childhood and occasionally even in infancy.

Osteocartilaginous exostoses exhibit wide variation in size and contour. The development of an overlying bursa is not uncommon, and, on occasion, the latter may contain rice bodies or calcified chondral bodies. The exostosis is invested by thickened fibrous periosteum beneath which there is a cap of hyaline cartilage, several millimeters in thickness. The lesion increases in size as a result of endochondral ossification and comes to a standstill when the growth zone is closed off by a thin plate of bone. Subsequently, the cartilage cap tends to involute, but remnants of it usually persist. These retain a latent capacity for reactivated growth, affording an explanation of the occasional development of peripheral chondrosarcoma in later life. Such chondrosarcomas develop relatively slowly and are not infrequently underdiagnosed as calcifying and ossifying osteochondromas when first observed. The incidence of chondrosarcomatous change in a solitary exostosis is substantially lower than it is in multiple exostosis and hardly seems to warrant mandatory extirpation as a routine preventive measure. When chondrosarcoma does develop, early recognition and wide surgical excision at the initial surgical intervention is of the utmost importance, if one is to obtain a cure.

References

1. Anderson, R. L., Jr., Popowitz, L., and Li, J. K.: An unusual sarcoma arising in a solitary osteochondroma, J. Bone Joint Surg. 51-A:1199, 1969.
2. Bethge, J. F. J.: Hereditäre multiple Exostosen und ihre pathogenetische Deutung, Arch. F. orthop. u. Unfall-Chir. 54:667, 1963.
3. Chiurco, A.: Multiple exostoses of bone with fatal spinal cord compression, Neurology 20:275, 1970.
4. Gokay, H., and Bucey, P. C.: Osteochondroma of the lumbar spine. Report of a case, J. Neurosurg. 12:72, 1955.
5. Jaffe, H. L.: Hereditary multiple exostosis, Arch. Pathol. 36:335, 1943.
6. Katzman, H., Waugh, T., and Berdow, W.: Skeletal changes following irradiation of childhood tumors, J. Bone Joint Surg. 51-A:825, 1969.
7. Keith, A.: J. Anat. 54:101, 1920.
8. Lichtenstein, L., and Jaffe, H. L.: Chondrosarcoma of bone, Am. J. Pathol. 19:553, 1943.
9. Orlow, L. W.: Die Exostosis bursata und ihre Bestehung, Deutsche Ztschr. f. Chir. 31:293, 1891.

Chapter 5

Solitary enchondroma of bone; enchondromatosis

This discussion deals with the common benign tumor that is composed of facets of mature hyaline cartilage and appears as a single lesion within the interior of some one bone.[5] Most often, it is one of the phalanges, especially of the hand, or a metacarpal bone that is the site of an enchondroma, but not infrequently it is a large limb bone, particularly the humerus or femur, and occasionally also the tibia. The innominate bones, too, are a frequent site for the development of cartilage tumors, although the latter are usually malignant, i.e., chondrosarcomas,[6] when first recognized. Cartilaginous tumors appearing in relation to ribs are almost invariably of the nature of osteocartilaginous exostoses.[4] Central chondromas of ribs and of the sternum are comparatively unusual in my experience, although such cases have been reported. The rare occurrence of enchondroma in a patella has likewise been described.[7] So-called enchondromas of the vertebral column have also been noted, but some of these, at least, appear actually to represent instances in which herniated intervertebral disc tissue was mistaken for neoplastic cartilage. For practical purposes, therefore, in dealing with solitary enchondroma of bone, one is concerned mainly with pertinent tumors arising within bones of the hand and occasionally of the foot, and within large limb bones. The former undergo malignant change only occasionally; I have seen material from three such cases within the past five years, all in finger phalanges of older adults. Enchondromas of long bones, on the other hand, not infrequently undergo malignant change, usually after a comparatively long quiescent interval, and this aspect will be considered presently.

Clinical features
Sex and age incidence

There appears to be no predilection for either sex. With respect to age incidence, the great majority of solitary enchondromas are encountered in patients between 10 and 50 years, and their observation in very young children appears to be exceptional.

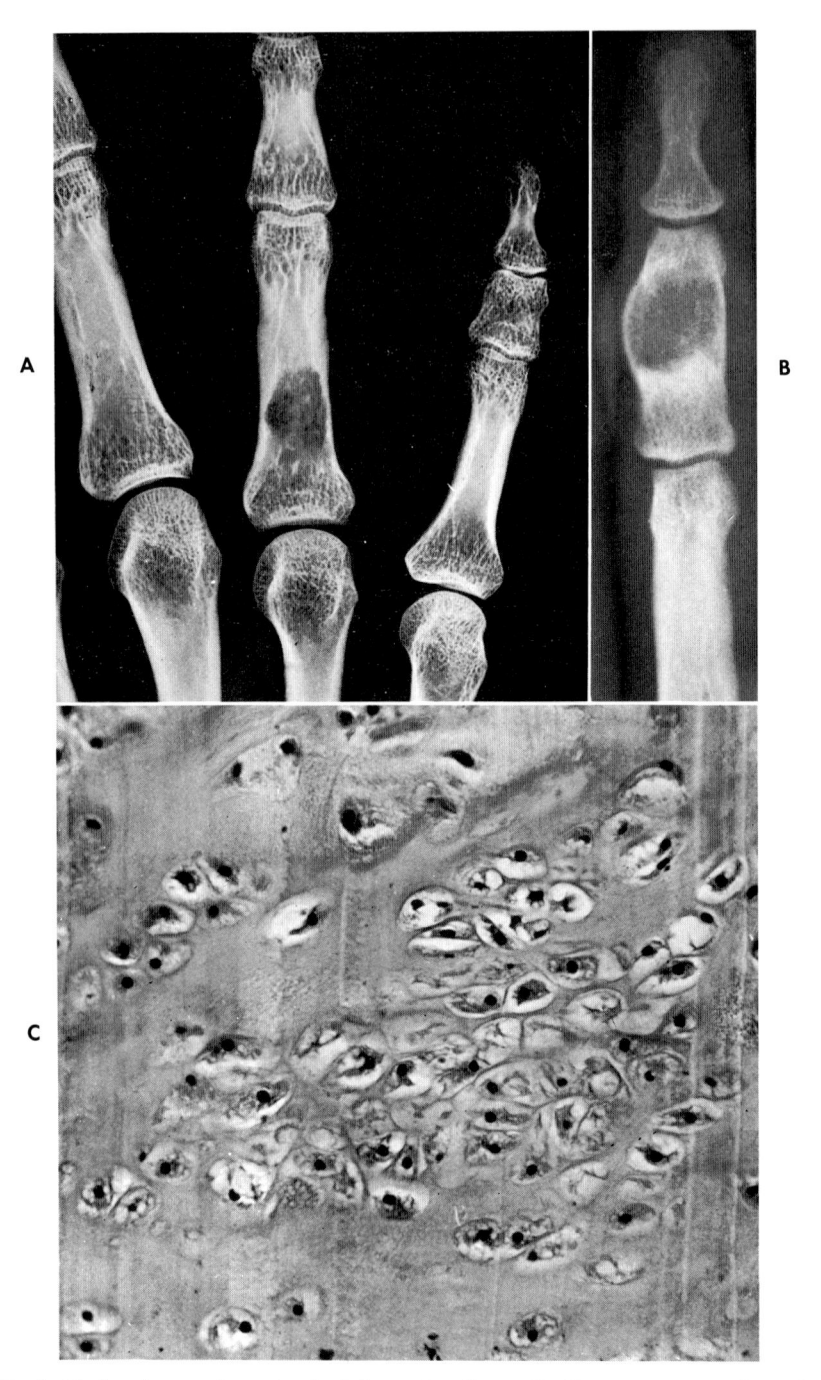

Fig. 5-1. **A**, Enchondroma of proximal phalanx of a finger. **B**, Roentgenogram of another enchondroma of a middle phalanx of a finger that has appreciably distended and thinned the overlying cortex. This particular lesion fails to show any clearly discernible calcific stippling. **C**, Photomicrograph of cartilage curetted from enchondroma illustrated in **A**. The cartilage-cell nuclei appear uniformly small and inconspicuous. (×260.)

Clinical history

From case histories taken as a whole, one gains the distinct impression that the tumor develops slowly and insidiously, although the clinical complaints may be of relatively short duration. A pertinent instance which may be cited is that of a physician with an enchondroma in the shaft of a femur; it had been discovered roentgenographically by chance seventeen years before it began to cause any difficulty. The physician eventually came to surgery only because the lesion became infected. In other instances, an injury to a limb bone, not necessarily a fracture, was responsible for pain, tenderness, and disability and directed attention to a heavily calcified and ossified enchondroma that must have been present for years. A rather common story in instances of phalangeal as well as metacarpal and metatarsal involvement is that the patient was unaware of anything wrong until a local trauma, often slight, was followed by pain and swelling, and a roentgenogram then revealed a rarefied lesion within the affected bone showing pathologic fracture of the attenuated overlying cortex. It is important to point out further that activated growth of an enchondroma may in itself be responsible for pain in the absence of any antecedent injury, and these cases in particular must be viewed with suspicion until biopsy or curettement rules out the possibility of early malignant change.

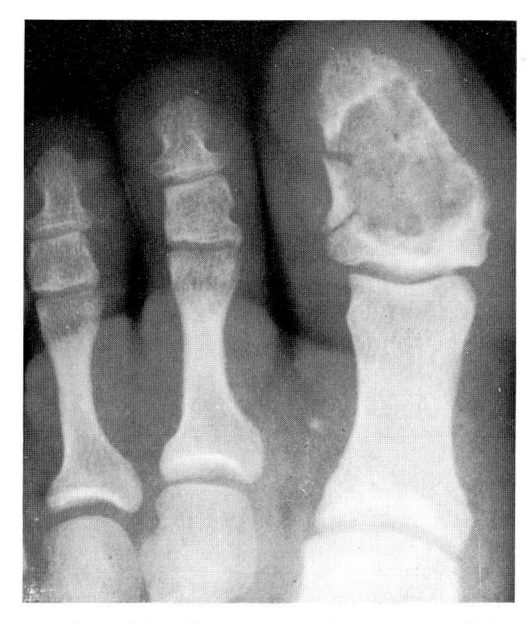

Fig. 5-2. Roentgenogram of an old enchondroma in the terminal phalanx of a large toe of a 44-year-old man. Infraction of the attenuated cortex at two points is attributable to a recent injury. There had been obvious enlargement of the toe prior to injury, however, and sections revealed indications of early chondrosarcomatous change. Amputation of the distal phalanx was performed.

32   Bone tumors
Roentgenographic picture

In phalanges, by far the most common site of localization, an enchondroma appears as a discrete, well-circumscribed, ovoid rarefaction shadow. It is usually located within the shaft of the phalanx at first, and as long as the epiphysis has not yet fused with the shaft, the former is not involved as a rule. Even after fusion has occurred, the end of the bone is not necessarily invaded. Whatever its position, the lesion may be situated centrally and fail to result in expansion of the bone, at least before it has attained appreciable size. More often, however, it is located somewhat eccentrically and causes some bulging and thinning of the overlying cortex, which is then prone to fracture. These eccentrically placed enchondromas are usually delimited internally by a thin sclerotized line. The rarefaction shadow cast by an enchondroma generally has a hazy, mottled appearance. It may be vaguely trabeculated, and frequently, though not invariably,

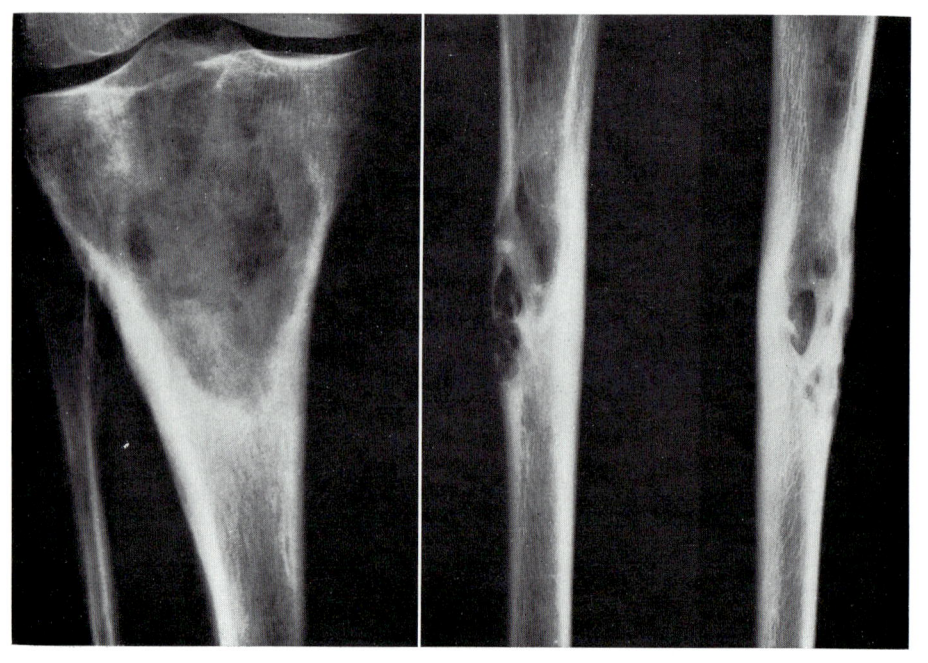

Fig. 5-3   Fig. 5-4

Fig. 5-3. Enchondroma in the proximal end of a tibia of a 50-year-old woman. The fuzzy mottling of the lesion reflects focal ossification. The patient had complained of dull pain in the knee region of at least three years' duration. When the lesion was curetted, it was found to be filled with blue-white, somewhat softened cartilage. Despite the clinical suspicion of malignancy, sections failed to show any clear-cut indications of chondrosarcomatous change that would justify a recommendation of ablation.

Fig. 5-4. Roentgenograms of another central cartilage tumor in a tibia of a 41-year-old man, biopsy sections of which showed evidence of early but definite malignant change justifying amputation. The same indications were present in a biopsy specimen obtained one year earlier, although their significance was not appreciated at the time.

presents dense stippled foci within it, reflecting spotty calcification and ossification.

In metacarpal and metatarsal bones, the roentgenographic changes produced by an enchondroma closely resemble those observed in phalanges. In these bones, however, the lesion is likely to be appreciably larger, as one might expect, and to result in more prominent bulging of the overlying cortex. Also, it seems to favor the distal rather than the proximal part of the shaft of the affected bone.

In the matter of roentgen interpretation, it may be stated in general that a circumscribed, rarefied, and expanded lesion of the character described occurring within a hand or foot bone is exceedingly likely to represent an enchon-

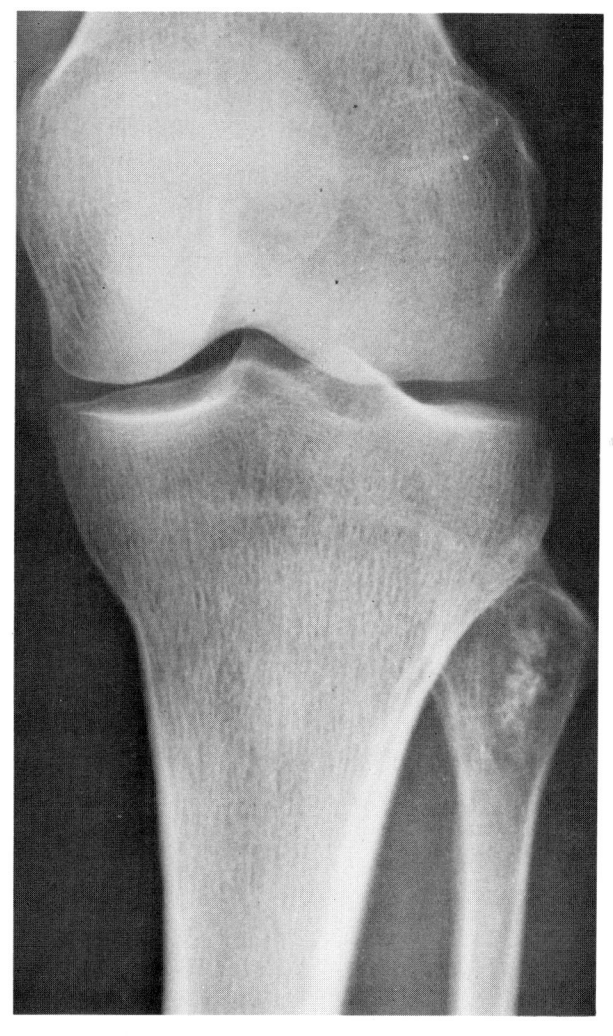

Fig. 5-5. Roentgenogram of an enchondroma in the head of a fibula, an unusual location. The patient was a woman of about 40 years of age.

droma, and if the lesion also exhibits calcific stippling, that impression becomes a virtual certainty (Fig. 5-1). There is a regrettable tendency on the part of some surgeons and even radiologists to refer loosely to such rarefied foci as "cysts." It should be noted, however, that genuine fluid-filled cysts, if they occur at all in hand bones, must be exceedingly rare. It is true that small inclusion cysts lined by squamous epithelium may be encountered occasionally in the distal portion of terminal phalanges of fingers,[2] but these are quite small and have a sharply outlined, punched-out appearance. Giant-cell tumors occasionally develop in metacarpal heads and rarely in phalanges, but they are not likely to be mistaken radiographically for enchondromas. Benign osteoblastoma, chondromyxoid fibroma, and aneurysmal bone cyst are additional lesions that may be encountered in hand or foot bones.

Much of what has been said concerning the roentgen appearance of enchondroma in hand and foot bones is applicable also to the lesion in long bones. The lesion in long bones, to be sure, is often more extensive and may at times involve a considerable part of the shaft, or even the entire shaft. Also, since the overlying cortical bone is relatively dense and thick, it may not be significantly expanded, or, if the cortex does bulge slightly, its expansion is likely to be limited to a small area. As noted, the presence of spotty or blotchy calcification or even of more delicate calcific stippling within the rarefied focus points definitely to enchondroma. In the absence of telltale calcification and ossification, however, the roentgenographic picture may be more ambiguous, and one must then consider as alternate possibilities a solitary focus of fibrous dysplasia, particularly if the lesion has appreciably expanded the affected bone area, and also solitary unicameral bone cyst, especially if the lesion involves the proximal shaft of the humerus. In such instances, only surgical exploration or biopsy will reveal the precise nature of the lesion that is present.

Pathologic observations

Since a solitary enchondroma is effectively treated by curettement, it is only occasionally that one has the opportunity to examine a tumor intact in its setting. One readily gathers, however, that the adjacent cortical bone is generally attenuated and often reduced to a thin shell if it comes from an area where the cortex has been bulged out, as is commonly the case when the lesion is in a phalanx or a metacarpal or metatarsal bone. On the other hand, when the cortex is not appreciably distended, as in the case of a lesion in a large limb bone, one may observe relatively little attenuation of the cortical bone. In any event, the endosteal surface of the cortex in the affected area is likely to show ridges and grooves from gradual erosion by the tumor tissue. There is usually no appreciable periosteal new bone reaction except at sites of infraction of the cortex.

The gross appearance of the neoplastic cartilage obtained by curettement from the interior of the lesion may vary considerably from case to case. Thus, the tissue from a lesion in a finger phalanx often resembles grains of boiled rice. In other instances, the lesional tissue consists largely of facets of bluish white, hyaline cartilage that is usually firm in consistency, but may be comparatively soft and even somewhat myxoid in places. In still others, it consists of bits of dull white cartilage intermingled with yellowish, gritty tissue representing heavily calcified and ossified cartilage. On the whole, calcification and ossification in an enchondroma seem best interpreted as an expression of aging or regression, and these changes are likely to be most pronounced in the lesions of long standing in limb bones, although they may also be a prominent feature in some of the older lesions in hand and foot bones.

On microscopic examination of an enchondroma, one observes that the cartilage tumor tissue is divided into facets or lobules of varying size. The connective tissue tracts between the facets of cartilage carry most of the blood vessels, in the vicinity of which calcification and ossification of cartilage are usually initiated. Enchondromas also vary considerably with respect to cellularity. Some are rather rich in cells and others are relatively poor, while still others show intermingled richly and poorly cellular areas. The intercellular ground substance is usually hyaline in large part or throughout. The cells within this hyaline matrix tend to lie within lacunae, many of which may be fairly large. A lacuna usually contains a single cartilage cell, though some may lodge two, and an occasional one a small nest of cells. In some areas the intercellular matrix may become edematous or even myxoid, in which case the cartilage cells, no longer surrounded by lacunae, tend to be multipolar or stellate in contour. It is the appearance of such modified fields that may cause certain enchondromas to be designated as myxomas or chondromyxomas.

In sections stained with hematoxylin and eosin, the ground substance will often appear dusty, reflecting the presence of calcareous granules within it. When calcification is more extensive, these granules will be rather conspicuous around the lacunae and also at the periphery of the cartilage lobules. Where calcification is particularly heavy, the cartilage cells may be found to have undergone necrobiosis or to have disappeared completely. Further, heavily calcified areas, particularly where they border on the interlobular vascular spaces, tend to undergo osseous metaplasia.

In the cytologic appraisal of the benignity of a central cartilage tumor, one should concentrate wholly on the cartilage-cell nuclei, selecting fields that are viable, not too heavily calcified, and remote from any fracture site that may be present. In such fields the cartilage cells of a benign tumor will be found consistently small. Their cytoplasm is generally pale and often more or less vacuolated, and its outlines are frequently indistinct. The cartilage-cell nuclei are likewise consistently small, and are roundish and dark staining. On scanning many preserved fields from as many parts of the tumor as possible, one may find very occasional cartilage cells that, though small, contain two nuclei, reflecting amitotic division. It should be emphasized, however, that some enchondromas contain practically no cartilage cells with double nuclei, and even those that do show only a few such cells in occasional fields. In summary, then, the extent of calcification and ossification, the character of the matrix, and the presence and size of the lacunae are of no practical significance. What stamps an enchondroma as benign cytologically is the fact that its viable cartilage cells are uniformly rather small and have single nuclei that are definitely not plump. While one does find, here and there, some cells (still small) with two nuclei, one does not find them regularly in all fields, even in small numbers (Fig. 5-1, C).

As noted, an enchondroma, especially in a long tubular bone, may occasionally undergo malignant transformation. The lesion may have been present as a benign growth for many years and may have been virtually symptomless during that time. Prior to its revivescence and malignant transformation, the enchondroma may even have become extensively calcified and ossified. The evolution of such a chondrosarcoma, though sometimes rapid, is usually a rather slow and insidious process. In this connection, it should be noted that the onset of persistent pain and spontaneous cortical perforation are ominous signs pointing to significant reactivated growth. Cytologic evidences of change in the direction of malignancy are detectable relatively early, but these are often rather subtle at first and present only in certain fields of the tumor. To recognize them, one has to have clearly in mind the characteristic cytologic pattern of the benign enchondroma as a standard and be on the alert for significant deviations from this pattern. If one finds, even in occasional areas, microscopic fields showing several or many binuclear cartilage cells, many cartilage cells with plump nuclei, and especially any cartilage cells, containing distinctly large or multiple nuclei, the tumor should no longer be regarded as a benign enchondroma. Eventually the histologic picture of such a tumor will become that of an obvious chondrosarcoma, but by that time the opportunity of obtaining a cure by radical surgery may have been lost. For pertinent case records emphasizing this important point, the reader is referred to Chapter 15 entitled "Chondrosarcoma of Bone."

Treatment and prognosis

Inasmuch as irradiation is not calculated to destroy cartilage tumors effectively, the treatment of choice for enchondroma of bone is surgical. This consists specifically of curettement, perhaps followed by chemical cauterization and, in addition, under appropriate circumstances, collapse of the distended part of the cortical wall and introduction of bone chips or insertion of a solid bone graft. Of some 14 phalangeal lesions studied by Jaffe and me,[5] a number were merely

---

Fig. 5-6. A, Roentgenogram of a central cartilage tumor situated in the neck and intertrochanteric region of a femur of a 20-year-old woman. The neoplasm has resulted in thinning and erosion of the cortex superiorly. From the roentgen picture alone it is hardly possible to venture the correct diagnosis with any assurance. B, Photomicrograph of a selected biopsy field showing (in its upper half) a focus of neoplastic cartilage in which the cartilage-cell nuclei are significantly enlarged and compacted. The finding of even an occasional field such as this suffices to establish a diagnosis of early chondrosarcoma. A six-year cure was obtained[8] without sacrificing the extremity through resection of the upper femur, placement of the autoclaved specimen as a graft, and fusion of the hip with the aid of massive tibial grafts. (×260.)

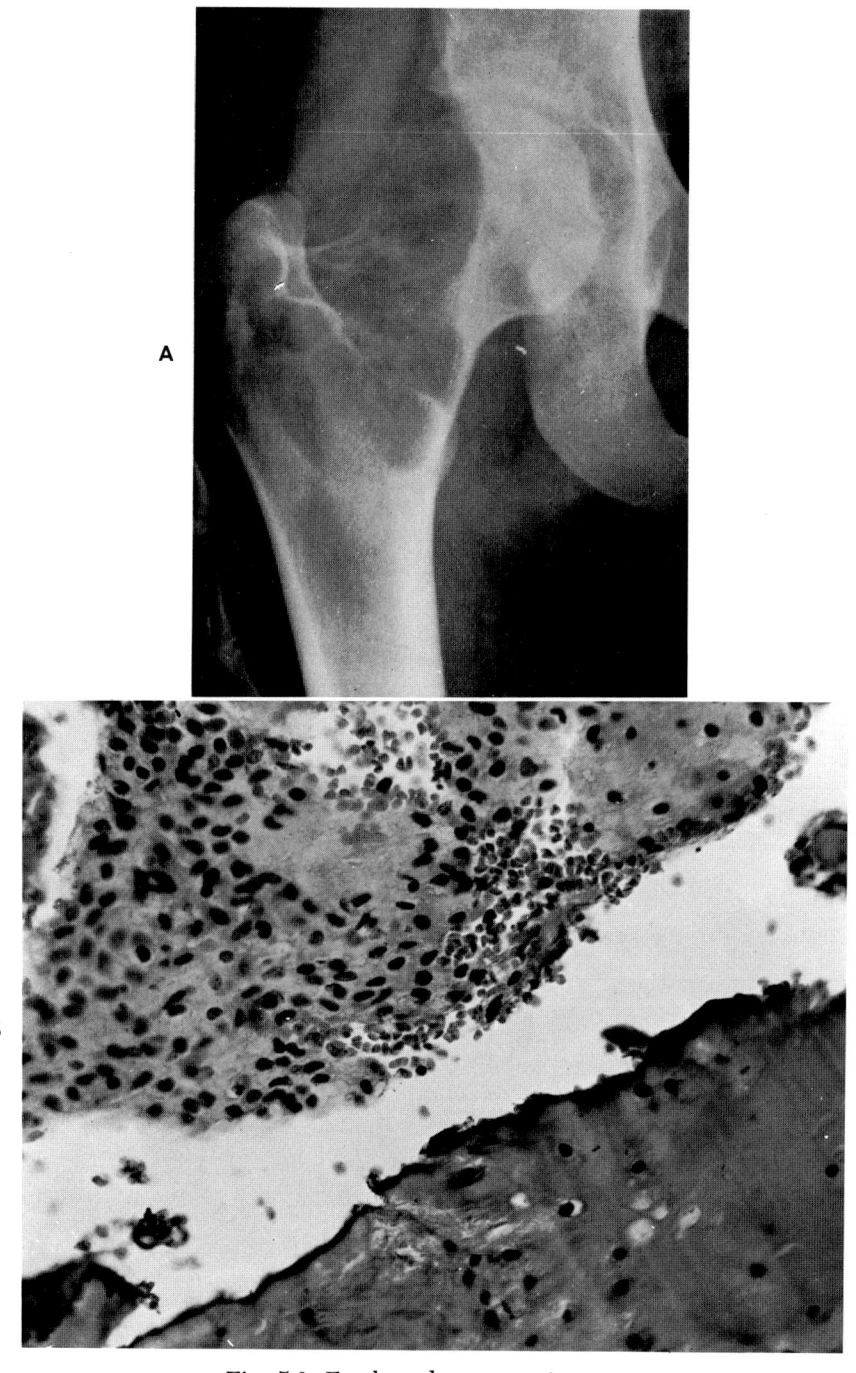

Fig. 5-6. For legend see opposite page.

curetted, some were curetted and cauterized, and some were curetted and filled with bone chips, with or without previous cauterization. No recurrences were noted in any of these cases, and healing was prompt and uncomplicated in all of them except one in which a course of preoperative radiation therapy had been given. The precise dosage used was not known, but the patient stated that she had received "ten x-ray treatments without benefit." Postoperatively in this case, the wound suppurated slightly and a number of the bone chips that had been inserted were sequestrated. One cannot, of course, be certain that this complication was attributable to the preoperative irradiation, although it is well known in general that heavily irradiated lesions in bone, which are subsequently operated upon, are particularly susceptible to infection.

Of some six lesions in metacarpal and metatarsal bones investigated, five were likewise treated by curettement, collapse of the cortical wall, and introduction of bone chips or a solid graft. In these cases, too, the postoperative course was uniformly favorable and there were no recurrences. The single exception noted was a case in which the entire metacarpal bone was extirpated apparently because the surgeon was impressed by the extensive involvement of this bone, although pathologically the lesion was entirely benign.

The same principles of surgical treatment were followed in some five of eight lesions of long tubular bones studied, again with uniformly good end results. Of the three remaining, one (a femoral lesion) had been treated elsewhere by resection of the lower end of the affected bone. Such treatment is obviously too radical for a solitary benign enchondroma, although the surgeon may have felt that by being drastic he was forestalling malignant transformation of the lesion. In another instance,[6] biopsy was followed ten months later by resection of the affected upper end of the humerus, since in the interval the lesion was persistently painful and showed roentgen evidence of further growth. It is interesting to note that sections of the periphery of this tumor showed evidence of early chondrosarcomatous transformation, although the periosteum had not yet been perforated at any point.

Skeletal enchondromatosis

One occasionally encounters patients who present central cartilage tumors in multiple sites, and this condition is usually designated as skeletal enchondroma-

---

Fig. 5-7. **A**, Photomicrograph of a representative field from an enchondroma of a tibia (biopsy specimen) in the case of a child with skeletal enchondromatosis (Ollier's disease) who also presented comparable lesions in the femur on the same side, resulting in deformity and appreciable shortening of the affected lower limb. The cartilage cells are more numerous than they are ordinarily in a solitary enchondroma, but their nuclei are not enlarged or otherwise significantly altered. (×65.) **B**, Roentgenogram from a case of enchondromatosis limited to the proximal and middle phalanges of the third finger of a hand. **C**, Another instance of limited Ollier's disease involving the radius, which is bowed (as well as some of the bones of the corresponding hand).

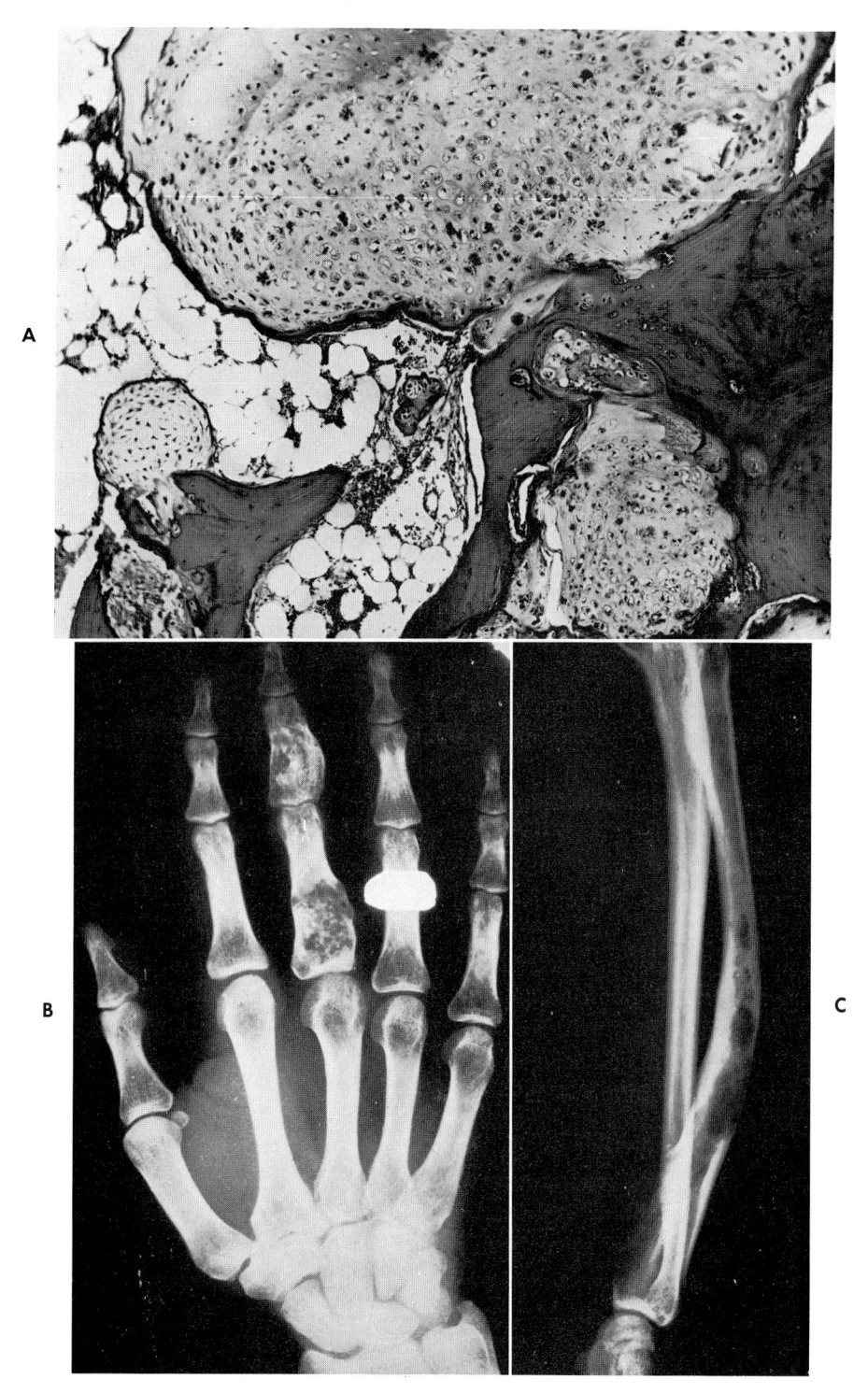

Fig. 5-7. For legend see opposite page.

tosis, being of the nature of a systematized developmental anomaly. Its clinical manifestations often appear early in childhood, and the skeletal lesions are sometimes associated with multiple hemangiomas of the skin, so-called Maffucci's syndrome (Fig. 5-11). Depending upon the severity of the condition, the enchondromas may be confined to the bones of a single digit, to several or all of the digits of one or both hands, to the bones of a single limb, usually a lower limb, or, if more extensive, may involve many bones in both upper and lower limbs. Even in the cases exhibiting widespread skeletal involvement, there is a strong tendency to unilateral or predominantly unilateral distribution, and these are often referred to as instances of Ollier's disease.[1] The latter eponym, incidentally, is often misapplied to instances of other conditions, particularly multiple exostosis.

Be that as it may, the important consideration to bear in mind in regard to skeletal enchondromatosis is that the individual lesions, as compared with solitary

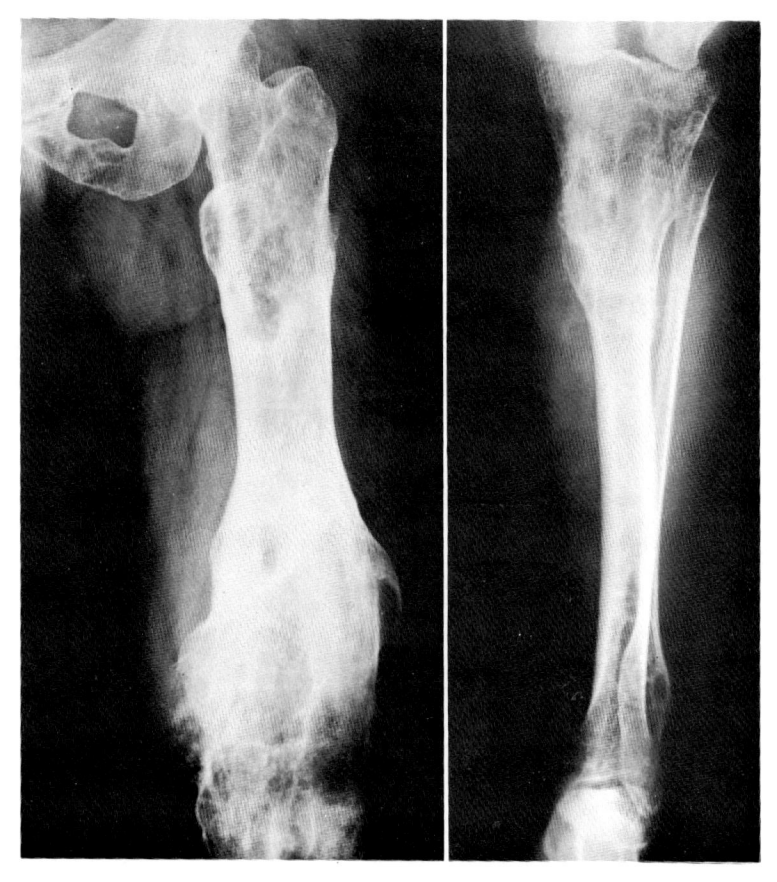

Fig. 5-8. Roentgenograms of another case of skeletal enchondromatosis (Ollier's disease) involving a lower limb. The patient was a young adult who had been aware of the condition since early childhood. Biopsy of the expanded lower femur failed to show evidence of malignant change.

enchondromas, appear more cellular histologically, exhibit a greater growth potential, and not infrequently exhibit a spurt of growth indicative of malignant change during adolescence or early adult life. When one has occasion to examine amputated limbs from such patients, it is not unusual to find evidence of chondrosarcomatous change developing in two or more tumor sites simultaneously. While the experience of any single observer is hardly extensive enough to have statistical validity, one gains the distinct impression that the hazard of chondrosarcoma in patients with skeletal enchondromatosis, even of moderate extent, is sufficiently great so that one has constantly to be on the alert for it. The grotesque pictures (in the older literature) of patients with enchondromatosis, exhibiting large protruding cartilage tumor masses on the hands and feet and occasionally in other sites, also furnish a convincing demonstration of the spontaneous tendency to malignant change in this remarkable condition.

It may be pertinent to emphasize that one must clearly distinguish such instances of skeletal enchondromatosis from multiple exostosis, just as one distinguishes a solitary enchondroma from an osteochondroma. In this connection,

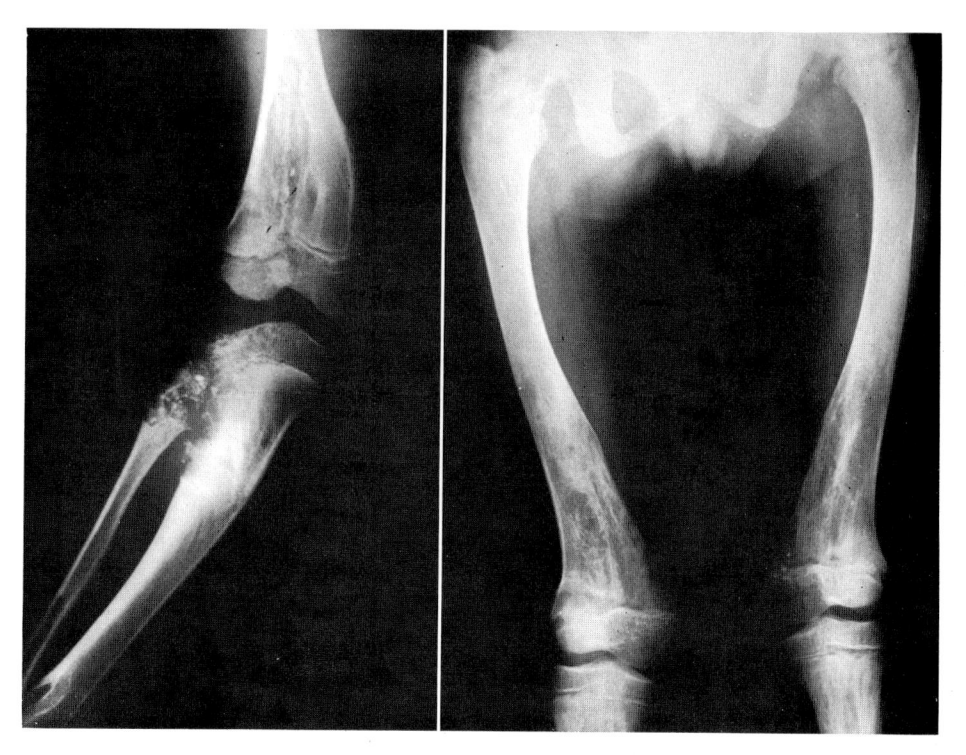

Fig. 5-9.   Fig. 5-10.

Fig. 5-9. Skeletal enchondromatosis (Ollier's disease) in a child, involving the lower femur and upper tibia and fibula.
Fig. 5-10. Skeletal enchondromatosis involving the large limb bones of both lower extremities in a child.

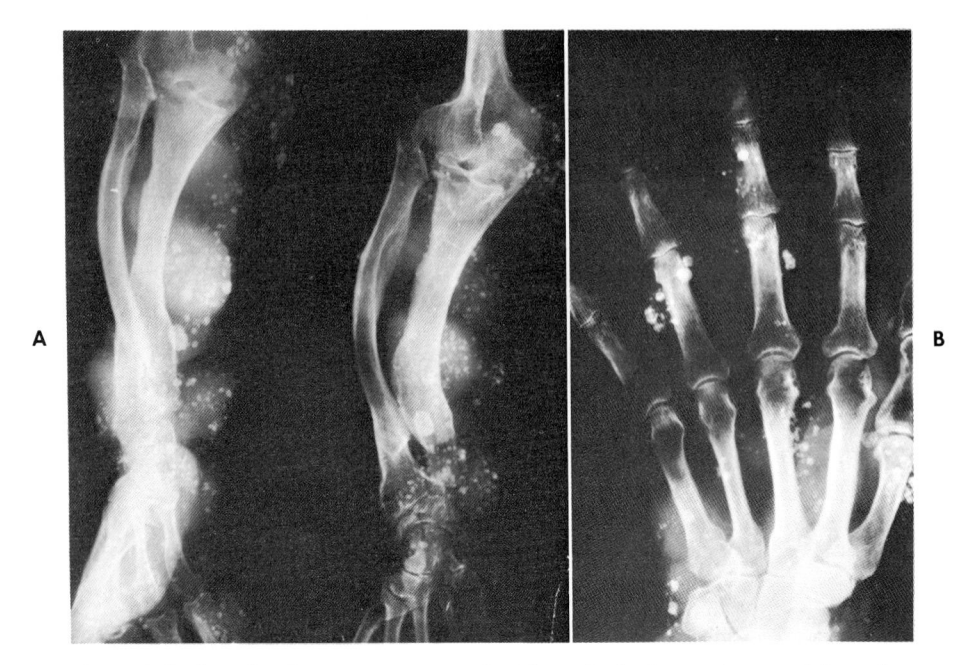

Fig. 5-11. Skeletal enchondromatosis associated with multiple hemangiomas of the soft parts (Maffucci's syndrome). This patient eventually developed chondrosarcoma of a scapula. (Courtesy Dr. Jorge Albores, Mexico City, Mexico.)

one must be aware that an enchondroma that has attenuated and has distended its overlying cortex may be mistaken by some for an exostosis and, conversely, an exostosis whose projection happens to overlap that of the shaft of the affected bone may simulate an enchondroma if only one roentgen view is examined. This consideration may perhaps account for the impression adhered to by some casual observers that the two conditions frequently coexist. Actually, I have never observed a single instance in which both peripheral and central cartilage tumors were present in the same patient. Nevertheless, certain French and Italian writers in recent years have advocated lumping skeletal enchondromatosis and multiple exostosis together under the head of "osteogenic disease," whatever that may mean. This tendency deserves to be deprecated, since it represents a backward step, blurring sharp and useful clinical distinctions that have a sound basis in pathologic anatomy. By the same token, one must deplore the practice, still adhered to by some writers, of indiscriminately bracketing the two conditions under the single head of dyschondroplasia.

Summary

The clinical, roentgenographic, and pathologic aspects of enchondroma of bone have been discussed. As its name implies, the lesion is a benign cartilaginous growth that develops in the interior of the affected bone. It has a predilection for limb bones, particularly the finger phalanges, the metacarpal and metatarsal bones, and the humerus and femur.

In relation to tubular bones, the lesion starts its development within the shaft and apparently within the metaphyseal region in particular. It may in time come to involve a considerable portion of the shaft. It may also extend into the adjacent or nearer epiphysis, though it is not likely to do so until after the epiphysis has fused with the shaft. An enchondroma developing within a large limb bone is not likely to distend the overlying cortex. In a hand or foot bone, however, it commonly does so, creating a bulge that can be readily detected clinically.

The lesion does not appear to be more common in one sex than in the other. Although the great majority of the patients are adolescents or younger adults when they present themselves for treatment, the tumor oftentimes seems clearly to be of rather long standing. The clinical complaints are generally mild and are usually referable to swelling of the affected part associated with some pain and tenderness. Many enchondromas come to clinical notice only after trauma has induced infraction of the distended cortex.

The roentgenographic picture is a valuable aid in the diagnosis of enchondroma. In dealing with enchondromas in large limb bones, the presence of radiopaque flecks or blotches representing foci of calcification and ossification often enables one to make the correct diagnosis even when the roentgenographic appearance of the lesion is otherwise ambiguous. In regard to pertinent tumors in phalanges and in metacarpal and metatarsal bones, there is a strong likelihood that one is dealing with an enchondroma if a fairly large area of rarefaction associated with thinning and bulging of the overlying cortex is observed. This is true even in the absence of spotty calcification, on the basis of the relative commonness of the lesion in these bones.

Enchondromas in hand and foot bones are, with few exceptions, innocuous and respond satisfactorily to conservative surgical treatment. This consists usually of curettement and filling of the defect with bone chips or insertion of a bone graft if the defect is large enough to warrant it. The benign character of such lesions is reflected cytologically in the fact that the great majority of the cartilage cells have a single nucleus that tends to be distinctly small in relation to the cell as a whole, and that the few cells that are binuclear likewise have small nuclei and are found only in occasional scattered fields.

An enchondroma, especially one in a long tubular bone, may occasionally undergo malignant transformation. Cytologically, in the early stages of this transition the lesion will deviate from the benign pattern just outlined in showing scattered fields containing many cartilage cells with plump nuclei, more than an occasional cell with two such nuclei, and even a number of cartilage cells with atypically large multiple nuclei. The prompt recognition of such early chondrosarcomas is of the utmost importance if one is to obtain a cure by radical surgery.

References

1. Bethge, J. F. J.: Die Olliersche Krankheit, Deutsch. Med. Wchnschr. 11:535, 1962.
2. Bissel, A. D., and Brunschwig, A.: Squamous epithelial bone cysts of the terminal phalanx and benign subungual squamous epithelial tumor of finger, J.A.M.A. 108: 1702, 1937.
3. Burack, P. I.: Ossifying enchondroma of head of humerus, Bull. Hosp. Joint Dis. 1:3, 1940.

4. Jaffe, H. L.: Hereditary multiple exostosis, Arch. Pathol. 36:335, 1943.
5. Jaffe, H. L., and Lichtenstein, L.: Solitary benign enchondroma of bone, Arch. Surg. 46:480, 1943.
6. Lichtenstein, L., and Jaffe, H. L.: Chondrosarcoma of bone, Am. J. Pathol. 19:553, 1943.
7. Stephenson, W. H.: Enchondroma of patella, Brit. J. Radiol. 26:156, 1953.
8. Thompson, V. P., and Steggall, C. T.: Chondrosarcoma of proximal portion of femur treated by resection and bone replacement: six year result, J. Bone Joint Surg. 38-A:357, 1956.

Chapter 6

Benign chondroblastoma of bone

Benign chondroblastoma is a tumor that was formerly identified as a giant-cell tumor variant, so-called, and specifically as the "cartilage-containing giant-cell tumor" (Kolodny), the "calcifying giant-cell tumor" (Ewing), or the "epiphyseal chondromatous giant-cell tumor" (Codman). In 1942, on the basis of a survey of nine cases of this peculiar tumor of bone, in collaboration with Jaffe,[11] I suggested the name "benign chondroblastoma of bone" as a more appropriate designation, holding that the lesion had no kinship whatsoever to genuine giant-cell tumor and that it should be regarded as a distinctive tumor in its own right, more logically classified among the benign tumors of bone derived from cartilage cells or cartilage-forming connective tissue. Since then, I[17] have had occasion to observe many additional cases, all of which have tended to substantiate the essential soundness of this concept. As for the significant clinical features of the tumor under discussion, we called attention particularly to its curious predilection for young patients, especially males whose ages fall within the second decade—an important point of differentiation from genuine giant-cell tumor,[12] which is observed only occasionally in patients under the age of 20 years. In recent years, I have observed a few instances of benign chondroblastoma in adults, but these are exceptional.[16] The roentgenographic picture of the tumor was described as that of a well-delimited, fuzzy or mottled, rarefied focus whose appearance and contour, considered in conjunction with its epiphyseal location and particularly the age and sex of the patient, might readily lead one familiar with the lesion to suspect the correct diagnosis, even before surgery.

Like Ewing, we were impressed by the regularly observed tendency to focal calcification within the lesional tissue, which constitutes a major feature of its cytologic pattern and affords a readily discernible cue to its recognition. Also, we observed, as had Codman, that the tumor regularly involves the epiphyseal end of a long bone, although by the time it comes to clinical notice, it may already have extended across the epiphyseal cartilage plate into the adjacent metaphyseal region. While Codman emphasized the occurrence of the tumor in the vicinity of the tuberosity of the upper end of the humerus (in keeping with his particular interest in lesions of the shoulder region), we found that it develops with greater frequency in the lower end of the femur and the upper end of the tibia and ap-

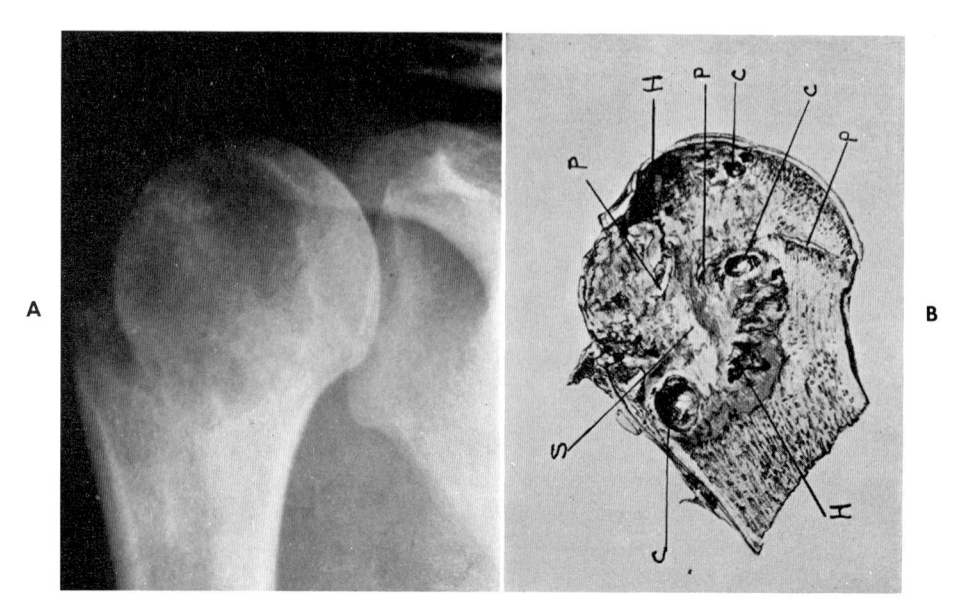

Fig. 6-1. A, Roentgenogram of a benign chondroblastoma developing in the upper end of a humerus, the site stressed by Codman. **B,** Photograph (reduced ⅔) of a coronally sectioned upper end of a humerus showing a pertinent tumor comparable to that illustrated in **A.** It involved the tuberosity and adjacent portions of the capital epiphysis. The letter notations have reference to remnants of the disrupted epiphyseal cartilage plate and to foci of hemorrhage, cystic softening, and fibrous replacement within tumor tissue. The patient was a 16-year-old boy in whom surgical resection was done on the mistaken premise that the tumor represented a sarcoma.

pears on occasion in the lower end of the tibia as well. We[17] have also observed a typical lesion that developed within the capital epiphysis and adjacent neck region of a femur (Fig. 6-4).

While the tumor is encountered commonly in the large limb bones, namely the femur, tibia, and humerus (in that order of frequency), it may develop occasionally in other centers of ossification. I have observed material from two tumors that arose in the glenoid rim of a scapula (Fig. 6-6), where secondary centers of ossification appear at puberty, and another unusual tumor in an iliac bone that apparently developed from the epiphyseal center of the inferior lateral spine of the ilium. Still another developed in an ischium and one other in a talus; both were in males 15 years of age.

Atypical benign chondroblastomas[4,16] may be encountered within bones of the foot and hand, as well as in large limb bones, and these will be considered further in the discussion on atypical chondroid tumors of bone.

In our survey of additional relevant papers, we pointed out that others had also encountered sporadic instances of the tumor, but, failing to appreciate its special features, had overdiagnosed it as chondrosarcoma[6,8,19] or even as osteogenic sarcoma.[14] An occasional case is still reported as a giant-cell tumor, and my correspondence indicates that some instances are still overrated by patholo-

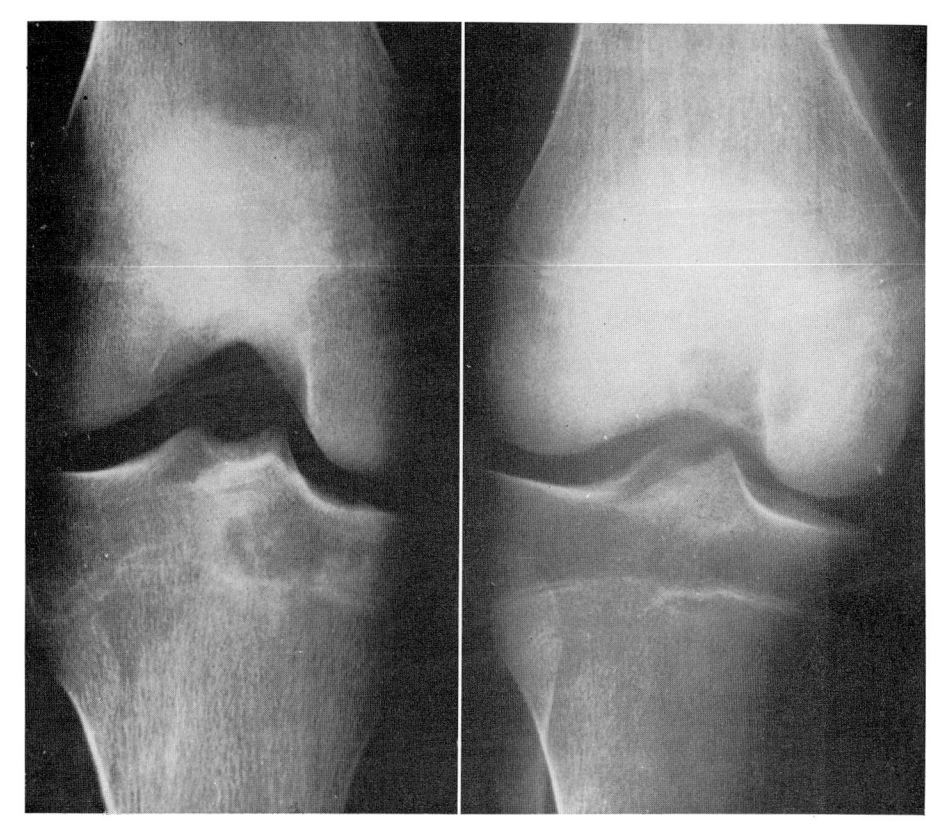

Fig. 6-2. Representative roentgenograms of two benign chondroblastomas situated in the upper epiphysis of the tibia and the lower epiphysis of the femur, respectively, their most common sites of localization.

gists as osteogenic sarcoma or chondrosarcoma, although this happens less often as times goes on.

Clinical features
Roentgenographic picture

Since gross specimens showing an entire tumor intact within its setting are seldom available, our knowledge concerning the manner in which the tumor develops, and its effect upon the surrounding bone, is largely gleaned from x-ray pictures of pertinent lesions. These show that the neoplasm tends to be round or ovoid in contour and, as noted, may be confined to part of an epiphysis, if still relatively small, or involve also part of the adjacent metaphysis, having already broken across the epiphyseal cartilage plate. When it involves the metaphysis as well, it may sometimes be so eccentrically located as to bulge out the overlying cortex without, however, destroying it. Actually, the tumor may vary in size from a small focus not much larger than an osteoid-osteoma nidus to one measuring as much as 6 cm. in greatest diameter. Whatever its size, its roentgeno-

48 *Bone tumors*

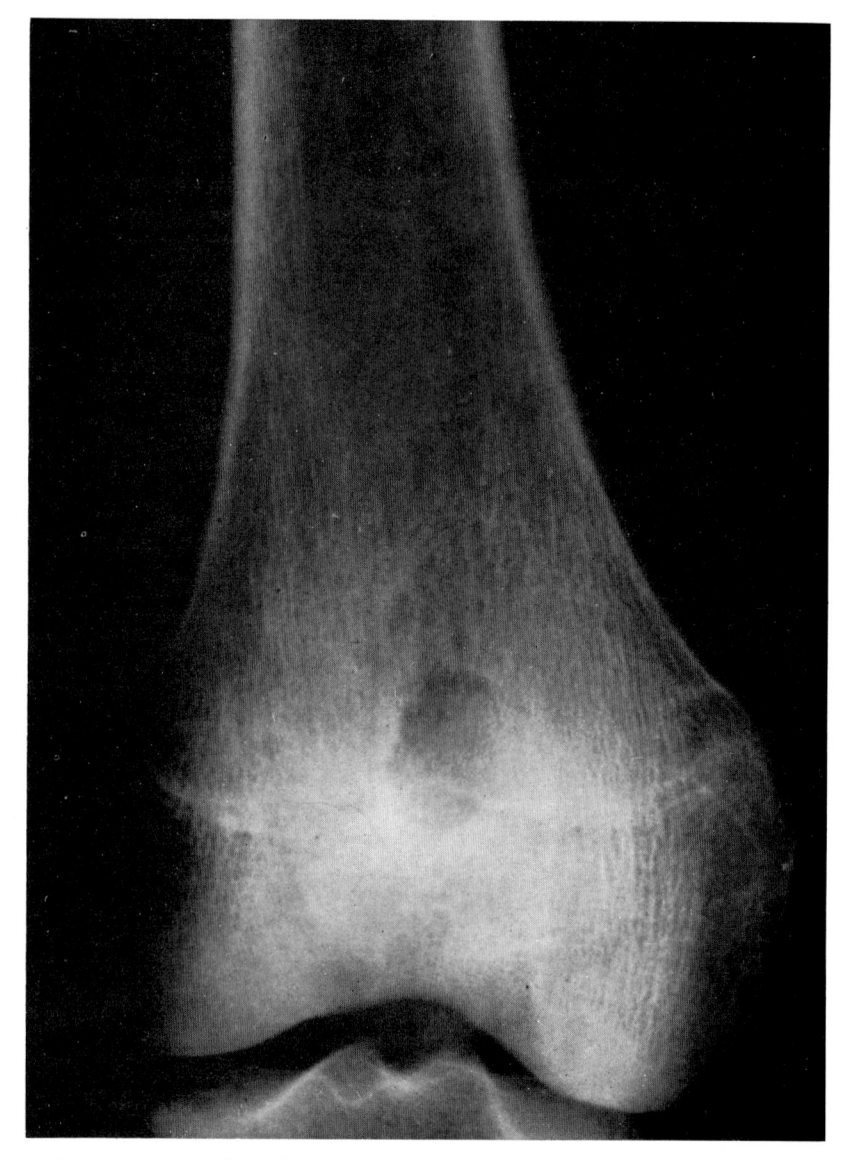

Fig. 6-3. Roentgenogram of another pertinent tumor in a 20-year-old man, originating in the lower epiphysis of a femur and extending into the metaphysis. The tumor has provoked some sclerosis of the surrounding spongy bone. The biopsy sections in this case were overdiagnosed as osteogenic sarcoma, and amputation was performed on the basis of this mistaken impression.

graphic appearance is that of a fuzzily mottled, rarefied focus that tends to be delimited by a well-defined, narrow, encircling line of sclerotized bone. The fuzzy mottling of its shadow reflects spotty calcification within the lesional tissue (Fig. 6-2).

With respect to the joint surface, the lesion frequently extends to the articular cartilage and may even protrude perceptibly into the joint. This is particularly

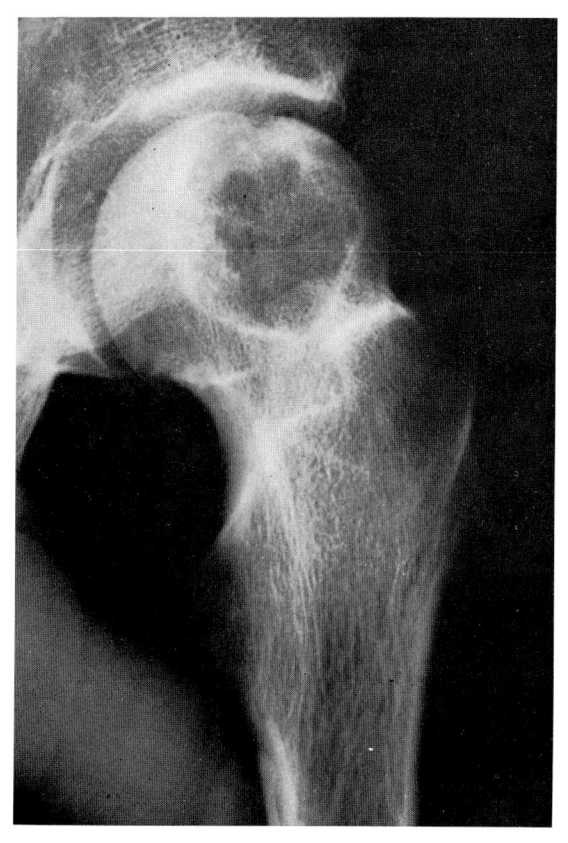

Fig. 6-4. Roentgenogram of a benign chondroblastoma situated within the head and neck region of the femur of a 20-year-old man. The lesion is fuzzily rarefied but well delimited and apparently extends to the articular cartilage of the head. Following thorough curettement and packing with bone chips, the patient made a rapid recovery and regained a full range of painless motion of the hip.

true of lesions bordering upon the knee joint, although even in the shoulder joint region, one may observe some destruction of the overlying articular cartilage.

Clinical complaints

The onset of the condition in the patients was insidious and the complaints had been present for some months before medical attention was sought. As in the case of most tumors of bone, some of the patients related their difficulty to some antecedent injury, but as many more gave no history of any relevant trauma. All of them referred their complaints to the affected joint region (knee, ankle, or shoulder), which was painful on motion, and more or less swollen and tender. With involvement of a lower extremity, limping was noted, as was some muscular atrophy of the affected side, and in some instances also, the presence of increased fluid in the neighboring joint.

50   Bone tumors

Pathology

Fortunately, only an occasional limb is ablated or resected upon the mistaken impression that the lesion represents a sarcoma, but when this does happen, one has the opportunity to study an entire intact specimen or, at least, a full section of it. One such resected humeral specimen has been described by Jaffe and me, and Phemister[19] has observed another. In the former, the tumor involved the tubercles, metaphysis, and an adjacent bit of the capital epiphysis of the humerus. The articular cartilage of the head was found preserved almost throughout, but did shown small marginal exostoses and a small defect in one area, filled in with connective tissue. In the cut section, the tumor measured 6 cm. in its long axis and 4 cm. across. The tumor tissue was sharply delimited from the neighboring uninvolved bone, and the delimiting margin was convexly lobulated. Within the limits of the tumor, one could clearly discern residual portions of the partially destroyed epiphyseal cartilage plate. Much of the tumor tissue was modified by cystic softening and hemorrhage. The relatively well-preserved tumor

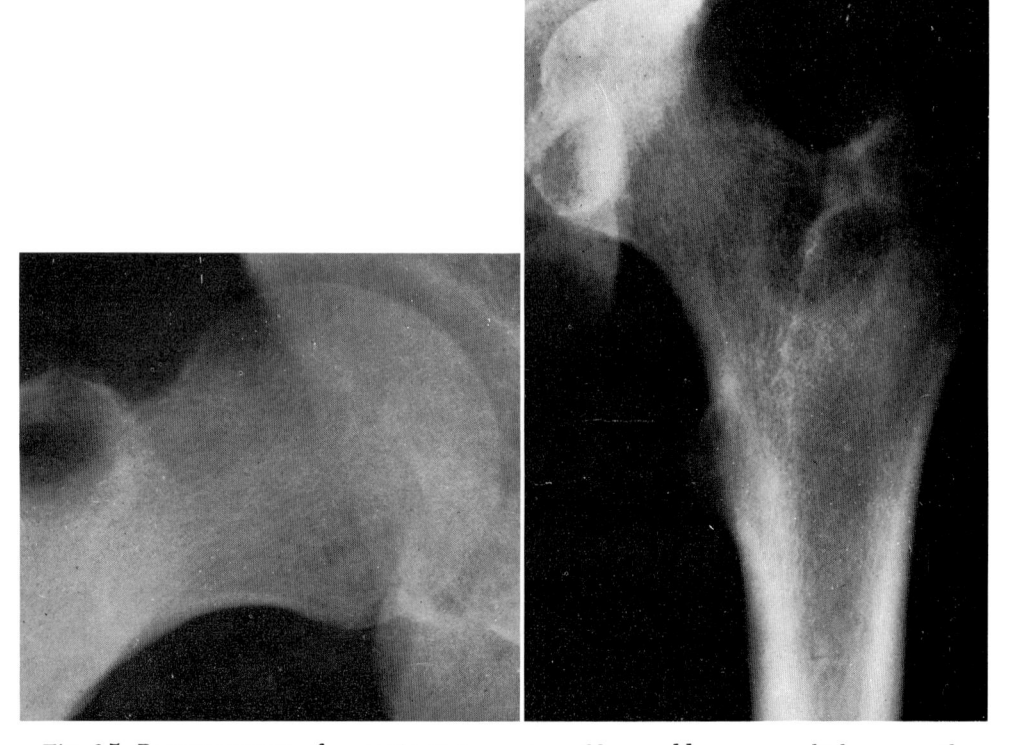

Fig. 6-5. Roentgenograms of a pertinent tumor in a 20-year-old woman, which apparently originated in the region of the greater trochanter, another unusual location for it. Positive identification of this tumor from the biopsy sections entailed some difficulty, but careful search revealed the presence of streaks of calcification within fields of necrotic tumor tissue. Satisfactory recovery and follow-up observation of the patient after curettement dispelled any lingering doubt that the tumor might represent a malignant neoplasm.

tissue was gray-brown in color and firm, or more yellowish and gritty from calcification within it (Fig. 6-1, B).

Ordinarily, of course, the surgical material available for study and diagnosis consists of small fragments obtained by curettement. In the interpretation of such material, it is essential for the pathologist to bear in mind that the cytologic pattern of the lesion frequently varies from specimen to specimen, and even in different fields of the same specimen, reflecting as it does, the evolutionary cycle of the lesion. Thus, the earliest phase is represented by cellular tumor fields composed of rather compact, roundish or polyhedral cells of moderate though variable size, with a relatively large nucleus, and sometimes more than one nucleus. Dispersed here and there, there may be a sprinkling of multinuclear giant cells, particularly where hemorrhage has occurred. These multinuclear cells (which account for much of the confusion of this lesion with giant-cell tumor of bone) are not constantly found and, even when present in scattered foci, do not seem to represent an integral part of the cytologic pattern (Fig. 6-8). The readily discernible clue to the diagnosis of benign chondroblastoma is the presence of focal areas of calcification throughout the cellular tumor tissue. Wherever this calcification is particularly heavy, the tumor cells swell and undergo degeneration and necrosis (after the manner of cartilage cells undergoing calcification preparatory to osseous transformation). Also, in the wake of necrosis, and as part of the reparative process, one observes resorption of calcific detritus, organization

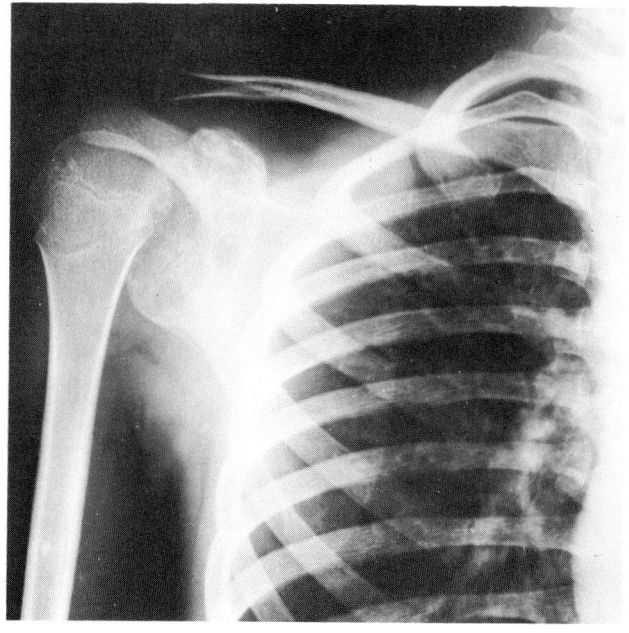

Fig. 6-6. Benign chondroblastoma in another unusual location, the glenoid of a scapula. The patient was a male adolescent.

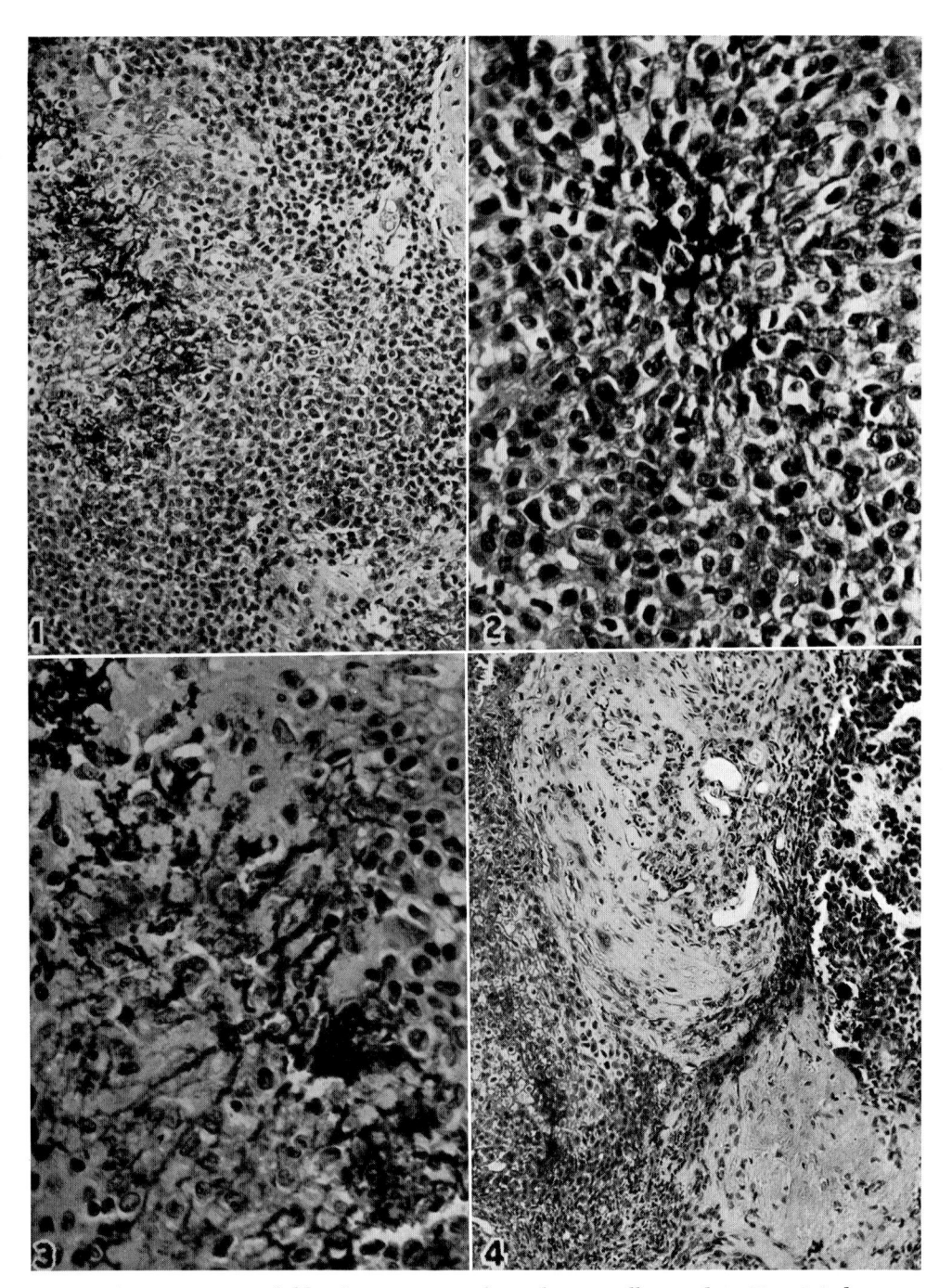

Fig. 6-7. Representative fields of tumor tissue from the case illustrated in Fig. 6-4 demonstrating the evolutionary cycle of the lesion. 1 through 4 show focal calcification within the cellular tumor tissue followed by degeneration and necrosis and, eventually, resorption of calcific detritus, and connective tissue replacement of necrotic fields leading to the formation of collagenous plaques often resembling osteoid or chondroid matrix.

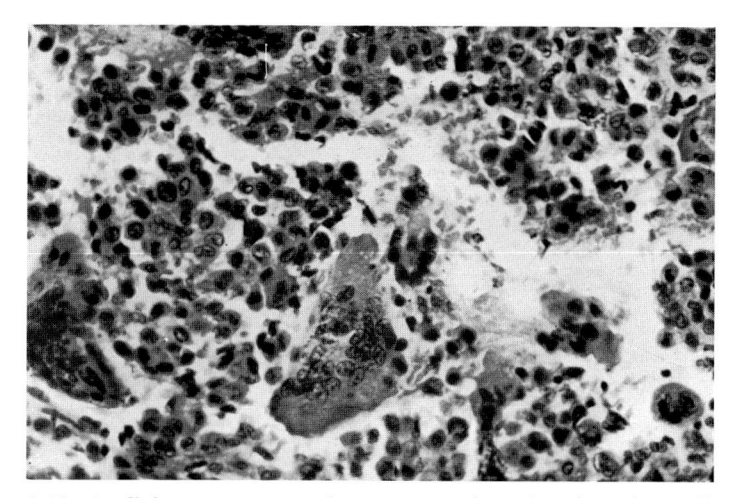

Fig. 6-8. A field of cellular tumor tissue showing a number of multinuclear cells within and about an area of blood extravasation. It is the appearance of such random fields that may cause the lesion to be mistaken at times for giant-cell tumor, although its cytologic pattern as a whole should hardly occasion any confusion. (See Fig. 6-7.)

of hemorrhage, and connective tissue replacement of necrotic fields. This connective tissue may ultimately assume the form of smaller or larger collagenous plaques, sometimes resembling chondroid, but more often osteoid, matrix. Finally, the latter may, in some few fields, go on to actual osseous transformation. It is the random intermingling of fields showing various phases of this sequence that often makes the composite cytologic picture seemingly complex (Fig. 6-7).

I have long held the view, at least as a working hypothesis in regard to pathogenesis, that the tumor may arise from an anomalous or accessory epiphyseal cartilage center that is stimulated to growth at the time of puberty by sex hormones or other unknown factors. Support for this view comes from a recent electron microscopy study by Welsh and Meyer[22] of two neoplasms in point, one in the region of the greater trochanter of a 10-year-old girl and the other in the head of a femur of an 18-year-old boy. From their examination, the conclusion was drawn that the tumor cells in each instance strongly resembled normal epiphyseal cartilage cells growing in tissue culture. In another comparable study, Wellman[21] recently drew the same inference.

Treatment and prognosis

Thorough curettement of the lesion and packing of the cavity thus created with cancellous bone chips appears to be the method of choice. As noted, this is likely to have been done in many instances, even before the diagnosis has been established on a histologic basis. Frozen section of a bit of the tumor tissue obtained at the time of operation should be sufficiently distinctive in its appearance to warrant an immediate impression in most cases, so that one need not wait upon paraffin sections to clarify the indications for definitive treatment. In those of our cases in which thorough curettement was carried out, the lesion healed without recurrence, and good function was restored. The end results in these cases were the same, whether or not the curettement had been followed by radiation therapy in moderate dosage. On the other hand, in a case in which the lesion was in a femur and merely a punch biopsy was taken, and the lesion subsequently was treated with heavy irradiation, a flexion contracture of the knee resulted, requiring arthrodesis for correction. On microscopic examination in this case, islands of viable tumor tissue were still recognizable in the osteoarticular shavings removed in the course of the knee fusion. Altogether, the weight of evidence seems to be against the necessity of irradiation and is certainly against very vigorous irradiation either with or without previous curettage.

The prospect of a cure and satisfactory restoration of function in patients properly treated is very good in our experience. This is in keeping with the observations of Codman, all of whose patients (nine in number) were well three to ten years after coming under treatment.

While the great majority of chondroblastomas respond satisfactorily to thorough curettement and go on to uneventful healing, it should be noted that occasional instances may manifest more aggressive behavior. I have knowledge of one case seen in consultation in which a tumor in point in the upper humerus recurred after curettement, necessitating a second procedure, and another case in which sections of the surgical specimen examined microscopically showed extension of tumor into periosteal connective tissue at a site where the cortex delimiting the tumor was defective. Another instance of local recurrence of a chondroblastoma (in the upper femur) after curettage and packing with bone chips has been published by Castleman.[1] The surgeon elected to replace the upper femur with a Moore prosthesis, and the patient was well and free of tumor eight years later. Coleman,[3] also, has reported an instance of chondroblastoma in a femoral condyle, which recurred within the joint and in the adjacent soft tissues following initial curettement; this patient was well some four years after last surgery. Similarly, in a case studied by Wellman[21] arising in a scapula, articular and soft tissue extension was noted, although this tumor had been neglected for twelve years and was as large as 15 cm. in greatest dimension. McBryde and Goldner[18] (in reporting recently on some eleven cases) have taken cognizance of these observations, admonishing surgeons to take pains to prevent spread of tumor and, if possible, avoid entering the neighboring joint.

Continuing, Kahn, Wood, and Ackerman[13] have observed an exceptional chondroblastoma originating in a femoral condyle, which recurred not only in the joint capsule (solitary nodule) but also spread via lymphatics around the knee joint, necessitating midthigh amputation. In this instance, the patient was apparently free of tumor eighteen months after ablation. The same authors[13] also reported a second unusual tumor in point (in the hip region); it spread locally despite multiple operations and eventually metastasized widely. This observation of spontaneous, frank malignant change is apparently unique in the literature to date. The case reported earlier by Hatcher[9] of chondrosarcomatous transformation at the site of a chondroblastoma seems clearly to represent an instance of postirradiation sarcoma.

It may be pertinent here to mention also that Geschickter and Copeland[7] have stressed the importance of distinguishing between benign chondroblastic tumors and "malignant chondroblastomas," though discussing them under a single head and implying that they have a common origin and possibly transitions. It seems to me that their malignant chondroblastomas so-called are actually frank chondrosarcomas readily distinguishable from benign chondroblastomas.

Summary

Benign chondroblastoma of bone is conceived of as a clinically and pathologically distinctive benign neoplasm that has no kinship to genuine giant-cell tumor, to which it has nevertheless been linked in the past as the so-called "calcifying" or "epiphyseal chondromatous" variant. It is my considered opinion that the neoplasm should be classified more logically among the tumors of bone derived from cartilage cells or cartilage-forming connective tissue. The tumor originates commonly within the epiphyseal end of a large tubular limb bone, though it frequently extends into the adjacent metaphyseal region. Specifically, the femur, tibia, and humerus are predilected (in that order), although the tumor may be encountered occasionally in other sites as well, as indicated. Also, in our experience, the tumor develops with remarkable consistency in young patients in the second decade and predominantly in males. Cytologically, tissue from a lesion may, in some fields at least, bear a superficial resemblance to giant-cell tumor of bone, especially if there has been hemorrhagic extravasation. However, the readily discernible cue to its recognition is the presence of focal areas of calcification. Where this is particularly heavy, the tumor cells undergo degeneration and necrosis, in the wake of which one also observes resorption of calcific detritus, organization of hemorrhage, and fibrous tissue replacement leading to the formation of dense collagenous plaques resembling chondroid or osteoid matrix.

Although this neoplasm of bone is rather uncommon, its recognition is nevertheless of practical importance, inasmuch as instances of it are sometimes overdiagnosed as chondrosarcoma or even osteogenic sarcoma, with the attendant recommendation of ablation.

The great majority of chondroblastomas respond satisfactorily to thorough curettement and go on to uneventful healing. An occasional one may recur locally after surgery, with or without soft tissue extension. Only a single instance of spontaneous, frank malignant change with metastasis has been recorded to date, and this complication would seem to be rare.

References

1. Castleman, B.: Case records of the Massachusetts General Hospital, N. Engl. J. Med. 271:94, 1964.
2. Codman, E. A.: Epiphyseal chondromatous giant cell tumors of the upper end of the humerus, Surg. Gynecol. Obstet. 52:543, 1931.
3. Coleman, S. S.: Benign chondroblastoma with recurrent soft tissue and intra-articular lesions: report of a case, J. Bone Joint Surg. 48:1554, 1966.

4. Coley, B. L., and Santoro, A. J.: Benign central cartilaginous tumors of bone, Surgery **22**:411, 1947.
5. Ewing, J.: The classification and treatment of bone sarcoma. In International Conference on Cancer. 1. Cont. (1928) Report of the International Conference on Cancer, Bristol, 1928, John Wright & Sons Ltd., pp. 365-376 (see p. 370).
6. Geschickter, C. F., and Copeland, M. M.: Recurrent and so-called metastatic giant cell tumor, Arch. Surg. **20**:715, 1930 (see p. 731).
7. Geschickter, C. F., and Copeland, M. M.: Chondroblastic tumors of bone: benign and malignant, Ann. Surg. **129**:724, 1949.
8. Hammerström, S.: Ein Fall von chondroblastischem Sarkom, Acta Radiol. **15**:668, 1934.
9. Hatcher, C. H.: The development of sarcoma in bone subjected to roentgen or radium irradiation, J. Bone Joint Surg. **27**:179, 1945 (see Case 1).
10. Hatcher, C. H.: Personal communication, Sept. 20, 1950.
11. Jaffe, H. L., and Lichtenstein, L.: Benign chondroblastoma of bone; a reinterpretation of the so-called calcifying or chondromatous giant cell tumor, Am. J. Pathol. **18**:969, 1942.
12. Jaffe, H. L., Lichtenstein, L., and Portis, R. B.: Giant cell tumor of bone; its pathologic appearance, grading, supposed variants and treatments, Arch. Pathol. **30**:993, 1940.
13. Kahn, L. B., Wood, F. M., and Ackerman, L. V.: Malignant chondroblastoma. Report of two cases and review of the literature, Arch. Pathol. **88**:371, 1969.
14. King, E. S. J.: An example of benign osteogenic sarcoma, Br. J. Surg. **19**:330, 1931.
15. Kolodny, A.: Bone sarcoma; primary malignant tumors of bone and giant cell tumor, Surg. Gynecol. Obstet. **44**(suppl. 1):1-214, 1927; Figs. 88, 98 (pp. 191, 202).
16. Lichtenstein, L., and Bernstein, D.: Unusual benign and malignant chondroid tumors of bone, Cancer **12**:1142, 1959.
17. Lichtenstein, L., and Kaplan, L.: Benign chondroblastoma of bone; unusual localization in femoral capital epiphysis, Cancer **2**:793, 1949.
18. McBryde, A., Jr., and Goldner, J. L.: Chondroblastoma of bone, Am. Surg. **36**:94, 1970.
19. Phemister, D. B.: Chondrosarcoma of bone, Surg. Gynecol. Obstet. **50**:216, 1930; p. 223.
20. Smith, D. A., Graham, W. C., and Smith, F. R.: Benign chondroblastoma of bone. Report of an unusual case, J. Bone Joint Surg. **44-A**:571, 1962.
21. Wellman, K. F.: Chondroblastoma of the scapula. A case report with ultrastructural observations, Cancer **24**:408, 1969.
22. Welsh, R. A., and Meyer, A. T.: A histogenetic study of chondroblastoma, Cancer **17**:578, 1964.

Chapter 7

Chondromyxoid fibroma of bone

Chondromyxoid fibroma, a comparatively late addition to the family of bone tumors, was described and christened by Jaffe and me[17,18] in 1948, on the basis of experience with eight cases of the lesion. Prior to this, it seems not to have been generally recognized as a distinctive neoplasm, although it appears likely that single instances were reported as enchondroma or myxoma and their malignant counterparts.[9,13,23] It is significant that the first two specimens in our own series were originally considered to be chondrosarcomas, and it was not until our entire chondrosarcoma material was surveyed[19] that the pathologic distinctiveness of these particular tumors was fully appreciated. It is true that the tumor presents certain cytologic features that may suggest malignancy to one who is unfamiliar with the lesion, but we have learned empirically that, with few exceptions, it is benign. A tendency to local recurrence in some instances in young children particularly has been noted,[21,22] necessitating further surgery for cure. Malignant change (to chondrosarcoma) has been recorded in one or two cases,[10,15] but this appears to be distinctly unusual, and I have not had occasion to observe it in my own experience.

Since the first edition of this book appeared, I have had the opportunity of observing material submitted for consultation from many additional patients, and my experience with this tumor now covers more than 50 cases altogether. Increasing awareness of it is evidenced also by the publication of an appreciable number of additional case reports within recent years.[8,14,15,20,21,22,26]

Chondromyxoid fibroma is a peculiarly differentiated tumor apparently derived from cartilage-forming connective tissue, which exhibits certain chondroid and also myxoid traits that hallmark the lesion cytologically. Basically, it is composed of spindle-shaped cells lying loosely in a myxoid intercellular matrix, which, as the tumor matures, may undergo substantial collagenization. The tissue of any particular specimen may also come to simulate cartilage tumor tissue in some or many fields, and in its gross appearance it likewise bears a certain resemblance to cartilage. However, the tumor is quite distinct from the common enchondroma, which is composed of facets of mature hyaline cartilage, and there is little room for confusion on that score. While chondromyxoid fibroma is not a particularly common neoplasm, its recognition is of some importance in that pathologically,

58   Bone tumors

as noted, it may be readily mistaken for sarcoma, especially chondrosarcoma and myxosarcoma, and, as such, treated more radically than is necessary.

Our original group of cases was put on record[18,19] mainly because of concern that pathologists encountering sporadic instances might overrate them as chondrosarcoma (or perhaps myxosarcoma). In recent years, the pendulum seems to have swung in the opposite direction, and I find that not a few pathologists indulge in wishful thinking and interpret frank chondrosarcomas (with myxoid matrix) as possible chondromyxoid fibroma.

Clinical features
Age and sex incidence

Most of the cases observed (approximately two-thirds) have been in comparatively young patients in the second and third decades. The remainder were in older adults, and I have seen but a single instance in a child below the age of 10 years. There appears to be no predilection for either sex.

Localization

The tumor is encountered most often in the lower extremity, particularly in the lower metaphysis of the femur, the upper metaphysis of the tibia, the lower

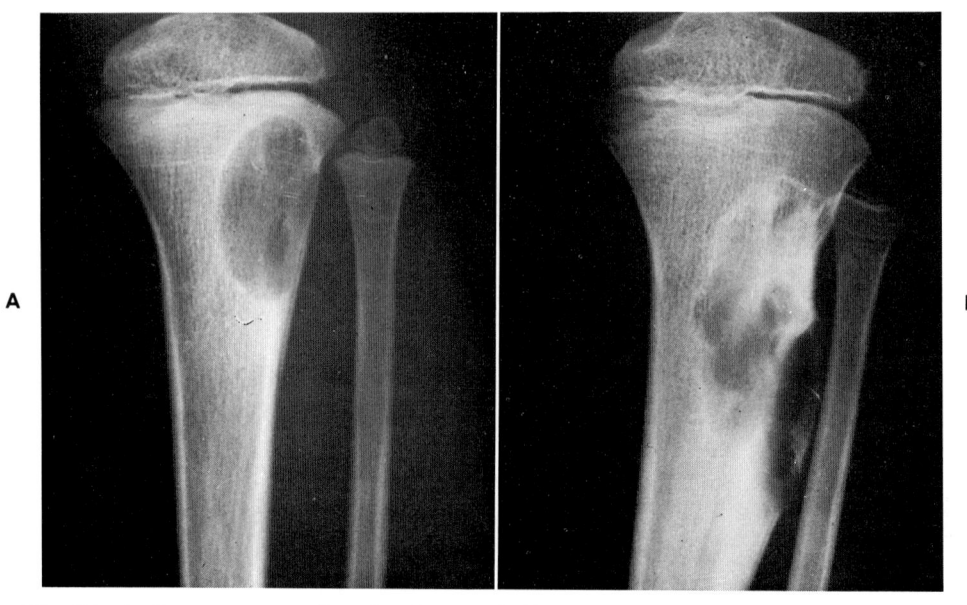

Fig. 7-1. **A**, Roentgenogram of a chondromyxoid fibroma in a young boy developing in the upper metaphysis of a tibia, a frequent site of localization. **B**, Recurrence of the tumor illustrated in **A**, after apparently inadequate curettement. Although this was disturbing clinically, the recurrent growth was sharply delimited internally by a zone of sclerotized bone, which was somewhat grooved or scalloped, and peripherally by a shell of cortical new bone. The surgeon elected to do a wide block excision, but thorough curettement and packing with bone chips would have sufficed for cure. This patient was entirely well and had good function of the affected limb when seen four years later.

end of the fibula, or in one or another of the foot bones (especially the metatarsals and calcaneus) or the hand bones (Fig. 7-3). In addition, a number have been observed in ribs and in the innominate bone, and an unusual case has been reported by Benson and Bass[2] that involved the vertebral column (at the level of D-1 to D-3). I have seen material from an unusual tumor in point located in the glenoid of a scapula (Fig. 7-6). An unusual, large tumor in point in the sternum has been reported by Teitelbaum and Bessone.[25] It seems probable that in time instances of it will be encountered in other sites as well.

Within the upper tibia and lower femur, the commonest sites of localization, the tumor was found in the metaphyseal area, as noted, not far from the neighboring joint. In these bones, the lesion was situated eccentrically, eroding and more or less destroying the overlying cortex. In the calcaneus the lesion was likewise eccentrically located in the volar portion of the body at some distance from the apophysis. In small tubular bones, such as the fibula or a metatarsal, the tumor may eventually occupy the entire width of the affected bone area and cause appreciable expansion of it.

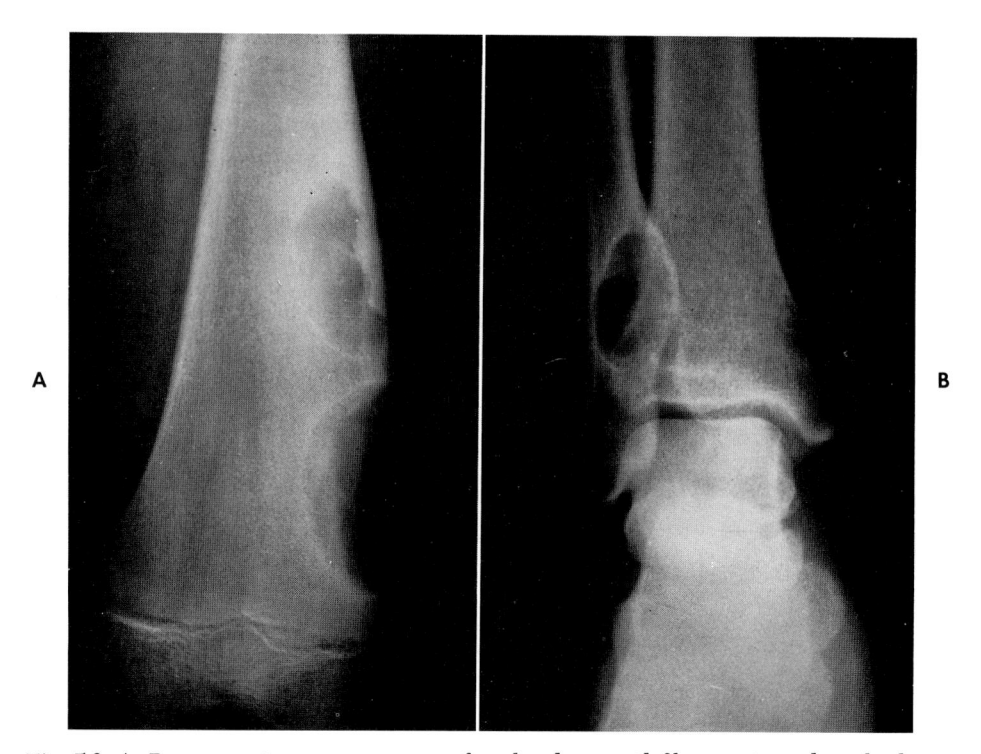

Fig. 7-2. **A**, Representative roentgenogram of a chondromyxoid fibroma situated in the lower shaft and metaphysis of a femur, another frequent site of localization. Tumors such as this are sometimes treated more aggressively than is required. **B**, Another chondromyxoid fibroma situated in the lower end of the fibula of a 30-year-old man. The lesion was known to have been present for eight years.

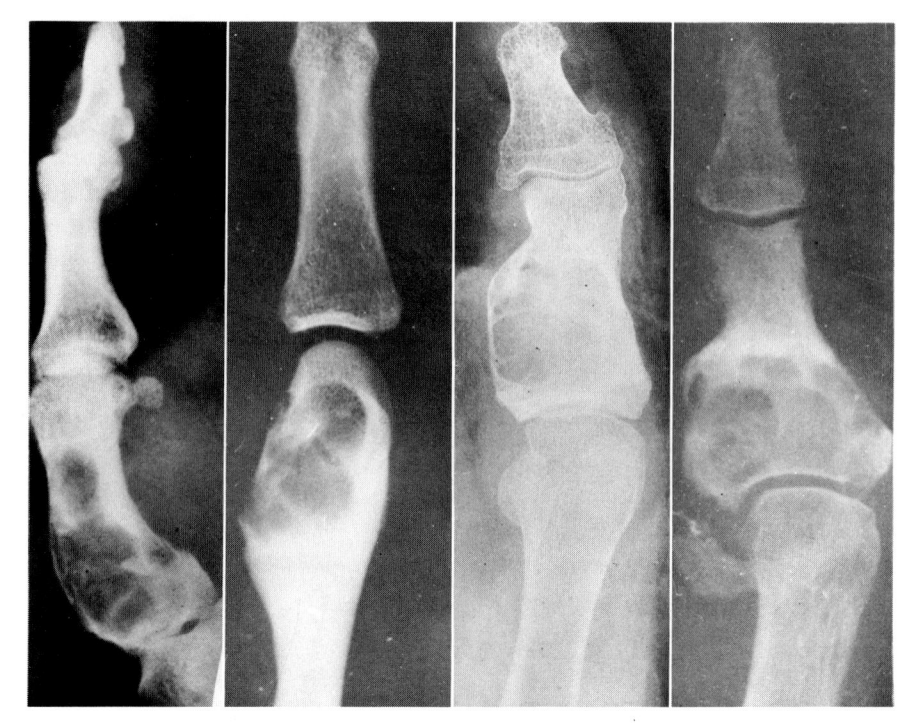

Fig. 7-3. Composite plate showing four chondromyxoid fibromas in metacarpals and phalanges. (Courtesy Professor E. F. Lascano, Buenos Aires, Argentina.)

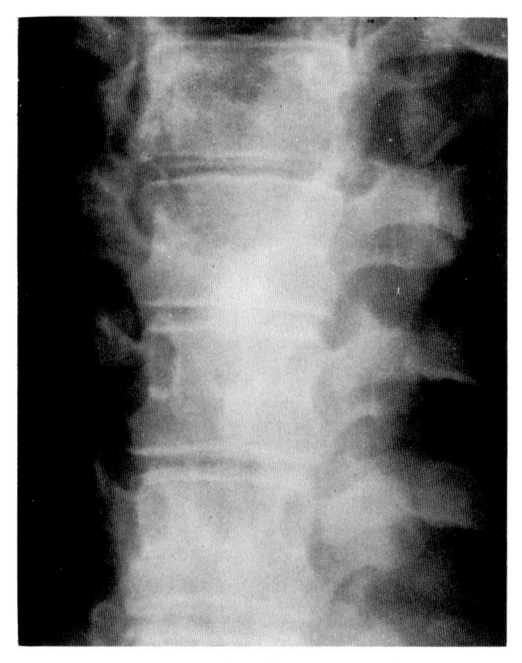

Fig. 7-4. Roentgenogram of an unusual chondromyxoid fibroma (reported by Benson and Bass) that involved the vertebral column at the level of D-1 to D-3, encroached upon the spinal canal, and caused symptoms of spinal cord compression. The symptoms were effectively relieved by surgery and supplementary x-ray therapy.

Chondromyxoid fibroma of bone 61

Clinical complaints

These were of no particular help in diagnosis, except insofar as they directed attention to the presence of a slowly developing lesion within the affected bone. The complaints were usually of some months' duration, if not longer, before the patients sought medical attention because of pain particularly on function of the

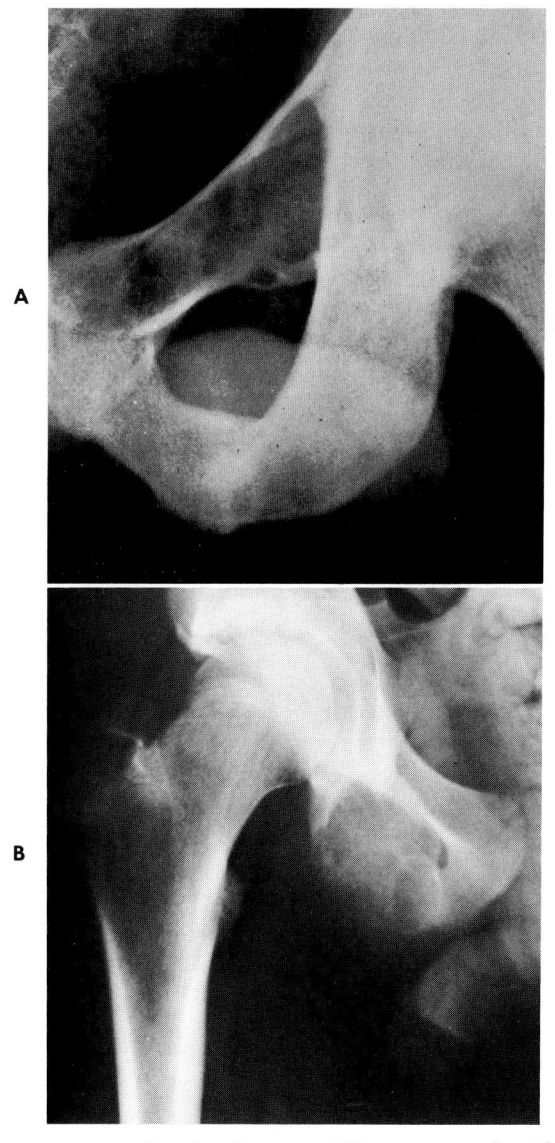

Fig. 7-5. A, Roentgenogram of a chondromyxoid fibroma situated within a pubic bone. Its cytologic picture is illustrated in Fig. 7-7, A. This roentgen film of the lesion as it appears in a flat bone lacks the distinctiveness of those illustrated in Figs. 7-1 and 7-2. B, Roentgenogram of another chondromyxoid fibroma in an ischium. Here again, the diagnosis was not suspected prior to tissue examination.

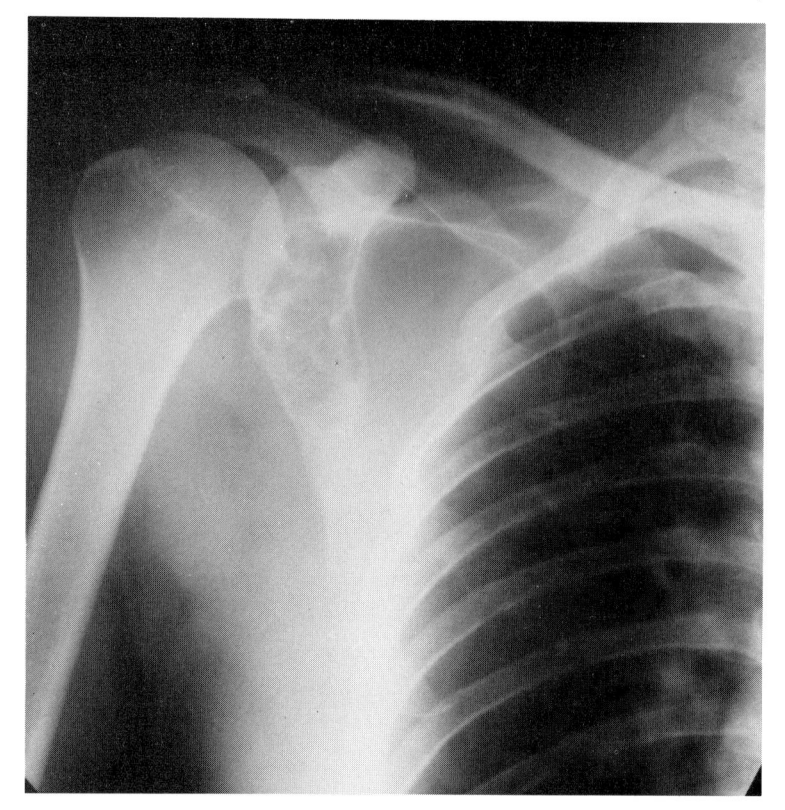

Fig. 7-6. Roentgenogram of another unusual chondromyxoid fibroma in the glenoid of a scapula. The patient was a 39-year-old man who had complained only of vague discomfort.

affected part, and, in most instances also, awareness of a palpable mass. In some of the cases observed, there was a history of a previous injury, but this is a story that one can elicit from a certain number of patients presenting virtually any bone tumor.

Gross pathologic features and their roentgenographic reflection

The tissue comprising a lesion of chondromyxoid fibroma is uniformly white, yellowish white, or tan in color, solid in texture, and rather firm but rubbery in consistency. While its appearance may suggest cartilage tumor tissue on casual inspection, it lacks the faceted pattern and blue-white luster of an enchondroma. It should be noted also that, despite the myxoid character of the intercellular matrix observed on microscopic examination, on gross examination the tissue does not appear at all slimy or mucinous.

The tumor completely replaces the bone at the site of development, and residua of the original spongy trabeculae are not usually found within it. Where it abuts on the cortex, it tends gradually to erode and destroy the latter, and the contour of the affected bone area becomes bulged. This expanded contour may be outlined, in part or throughout, by a thin shell of periosteal new bone. Where a delimiting cortical shell is absent, the tumor is still confined by the periosteum and the overlying parosteal connective tissue, and ordinarily it exhibits no tendency to be invasive. Internally, when the tumor does not extend across the entire width of the bone, it is bordered, as a rule, by a clearly outlined bed of sclerotized and often distinctly notched osseous tissue.

These gross features of the lesion are reflected in its roentgenographic appearance. It should be noted that the tumor may attain appreciable size, although occasionally it is discovered while still quite small. Among the tumors I have observed, there were some measuring as much as 7 or 8 cm. in length and 4 or 5 cm. across. Within a large limb bone, as indicated, the tumor tends to be eccentrically located in the metaphyseal area and does not ordinarily encroach upon the bone end. The contour of the tumor may appear round, but is more often ovoid, and its long axis coincides with the long axis of the affected bone. The area occupied by the lesion appears relatively radiolucent. The external border of such a tumor, as noted, tends to be outlined by a more or less expanded, delicate shell of periosteal new bone, although the latter may be defective in places. Its internal border is outlined by a well-defined, oftentimes scalloped, sclerotized line. The grooved and notched character of this perifocal bone may also cause the projection of the lesion to appear pseudotrabeculated. Altogether, these features tend to give the lesion a rather distinctive appearance that enables one to recognize it even before surgery (Figs. 7-1 and 7-2). When the tumor is still comparatively small, however, or when it presents in a rib or in a foot bone as an expanded lesion extending across the entire width of the affected bone, it is more difficult to identify. In such instances, though one may still suspect its presence, one would also have to consider such alternatives as a solitary focus of fibrous dysplasia, enchondroma, and possibly aneurysmal bone cyst. More detailed consideration of these problems from the radiologist's point of view may be found in articles by Turcotte, Pugh, and Dahlin[26] and by Feldman, Hecht, and Johnston.[7]

Microscopic appearance

The cytologic picture presented by any particular lesion of chondromyxoid fibroma varies somewhat with its age or what one may regard as its degree of maturation. In general, increasing maturity appears to be reflected in progressive collagenization of the intercellular matrix of the lesion. In some instances the matrix acquires a chondroid appearance as well. Be that as it may, the basic cytologic pattern is that of fields of tumor cells of spindle or multipolar shape rather loosely dispersed within a myxoid intercellular matrix. This lesional tissue tends to be demarcated into pseudolobules by narrow, vascularized, curving bands of more compacted tumor cells. Within these myxoid fields, the tumor cells, on the whole, have indistinct cytoplasmic borders, although many of them show branching fibrillar processes. The cell nuclei, as indicated, are for the most part spindle shaped, ovoid, or multipolar and stand out prominently. The supporting connective tissue is somewhat vacuolated and has a bluish hue when stained with hematoxylin. When sections are stained for the demonstration of mucin, the intercellular matrix does not give the mucin response, and it seems probable that the myxoid character of the matrix is attributable to its aqueous content rather than mucin (Fig. 7-7).

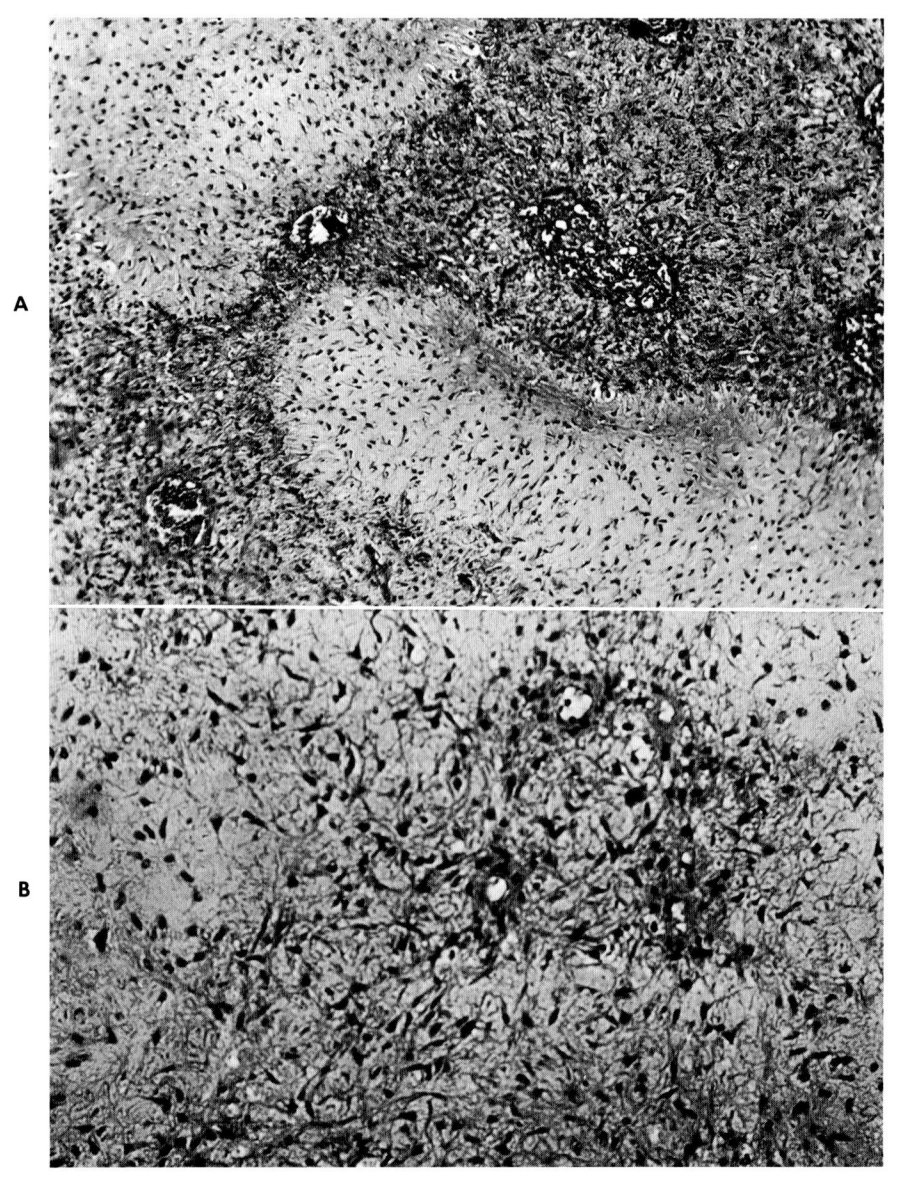

Fig. 7-7. **A** and **B**, Photomicrographs showing the general cytologic pattern of the tumors illustrated roentgenographically in Figs 7-4 and 7-5, respectively. The spindle-shaped tumor cells are loosely dispersed in a myxoid intercellular matrix. There are also occasional fields, **A**, which have acquired a chondroid appearance. (×100.)

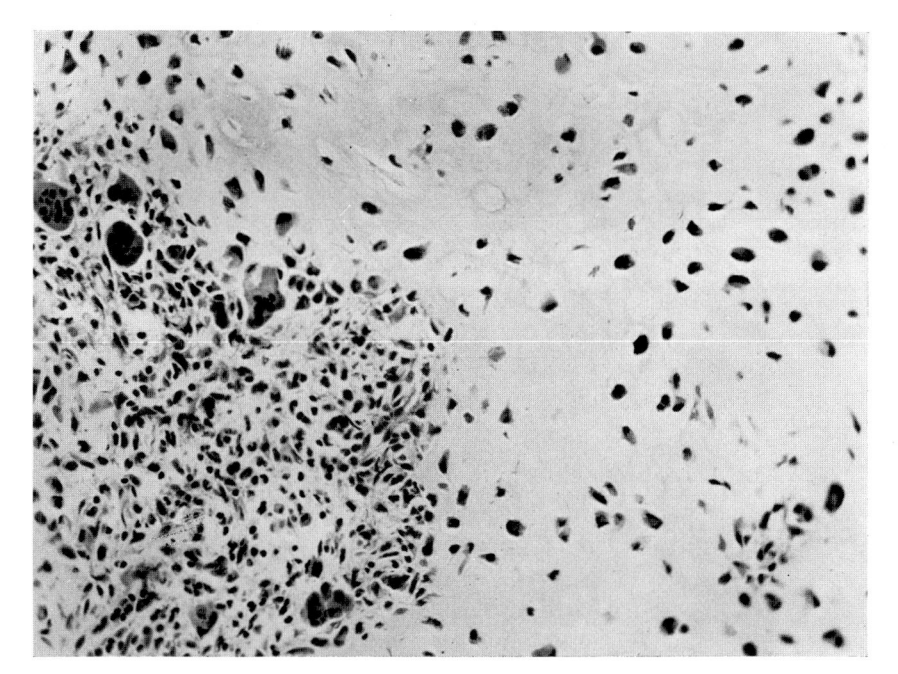

Fig. 7-8. Photomicrograph of another pertinent lesion showing the presence of several multinuclear cells within a tract of supporting connective tissue, though not within the lesional tissue proper. It is the appearance of such fields that may cause the lesion to be interpreted as a peculiar giant-cell tumor. (×135.)

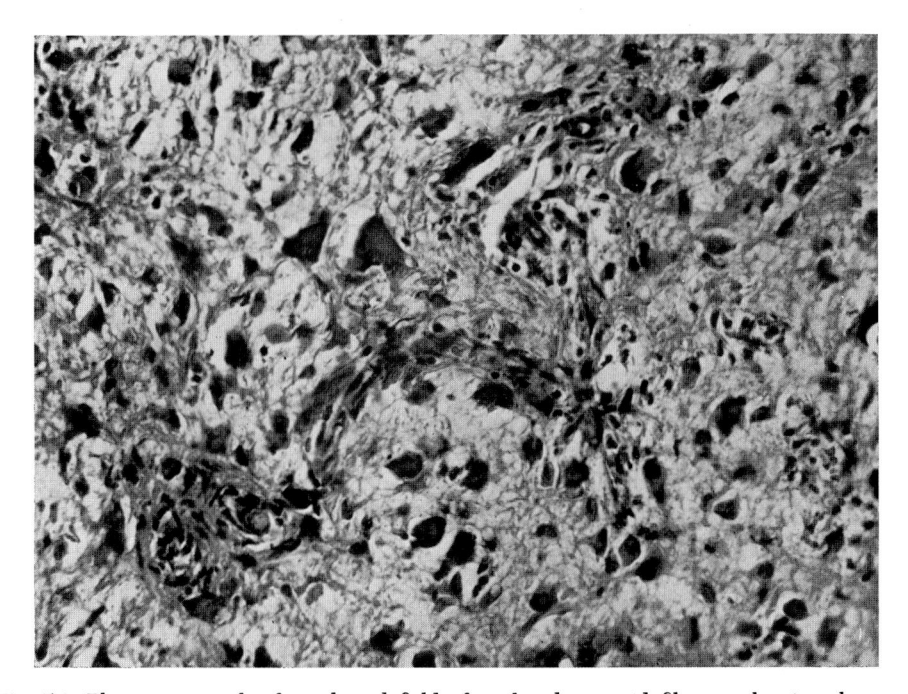

Fig. 7-9. Photomicrograph of a selected field of a chondromyxoid fibroma showing the presence of numerous ominous-looking multinuclear cells. The latter should not be regarded as an indication of malignancy; this particular tumor was actually quite indolent in its growth. (×275.)

At the periphery of the pseudolobules particularly, one is likely to find more compacted tumor cells with prominent nuclei. Some or even many of these cells may present large, plump nuclei, strikingly hyperchromatic nuclei, or atypical large double or multiple nuclei, creating an unduly ominous impression, if one is unfamiliar with the lesion (Fig. 7-9). In this vicinity also, and especially around the blood vessels within tracts of supporting connective tissue, one may observe evidence of blood extravasation and the presence of occasional multinuclear giant cells and hemosiderin-laden macrophages, along with a number of small mononuclear cells and polymorphonuclear leukocytes. Here also, there may be macrophages containing sudanophilic droplets and occasional small nests of foam cells. It should be noted that the presence of multinuclear cells within the connective tissue framework may sometimes cause the lesion to be mistaken for giant-cell tumor, even though the cytologic pattern of the lesion as a whole is quite at variance with that of genuine giant-cell tumor. To cite a case in point, the neoplasm illustrated by Willis[27] as a "chondromatous osteoclastoma" is undoubtedly an instance of chondromyxoid fibroma (Fig. 7-8).

In the more mature tumors, while a tendency toward lobular arrangement may still be maintained, one observes evidence of appreciable collagenization of the intercellular matrix, either focally or throughout. In such areas, a loose network of crisscrossing collagen fibers can be demonstrated by appropriate stains. In some lesions, these collagen fibers are interwoven into a compact mat, and smaller or larger hyaline patches may develop. In an occasional lesion, a few small foci of calcification and ossification may be noted, but this is likely to be an inconspicuous feature. In the older tumors, also, the matrix tends to take on a chondroid appearance in places, and in such fields many of the tumor cells come to lie in lacunae, so that the area as a whole acquires a certain resemblance to cartilage. This chondroid appearance, considered in conjunction with the presence of tumor cells with prominent hyperchromatic nuclei and cells with two or more nuclei, accounts for the fact that chondromyxoid fibroma is often mistaken for chondrosarcoma by pathologists who are not familiar with the lesion (Fig. 7-9). By the same token, when the intercellular matrix is predominantly myxoid rather than chondroid, one can readily understand how a diagnosis of myxosarcoma might be entertained. It should be emphasized, however, that in spite of any seemingly ominous cytologic features that may be present, the biologic behavior of the neoplasm is that of a benign tumor. Metaphorically speaking, chondromyxoid fibroma of bone is a neoplasm whose bark is worse than its bite.

It remains to consider in passing the question of the possible relationship of chondromyxoid fibroma to so-called myxoma of bone. This is rather difficult to answer, particularly since the existence of a pure myxoma of bone (outside of jaw bones) analogous to myxoma (or myxosarcoma) of skeletal soft parts has not been firmly established. It is almost impossible, for instance, to determine from the papers of Bloodgood, dealing ostensibly with "myxoma of bone," precisely what the tumors described actually represent, although it is my impression that the more aggressive ones may well have been chondrosarcomas exhibiting secondary myxoid change. Viewing the question from an academic standpoint, if one defines myxoma as a mesenchymal connective tissue neoplasm of soft, slimy appearance, containing abundant mucin within its ground substance, then chondromyxoid fibroma fails to meet these criteria. Further, if one compares the tissue of a chondromyxoid fibroma with that of an umbilical cord, one finds but little resemblance between them. Nevertheless, it would appear that the tumor under discussion is sometimes misinterpreted as a myxoma of bone, and it is interesting to note that at least one of the tumors reported by Bloodgood[3] under that head seems to be a case in point. This applies also to the instance reported by Bauer and Harrell[1] in the lower metaphysis of the femur of a 12-year-old boy. The five cases reported by Scaglietti and Stringa[22] as "myxoma of bone in children" would seem to represent instances of chondromyxoid fibroma in children below the age of 10, which grew more rapidly and had a greater tendency to recurrence after curettage, as compared with comparable tumors in older patients.

Treatment and prognosis

In keeping with the clinically benign behavior of the tumor (in all but a few instances), surgical treatment should be conservative, either thorough curettement (encompassing all the peripheral facets or pockets) or en bloc resection, if this is preferred. In the great majority of instances, at least in adolescents or adults, this should result in cure. Occasionally, local recurrence may be observed following inadequate removal of the tumor, necessitating a second surgical procedure (Fig. 7-1). The experience of Scaglietti and Stringa[22] and of Ralph[21] strongly suggests that, in children below the age of 10 or perhaps 15 years, the tumor may have greater growth potential and, concomitantly, a greater tendency to local recurrence after initial curettement. Another noteworthy example of unusual local aggressiveness that I have seen is a tumor in point in a proximal toe phalanx, which recurred twice after curettement and then seeded the soft parts locally after phalangectomy (and replacement by graft), so that a ray amputation was done eventually, about two years after initial surgery. The recurrent tumor still looked like chondromyxoid fibroma cytologically, and, in retrospect, there was no way to anticipate from the original specimen that this tumor would prove to be aggressive.

It should be noted also that Iwata and Coley[15] have reported malignant change (to low-grade chondrosarcoma) in one of their cases. This particular tumor developed in the upper fibula of a 17-year-old boy, recurred after curettement, and apparently changed its pathologic character in the course of a second recurrence. It did not metastasize, however. Incidentally, the experience cited by Jaffe[16] has reference to the same case. Gilmer and associates[10] also state that they have observed chondrosarcomatous change in one case, but give no details. Feldman, Hecht, and Johnston[7] have cited several other instances in the literature of ostensible malignant transformation, but their reliable appraisal is difficult without recourse to original material. Some of them, at least, may well have been sarcomas to begin with.

Summary

The tumor designated as chondromyxoid fibroma of bone seems not to have been generally recognized prior to 1948 as a distinctive neoplasm, although it appears likely that single instances of it were reported as enchondroma or myxoma and their malignant counterparts. An occasional instance may also be mistaken for an unusual giant-cell tumor. Our intrepretation of the lesion is that of a peculiarly differentiated connective tissue tumor exhibiting in the course of its evolution certain chondroid and also myxoid traits that hallmark the lesion cytologically. It is composed basically of cells lying loosely in a myxoid intercellular matrix that, as the tumor matures, may undergo substantial collagenization. The tissue of any particular tumor may also come to simulate cartilage tumor tissue in some or many fields, and in its gross appearance it likewise bears a certain resemblance to cartilage. There are, however, distinct differences between the appearance of this tumor and that of the common garden variety of enchondroma. The presence of smaller or larger numbers of tumor cells exhibiting nuclear atypism may cause the lesion to appear more ominous than we know it to be, explaining why it is sometimes overdiagnosed as a malignant tumor and, particularly, as chondrosarcoma.

My total experience to date with this tumor comprises some 50 cases, and increasing awareness of it is evidenced also by the publication of an appreciable number of case reports recently. The tumor is encountered most often in one or another bone of a lower limb, although instances have been observed in the hand bones, the scapula, the ribs, the innominate bone, and the vertebral column as well. Most of our patients were adolescents or young adults, though some were older. The lesion, as a rule, evolves slowly and is often of some months' or even several years' standing before surgical treatment is sought. Within the femur and tibia, the commonest sites of localization, the lesion was found consistently in the metaphyseal area adjacent to the knee joint and was eccentrically located. The roentgenographic picture has a certain distinctiveness, at least when the lesion is in a large limb bone and has attained appreciable size, although its differentiation at times from aneurysmal bone cyst, enchondroma, or a focus of fibrous dysplasia may be difficult without tissue examination. The tumor is apparently benign and in the great majority of instances can be cured by thorough curettement. A tendency to local recurrence in some instances, in young patients particularly, has been noted, necessitating further surgery for cure. Malignant change (to chondrosarcoma) has been recorded in a few instances, but this appears to be distinctly unusual. While the tumor is not a particularly common one, its recognition is of some importance in that, pathologically, it may be readily mistaken for a sarcoma, especially chondrosarcoma or myxosarcoma, and, as such, treated more radically than is necessary.

References

1. Bauer, W. H., and Harrell, A.: Myxoma of bone, J. Bone Joint Surg. 36-A:263, 1954.
2. Benson, W. R., and Bass, S., Jr.: Chondromyxoid fibroma; first report of occurrence of this tumor in vertebral column, Am. J. Clin. Pathol. 25:1290, 1955.

3. Bloodgood, J. C.: Bone tumors; myxoma, Ann. Surg. 80:817, 1924.
4. Copello, O.: Mixoma del metatarsiano, Bol. y trab. de la Soc. de cir. de Buenos Aires 19:1151, 1935.
5. Dahlin, D. C., Chondromyxoid fibroma of bone, with emphasis on its morphological relationship to benign chondroblastoma, Cancer 9:195, 1956.
6. Dahlin, D. C., Wells, A. H., and Henderson, E. D.: Chondromyxoid fibroma of bone; report of two cases, J. Bone Joint Surg. 35-A:831, 1953.
7. Feldman, F., Hecht, H. L., and Johnston, A. D.: Chondromyxoid fibroma of bone, Radiology 94:249, 1970 (extensive bibliography).
8. Frank, W. F., and Rockwood, C. A., Jr.: Chondromyxoid fibroma: review of the literature and report of four cases, South. Med. J. 62:1248, 1969.
9. Freund, E.: Unusual cartilaginous tumor formation of skeleton, Arch. Surg. 33:1054, 1936 (Case 1).
10. Gilmer, W. S., Jr., Higley, G. B., Jr., and Kilgore, W. E.: Atlas of bone tumors including tumorlike lesions, St. Louis, 1963, The C. V. Mosby Co., p. 36.
11. Goorwitch, J.: Chondromyxoid fibroma of rib; report of an unusual benign primary tumor, Dis. Chest 20:186, 1951.
12. Hadders, H. N., and Oterdoom, H. J.: Fibroma Chondromyxoides Ossis, Ned. Tijdschr. Geneeskd. 98:555, 1954.
13. Herfarth, H.: Ein zentrales Myxom der Tibia, Arch. klin. Chir. 170:283, 1932.
14. Hutchison, J., and Park, W. W.: Chondromyxoid fibroma of bone, report of a case, J. Bone Joint Surg. 42-B:542, 1960.
15. Iwata, S., and Coley, B. L.: Report of 6 cases of chondromyxoid fibroma of bone, Surg. Gynecol. Obstet. 107:571, 1958.
16. Jaffe, H. L.: Tumors and tumorous conditions of the bones and joints, Philadelphia, 1958, Lea & Febiger, p. 210.
17. Jaffe, H. L., and Lichtenstein, L.: Chondromyxoid fibroma of bone; a distinctive benign tumor likely to be mistaken especially for chondrosarcoma, Arch. Pathol. 45:541, 1948.
18. Lichtenstein, L.: Chondromyxoid fibroma of bone (Abstr.), Am. J. Pathol. 24:686, 1948.
19. Lichtenstein, L., and Jaffe, H. L.: Chondrosarcoma of bone, Am. J. Pathol. 19:553, 1943 (see pp. 567-568 and Fig. 26).
20. Pritchard, R. W., Stoy, R. P., and Barwick, J. T. F.: Chondromyxoid fibroma of the scapula, J. Bone Joint Surg. 46-A:1759, 1964.
21. Ralph, L. L.: Chondromyxoid fibroma of bone, J. Bone Joint Surg. 44-B:7, 1962.
22. Scaglietti, O., and Stringa, G.: Myxoma of bone in childhood, J. Bone Joint Surg. 43-A:67, 1961.
23. Soubeyran, P.: Rev. Chir. 29:239, 588, 1904.
24. Stradford, H. T.: Chondromyxoid fibroma of bone, Bull. Charlotte Memorial Hosp. 3:7, 1948.
25. Teitelbaum, S. L., and Bessone, L.: Resection of a large chondromyxoid fibroma of the sternum, J. Thorac. Cardiovasc. Surg. 57:383, 1969.
26. Turcotte, B., Pugh, D. G., and Dahlin, D. G.: The roentgenographic aspects of chondromyxoid fibroma of bone, Am. J. Roentgenol. 87:1085, 1962.
27. Willis, R. A.: Pathology of tumours, London, 1948, Butterworth & Co., Ltd., p. 684, and Fig. 329.

Chapter 8

Unusual benign and malignant chondroid tumors of bone

It has become increasingly apparent that, apart from classical benign chondroblastoma and chondromyxoid fibroma, there is a gamut of peculiar tumors of bone, that, for convenient reference, may be designated as chondroid. These tumors frequently manifest striking individual variation, but they exhibit common subtle or more obvious indications of cartilage-forming connective tissue derivation. In 1959 we[12] published our provisional impressions based upon study and analysis of 25 such neoplasms. Since then I have collected material from some 40 or more additional tumors in point, which will be the subject of a later report. The remarkable size of this collection can be attributed to the fact that they were submitted for consultation and came from many different sources both here and abroad. As the qualifying adjective "chondroid" implies, these tumors were not at all composed of full-fledged hyaline cartilage, as seen in enchondroma or the usual chondrosarcoma. In fact, some were composed essentially of poorly differentiated spindle connective tissue showing only focal areas of cartilage or chondroid matrix microscopically. Others had apparently reached an early chondroblastic stage of differentiation, and these constitute a small but clinically significant group that will be discussed later. Even the more differentiated ones that had some resemblance to either benign chondroblastoma or chondromyxoid fibroma differed sufficiently from their classical prototypes, so that their precise interpretation presented a problem initially.

Investigation of this composite group of chondroid neoplasms of bone, some of which proved to be benign and others, malignant, took us into a largely unexplored field. It was only after pathologic survey of all of them (and a good deal of preliminary sorting) that some logical grouping and better appreciation of individual variation became possible. Similarly, it was only through clinical follow-up observations that we gained reliable insight into the potential seriousness, or the lack of it, of each of the groups to be discussed presently. Trustworthy appraisal would hardly have been feasible from cytologic analysis alone, since arbitrary criteria for malignancy applied indiscriminately may be based upon false premises. It should be clearly stated, however, that the opinions and conclusions expressed are necessarily tentative and subject to empirical confirmation by more extensive data. They are presented with a view to recording some useful precedents and providing a convenient framework of reference within which further observations may be charted.

Our provisional classification of these unusual chondroid tumors (other than classical benign chondroblastoma and chondromyxoid fibroma) appears to parallel, in a general way, the embryologic developmental sequence observed in the formation of cartilage[6] from spindle-cell mescenchyme, through an intermediate chondroblastic stage, and, finally, to more clearly defined or differentiated cartilage-like tissue. Specifically, there were four among them (three located in bones of the foot and one in a femoral condyle) that were composed essentially of rather cellular or more collagenized spindle connective tissue showing only focal chondroid fields as the sole clue to diagnosis. These did not exhibit any malignant potentiality, although the available follow-up data bearing on this point were really inconclusive. The original series also included two frankly malignant mesenchymal tumors showing focal chondroid differentiation. As previously noted,[10] these presented initially in the calvarium and vertebral column respectively and subsequently appeared in other bones, apparently reflecting multicentric origin rather than metastasis. They would seem to represent a comparatively rare, primitive or mesenchymal type of chondrosarcoma that tends eventually to spread over the skeleton. Continuing, there was another group of four comparable tumors (three situated in foot bones and one in a finger phalanx) that were composed throughout of columns and nests of rounded cells, interpreted as early chondroblasts, enveloped in a more or less myxoid matrix. Their cytologic pattern has led some pathologists to regard them initially as "chordoid" (i.e., reminiscent of chordoma) or as "mixed tumors" (in the mistaken belief that the tumor cells were of epithelial nature). Be that as it may, they all proved in time to be locally invasive neoplasms, apparently of low-grade malignancy, although eventually requiring amputation, and we are inclined to interpret them as representing a special chondroblastic type of chondrosarcoma that is not prone to metastasize. Its multicentric counterpart, unique in our experience, was observed in a single instance, in which comparable tumor foci were encountered in the scapula and in a number of ribs.

The remaining 14 tumors in this survey were more clearly differentiated, but were unusual for one reason or another; as such, they were readily recognizable as apparently benign chondroid tumors, although their precise classification beyond that had been somewhat puzzling initially. In order to appreciate these subtleties better, the neoplasms in point were reviewed against the background of an appreciable number of tumors in our files representing fully evolved and altogether typical instances of benign chondroblastoma and chondromyxoid fibroma. It is noteworthy that no aggressive or multicentric tumors were observed in this category. Included among them were five tumors that we interpreted as atypical benign chondroblastomas, the cytologic peculiarities of which (discussed further on) were such as to prompt some pathologists to designate a number of them as "enchondromatous giant-cell tumors." Three of these tumors were situated in an astragalus, a calcaneus, and a finger phalanx, respectively, while two were in the proximal humerus. Interestingly enough, all of them were encountered in comparatively young male patients between the ages of 10 and 21 years. There were two additional unusual benign chondroblastomas in adults that stood out from the others, exhibiting occasional fields suggestive of chondromyxoid fibroma. Along another line of differentiation there were three neoplasms that, though clearly discernible as chondromyxoid fibromas, appeared somewhat different from the general run of such tumors in that they were more cellular and contained fields of undifferentiated cells that, for convenient reference, may be designated as reserve cells. Finally, there were four additional atypical chondromyxoid fibromas that deserve special mention since they presented more or less conspicuous focal calcification not ordinarily seen in such tumors. Although they are apparently of no great clinical significance, it seems worthwhile in the interest of clarity to highlight these deviations from the usual pattern and, by inference, to stress the close pathologic relationship between benign chondroblastoma and chondromyxoid fibroma.[3] As noted,[11] however, there are valid reasons for maintaining the separate identity of fully evolved tumors of the nature of benign chondroblastoma and chondromyxoid fibroma, and any attempt to lump them together indiscriminately because of occasional overlapping cytologic features is, in our opinion, to be deprecated.

Of clinical interest is the fact that as many as 12 of the 22 solitary tumors in this series were encountered in bones of the foot, specifically, the calcaneus, astragalus, metatarsals, and toe phalanges. Of the remainder, some seven were observed in large limb bones; specially, the distal femur, the proximal humerus, and the distal ulna (these were mainly instances of atypical chondroblastoma or chondromyxoid fibroma). Only three were encountered in bones of the hand

---

Fig. 8-1. **A**, Roentgenogram showing initial appearance of this poorly differentiated chondroid tumor in a second metatarsal bone. It was interpreted clinically as an enchondroma. **B**, "Recurrent" lesion some months later, requiring a second, more thorough curettement. **C**, Photomicrograph of a selected field in the specimen seen in **B**, showing a focus of hyaline cartilage developing within a rather cellular, spindle-cell stroma, which dominated the cytologic picture elsewhere. Giant-cell macrophages are prominent within vascular spaces and at the periphery of the cartilage field. (×310.) **D**, Roentgenogram of another poorly differentiated chondroid tumor situated in the posterior volar portion of the calcaneus of a 60-year-old woman. (Its appearance is not unlike that of a chondromyxoid fibroma.) **E**, Photomicrograph of a representative field of the tumor illustrated in **D**, showing a random small chondroid patch within a cellular, mesenchymal spindle-cell stroma. Such areas of chondroid differentiation were inconspicuous and required some search for their detection. (Azure A stain; ×310.) **F**, Roentgenogram of still another poorly differentiated chondroid tumor replacing the entire proximal phalanx of a large toe of a 39-year-old man. Although the involved phalanx is strikingly deformed from compression and broadening, the tumor is still contained within a shell of cortical new bone. **G**, Photomicrograph of the tumor illustrated in **A**, showing foci of calcified chondroid matrix within a spindle-cell stroma (not unlike that seen in **E**). (×310.)

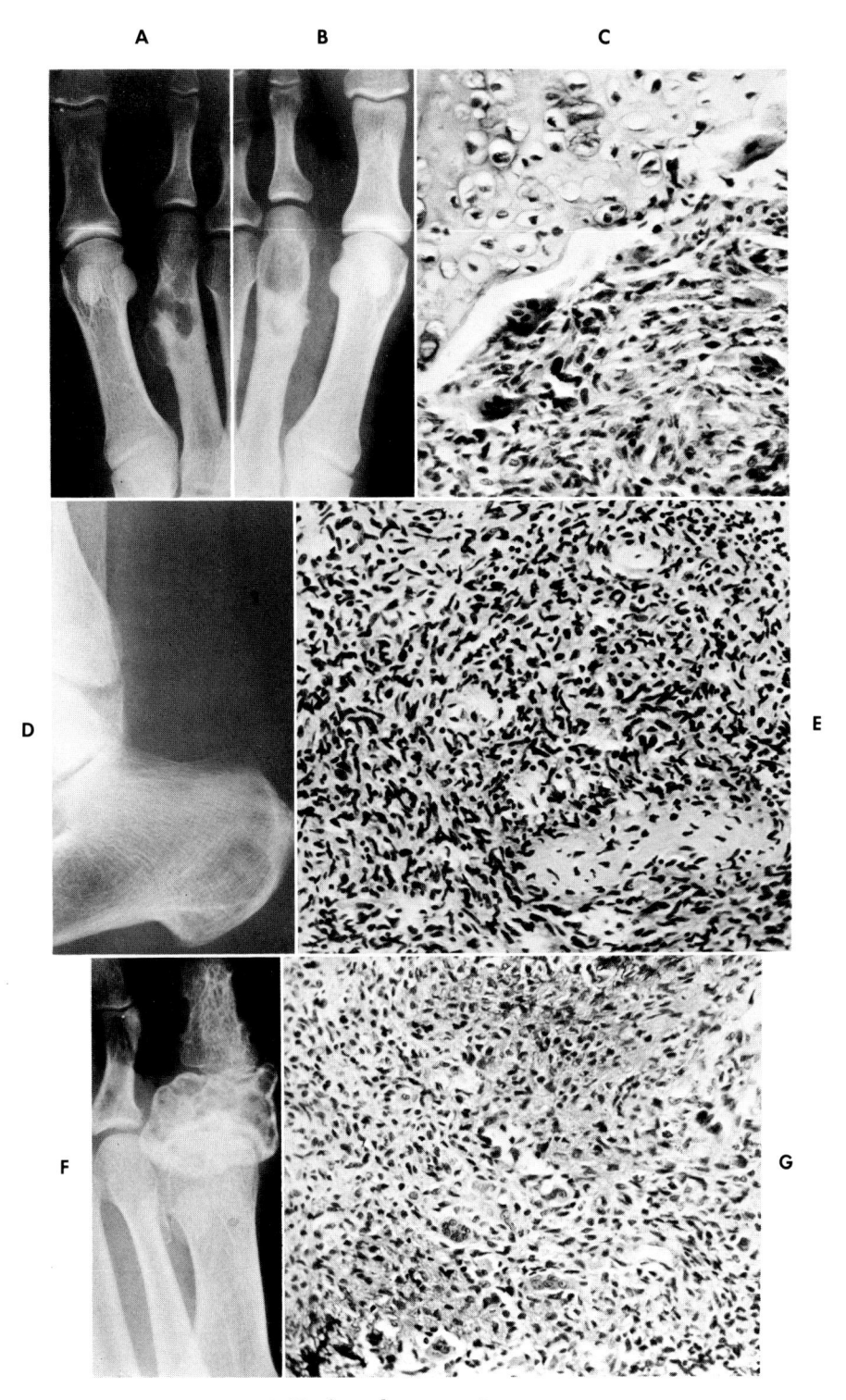

Unusual benign and malignant chondroid tumors of bone 73

Fig. 8-1. For legend see opposite page.

(unlike the common enchondroma, composed of mature hyaline cartilage, that predilects finger phalanges, and metacarpals). With reference to age incidence, the patients were adults, with the apparently significant exception of those presenting atypical chondroblastomas with giant-cell fields, who, as noted, were between the ages of 10 and 21.

The remainder of this discussion will be devoted to more detailed consideration of the major groups outlined above.

Poorly differentiated chondroid tumors

Some four neoplasms were placed in this category, and, as noted, they were situated in a metatarsal bone, the calcaneus, the proximal phalanx of a large toe, and the distal metaphysis of a femur, respectively. The patients were all adults, whose ages ranged between 20 and 60 years. The roentgenograms showed a well-defined, radiolucent defect in each instance. From its location and general appearance one could suspect a cartilage tumor of some sort, but the picture lacked distinctiveness, otherwise.

As indicated, these tumors were composed cytologically of compact spindle connective tissue cells, appearing more mesenchymal than fibroblastic, the nature or potentiality of which could be inferred only from the finding of random patches or more prominent fields of cartilage matrix within the connective tissue. Although they exhibited striking individual variation, we have nevertheless bracketed them together in the belief that they represent related neoplasms composed of poorly or partially differentiated cartilage-forming connective tissue, reminiscent of precartilage mesenchyme. This connective tissue may be sufficiently cellular as to create a somewhat ominous impression. It also exhibits a prominent content of giant-cell macrophages, mainly within vascular channels or areas of blood extravasation, as well as a tendency to marked collagenization in places. As for the fields of cartilage differentiation, these may be chondroid (exhibiting slight tinctorial metachromasia with azure A or methylene blue stains) or more hyaline and partially calcified (Fig. 8-1).

With reference to prognosis, the available follow-up data are limited by pertinent circumstances, but as far as they go, they have not indicated any aggressive behavior on the part of the tumors in point.

Mesenchymal chondrosarcoma

As indicated, we have observed material from two comparable extraordinary neoplasms composed of a compact, richly cellular, primitive-looking, stubby spindle-cell stroma exhibiting chondroid differentiation in places. Many of the sections contained no cartilage fields whatsoever, and from these alone one could hardly venture any definitive diagnosis beyond that of some mesenchymal sarcoma. Clinically, it is relevant that in each instance the tumor presented initially in a single bone site and, after a comparatively long interval, appeared in other bones and eventually spread over the skeleton. What little visceral spread was observed seemed clearly to be terminal and minimal in extent. We are inclined to interpret these remarkable tumors as being derived from cartilage-forming mesenchyme and, in all probability, having a multicentric origin. As such, they represent a comparatively rare, special type of primitive or mesenchymal chondrosarcoma (Fig. 8-2).

The first case was that of a 26-year-old man whose first major difficulty was paraplegia from extradural cord compression at the site of a tumor in T-4 and T-5, although for two to three years previously he had complained of pain across the chest that occasionally radiated into the lower extremities. Thoracotomy was performed, and decompression was accomplished by the removal of some 40 grams of tumor tissue. The patient did fairly well for a year thereafter and then developed multiple bone lesions elsewhere (parietal and occipital bones

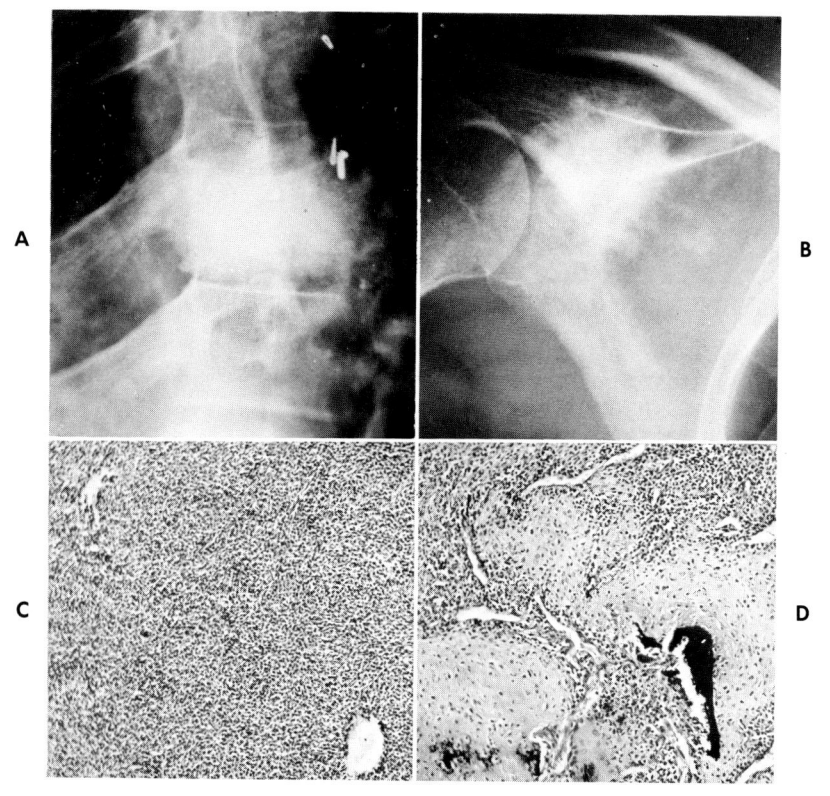

Fig. 8-2. A, Roentgenogram showing the initially presenting tumor within the fourth dorsal vertebra in the first case of multicentric mesenchymal chondrosarcoma described. As noted, this eventually caused extradural cord compression, requiring thoracotomy and partial excision of the tumor for relief. The radiopacity of the lesion reflects calcification of chondroid matrix. (See Fig. 8-1, F.) B, Roentgenogram of another similar tumor in the scapula of the patient in A, one of many such skeletal foci that appeared within the ensuing two years. C, Photomicrograph of tumor tissue excised from the neoplasm illustrated in A, showing the picture of a primitive or mesenchymal sarcoma, composed of uniform small spindle cells. The clear spaces represent blood channels. (×135.) D, A random field of the specimen seen in C, showing within this mesenchymal stroma smaller and larger chondroid foci, many of which are calcified. (×135.)

of the calvarium, sternum, sacroiliac bones, and scapula). Biopsy of a number of these showed the same cytologic picture. The patient died in a cachectic state a little more than two years after the initial operation. Autopsy showed the skeleton to be riddled with tumor; no lymph node extension was observed, and otherwise there were only scattered, minute tumor foci in the lungs, liver, and kidney, apparently reflecting terminal spread.

The second case was that of a 22-year-old woman who presented initially with a tumor in the parietal bone, compressing the contiguous cerebral cortex and requiring craniotomy for relief. She remained ostensibly well for as long as nine years thereafter, except for rare convulsive seizures, and then developed manifestations of extradural cord compression. Laminectomy disclosed a tumor in the body of T-3, extending anteriorly into the mediastinum, and this was substantially destroyed with the aid of cauterization. The patient also recovered from this operation, only to develop a third tumor in a femoral condyle, for which amputation was done. It was learned on follow-up that she died several years later (twelve years after treatment of the initially presenting tumor in the calvarium), presumably from further skeletal dissemination, although, unfortunately, no autopsy was performed. Without launching into details, suffice it to state that tissue from all three tumors presented the same cytologic pattern, which was entirely comparable to that observed in the preceding case and also interpreted as that of a peculiar, slowly evolving, multicentric mesenchymal sarcoma showing partial chondroid differentiation, or, expressed more succinctly, a multicentric mesenchymal chondrosarcoma.

This past year, I had occasion to see the sections and roentgenograms of two additional mesenchymal chondrosarcomas, one in an iliac bone and the other in the vertebral column, but too little time has elapsed for their full story to unfold. That malignant cartilage tumors of this peculiar histologic type are not as rare as one might suppose is evidenced in the article by Dahlin and Henderson[4] in which ten such tumors were presented, all but one from the files of the Mayo Clinic. These neoplasms developed in many different sites and the patients were all adults. The authors emphasize the tendency to metastasis in unusual locations, sometimes after remarkable delay.

Chondroblastic sarcoma

Four other neoplasms in this series had much in common and fell into the same category of slowly growing, locally invasive, low-grade chondroblastic sarcoma, one that seems to be unfamiliar to most clinicians and pathologists. Three of the instances in point were encountered in foot bones (the astragalus, calcaneus, and a metatarsal bone) and the fourth, in a finger phalanx. The patients were all adults of varying ages. The roentgen picture, at the outset at least, was that of a circumscribed rarefied defect, so that conservative surgery was employed initially. The sequence of events thereafter was recurrence, necessitating one or more additional unsuccessful attempts at extirpation, and eventually, after one or two or several years, amputation of the affected part when the tendency

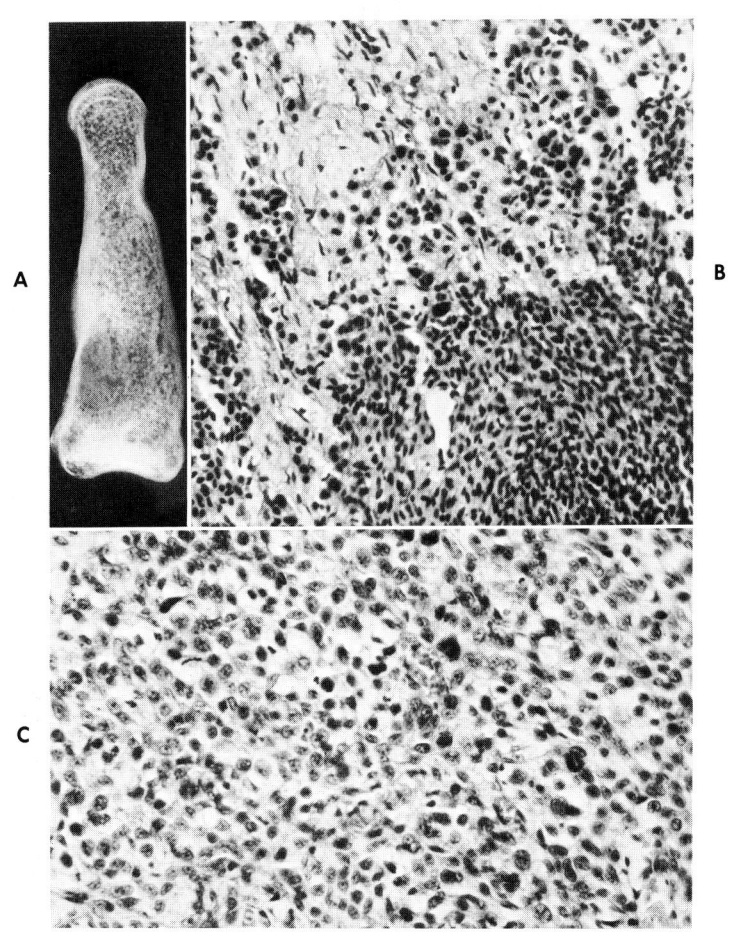

Fig. 8-3. A, Roentgenogram (enlarged from a Kodachrome reproduction) of a tumor in the middle phalanx of a third finger of a 26-year-old man, which we interpreted as a low-grade chondroblastic sarcoma. The circumscribed rarefied defect toward the base of the phalanx reflects the second recurrence of this tumor, for which amputation was performed. B, Photomicrograph of a selected field from the initial specimen of the tumor illustrated in A. Note (in the lower right-hand corner) an area of compact undifferentiated spindle cells and, issuing from it, columns of more discrete, rounded cells, which we interpret as young chondroblasts. The ground substance here was somewhat basophilic. Elsewhere, there were irregular patches of distinct chondroid matrix. (H & E stain; ×310.) C, Photomicrograph of a representative field of the recurrent tumor in the amputation specimen illustrated in A. The neoplasm has become dedifferentiated and manifests loss of chondroid matrix, increased cellularity, and some enlargement of the cells, as well as more than occasional multinucleated tumor cells. From this pattern alone, without recourse to the earlier specimens, it would be difficult to venture any definitive diagnosis. (×130.)

78 Bone tumors

to local invasion well beyond the confines of the bone of origin became quite obvious. The period of follow-up observation after ablation in our cases does not extend beyond a few years, but we have no information to indicate that distant metastasis through hematogenous spread took place in any of the instances cited.

The instructive case reported by Durbin and Smith in 1955[5] appears to be

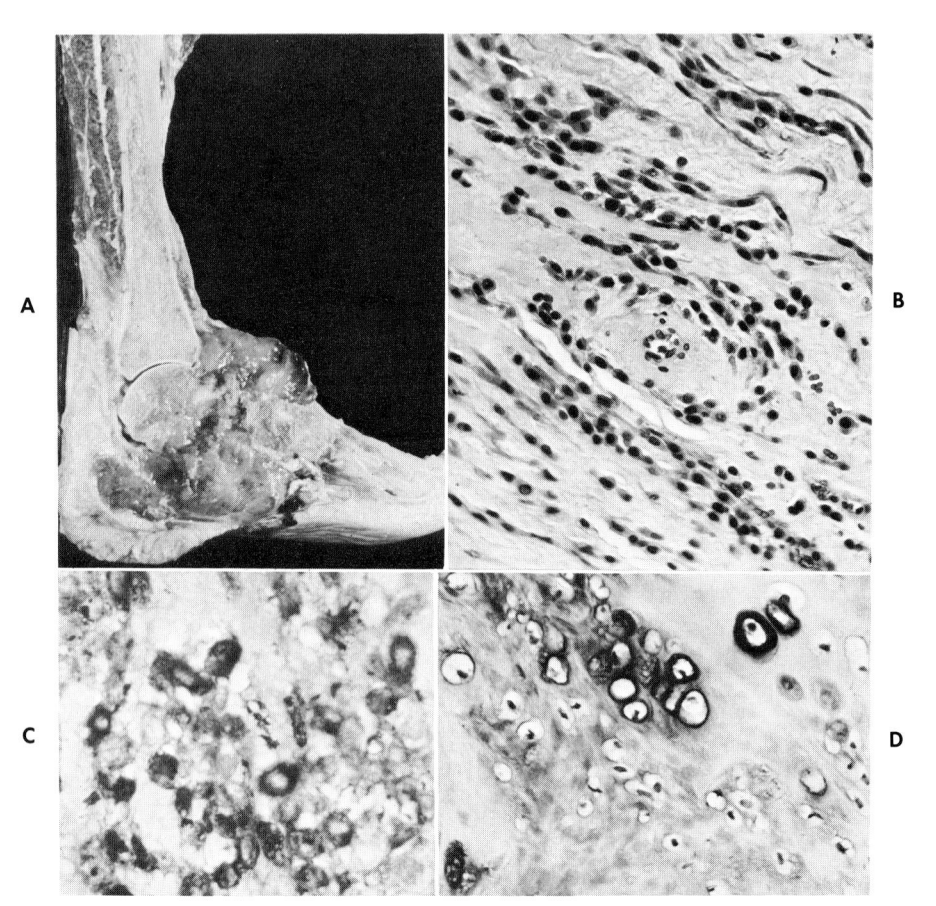

Fig. 8-4. A, Photograph (reduced) of a sagittal section through the amputated leg, showing the spread of tumor (originating in the os calcis) through the tarsal bones, around the ankle joint, and into the ulcerated skin on the dorsum of the foot. The interval between the initial conservative operation and amputation was five years. B, Photomicrograph of a representative field of this recurrent and locally invasive tumor interpreted as a low-grade chondroblastic sarcoma that originated in a calcaneus. Note the distinctive pattern of columns of tumor cells within a loose myxoid ground substance. In hematoxylin and eosin–stained sections, the bright acidophilic cytoplasmic stain of these cells contrasted sharply with the basophilic matrix. (×250.) C, Higher magnification of the tumor cells illustrated in B, stained with periodic acid–Schiff and intended to show the presence of coarse Schiff-positive cytoplasmic granules. (These were more clearly demonstrated in the slides.) (×590.) D, A random field of the tumor illustrated in C (found after prolonged search) showing unmistakable focal cartilage differentiation. (×310.)

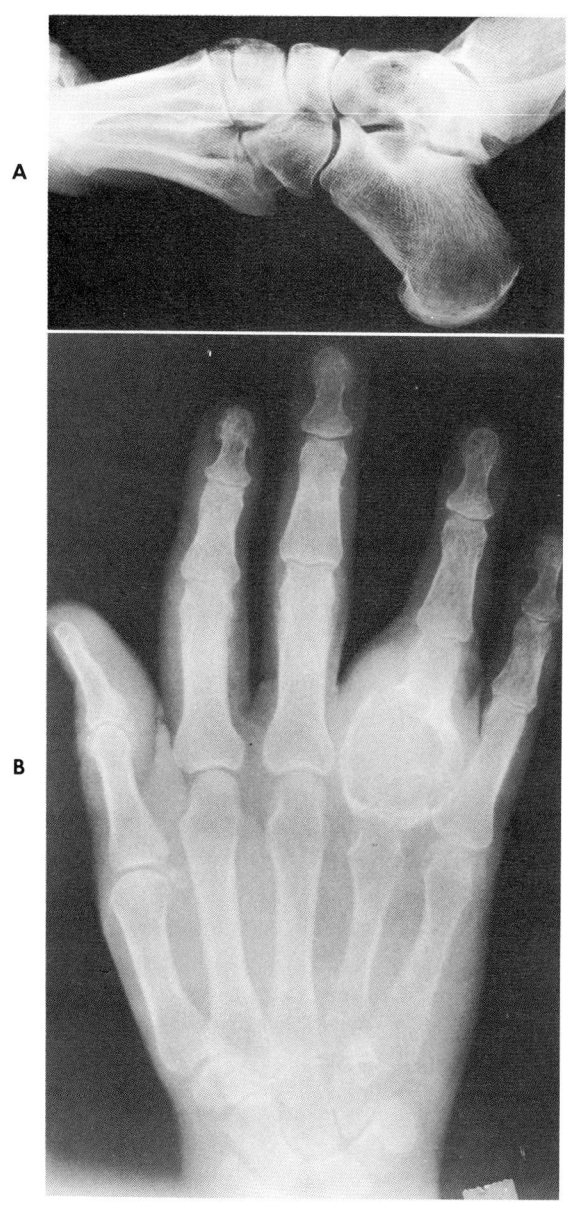

Fig. 8-5. **A,** Roentgenogram showing a well-defined, though not sharply circumscribed, rarefied defect in an astragalus of a young adult woman, reflecting the initial appearance of still another chondroblastic sarcoma. This was treated originally by curettement, and amputation was performed some two years later, after recurrence. The patient ambulates with a prosthesis and was known to be well four years after amputation. **B,** Roentgenogram of another chondroblastic sarcoma, presenting as an unusual expanded lesion in a proximal finger phalanx of a man of 62. The finger was amputated proximal to the tumor.

another in point. It is particularly interesting in that fully seven years elapsed after the initial appearance of the tumor before its insidiously malignant character was clearly recognized. Incidentally, a tumor transplant developed in the tibia of this patient, at a site from which cancellous bone had been removed for packing the calcaneal defect. With reference to the paper by Copeland and Geschickter[2] on malignant chondroblastic tumors of bone, it is difficult to surmise precisely what they had in mind, even after repeated perusal of their discussion, but in any event it seems clear that they were not dealing with the neoplasms discussed here as chondroblastic sarcoma (Fig. 8-5, *B*).

The cytologic picture, though varying somewhat from case to case, is sufficiently distinctive in its salient aspects to be readily recognizable if one is familiar with it. These tumors are composed characteristically of strands or cords of cells, or more compact nests of them with well-defined cytoplasmic borders and distinctly acidophilic cytoplasm, growing in a manner reminiscent of chordoma. The cell nuclei are of rounded or ovoid contour, sometimes vacuolated, of somewhat variable size, and often binuclear. Occasional nuclei may be hyperchromatic, distinctly larger than the average run, and sometimes multinuclear. The ground substance, in places or throughout, tends to be distinctly basophilic and myxoid in appearance, as well as pseudolobular in configuration. Against this background the dispersed acidophilic cords of tumors cells stand out sharply. In some places this matrix takes on a chondroid appearance, and within such fields the tumor cells are lodged within lacunar spaces. Inconspicuous patches of frank hyaline cartilage matrix were demonstrated in one of the cases, but only after careful search. In another of the tumors, which seemed relatively less differentiated, we could trace transitions between the characteristic cords or columns of tumor cells and fields of more compact, stubby, spindle-shaped mesenchymal cells (apparently precartilage mesenchyme). Altogether, we are inclined to interpret the basic tumor cells as young chondroblasts (which do not yet exhibit any focal calcification) and the tumors in point as low-grade chondroblastic sarcomas, different biologically and cytologically from conventional chondrosarcoma and showing a consistent tendency to insidious local invasion, but little or no disposition toward early metastasis (Figs. 8-3 to 8-5, *A*).

Multicentric chondroblastic sarcoma

That low-grade chondroblastic sarcoma, as described in the preceding section, may have its multicentric counterpart (even as the mesenchymal chondroid tumors do on occasion) is evidenced by an unusual case that is unique in our experience, and for which we can find no precedent in the literature. This patient was a 40-year-old woman who presented with a tumorous defect in a scapula and many similar lesions in the ribs bilaterally that were known to have been present for at least three years (Figs. 8-6, *A* and *B*). Two separate rib lesions were biopsied (three years apart). They both showed the same picture, that of short cords of cells with prominent nuclei and strongly acidophilic cytoplasmic streamers loosely dispersed in a basophilic, rather myxoid matrix (Fig. 8-6, *C*).

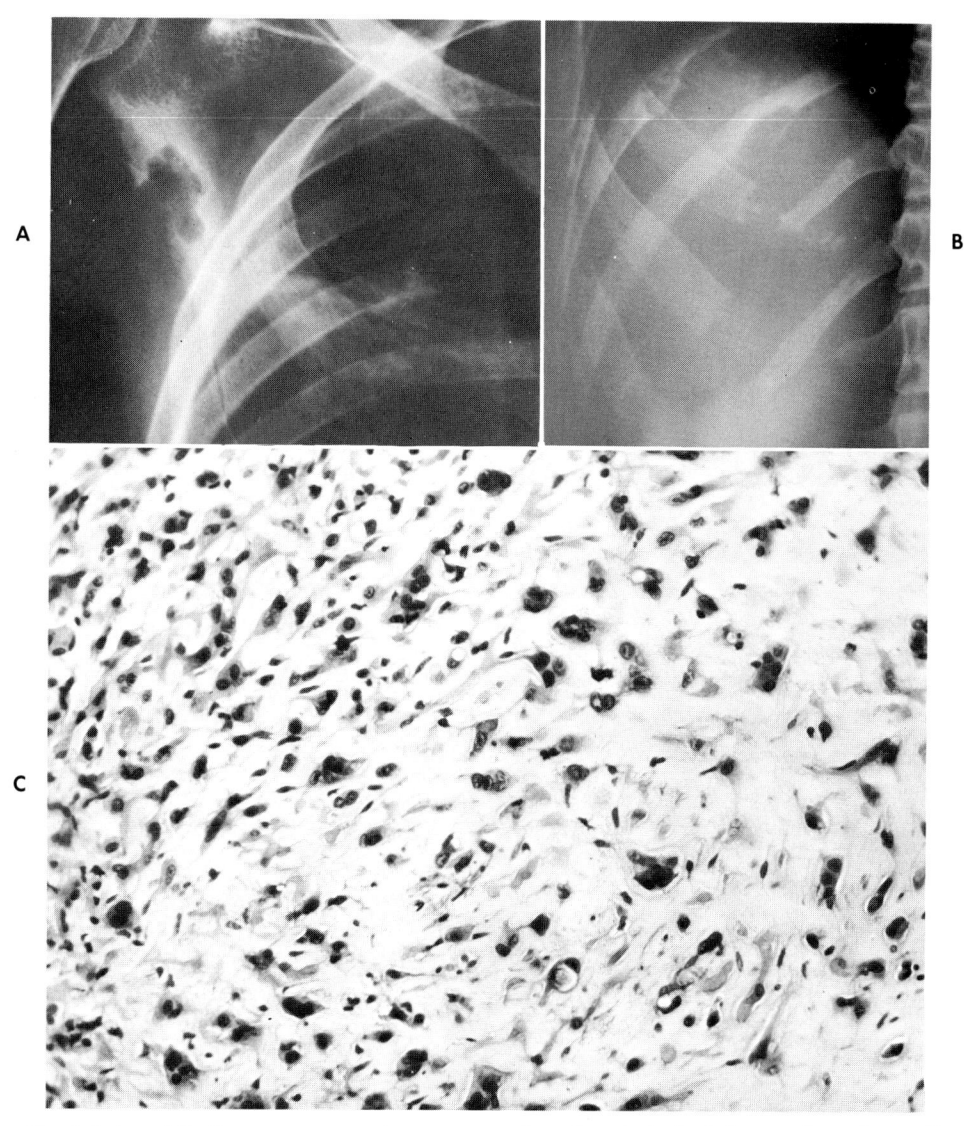

Fig. 8-6. **A** and **B**, Roentgenograms showing a number of eroded rib defects and another well-demarcated lesion along the lateral border of the scapula of a 40-year-old woman. Biopsy of one of the rib lesions in 1955 and of another in 1958 showed the presence of a chondroid tumor that we interpret as a low-grade chondroblastic sarcoma developing in multiple skeletal foci. **C**, Photomicrograph of a representative field in the biopsy specimen of one of the rib lesions illustrated in **B**, showing short cords of tumor cells (with strongly acidophilic cytoplasm) dispersed in a matrix that was somewhat basophilic. This pattern resembles that shown in Fig. 8-4, *B*, and differs from it only in that the tumor cells are appreciably larger and exhibit greater nuclear atypism. Other fields showed early extension of tumor through the eroded rib cortex into the attached muscle bundles. (×250.)

As noted, this cytologic picture differed from that of the tumors described under the heading of chondroblastic sarcoma only in that the tumor cells were appreciably larger and exhibited greater nuclear atypism—the basic pattern was the same.

Atypical benign chondroblastoma

The better differentiated and relatively more mature range of the chondroid tumors surveyed here is represented by some 14 neoplasms, half of which were designated as atypical benign chondroblastoma, for convenient classification, and the other half as atypical chondromyxoid fibroma. To the best of our knowledge, these tumors responded well to conservative surgical treatment, and the emphasis upon "atypical" has reference to more or less subtle cytologic deviations from the conventional pattern of the tumors in question, rather than to any significant difference in their clinical behavior. By way of maintaining perspective, it should be emphasized further that for every "atypical" benign chondroblastoma there are probably 10 or more (an educated guess) that start in the epiphyses of large limb bones of teen-agers and exhibit the usual, now well-familiar cytologic pattern.[7,12] On the other hand, better insight into their nature helps to explain certain instances of benign chondroblastoma previously reported[1] in bones other than large limb bones (notably, bones of the foot and hand), as well as in older adult patients.

Of the seven tumors classified as atypical benign chondroblastoma, two were situated in bones of the foot (astragalus and calcaneus), one in a finger phalanx, and four in large limb bones (three in the upper humerus and one in the distal end of a femur). Of this number, five (including those in the foot and hand, as well as two in the proximal humerus) apparently constituted a distinct subgroup, and, following the usual trend of chondroblastoma in general, the patients were all boys and young men whose ages ranged from 10 to 21 years. In all but one of these five instances, the initial impression of the examining pathologist was chondroblastoma, although he was sufficiently uncertain about the interpretation of one or another unusual cytologic feature to seek another opinion. In one such instance, the local consultants were unduly impressed by tumor recurrence after inadequate surgical treatment (thorough curettement was not done initially) and ventured an opinion of low-grade osteogenic sarcoma. Two other tumors in point were submitted to the Armed Forces Institute of Pathology for review, and the impression recorded there was "enchondromatous giant-cell tumor." This problem is nomenclature and our views on the inappropriateness of the latter designation will be considered presently (Fig. 8-7).

Without launching into a detailed account of the individual tumors in point, their cytologic aberrations from the familiar normal pattern of benign chondroblastoma[12] (that of closely approximated, uniform, rounded chondroblasts exhibiting focal calcification and the resulting organization of calcified necrotic tumor fields) may be stated as follows. In some instances the chondroblasts were perceptibly larger and showed an appreciable number of mitoses, and in some

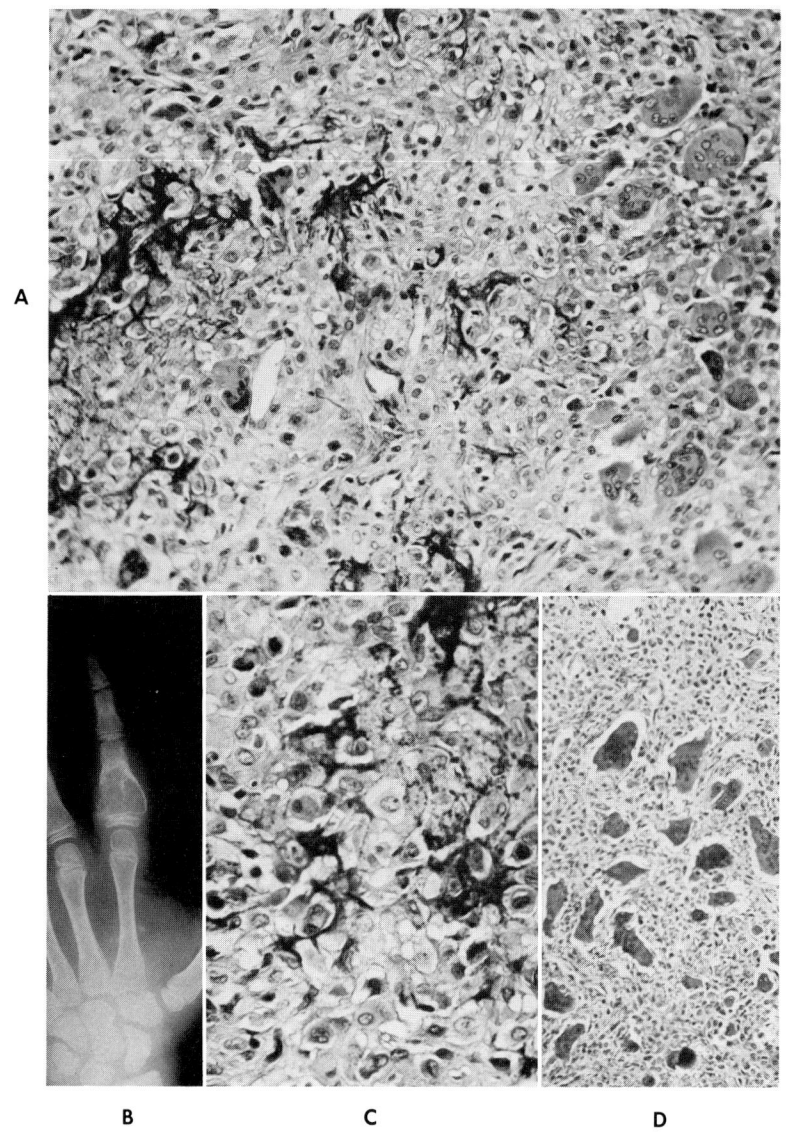

Fig. 8-7. A, Photomicrograph of an atypical chondroblastoma (in a calcaneus) showing conspicuous focal calcification as well as prominent giant-cell reaction on the right (in proximity to an area of blood extravasation). (×170.) B, Roentgenogram (reduced) of a circumscribed tumor in the proximal phalanx of a finger, which also proved to be an atypical benign chondroblastoma. Follow-up more than four years later showed an excellent clinical result. C, Photomicrograph of a selected field of the tumor illustrated in B, showing conspicuous calcification in a field of chondroblasts. (×250.) D, Another field of the tumor in B (called "enchondromatous giant-cell tumor" by some observers) showing prominent giant-cell reaction. Closer scrutiny shows these cells to be lodged within vascular spaces, and they would appear to represent skeletal giant-cell macrophages rather than a significant integral component of the tumor. (×135.)

places they were more elongated or spindle shaped. In other instances there were relatively large and conspicuous fields of chondroid matrix, not necessarily associated with calcification and necrosis of tumor tissue, and these sometimes showed focal secondary ossification. Finally, in a number of instances giant cells were inordinately prominent, especially in the vicinity of blood extravasation, within and about vascular spaces, and around the periphery of fields of mineralized chondroid matrix. To give these giant cells (for the most part, multinuclear skeletal macrophages) a position of major, if not dominant, importance, as is implied in the designation of giant-cell tumor, however qualified, is to distort the picture as a whole. In effect this reverts to the once useful but now outdated concept of chondromatous giant-cell tumor, so-called, stemming from Kolodny, Ewing, and Codman.

The two remaining atypical benign chondroblastomas attracted attention because they presented scattered fields of myxoid (or chondromyxoid) matrix in which the tumor cells had a spindled orientation, reminiscent of chondromyxoid fibroma. In keep with this "hybrid" tendency, it is interesting to note that in both instances the patients were not teen-agers, but adults, 37 and 44 years of age, respectively. It should be emphasized, however, that the basic dominant cytologic pattern of these neoplasms was that of chondroblastoma, as evidenced by fields of massed, rounded chondroblasts exhibiting conspicuous focal calcification. Secondary giant-cell reaction was not at all a prominent feature, being observed only in sites of hemorrhage and, occasionally, at the periphery of a patch of mineralized matrix. Incidentally, in one of the cases, the initial impression of the examining pathologist was that of possible chondrosarcoma (Fig. 8-8).

Atypical chondromyxoid fibroma

For convenient orientation, the conventional cytologic pattern of chondromyxoid fibroma may be concisely described as that of fields of tumor cells of spindle or multipolar shape, loosely dispersed within a myxoid intercellular matrix. This lesional tissue may in places acquire a chondroid appearance, and

---

Fig. 8-8. **A**, Roentgenogram of an unusually large benign chondroblastoma taken after the patient (then 20 years of age) had sustained a pathologic fracture. Punch biopsy at the time was interpreted as showing "giant-cell tumor." **B**, Roentgenogram of the tumor illustrated in **A**, taken three years later, showing calcific mottling not previously in evidence. Because of the large size of the tumor, a suspicion of sarcomatous change was entertained clinically, but this was not supported by the biopsy sections. **C**, Roentgenogram of still another expanded, but well-delimited, atypical benign chondroblastoma in the lower femur of a 44-year-old man. Although this tumor involves part of the old epiphyseal region, its appearance otherwise could pass for that of a chondromyxoid fibroma. Surgical treatment was conservative, and the patient was well, without local recurrence, two years later. **D**, Photomicrograph of a selected field of an unusual benign chondroblastoma originating in the region of the capital humeral epiphysis (the site stressed by Codman) of a 37-year-old man. Note a field of chondroblasts in the upper portion of the figure and a patch of chondromyxoid matrix in the lower portion. Elsewhere in this tumor there were fields showing typical focal calcification. (×300.)

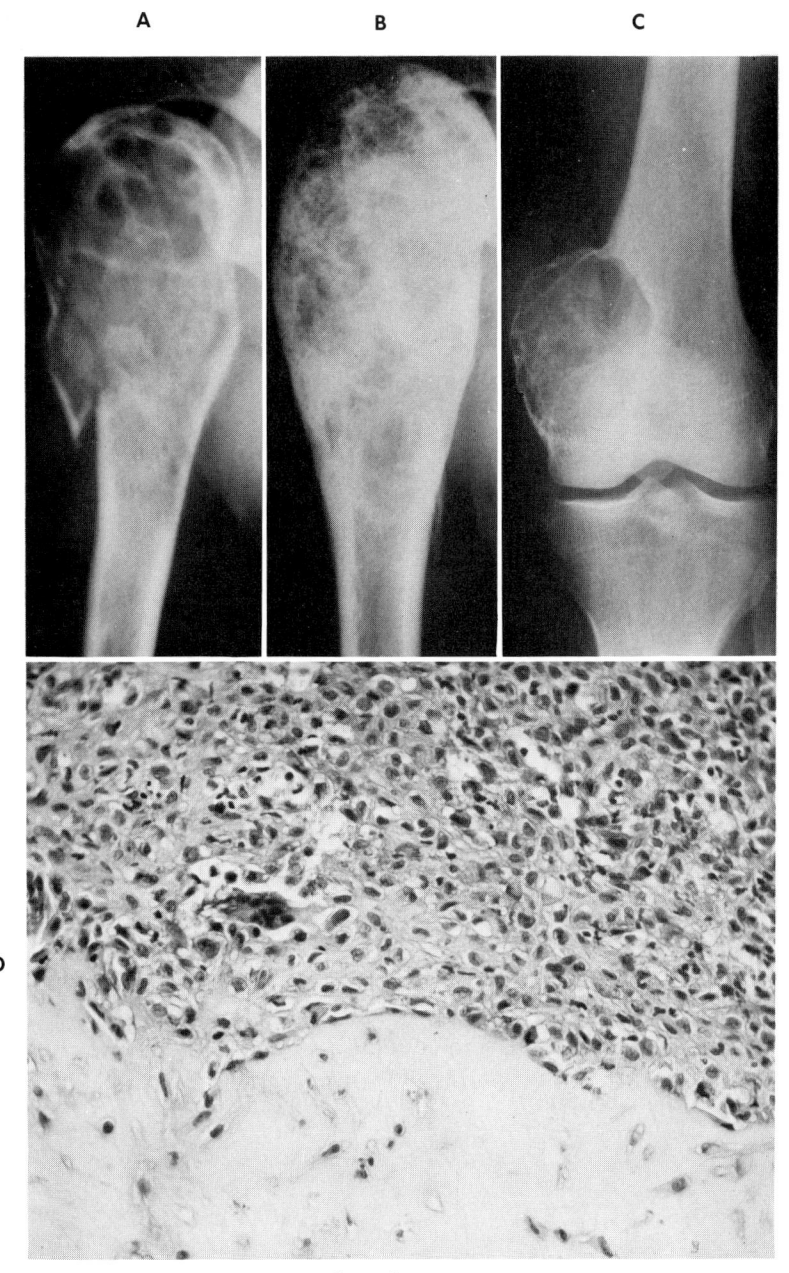

Unusual benign and malignant chondroid tumors of bone 85

Fig. 8-8. For legend see opposite page.

it tends also to be demarcated into pseudolobules by narrow, vascularized curving bands of more compacted tumor cells.[8,9] The seven tumors classified as atypical chondromyxoid fibroma had sufficient resemblance to the conventional pattern for this to be clearly recognized by all but two of the examining pathologists who submitted their material for opinion. Incidentally, it is gratifying that none of them initially ventured an opinion of chondrosarcoma or myxosarcoma (a common trap some years ago when the nature and clinical behavior of chondromyxoid fibroma was not as yet well recognized). On the other hand, the instances in point showed a cytologic picture that deviated from the usual pattern, as described, in a number of noteworthy respects, which will be indicated presently. It should be emphasized at the outset, however, that these cytologic variations are not of any clinical importance apparently, for the available follow-up data indicated that the patients in question obtained a good result without local recurrence after definitive conservative surgery—the periods of observation ranged up to four and one-half years. It may be added that the patients were all adults (of both sexes) whose ages ranged from 22 to 54 years. As for localization, four of the tumors were encountered in bones of the foot (toe phalanx, two; metatarsal, one; calcaneus, one), one in a metacarpal, and two in limb bones (lower femur, one; distal ulna, one).

The tumors in point were interpreted as falling into two distinct subgroups: those that appeared to be not fully differentiated and those that showed focal calcification, not ordinarily observed in chondromyxoid fibroma. The former, three in number, manifested less distinct pseudolobulation or none at all, greater cellularity on the whole, and, more particularly, fields of compact undifferentiated cells with large, pale, round or ovoid nuclei, which may be regarded as reserve cells. The remaining four tumors were unusual in that they showed focal calcification in a lattice pattern, or in a more widespread streaky fashion, or in

---

Fig. 8-9. **A,** Roentgenogram of an expanded tumor in the distal phalanx of the right hallux of a 22-year-old woman, which proved to be an atypical chondromyxoid fibroma. She had complained of pain for three months and of swelling for a much longer time. Surgical treatment consisted of excision of the distal phalanx. **B,** Roentgenogram of another atypical chondromyxoid fibroma replacing and expanding the proximal phalanx of a third toe of a 27-year-old man, who had complained of swelling and pain for about one and one-half years. Its tendency to conspicuous focal calcification is clearly reflected in the figure. **C,** Roentgenogram of still another atypical chondromyxoid fibroma, in this instance in the distal end of a femur in a 29-year-old young man. Its outline is well defined and somewhat scalloped. Anteriorly, the thin shell of cortical bone is still intact; posteriorly, it is defective, but the tumor is delimited by a faintly outlined, imperfect shell of periosteal new bone. **D,** Photomicrograph of a representative field of the tumor seen in **C,** showing prominent streaky calcification within a chondromyxoid matrix. (×310.) **E,** Photomicrograph of a representative field of an atypical chondromyxoid fibroma, showing a pattern of heavy focal calcification. (This tumor was situated in the distal ulna of a 47-year-old man, who had complained of gradual enlargement and tenderness for several months. The involved distal end of the ulna was resected and bone grafts used for reconstruction. Follow-up more than four years later showed a satisfactory clinical result.) (×250.)

the form of heavier, blotchy deposits. This feature is, of course, reminiscent of benign chondroblastoma, and it is understandable that the tumors in question might be regarded by some as hybrid or combination forms.[3] With a view to keeping the nomenclature as simple as possible, we prefer to designate them as "atypical chondromyxoid fibromas showing focal calcification" inasmuch as their basic pattern was that of chondromyxoid fibroma (Fig. 8-9).

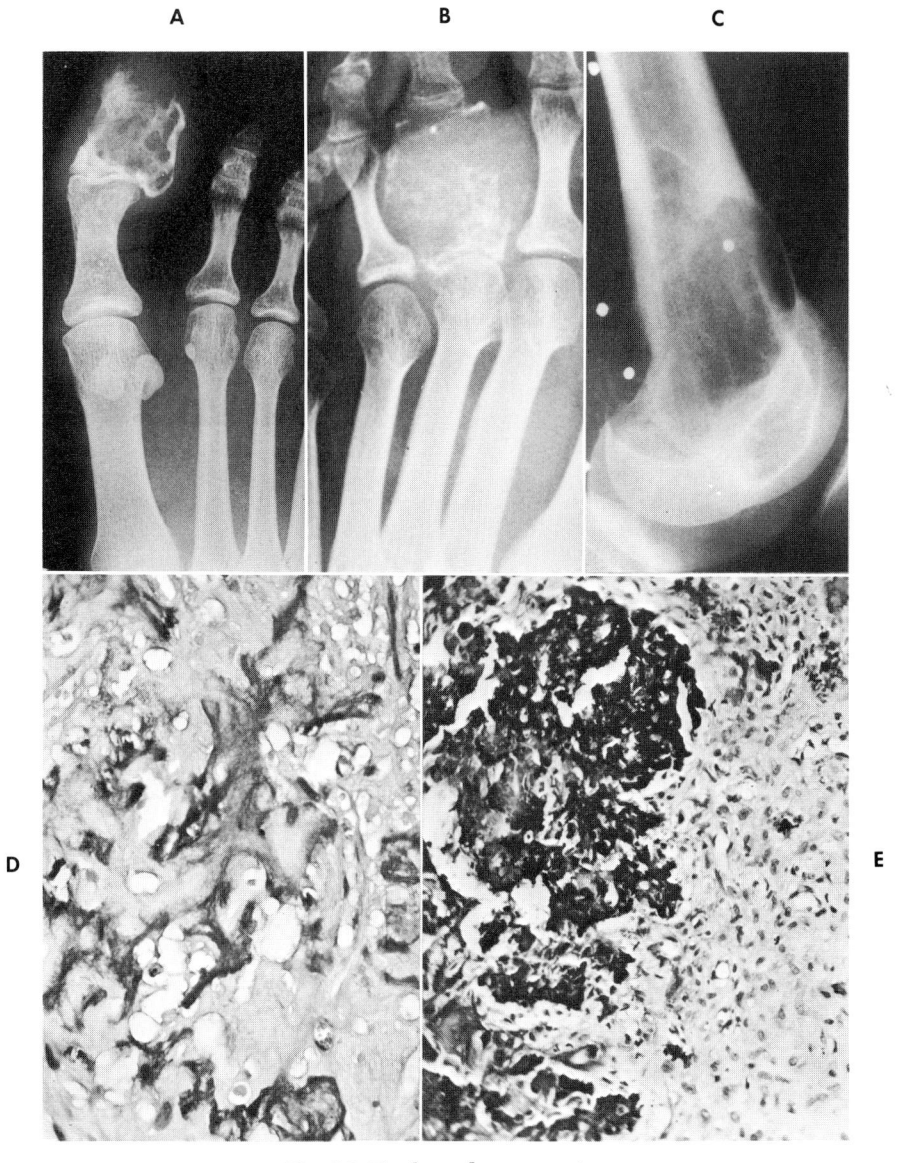

Fig. 8-9. For legend see opposite page.

Summary

This chapter presents a pathologic survey of a composite collection of 25 unusual and largely unfamiliar chondroid tumors of bone. Consideration also is given to some of the clinical implications. One group of these neoplasms was provisionally classified as poorly differentiated or mesenchymal cartilage tumors. Of these, only the multicentric ones were obviously malignant. Another clinically important group was interpreted as low-grade chondroblastic sarcoma, which showed a consistent tendency to recurrence after conservative treatment and insidious local invasion that eventually required amputation, but little or no disposition toward metastasis. This neoplasm, too, has its multicentric counterpart, although it is rarely encountered. The remainder, constituting a majority of those discussed, were designated as either atypical benign chondroblastoma or atypical chondromyxoid fibroma. The variations of the cytologic pattern of these mavericks from that of their classical prototypes are discussed in some detail.

References

1. Coley, B. L., and Santoro, A. J.: Benign central cartilaginous tumors of bone, Surgery 22:411, 1947.
2. Copeland, M. M., and Geschickter, C. F.: Chondroblastic tumors of bone; benign and malignant, Ann. Surg. 129:724, 1949.
3. Dahlin, D. C.: Chondromyxoid fibroma of bone, with emphasis on its morphological relationship to benign chondroblastoma, Cancer 9:195, 1956.
4. Dahlin, D. C., and Henderson, E. C.: Mesenchymal chondrosarcoma. Further observations on a new entity, Cancer 15:410, 1962.
5. Durbin, F. C., and Smith, G. S.: Chondromatous tumour of calcaneus, J. Bone Joint Surg. 37-B:584, 1955.
6. Ham, A. W.: Histology, ed. 3, Philadelphia, 1957, J. B. Lippincott Co., pp. 248-249.
7. Jaffe, H. L., and Lichtenstein, L.: Benign chondroblastoma of bone; reinterpretation of so-called calcifying or chondromatous giant cell tumor, Am. J. Pathol. 18:969, 1942.
8. Jaffe, H. L., and Lichtenstein, L.: Chondromyxoid fibroma of bone; distinctive benign tumor likely to be mistaken especially for chondrosarcoma, Arch. Pathol. 45:541, 1948.
9. Lichtenstein, L.: Chondromyxoid fibroma of bone (Abstra.), Am. J. Pathol. 24:686, 1948.
10. Lichtenstein, L.: Diseases of bone, N. Engl. J. Med. 255:427, 1956.
11. Lichtenstein, L.: Bone tumors, ed. 2, St. Louis, 1959, The C. V. Mosby Co., pp. 82-83.
12. Lichtenstein, L., and Bernstein, D.: Unusual benign and malignant chondroid tumors of bone. A survey of some mesenchymal cartilage tumors and malignant chondroblastic tumors, including a few multicentric ones, as well as many atypical benign chondroblastomas and chondromyxoid fibromas, Cancer 12:1142, 1959.

Chapter 9

Osteoid-osteoma

The concept of osteoid-osteoma, once controversial, has now won general acceptance, and any questions that remain are of greater academic than practical import. Osteoid-osteoma was first described as a distinctive benign osteoblastic tumor by Jaffe[9] in 1935 in a paper reporting five relevant instances developing within spongy bone. Subsequently Jaffe and I[12] observed that the same lesion also frequently developed in relation to the cortices of the shafts of long bones and that, when it did so, it provoked remarkable sclerosis of the surrounding cortex out of proportion to the small size of the nidus. Such cases had previously been commonly misclassified (and still are, though less often) as instances of cortical bone abscess or of sclerosing nonsuppurative osteomyelitis. Incidentally, it was never maintained that there was not a sclerosing form of osteomyelitis (Garré's osteomyelitis), but only that some or many cases, so-called, proved on closer scrutiny to be instances of osteoid-osteoma. The report of this further experience with the lesion was published in 1940 and dealt with 33 cases in all. The relative frequency of the lesion was further demonstrated by the fact that in 1945 Jaffe[10] was able to report on 62 proved cases, and the tally at present exceeds 150. Additional observations of value on sizable groups of cases have now been reported from many centers.

In fact, the condition has become so familiar to medical men generally that the only cases about which I am consulted nowadays are either those in which there was recurrence of symptoms after incomplete removal, or those in which the nidus was fragmented in the course of surgical extirpation and the examining pathologist failed to recognize the distinctive character of one or more of the fragments present in the sections.

It is interesting to note by way of historical perspective that the concept met with a good deal of resistance at first from a number of orthopedists and radiologists reluctant to give up the idea of a low-grade infection as a basis for the condition,[2] but it gradually won over as stout adherents[4,8,17,20,21,23] all but a few die-hard skeptics.[1] At the present time, even those who have some reservation as to whether the lesion represents a genuine neoplasm readily accept the fact that it is highly distinctive and clearly recognizable roentgenographically and pathologically. It is freely admitted that there are still a number of questions not as yet possible to answer satisfactorily, but these do not relate to the identity of the lesion. Why is the lesion so small, as a rule? Why it is so often painful? What would happen to the lesion ultimately if it were left undisturbed? What is the effect of x-ray irradiation upon it?

An osteoid-osteoma may be defined as an oval or roundish tumorlike nidus that is composed of osteoid and trabeculae of newly formed bone deposited within a substratum of highly vascularized osteogenic connective tissue. The lesion, even when it is fully evolved, usually does not exceed a centimeter in its greatest dimension. My recent experience has shown, however, that an osteoid-osteoma may occasionally attain a substantially large size (up to 5 or 6 cm. in greatest dimension). These will be considered later (Figs. 9-7 and 9-8). It may develop either within the spongiosa, often at or near an articular surface, or in relation to the cortex of the affected bone. In the latter situation, the lesion may be located within the cortex or abut against its inner surface. When it develops within a spongy bone area, it provokes merely a thin rim of reactive sclerosis around it, but when it develops in relation to the cortex of a long bone, for some reason or other, one commonly observes a perifocal zone of dense sclerotized cortical bone extending for a considerable distance beyond the osteoid-osteoma per se.

The lesion may be encountered in young children but is seen more often in adolescents and young adults. It is distinctly uncommon beyond the age of 30 years. The site of the lesion was found to be a tibia or a femur in about half of the cases. Involvement of other bones in the lower extremity, particularly the foot bones, is also fairly common. Less common, though by no means unusual, is localization in a bone of an upper limb or in the vertical column (usually the arch rather than a body).[15,16] I have seen an instance in a rib (the twelfth) of a young woman who had complained of pain in that site for three to four years, and also another in the twelfth rib of a 6-year-old boy. A noteworthy instance has been described as occurring in a mandible, but to my knowledge the lesion has not as yet been observed in the calvarium.

It may be mentioned here that Lapidus and Salem[13] reported a case in which it is claimed from the roentgen findings that two separate osteoid-osteoma lesions were present in a femur. However, the identity of only one of these lesions was established by pathologic examination. Another presumptive case reported from Upsala, Sweden, as bilateral symmetrical osteoid-osteoma appeared to me on review of the available sections to be an instance of bilateral osteoperiostitis, provoking localized cortical thickening.

Diagnosis
Clinical complaints

The duration of symptoms at the time the patient seeks treatment usually varies from about six months to two years. I am familiar with a case in which the complaints were of fully seven years' duration, and it is interesting to note that the osteoid-osteoma removed from this patient, with prompt and complete relief as usual, showed no indication whatsoever of spontaneous involution. The major complaint referable to the tumor is pain, mild and occasional at first but increasing in persistence and severity, so that ultimately it often keeps the patient awake at night. It is noteworthy also that this bone pain is often relieved by aspirin. Very occasional osteoid-osteomas may fail to provoke this pattern of bone pain.[14] Schulman and Dorfman,[22] using silver stains, demonstrated nerve fibers within the nidus of osteoid-osteomas in a high percentage of the cases studied. Local swelling may become apparent in some instances, and, in most, a sharply localized point of exquisite tenderness over the painful area can be demonstrated. Only rarely does one note slight local heat and redness, and in none of our cases was there a history of a febrile episode in connection with the lesion.

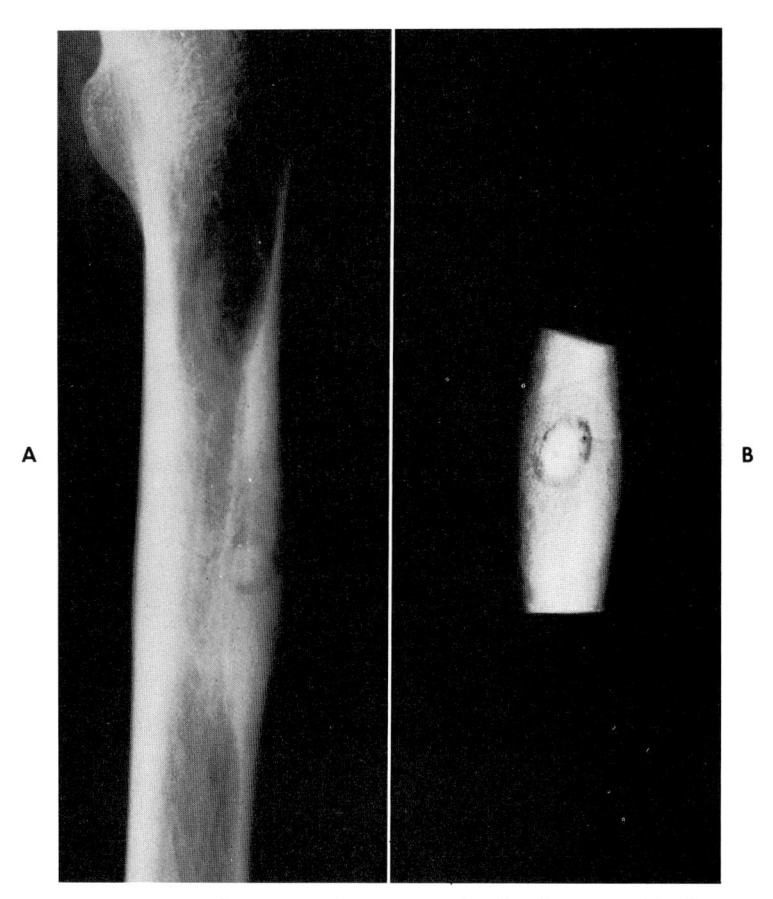

Fig. 9-1. A, Roentgenogram of an osteoid-osteoma nidus developing within the cortex of the shaft of a femur. The lesion, though comparatively small, has provoked considerable perifocal cortical thickening. B, Roentgenogram of the surgically excised cortical block incorporating the lesion. The latter is relatively radiopaque, and the thin lucent halo around it marks its junction with the surrounding thickened cortex.

Roentgen diagnosis

The diagnosis of osteoid-osteoma is not difficult usually if one is familiar with its clinical peculiarities, and if it has advanced sufficiently in its evolution to be clearly demonstrable roentgenographically. In occasional instances, the development of distressing pain may antedate the clear demonstration of the offending lesion in roentgenograms of the affected part (e.g., an astragalus or calcaneus) by some months or even a year or more. In such instances, the patients may be regarded for a time as malingerers or psychoneurotics. There may also be some lag in the recognition of a nidus that develops beneath the articular cartilage of a long bone or of one that is situated within a facet or a lamina of a vertebral body. In a pertinent case presenting a characteristic roentgen picture, the osteoid-osteoma nidus appears as a small, oval or roundish focus that is usually relatively radiolucent, but may occasionally be radiopaque. The shadow of this nidus is

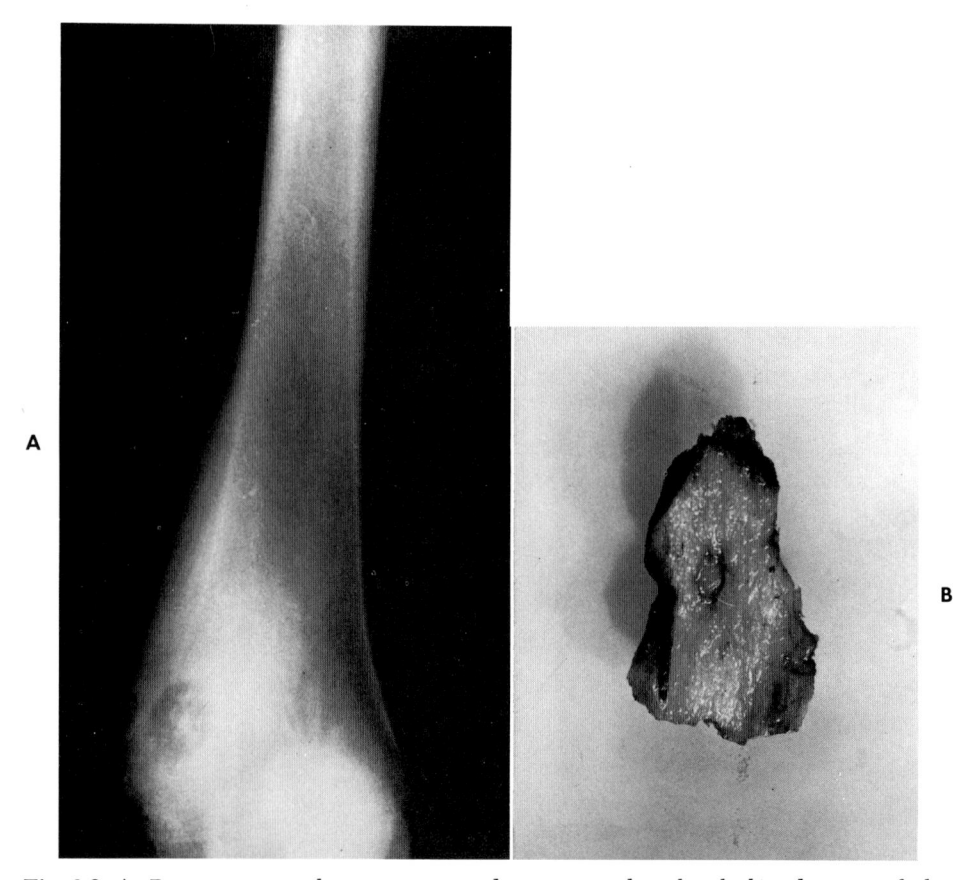

Fig. 9-2. **A,** Roentgenogram showing an osteoid-osteoma within the thickened cortex of the lower femur (of a young man who had complained of persistent, distressing localized pain in that area). Although the original x-ray film (received from abroad) was of rather poor quality, the offending osteoid-osteoma nidus can be clearly visualized. **B,** Photograph (natural size) of a surgically extirpated block of thickened cortical bone from a comparable case, showing an encoffined small ovoid lesion of osteoid-osteoma.

often, though by no means regularly, surrounded by a more or less dense shadow reflecting the reactive sclerosis of the neighboring bone. This sclerotized zone around the nidus may be only a narrow ring, or it may spread for several centimeters about the lesion, even when the latter is situated in the spongiosa. If the lesion develops within or just beneath a shaft cortex, the perifocal densified area may extend for several inches above and below the lesion. Further, the thickening of the cortex may be found to extend for a considerable distance around the circumference of the affected shaft area, tending to obscure the small lesion that provokes it. In such cases, overexposing the film and coning down on the affected area in various planes may enable one to discern the central nidus more readily, although in occasional instances in which the latter is relatively radiopaque even this procedure is not successful.

The major problem in differential diagnosis is to distinguish between osteoid-osteoma and the occasional instance of relatively small, intracortical bone abscess

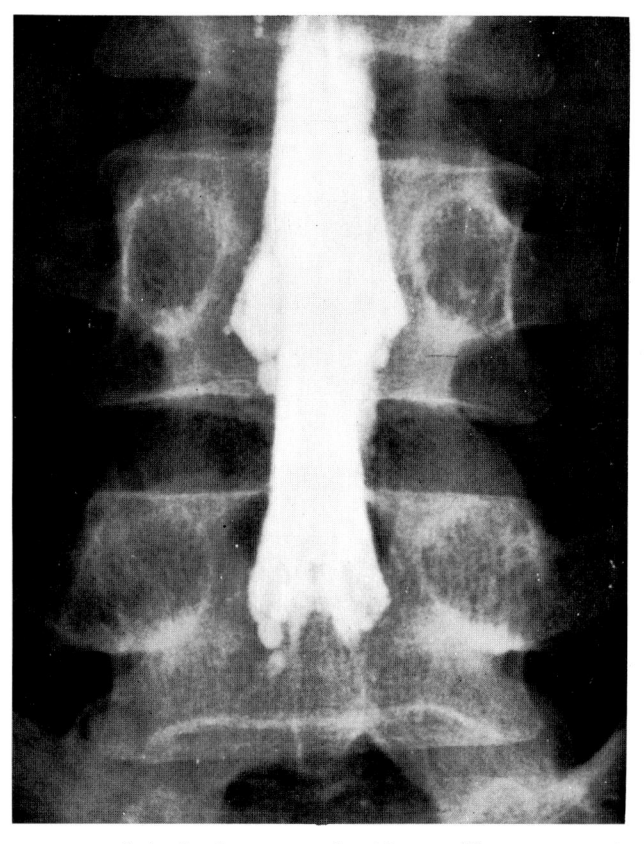

Fig. 9-3. Roentgenogram of the lumbar spine of a 22-year-old man presenting a sciatic syndrome clinically for over two years and distressing low back pain for one year. Surgical exploration revealed the presence of a circumscribed, globular osteoid-osteoma focus, 7 mm. in diameter (clearly visualized in the roentgenogram) situated within the inferior facet of the fifth lumbar vertebra. Its removal resulted in complete relief of pain.

94   Bone tumors

that may simulate it. On occasion also, it may be difficult on the basis of the roentgen picture alone to distinguish osteoid-osteoma from chronic sclerosing osteomyelitis. In such cases, one must take into consideration the clinical findings as well, and there may be no definitive answer until after pathologic examination of the surgical specimen.

Pathology

When an osteoid-osteoma in a spongy bone area is removed intact in its setting, or at least removed without fragmentation or crumbling, it stands out

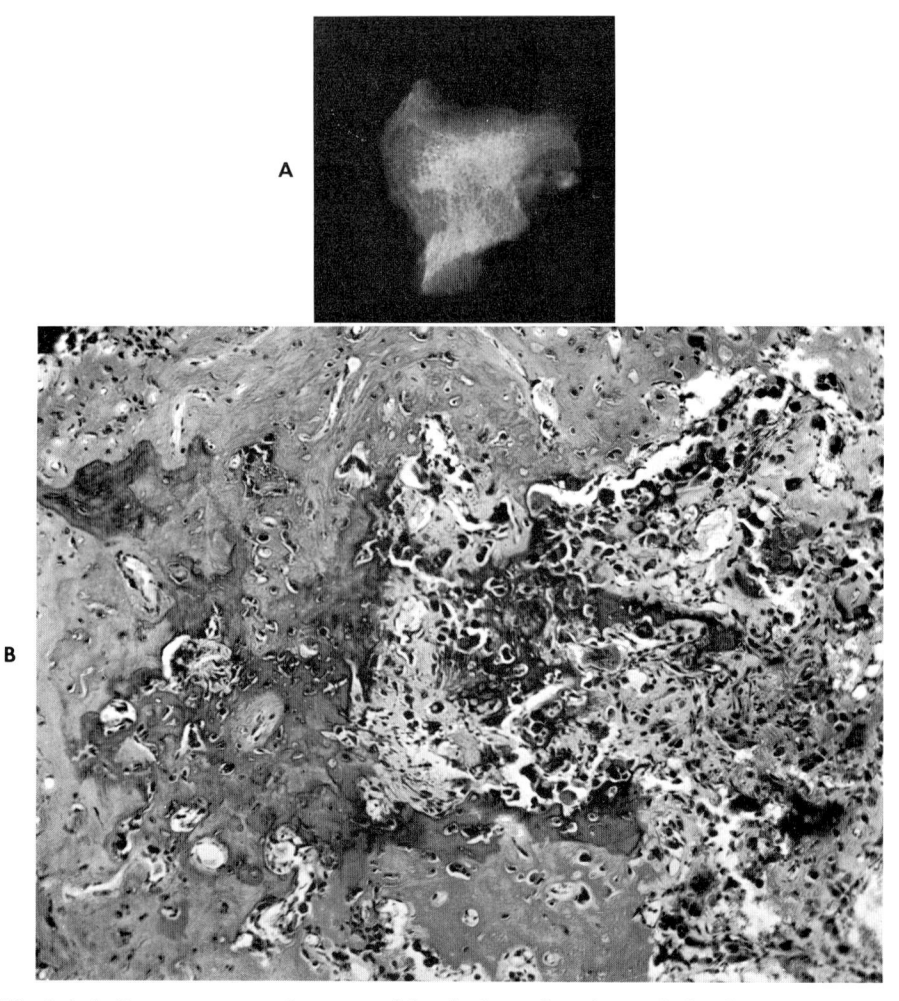

Fig. 9-4. **A**, Roentgenogram of a resected head of a radius that includes the major portion of an osteoid-osteoma. This was not visualized in the clinical films because the bones of the elbow were heavily overlaid by periosteal new bone resulting from an injury. The surgical procedure afforded prompt relief of pain. **B**, Photomicrograph of a field of the osteoid-osteoma illustrated in **A**, which is still composed largely of osteoid undergoing calcification and conversion to atypical bone. (×70.)

strikingly in the gross as a circumscribed reddish bony focus. When a thickened cortical bone block containing a nidus in its interior is excised, serial slices made preferably with a band saw will reveal the encoffined nidus in one or two of the blocks (Fig. 9-5, A). The lesion is very likely to be situated at the junction of the new and old cortex, or somewhat deeper toward the medullary cavity. When the nidus has been broken up into small fragments (by a chisel or curette), the fragments may be mistaken for bits of granulation tissue, although they can be clearly identified as portions of an osteoid-osteoma by an experienced observer on microscopic examination (Fig. 9-9).

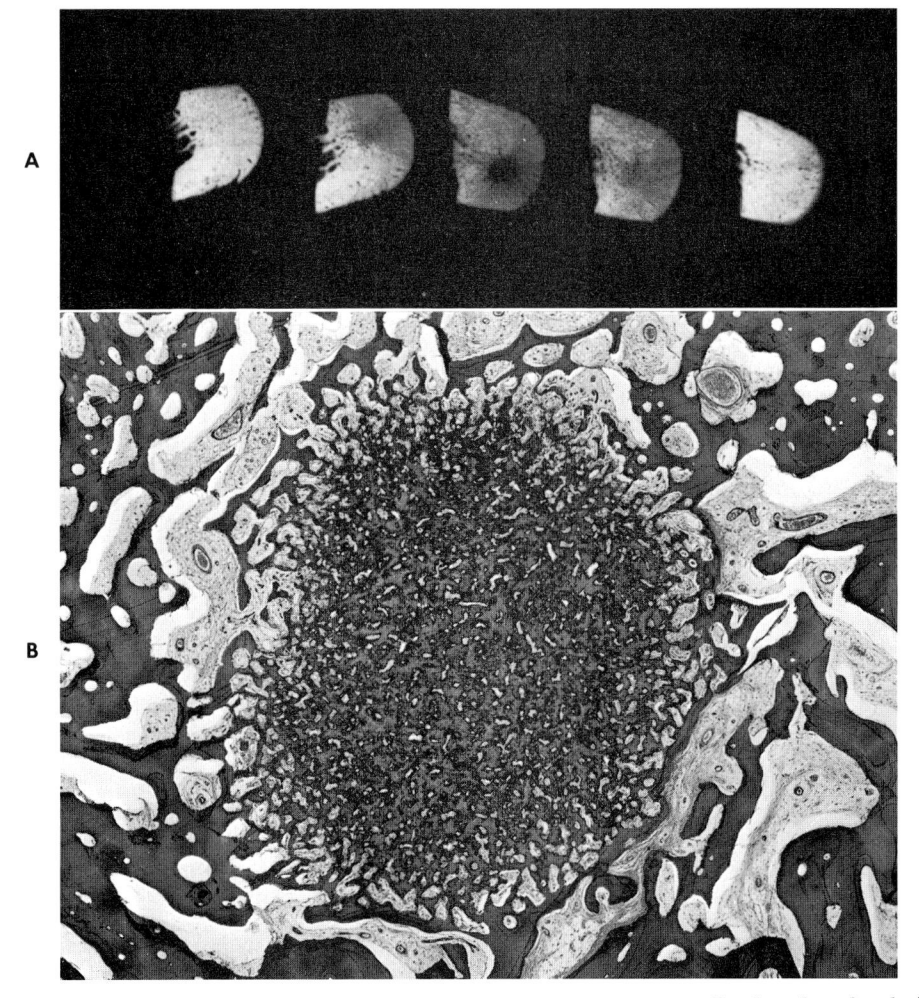

Fig. 9-5. A, Roentgenogram of serial slices of an osteoid-osteoma encoffined within the thickened cortical bone of the shaft of a femur. The specimen was excised en bloc and sectioned with a band saw. B, Photomicrograph of the osteoid-osteoma nidus illustrated in A. It is composed of irregularly calcified osteoid and new bone.

96   Bone tumors

In microscopic sections the lesion stands out sharply as a circumscribed focus of osteoid and more or less calcified, atypical bone developing within a background of richly vascular, osteoblastic connective tissue. Some lesions are composed in large part of compact osteoid. In other lesions, apparently the older ones, these sheets of osteoid have already been split up and remodeled into trabeculae, which become calcified and converted to atypical bone. This is essentially the picture of the fully evolved lesion. On the other hand, it has been rather difficult from the material available to trace satisfactorily the genesis of the lesion from the very beginning, and the earlier stages of its evolution require further clarification. This much we do know, however. We have observed a number of pertinent specimens from cortical locations, particularly which indicate that, initially at the site in the cortex where the lesion is developing, a peculiar condensation and an intense reconstruction and vascularization of the original cortical bone set in. The latter is soon substantially resorbed, though perhaps not completely, and is replaced by highly atypical osseous tissue, deposited ap-

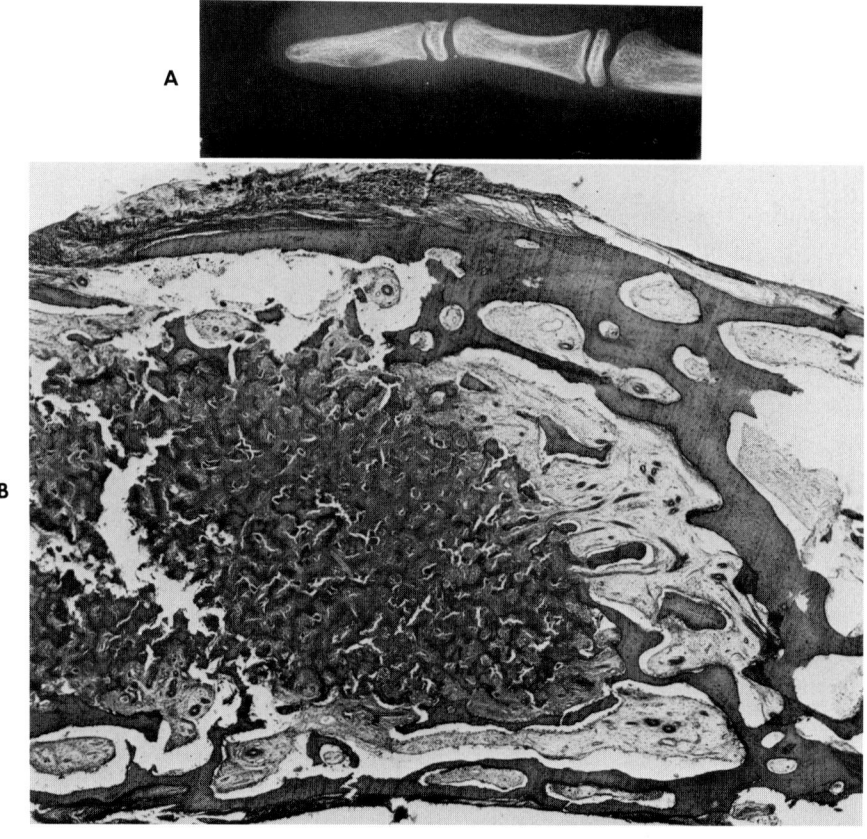

Fig. 9-6. **A,** Roentgenogram of a small osteoid-osteoma developing beneath the cortex of the distal phalanx of a fifth finger of a 14-year-old boy who had complained of pain for about a year. The circumscribed dense nidus is surrounded by a radiolucent halo. **B,** Photomicrograph showing the topography of the osteoid-osteoma illustrated in **A.** (×20.)

parently by the osteogenic connective tissue carried in along with the blood vessels that are invading the area. While this focus of bone is undergoing creeping replacement and reconstruction, the overlying periosteum may be depositing a thick layer of new bone, the architecture of which is rather normal aside from its condensation. Within this reactive new cortical bone, one may observe small focal collections of lymphocytes in the immediate vicinity of the nidus, but this feature apparently reflects nothing more than an expression of chronic irritation.

As to the interpretation of the lesion of osteoid-osteoma, we still feel confident on the basis of the additional experience we have had since 1940 in affirming that this peculiar lesion of bone is unique, and that it does not represent a response to infection. The evidence against the idea that osteoid-osteoma may have an infectious-inflammatory basis will not be repeated here, and for a detailed analysis of that question the reader is referred to our article published in 1940.[12] In it we also explain why we do not believe that the osteoid-osteoma lesion represents a peculiar healing or reparative form of some other familiar lesion, or that

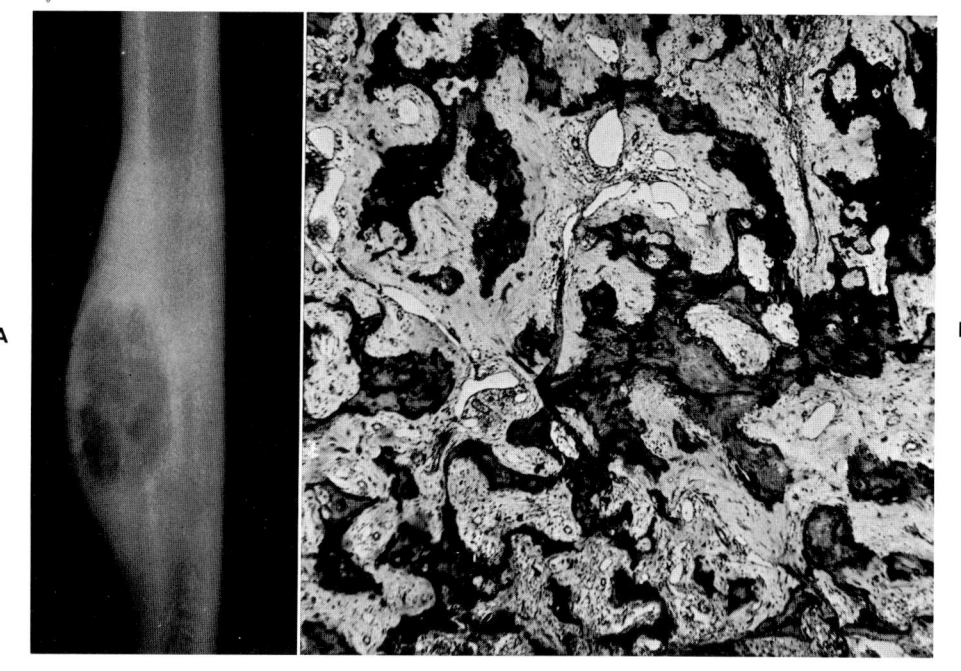

Fig. 9-7. **A**, Roentgenogram of an osteoid-osteoma of unusual size, which has provoked marked cortical thickening of the shaft of the humerus. The patient was a 20-year-old young man who had complained of dull aching pain, as well as swelling, of the affected arm. In the clinical roentgenograms, the lesion proper measured as much as 5 cm. in its long axis. Surgical treatment consisted of thorough curettement through a large cortical window, which effected complete lasting relief of symptoms. **B**, Photomicrograph of a selected field of the lesion illustrated in **A**, showing heavily calcified, large irregular patches of osteoid. Other fields showed a more conventional, readily discernible picture of osteoid-osteoma, remarkable only in that its connective tissue was inordinately vascular. (×40.) (From Lichtenstein, L.: Benign osteoblastoma, Cancer 9:1044, 1956.)

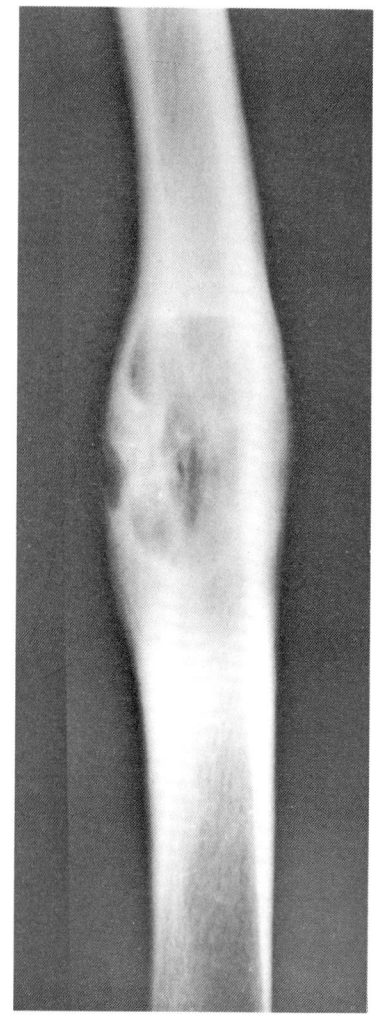

Fig. 9-8. Roentgenogram of another osteoid-osteoma of "giant" size in the shaft of a femur, resembling the one illustrated in Fig. 9-7.

it originates from an embryonic rest. Altogether, we have been led both by the process of elimination and by consideration of the anatomic characteristics of the lesion itself to the conclusion that it is best interpreted as a neoplasm and specifically as a peculiar benign tumor of bone of osteoblastic connective tissue derivation.

Added support for this concept comes from the observation of a number of remarkably large osteoid-osteomas, one of which (in the shaft of a humerus of a young adult) measured as much as 5 cm. in its long axis (Fig. 9-7). I have also observed a comparable osteoid-osteoma in the shaft of a femur, which measured more than 6 cm. in its long axis (Fig. 9-8). Another comparable instance

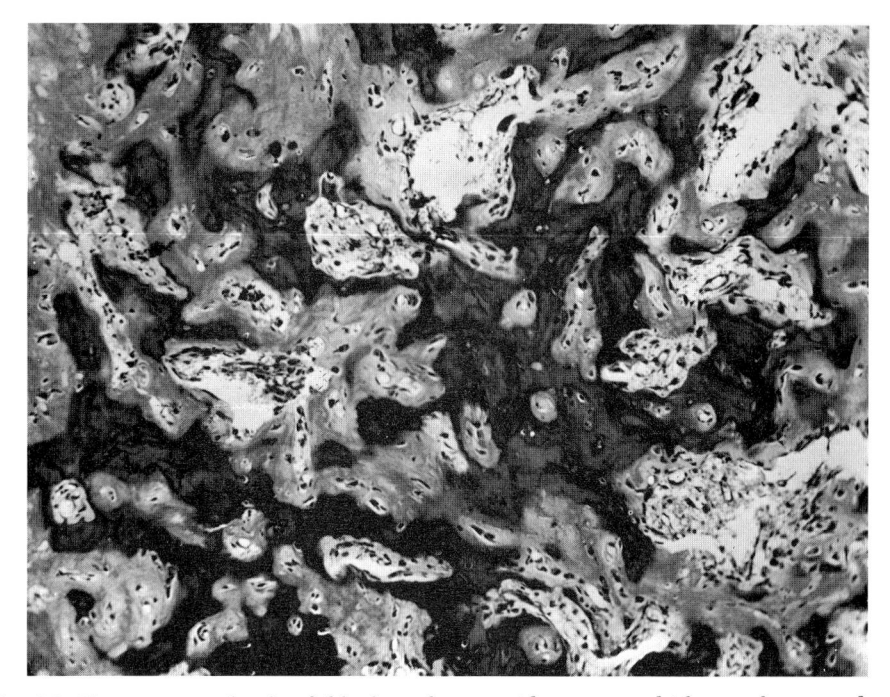

Fig. 9-9. Photomicrograph of a field of another osteoid-osteoma, which was fragmented and removed piecemeal by curettement, rather than excised en bloc. Patches of osteoid are undergoing irregular heavy calcification and conversion to atypical bone and show also invasion by tracts of rather vascular, osteoblastic connective tissue. The identification of a lesion such as this hinges on the ability of the pathologist to recognize its distinctiveness.

was encountered in the lamina of a lumbar vertebra of a child. Incidentally, the designation of giant osteoid-osteoma for these lesions of remarkable size might be appropriate, and it seems unfortunate that Dahlin applied this name to the category of tumors we now call benign osteoblastoma.

Still another cogent argument for the tumorous nature of osteoid-osteoma can be based upon the strong cytologic resemblance of *some* lesions of osteoid-osteoma, in part or substantially throughout, to certain instances of benign osteoblastoma, the neoplastic nature of which can hardly be disputed (Chapter 10). On the other hand, the categorical statement of Byers[3] that the two are histologically indistinguishable except for size hardly seems justified. The variable cytologic patterns of the osteoblastomas illustrated in Figs. 10-8, *B* to *D* and 10-9 are quite different from that of osteoid-osteoma.

Treatment and prognosis

As noted, surgical removal of the lesion will effect almost immediate and lasting relief. In none of our cases in which the lesion was completely removed surgically was there any recurrence, and invariably the pain caused by the lesion disappeared with dramatic promptness. The nidus and some of the surrounding bone may be removed by curettement, but this should be thorough, since otherwise there is danger of recurrence of the complaints. If the osteoid-osteoma nidus is missed on surgical intervention (e.g., one situated deep within the neck or intertrochanteric region of a femur may be difficult to localize), pain will recur after a short interval, and increasing perifocal sclerosis will manifest itself. For this reason, it is strongly advised that x-ray control be utilized to aid in effective localization and to make certain before the operation is concluded that the osteoid-osteoma nidus has actually been removed. In the case of lesions embedded within thickened shaft cortices we have been advocating block resection whenever possible, in order to obtain the nidus intact in its setting for more complete and satisfactory pathologic examination. However, it is not essential for clinical cure to remove all of the thickened perifocal bone or even a substantial part of it. When such a case is explored, it may be helpful in the matter of localization to bear in mind that the osteoid-osteoma focus is likely to be situated directly beneath the point of greatest convexity of the thickened cortical surface.

The ultimate fate of an untreated lesion is not known, although we have seen a number of cases in which the clinical complaints were of several years' duration (in one instance as long as seven years) and in which the nidus eventually removed at surgery showed no indication of change in the direction of involution. Also, we have little relevant information in regard to the possible effectiveness of irradiation in the treatment of osteoid-osteoma. In a case cited by Jaffe,[10] x-ray irradiation (2,000 r, total dose) of a pertinent lesion in the humerus of a 15-year-old boy afforded relief for three years, but recurrence of pain eventually necessitated surgical excision. It seems to me that this modality should be reserved for lesions in surgically inaccessible sites (e.g., in the upper cervical spine).

Summary

The lesion designated as osteoid-osteoma is a highly distinctive one and seems best interpreted as a peculiar benign tumor of osteoblastic derivation. The condition is not uncommon, and our experience with it now exceeds 100 cases. It is encountered mainly in older children, adolescents, and young adults below the age of 30 years. Although it may affect almost any bone, it has a predilection for the bones of the lower extremity, especially the femur and tibia. It is a roundish or ovoid lesion that usually does not exceed a centimeter in its greatest dimension, although I have observed some that were substantially larger. It may develop in the spongiosa or in the cortex of the affected bone, and it stands out from the surrounding osseous tissue as a sharply delimited nidus. This is usually composed of osteoid and more or less calcified atypical new bone that can be seen to have developed out of a rather vascular osteogenic connective tissue. When an osteoid-osteoma develops in the spongiosa, a narrow or even fairly wide zone of the surrounding spongy osseous tissue usually becomes densified and sclerotic. When it develops within or just beneath the cortex, the latter tends to become markedly thickened, mainly through periosteal new bone formation, and if the lesion develops in the cortex of a long bone, as it often does, the reactive cortical thickening may be very striking and out of proportion to the size of the offending nidus.

The diagnosis of osteoid-osteoma is not difficult in most instances if one is familiar with its clinical peculiarities and if the lesion has advanced sufficiently in its evolution to be clearly demonstrable roentgenographically. In interpreting the roentgenographic films in a case of osteoid-osteoma, one must remember that there are two aspects—that of the lesion proper and that of the reaction which it has provoked around it. The osteoid-osteoma proper is usually indicated by a relatively radiolucent area, although, if it has become substantially calcified and ossified, it may appear as a relatively radiopaque nidus. One may have difficulty in clearly distinguishing the osteoid-osteoma shadow in the cortex of a long bone if the reactive cortical thickening is considerable or if the lesion has become ossified, since its shadow may then be dominated by that of the thickened cortex. Because the roentgenographic study has these two aspects, a case of osteoid-osteoma in a spongy bone area may be mislabeled as chronic osteomyelitis with bone abscess or with an annular sequestrum. Similarly, a case of osteoid-osteoma in the shaft of a long bone may be mislabeled as sclerosing nonsuppurative osteomyelitis of Garré or intracortical bone abscess.

The presenting symptoms clinically are localized tenderness and pain, usually of at least several months' duration, which may be persistent and severe enough to awaken the patient at night. The clinical findings do not point to an infectious-inflammatory basis for the disorder. Complete surgical excision of the osteoid-osteoma proper, with or without some of the surrounding bone, results in clinical cure with prompt and often dramatic relief of distressing pain. Following incomplete removal of an osteoid-osteoma (usually in a site where accurate localization is difficult), one may expect only temporary relief, followed by return of pain requiring a second exploration. In no case in which the lesion was completely removed surgically has there been a recurrence.

References

1. Brailsford, J. F.: Chronic Sub-periosteal abscess, Brit. J. Radiol. 15:313, 1942; Brailsford, J. F.: Radiology of bones and joints, ed. 3, Baltimore, 1944, Williams & Wilkins Co., p. 373.
2. Brown, R. C., and Ghormley, R. K.: Solitary (eccentric) cortical abscess in bone, Surgery 14:541, 1943.
3. Byers, P. D.: Solitary benign osteoblastic lesions of bone. Osteoid osteoma and benign osteoblastoma, Cancer 22:43, 1968.
4. Coley, B. L., and Lenson, N.: Osteoid-osteoma, Am. J. Surg. 77:3, 1949.
5. Foss, E. L., Dockerty, M. B., and Good, C. A.: Osteoid-osteoma of the mandible. Report of a case, Cancer 8:592, 1955.
6. Goidanich, I. F., and Zanasi, R.: Osteoma osteoide ed Osteomielite sclerosante: due entità chiniche definite e distiute, Chir. d. org. di movimento 43:427, 1956.
7. Golding, J. S. R.: The natural history of osteoid-osteoma; with a report of twenty cases, J. Bone Joint Surg. 36-B:218, 1954.
8. Jackson, A. E., Dockerty, M. B., and Ghormley, R. K.: Osteoid osteoma: a clinical study of 20 cases, Mayo Clin. Proc. 24:380, 1949.
9. Jaffe, H. L.: Osteoid-osteoma: a benign osteoblastic tumor composed of osteoid and atypical bone, Arch. Surg. 31:709, 1935.
10. Jaffe, H. L.: Osteoid-osteoma of bone, Radiology 45:319, 1945.
11. Jaffe, H. L.: Tumors and tumorous conditions of the bones and joints, Philadelphia, 1958, Lea & Febiger, p. 94.

12. Jaffe, H. L., and Lichtenstein, L.: Osteoid-osteoma: further experience with this benign tumor of bone, with special reference to cases showing the lesion in relation to shaft cortices and commonly misclassified as instances of sclerosing nonsuppurative osteomyelitis or cortical-bone abscess, J. Bone Joint Surg. 22:645, 1940.
13. Lapidus, P. W., and Salem, E. P.: Osteoid-osteoma. Report of a case with probable double lesion, Arch. Surg. 58:318, 1949.
14. Lawrie, T. R., Aterman, K., and Sinclair, A. M.: Painless osteoid-osteoma. Report of two cases, J. Bone Joint Surg. 52-A:1357, 1970.
15. Maclellan, S. J., and Wilson, F. C., Jr.: Osteoid osteoma of the spine. A review of the literature and report of six new cases, J. Bone Joint Surg. 49-A:111, 1967.
16. Mayer, L.: The surgery of osteoid osteoma, Bull. Hosp. Joint Dis. 12:174, 1951.
17. McKeever, F. M.: Osteoid-osteoma, West. J. Surg. 58:213, 1950.
18. Morrison, G. M., Hawes, L. E., and Sacco, J. J.: Incomplete removal of osteoid-osteoma, Am. J. Surg. 80:476, 1950.
19. Paus, B. C., and Kim, T. K.: Osteoid osteoma of the spine, Acta Orthop. Scand. 33:24, 1963.
20. Pines, B., Lavine, L., and Grayzel, D. M.: Osteoid-osteoma. Etiology and pathogenesis, report of 12 new cases, J. Internat. Coll. Surgeons 13:249, 1950.
21. Pritchard, J. E., and McKay, J. W.: Osteoid-osteoma, Can. Med. Assoc. J. 58:567, 1948.
22. Schulman, L., and Dorfman, H. D.: Nerve fibers in osteoid-osteoma, J. Bone Joint Surg. 52-A:1351, 1970.
23. Sherman, M. S.: Osteoid-osteoma. Review of the literature and report of 30 cases, J. Bone Joint Surg. 29:918, 1947.

Chapter 10

Benign osteoblastoma

In this section I have attempted to delineate more clearly the pathologic nature and appropriate treatment of certain benign tumors of bone of osteoblastic derivation, other than osteoid-osteoma and osteoma so-called. Their recognition is of practical importance in that they may be mistaken for malignant tumors, especially osteogenic sarcoma, and, as such, treated more aggressively than is required. I have had occasion within recent years to observe material from as many as 37 pertinent instances encountered in long bones, the vertebral column, and other sites that will serve as the basis for discussion.

The first series of cases I designated as benign osteoblastoma was reported in *Cancer*[13] in 1956, and a summary of this article appeared earlier that year in *The New England Journal of Medicine*.[16] Almost coincidentally, but independently, an article by Jaffe[8] was published in which the same name was used and essentially the same views were expressed concerning the pathologic characteristics of this tumor. A second larger series of some 20 cases was reported by Sawyer and myself[17] in 1964. Considerable interest in the subject has been evinced, and an appreciable number of additional case reports have appeared.[2,4,7,18,21,22,24] Also noteworthy is a detailed analysis of the roentgenograms of many published reports of benign osteoblastomas, as well as of several new ones, by Pochaczevsky, Yen, and Sherman.[20] Finally a wealth of pertinent clinical and pathologic data is contained in a well-illustrated article by Goidanich and Battaglia,[5] reporting on 14 cases.

These benign osteoblastic tumors include the ones previously called "osteogenic fibroma," as well as those referred to provisionally as "other osteoid-tissue–forming tumors" in my original classification of primary tumors of bone. I have come to feel that for all practical purposes they comprise a single category of benign osteoid- and bone-forming tumors that may be appropriately designated as benign osteoblastoma. Most of the tumors reported by Dahlin and Johnson[3] under the heading of "Giant Osteoid Osteoma" are undoubtedly cases in point (benign osteoblastomas), although a few may be plausibly interpreted as genuine osteoid-osteomas, particularly the smaller lesions provoking a sclerotic reaction around them. Their proposed name for the tumor does not appeal to me, if only for the reason that the concept of classical osteoid-osteoma has become too firmly established and useful to be vitiated by the inclusion of other tumors differing in a number of essential respects, clinically and radiologically, as well as pathologically. If the designation of giant osteoid-osteoma is to have any usefulness within the present framework of reference, it might apply rather in a literal sense to the genuine osteoid-osteomas of unusual size that one encounters occasionally. As previously noted, I have had the opportunity to observe several such remarkably large osteoid-osteomas (Figs. 9-7 and 9-8).

The tumors in point exhibit appreciable variation in cytologic detail (Figs. 10-7 to 10-9), which will be considered further on, but their common basic pattern is readily recognizable if one becomes familiar with it. The important thing is to avoid being confused by their content of multinuclear cells, mainly osteoclasts about trabeculae of osteoid and new bone, and to recognize clearly that their richly, vascular, osteoblastic connective tissue stroma is not that of a sarcoma.

Clinical features
Age and sex incidence

In our case material, two-thirds of the patients were children or teen-agers. The remainder were adults, the oldest, 78 years of age. Sex difference is apparently not great enough to be meaningful.

Localization

In general, it appears that the tumor occurs with greatest frequency in limb bones (including those of the hand and foot), the vertebral column, and the calvarium, but it has been encountered in other bones as well, e.g., ribs, scapula, and innominate bone. Of the large limb bones, the tumor has a predilection for the bones of the lower extremity and particularly the femur and tibia are predilected. In our combined group of 37 cases, tumors in large limb bones and in

---

Fig. 10-1. **A**, Roentgenogram of a benign osteoblastoma situated in the lower end of a radius in an adult. It has expanded and attenuated the overlying cortex but is well delimited by a delicate shell of periosteal new bone, while its internal border is sharply outlined by a sclerotized line. The clinical symptoms were of at least two years' duration. **B**, Roentgenogram of another osteoblastoma (in a 6-year-old child that has expanded the spinous process and encroached upon the body of C-4). The expanded portion of the tumor is well outlined peripherally. **C**, Roentgenogram of a benign osteoblastoma situated eccentrically in the lower metaphysis of the femur of a 14-year-old girl who had complained of pain for several months. Like the tumor illustrated in **A**, it is delimited peripherally by a thin shell of periosteal new bone and internally by a sclerotized border. The sections were interpreted by one consultant pathologist as showing a giant-cell tumor and by another as a sarcoma, with the recommendation of amputation. The lesion was treated by curettement and packing with bone chips, and, at the last follow-up eight months later, the patient had made a complete recovery. **D**, Roentgenogram of a tumor that has markedly expanded the base and proximal shaft of a fifth metatarsal bone and shows fine radiopaque stippling, reflecting new bone formation. (From Lichtenstein, L.: Benign osteoblastoma, Cancer 9:1044, 1956.)

Benign osteoblastoma 105

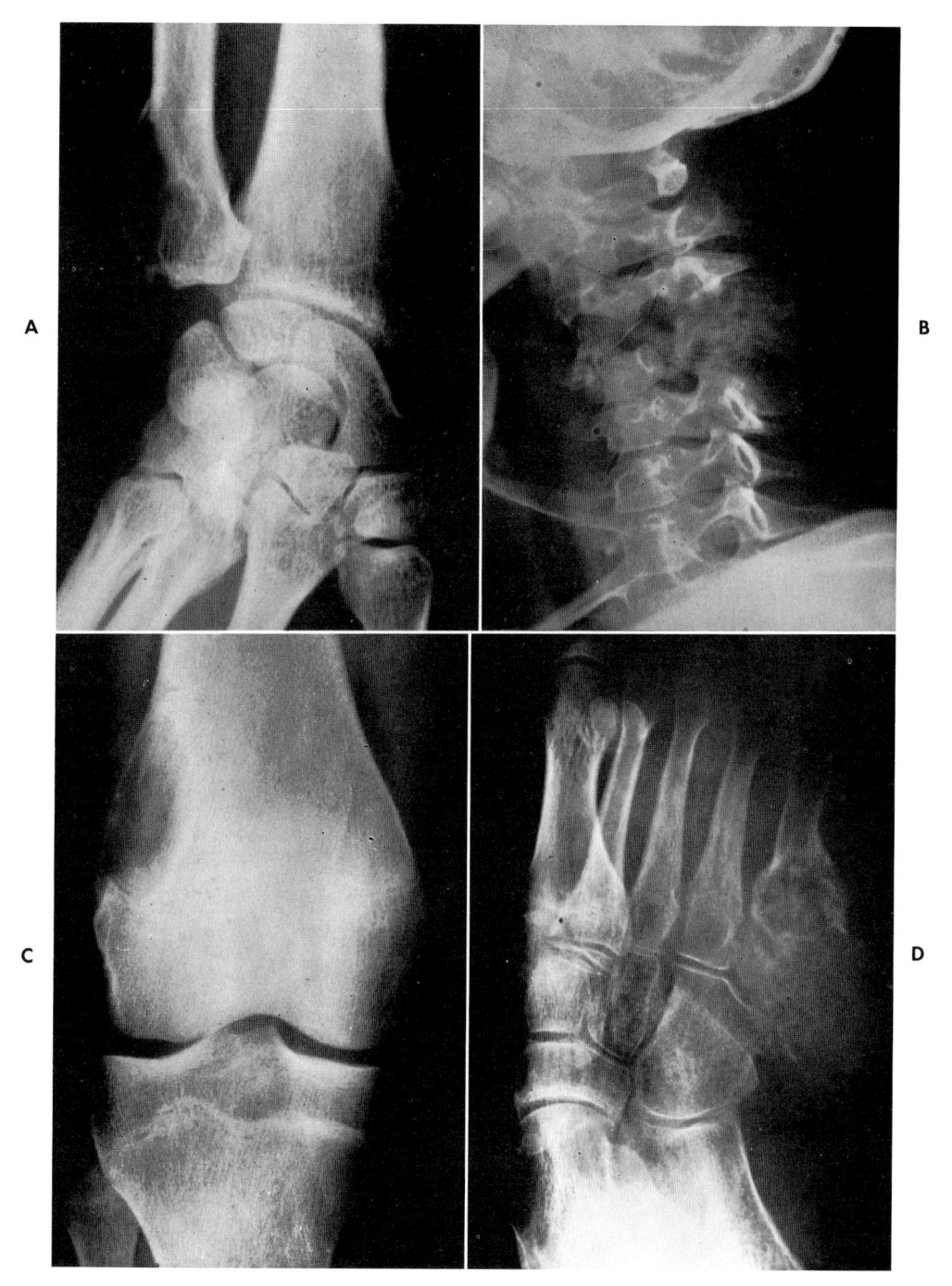

Fig. 10-1. For legend see opposite page.

106   Bone tumors

the vertebral column account for fully 60%, those in the calvarium, 20%, and those in the hand and foot bones together, about 18%.

Clinical complaints

The major complaints were pain, often of insidious onset, and/or palpable, slightly tender swelling that increased perceptibly under observation. On the whole, the clinical findings in themselves were not sufficiently distinctive to be of much help in differential diagnosis. The pain was not of the type commonly encountered with osteoid-osteoma in that it did not tend to awaken the patient at night or to be relieved especially by aspirin. The duration of symptoms prior to surgery ranged from a few months to as long as two years.

It is noteworthy that the lesions developing in the neural arch of a vertebra (rather than its spinous process) gradually induced compression of the spinal cord, manifested by weakness and eventually paraplegia that required surgical intervention for relief. This complication was also noted in two comparable instances reported by Golding and Sissons.[6] Incidentally, their first tumor was regarded provisionally as an osteogenic sarcoma and, as such, was heavily irradiated (total dosage of 5,000 r), while the second also received as much as 3,600 r postoperatively on the mistaken premise that it represented a giant-cell tumor (osteoclastoma).

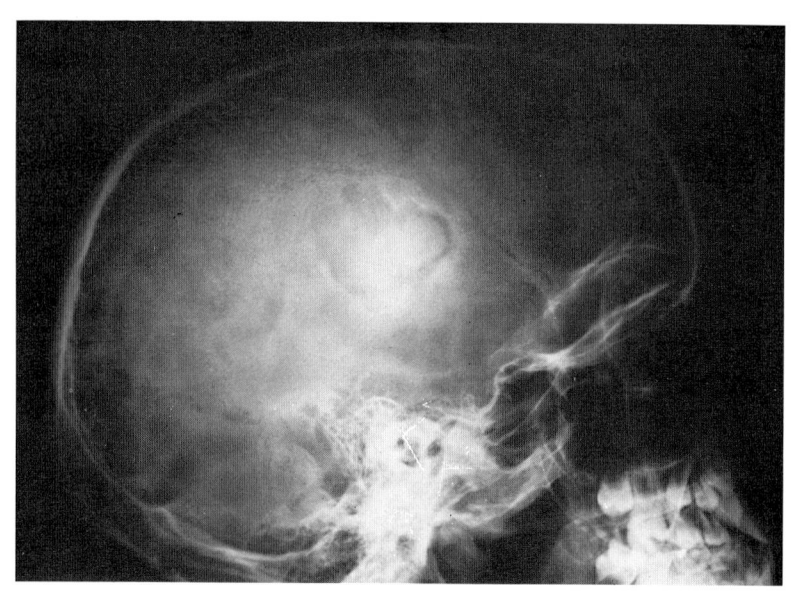

Fig. 10-2. Roentgenogram of a circumscribed tumor in the right temporal bone of a 9-year-old girl that had slowly increased in size over a period of two years. It had provoked slight reactive sclerosis around most of its periphery. The tumor measured 3.5 cm. in its greatest dimension and 2.5 cm. in thickness and was found at surgical exploration to have expanded both tables of the calvarium. The patient was entirely well at the last follow-up, thirteen months after local excision. (From Lichtenstein, L.: Benign osteoblastoma, Cancer 9:1044, 1956.)

Roentgenographic picture

For convenient orientation a number of representative roentgenograms are illustrated in Figs. 10-1 to 10-5. While they tend to convey the impression of a benign neoplasm, the picture as a whole is not nearly so distinctive as that of some other benign tumors of bone. This much seems clear, however. Irrespective of size and location, the tumor tends to be well circumscribed. When it has attenuated and expanded the overlying cortex, as it often does, it is still delimited by a delicate shell of periosteal new bone. Incidentally, in no instance observed was there pronounced cortical new bone formation surrounding the lesion, as occurs with osteoid-osteoma arising within or beneath the cortex of a large limb bone (Fig. 9-7). Along its internal border, the tumor tends to be delimited by a sclerotized margin, testifying to its relatively slow rate of growth. The lesion

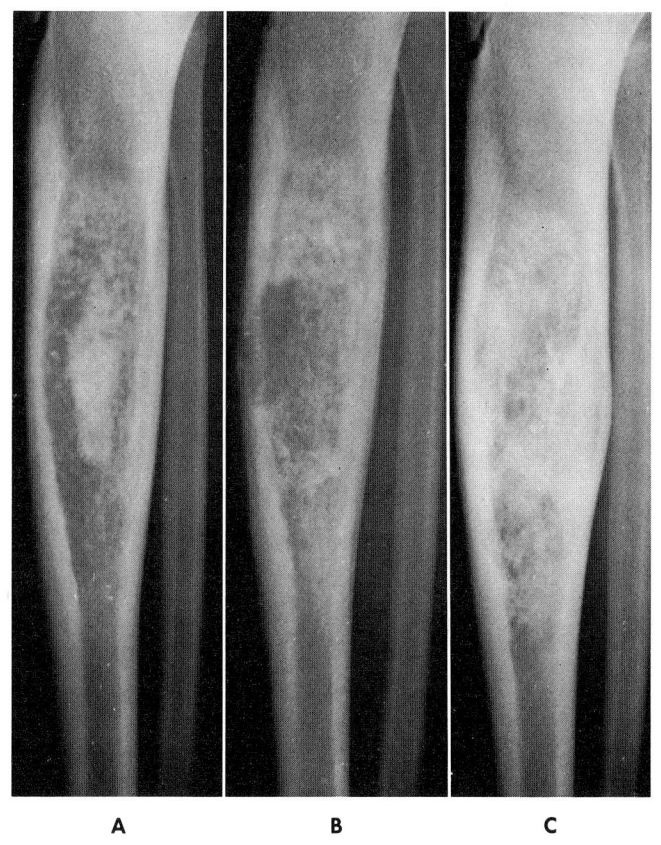

Fig. 10-3. A, Roentgenogram of another benign osteoblastoma in the shaft of the tibia of a 12-year-old girl; this osteoblastoma is somewhat unusual in that it presents a large central bony focus. B, The latter was excised (with the thought that it might represent an osteoid-osteoma), but the lesion was otherwise not disturbed. C, Follow-up roentgenogram taken fourteen months later shows restoration of a good, thick intact cortex and no increase in the size of the residual tumor by actual measurement. Photomicrographs of this tumor are illustrated in Fig. 10-8, B and C. (From Lichtenstein, L.: Benign osteoblastoma, Cancer 9:1044, 1956.)

108 Bone tumors

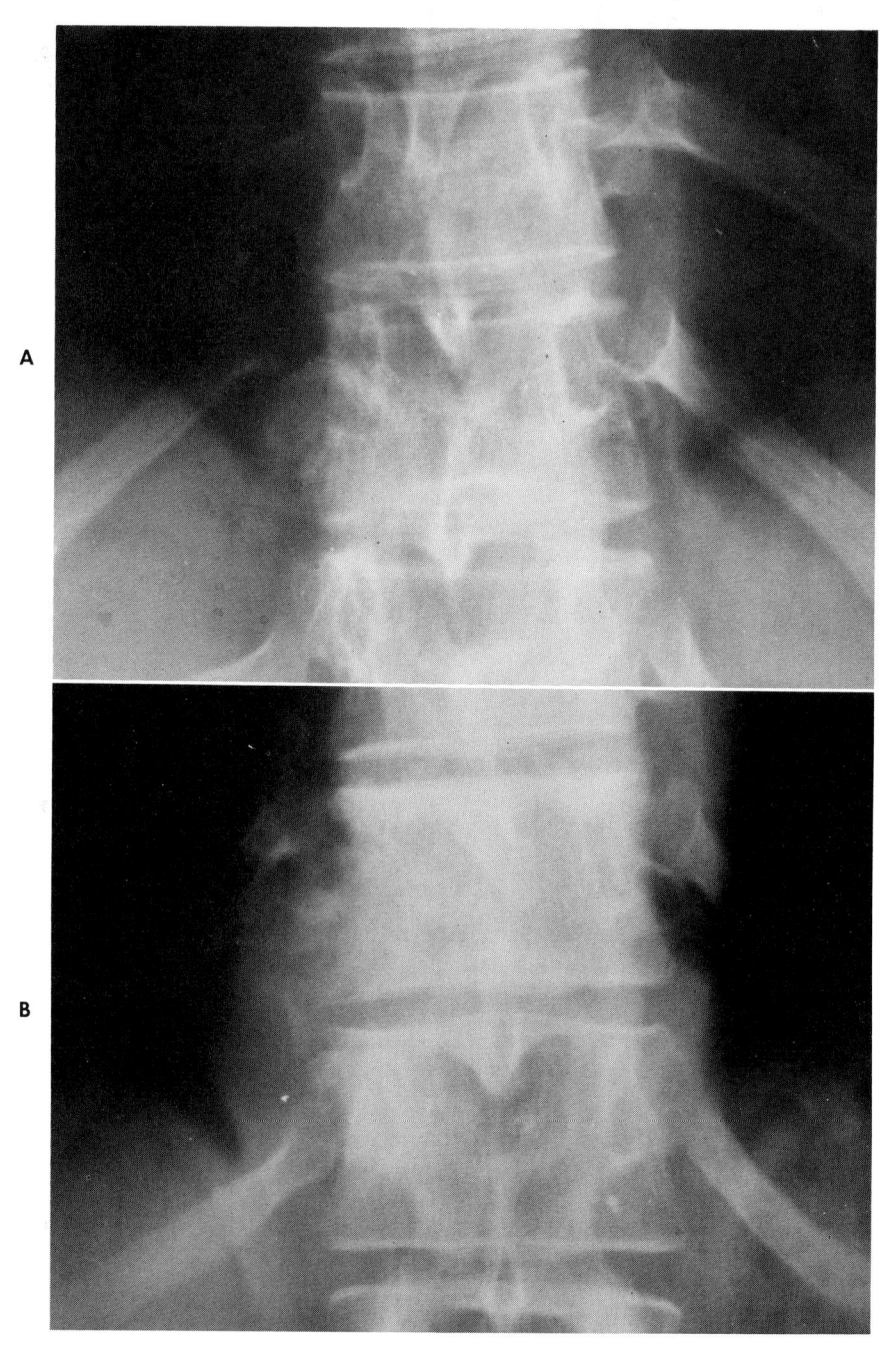

Fig. 10-4. **A,** Roentgenogram of a benign osteoblastoma producing a defect in the lamina and pedicle of the eleventh thoracic vertebra. The patient, a 20-year-old man, had complained of back pain for seven months. At surgical exploration, partial removal by curettement was done, with some relief of symptoms. No supplementary x-irradiation was given. **B,** Recurrent tumor about one year later, producing a paravertebral mass, somewhat more radiopaque than the original defect. This time curettement was supplemented by roentgen irradiation.

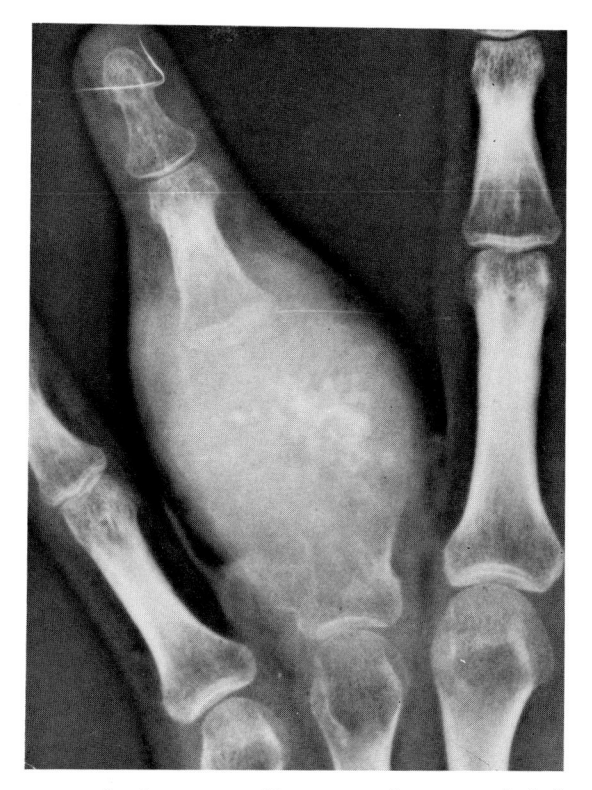

Fig. 10-5. Roentgenogram of a benign osteoblastoma in the proximal phalanx of a ring finger showing radiopaque stippling reflecting irregular calcification of osteoid. Ray amputation was done.

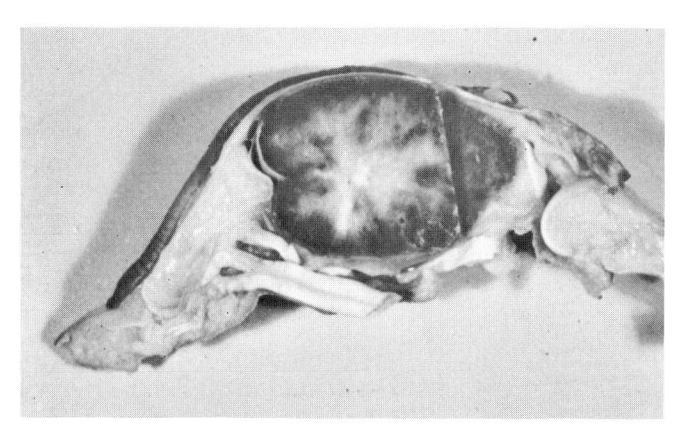

Fig. 10-6. Sagittal section of another benign osteoblastoma in the proximal phalanx of a finger, for which a ray amputation was done. The tumor was well circumscribed and its expanded portion was delimited by a delicate, imperfect shell of cortical new bone. The darker areas within it reflect congestion and extravasation of blood.

itself may be essentially radiolucent or, on the other hand, exhibit soft or somewhat harder radiopaque mottling (depending upon the extent of focal calcification of osteoid and its conversion to bone). The instance in the shaft of the tibia illustrated in Fig. 10-3 is exceptional in that it presents a large ovoid nidus of dense bone in its interior. Incidentally, tumors that have been irradiated (in the vertebral column, for example) tend to become intensely radiopaque after some months.

Pathologic features
Gross appearance

The few available intact gross specimens (obtained by resection or amputation, rather than curettement) indicate, as had been surmised from roentgenograms, that the tumor is well circumscribed. This is also borne out in the published illustrations of other contributors.[3,5,24] When it has expanded the bone, it is still delimited by a shell of cortical new bone or, if the latter is defective, by thickened periosteal connective tissue (Fig. 10-6). With reference to tumors in the calvarium particularly, it is relevant to note that they may expand the inner, as well as the outer, table, and cause adherence of the dura and localized compression or depression of the underlying cerebral cortex. Whatever its localization, the lesion in the gross usually appears reddish, more or less gritty, and is likely to be quite vascular, so that hemostasis at the time of surgery may be effected with some difficulty.

Microscopic findings

The microscopic picture, though showing a number of varying patterns, is sufficiently distinctive in its salient aspects to be readily recognized, if one is familiar with it, and to be distinguished from that of osteogenic sarcoma and giant-cell tumor in particular. As Dahlin emphasized, some benign osteoblastomas have sufficient resemblance to osteoid-osteoma to strongly suggest that they may be related, but this is not true of all, or even most of them. Some show a much more irregular pattern of osteoid deposition and calcification, becoming quite unusual and striking at times, and the picture may vary from one field to another. Focal calcification of osteoid in these circumstances may be quite heavy (Fig. 10-9, *B*). In other tumors one may observe dense sheets of osteoid and irregularly calcified new bone with little intervening connective tissue stroma; we have observed this in several tumors in the calvarium particularly. Still other benign osteoblastomas apparently develop through the growth of focal nodular aggregates of osteoblasts in different stages of maturation and tend to be multicentric (Fig. 10-9, *A*). Such proliferating osteoblasts at the height of their activity may be impressively large, but they are uniform in appearance and exhibit neither nuclear atypism nor mitotic figures that might suggest a diagnosis of osteogenic sarcoma. Calcification may be observed rather early as delicate or coarser streaks within these nests of proliferating osteoblasts. This seems often to precede the deposition of mineralized matrix.

Benign osteoblastoma 111

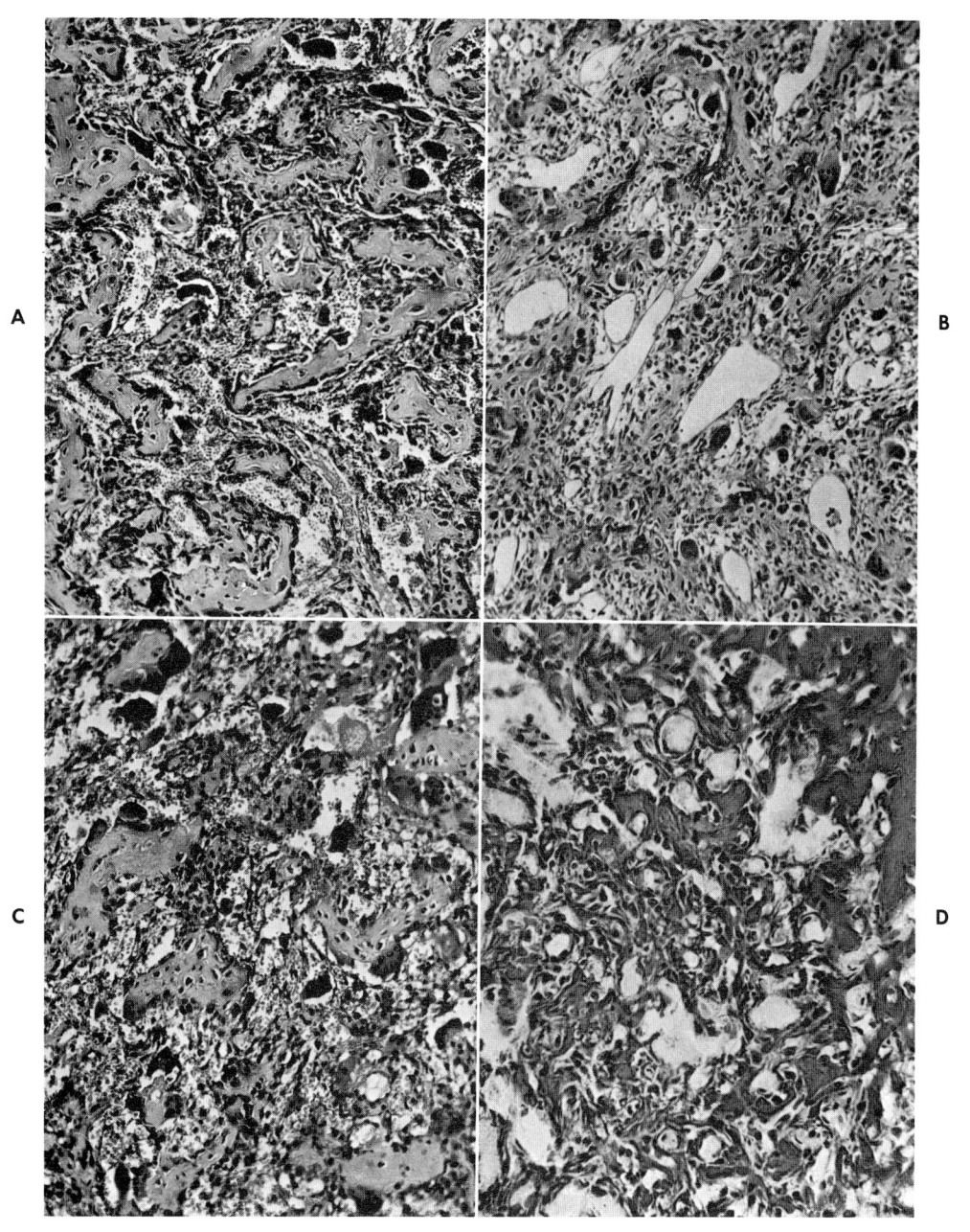

Fig. 10-7. A, B, and C, Representative photomicrographs of a number of benign osteoblastomas showing in common rather orderly deposition of trabeculae of osteoid and new bone within a richly vascularized background of osteoblastic connective tissue. Multinuclear macrophages, mainly osteoclasts, are prominent here and may suggest giant-cell tumor to an inexperienced observer. (×110, ×110, and ×160, respectively.) D, Photomicrograph of another tumor showing extensive deposition of only partially reconstructed osteoid as its salient feature. Tumors such as this may be mistaken for osteogenic sarcoma, even though their stroma is hardly that of a malignant neoplasm. (×200.) (From Lichtenstein, L.: Benign osteoblastoma, Cancer 9:1044, 1956.)

Whatever the pattern of osteoid and bone formation may be in any given tumor, and this may differ rather widely, as noted, the stroma is quite vascular as a rule and may exhibit conspicuous extravasation of blood. Where the stroma is more fibrocystic, it is still permeated by many small blood vessels. Also within this stroma, and especially around the periphery of fields of mineralized matrix, whether or not these are calcified, one may observe numerous giant-cell macrophages. These need not be construed as suggesting giant-cell tumor, if one bears in mind that a previously untreated giant-cell tumor that has not sustained a pathologic fracture does not contain abundant osteoid and new bone, as a rule.

Differentiation from other lesions

It has already been intimated that the cytologic pattern of a number of the tumors studied (Fig. 10-8, A), though by no means all, was sufficiently reminiscent of osteoid-osteoma to suggest a close pathologic relationship. Incidentally, this cytologic resemblance would seem to lend support to the view that osetoid-osteoma represents a genuine benign neoplasm of bone. It should be emphasized, however, that benign osteoblastomas differ from classical osteoid-osteoma in that they are substantially larger, are not of sharply defined spherical or ovoid contour, do not present a roentgen-ray picture remotely suggestive of osteoid-osteoma, and do not induce the characteristic history of persistent localized bone pain associated with that lesion. Conceived in a very broad sense, osteoid-osteoma and so-called osteoma (of the orbit and paranasal bones, particularly) may be regarded as special types of benign osteoblastoma. As indicated, however, there are distinct advantages to retaining their separate established identities, although they may well represent related members of the same family of benign tumors of osteoblastic derivation.

It may be relevant here to consider the appropriate classification of certain benign osteoid- and bone-forming tumors that provoke marked cortical thickening. When such a tumor is enveloped by sclerotized bone, we prefer to designate it as an osteoid-osteoma, rather than benign osteoblastoma, even though it may be substantially larger than the conventional ones developing within or just

---

Fig. 10-8. **A,** Photomicrograph of still another tumor showing a pattern reminiscent of osteoid-osteoma. This particular lesion was a thumb-shaped gritty tumor, measuring 3.5 cm. in length, that had compressed the spinal cord extradurally at the level of D-2. (×100.) **B,** Photomicrograph of a selected field of the tumor in the tibia illustrated in Fig. 10-3. The trabeculae of atypically calcified new bone here have a more irregular pattern. (×150.) **C,** A relatively cellular field of the tumor illustrated in **B,** showing compact round or ovoid stromal cells that have as yet laid down but little osteoid matrix. These cells, however, are relatively small and essentially uniform and, as such, are not calculated to create the impression of a sarcoma. (×340.) **D,** Photomicrograph of a representative field of another pertinent tumor (in the calvarium) showing relatively cellular osteoblastic stroma. The osteoblasts between and about trabeculae of calcifying osteoid are distinctly plump but quite uniform, and the soundness of the impression of a benign tumor was borne out by the clinical result. (×210.) (From Lichtenstein, L.: Benign osteoblastoma, Cancer 9:1044, 1956.)

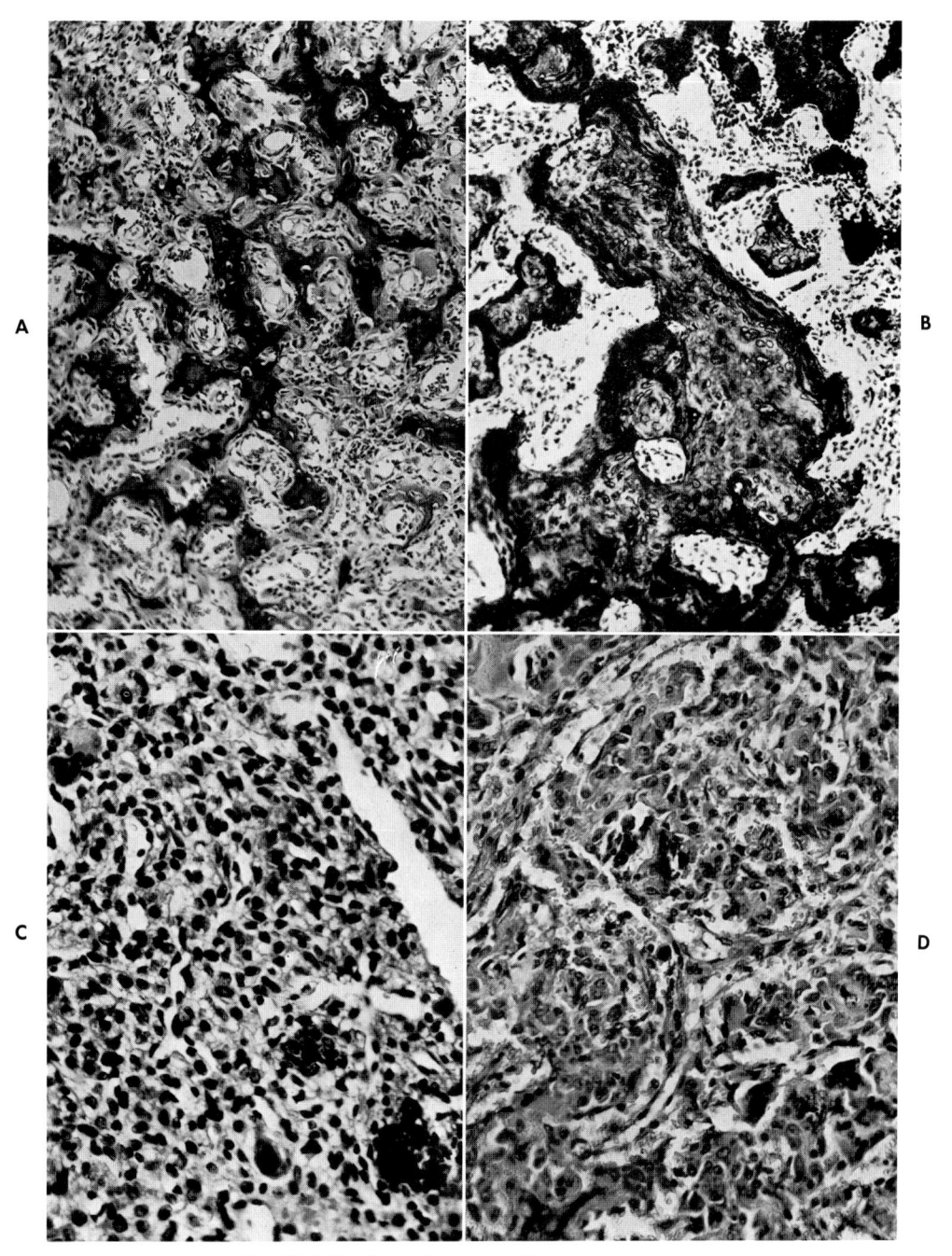

Fig. 10-8. For legend see opposite page.

beneath the cortex of a large limb bone.[10] By this criterion the instance illustrated as Fig. 2 in the paper by Dahlin and Johnson,[3] and several illustrated as Figs. 23, 34, 37, and 38 in the paper by Goidanich and Battaglia,[5] might plausibly be interpreted as osteoid-osteomas. Further, one occasionally encounters tumors closely resembling classical osteoid-osteoma (clinically, radiologically, and pathologically), which are of exceptional size, measuring as much as 5 to 6 cm. in their

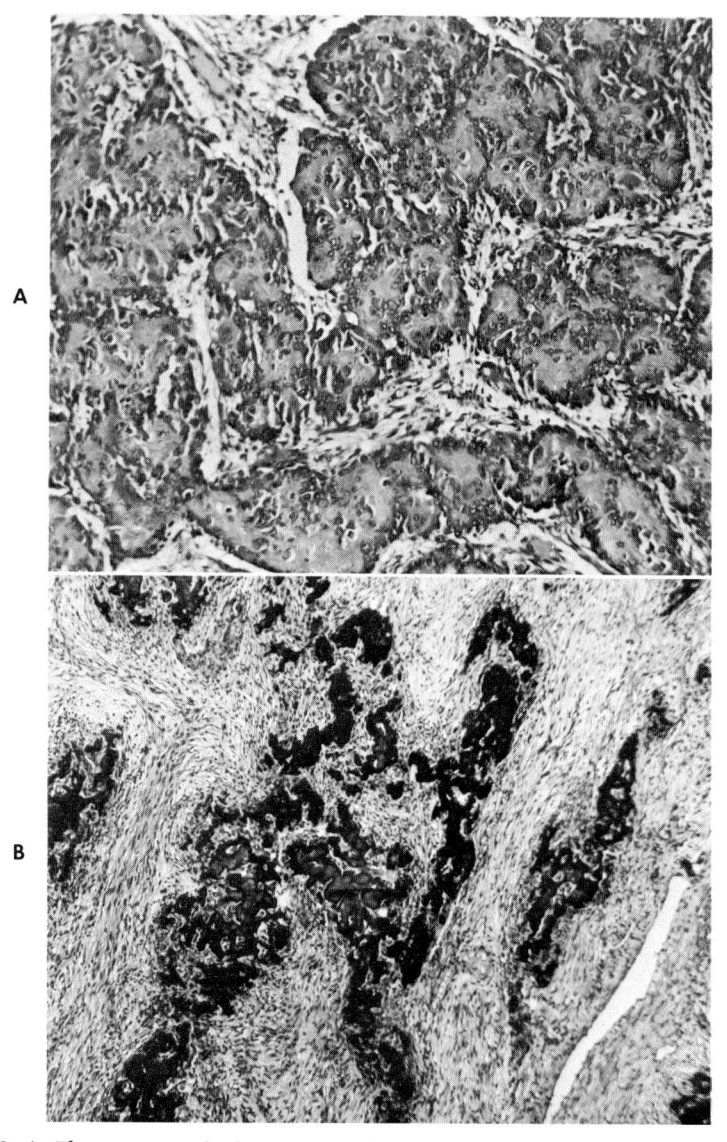

Fig. 10-9. **A**, Photomicrograph showing a multicentric pattern of osteoblasts that are forming osteoid matrix. (×120.) **B**, Photomicrograph (of a tumor in the humerus of a child) showing foci of osteoblasts heavily impregnated by calcium. The intervening stroma is rather fibrocytic. (×120.)

long axis. One such unusual instance in the sclerotized cortex of the shaft of a humerus was illustrated as Fig. 9-7. Another one of unusual size, which we have observed, developed in the thickened shaft of a femur and is illustrated as Fig. 9-8. As previously indicated,[17] the designation of giant osteoid-osteoma for such tumors of remarkable size seems not inappropriate, although unfortunately Dahlin and Johnson applied this name to the whole category of osteoid- and bone-forming tumors that we now call benign osteoblastoma.

Fibrous dysplasia

Although there has been a tendency in the past to label some solitary lesions of fibrous dysplasia showing appreciable new bone formation, especially in jaw bones, as "fibrous osteoma" or "ossifying fibroma" (benign osteoblastoma in the present terminology), their accurate differentiation microscopically should not occasion much difficulty. Lesions of fibrous dysplasia are on the whole more fibrous and less vascular and their trabeculae of new bone, being formed by metaplasia of the connective tissue, are not rimmed by ostoblasts, as are lesions of benign osteoblastoma (Figs. A-6 to A-8).

Giant-cell tumor

As for differentiation from giant-cell tumor cytologically (apart from distinct clinical differences), this might conceivably be a problem if one is dealing with a needle aspiration biopsy, but not otherwise. Suffice it to reiterate that the irregularly dispersed multinuclear cells observed represent osteoclasts or macrophages in proximity to blood vessels or within fields of blood extravasation, rather than syncytial tumor cells. Moreover, prominent osteoid and bone formation is not an integral feature of genuine giant-cell tumor.

Osteogenic sarcoma

The distinction between benign osteoblastoma and osteogenic sarcoma may prove troublesome at times, if one attempts to base opinion upon a small biopsy specimen without benefit of the roentgenograms and good clinical orientation— a practice that should be heartily discouraged in general. As noted, an occasional benign osteoblastoma may present a relatively compact stroma, but the cells appear quite uniform and the intercellular matrix is deposited in a rather orderly trabecular pattern, as a rule. If one observes irregular heavy columns or long crisscrossing streamers of osteoid or new bone or both, one must then be circumspect about the strong possibility of osteogenic sarcoma. Also, if any tumor cartilage is present, the lesion is likely to be something other than benign osteoblastoma. Altogether, the distinction should not be a difficult one to make. That the problem is not an academic one, however, is evidenced by the fact that the tumor illustrated in Fig. 10-1, *C* was interpreted as a sarcoma by one consultant who examined the sections, while the tumor illustrated in Fig. 10-1, *D* was thought to be malignant by about 60% of the pathologists who saw it at a state-wide slide conference.[25]

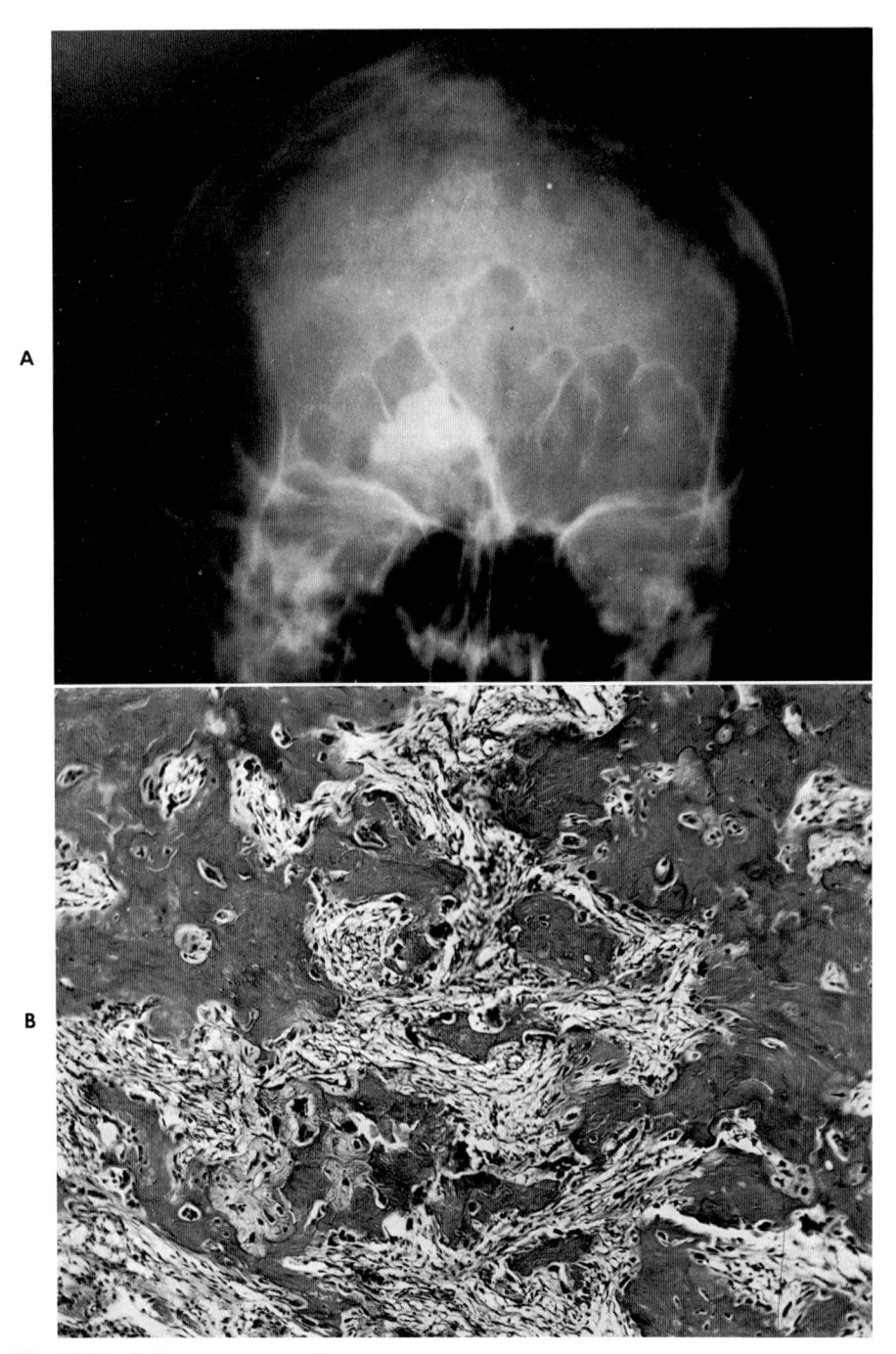

Fig. 10-10. A, Roentgenogram showing an osteoma, so-called, protruding into a frontal sinus. **B,** Photomicrograph of a representative field of the osteoma of the calvarium illustrated in **A,** showing prominent formation of plaques and trabeculae of new bone within an osteoblastic connective tissue matrix. (×100.)

Treatment and prognosis

Surgical treatment should be conservative, in keeping with the benign character of the tumor. When the latter is of relatively small or moderate size, thorough curettement and packing with bone chips appears to be the procedure of choice. Also, when the tumor is situated in the calvarium, conservative curettement or resection should suffice for clinical cure, and there appears to be no necessity for sacrificing any wide margin of surrounding intact bone or resorting to supplementary irradiation. When the tumor is located in a spinous process of a vertebra, local excision is calculated to give a satisfactory clinical result. In dealing with a lesion in the neural arch of a vertebra that has induced weakness or paraplegia, one must at least excise the tissue responsible for extradural compression of the spinal cord or its nerve roots, although it may be difficult, if not hazardous in this situation to effect complete removal.

The limited growth potential of the neoplasm is convincingly demonstrated by the sequence of events in the instance of the shaft of the tibia illustrated in Fig. 10-3. In this case, because of the extent of the lesion and uncertainty as to its nature, the surgeon elected to do only a limited biopsy and to remove the radiopaque focus in the interior of the lesion (thought possibly to represent an osteoid-osteoma nidus), without attempting thorough curettement. Despite only partial extirpation, roentgenograms taken 14 months later showed reconstruction of the cortical defect, without measurable increase in the size of the lesion.

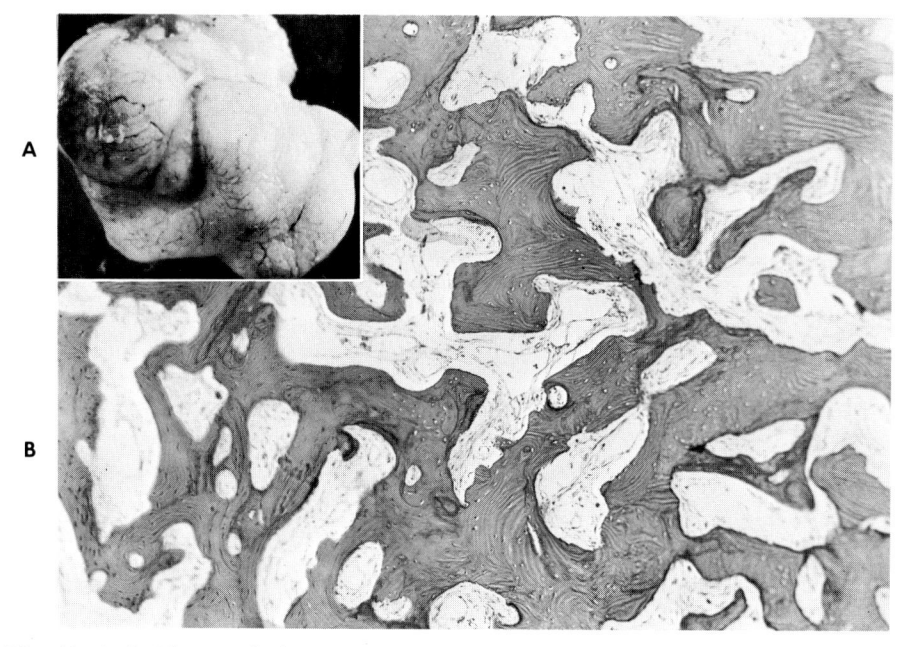

Fig. 10-11. **A,** Photograph (2½ times natural size) of an osteoma protruding into the frontal sinus. Specimen was obtained during autopsy. **B,** Photomicrograph of the osteoma illustrated in **A.** It is composed of mature, reconstructed, irregular trabeculae of bone. (×48.)

In nine of the eleven cases originally presented, follow-up data were obtained covering intervals ranging from seven months to three years after surgical treatment. In none of these was local recurrence noted roentgenographically, and the clinical results were correspondingly satisfactory. It is significant that this favorable trend was noted also in the relevant cases reported by Dahlin and Johnson, in many of which the follow-up observations covered a much longer period, ranging up to nineteen years.

In our second series,[17] we had follow-ups in half of the 20 cases cited, ranging from 1 to 5 years. In seven of these, the period of postsurgical observation covered from four to five years or more. In not a single instance was local recurrence noted (even in those treated by curettement), and the patients were all reported to be doing well and to be symptom free.

Of particular interest is a long-term follow-up in one of the cases reported in my original series,[13] that of an 18-year-old boy in whom the tumor had involved the laminae and pedicles of L-1 and L-2 and impinged upon the spinal roots. In this case, there had been local recurrence of the bone-forming neoplasm and return of symptoms nine years after laminectomy and piecemeal incomplete removal of a moderate-sized tumor, followed by roentgen-ray irradiation. Partial extirpation of the recurrent tumor accomplished decompression and relief of symptoms as readily as it had initially. At the time there was some concern about the eventual outcome, and it is interesting and reassuring therefore to note the subsequent course of events. Three years later the patient again required reoperation, followed once more by irradiation, but at last report he was clinically well and working, fully sixteen years after his original operation.

Malignant change in osteoblastoma

It has become apparent within the past several years that occasional osteoblastomas may undergo malignant change and spread well beyond the confines of the original growth. A notable instance in point was reported by Mayer,[18] that of an osteoblastoma in an acetabulum which recurred after nine years and produced a mass the size of a child's head, occupying the entire pelvis. The same author also elicited, through correspondence,[19] information concerning several other as yet unreported tumors that seem to be comparable. Through the courtesy of Dr. Deffebach, I have also seen material from an osteoblastoma in a distal tibia that manifested malignant change (to osteosarcoma) seven years after original surgery. This neoplasm not only invaded the adjacent soft parts, but also metastasized to the lungs.

Viewed in perspective against our total backlog of experience with osteoblastoma to date, this unfortunate complication would seem to have a relatively low, but significant incidence, although this impression is, of necessity, provisional, pending further information. One must be critical, however, in interpreting relevant instances; if an osteoid-and-bone–forming tumor is aggressive from the beginning, it is very likely to represent an osteogenic sarcoma, rather than osteoblastoma.

One other comment in regard to nomenclature is indicated here. Because of the observations cited, the appropriateness of the qualifying adjective *benign* in the designation of benign osteoblastoma has been questioned. However, until it is demonstrated that malignant change occurs more frequently than seems to be the case at present, I prefer to retain the original name. This was intended to highlight the distinction from osteogenic sarcoma, which, pathologically speaking, is a malignant osteoblastoma.

Summary

This section attempts to delineate the pathologic nature and appropriate treatment of certain benign osteoblastic tumors, other than classical osteoid-osteoma and osteoma so-called, on the basis of experience with 37 pertinent instances encountered in long bones, the vertebral column, and many other sites. The name "benign osteoblastoma" is employed to designate appropriately this category of osteoid- and bone-forming tumors, including those previously called "osteogenic fibromas," among others. Their recognition is of particular importance in that they may be mistaken for giant-cell tumor or osteogenic sarcoma and, as such, treated more aggressively than is required.

These benign osteoid- and bone-forming tumors are encountered most often in children or teen-agers, particularly in limb bones, the vertebral column, and the calvarium. The roentgenographic picture may not be sufficiently distinctive to permit accurate identification. In some lesions, the microscopic picture may resemble that seen in osteoid-osteoma; in others, there may be a variety of additional distinctive patterns that have been illustrated.

When an osteoid- and bone-forming lesion provokes marked reactive osteosclerosis around it, I prefer to designate it as an osteoid-osteoma, rather than benign osteoblastoma, even though it may be substantially larger than the usual osteoid-osteoma.

In two cases that we have observed,[17] the tumor developed eccentrically on the surface of a long bone, rather than in its interior. These two tumors are unusual in our experience, and they were interpreted provisionally as the periosteal counterpart of benign osteoblastoma.

Surgical treatment should be conservative, in keeping with the benign character of the tumor. In the treatment of benign osteoblastoma in the vertebral column impinging on the spinal cord or its nerve roots, the surgeon should be content to accomplish decompression, promptly followed by roentgen irradiation.

It should be noted that occasional osteoblastomas may undergo malignant change after some years and spread well beyond the confines of the original growth. This complication would seem to have a relatively low, but significant incidence.

References

1. Ackerman, L. V., and Spjut, H. J.: Tumors of bone and cartilage. In AFIP Fascicle 4—Section II, Atlas of tumor pathology, Washington, D. C., 1962 (see pp. 87-89 and Figs. 94, 95, 98, 99, and 100).
2. Bethge, J. F. J.: Benignes Osteobastom, Chirurg. 34:121, 1963.

3. Dahlin, D. C., and Johnson, E. W., Jr.: Giant osteoid osteoma, J. Bone Joint Surg. 36-A:559, 1954.
4. Giannestras, N. J., and Diamond, J. R.: Benign osteoblastoma of the talus. A review of the literature and report of a case, J. Bone Joint Surg. 40-A:469, 1958.
5. Goidanich, I. F., and Battaglia, L.: Osteoblastoma (Fibroma Osteogenetico). Neoplasia Benigna di Tessuto Osteoblastico. Studio clinico, radiographico ed anatomopathologico di 14 casi, Chir. d. org. di movimento (Fasc. 5) 46:353, 1959.
6. Golding, J. S. R., and Sissons, H. A.: Osteogenic fibroma of bone; a report of two cases, J. Bone Joint Surg. 36-B:428, 1954.
7. Guy, R., Lafond, G., Gagnon, P. A., Raymond, O., and Bourgeois, J.: L'Osteoblastome Benin (Fibroma osteogenique l'osteome osteoide geant), Union Med. Can. 88:666, 1959.
8. Jaffe, H. L.: Benign osteoblastoma, Bull. Hosp. Joint Dis. 17:141, 1956.
9. Jaffe, H. L.: Tumors and tumorous conditions of the bones and joints, Philadelphia, 1958, Lea & Febiger, pp. 107-116.
10. Jaffe, H. L., and Lichtenstein, L.: Osteoid-osteoma: further experience with this benign tumor of bone with special reference to cases showing the lesions in relation to shaft cortices and commonly misclassified as instances of sclerosing nonsuppurative osteomyelitis or cortical bone abscess, J. Bone Joint Surg. 22:645, 1940.
11. Jaffe, H. L., and Mayer, L.: An osteoblastic osteoid tissue-forming tumor of a metacarpal bone, Arch. Surg. 24:550, 1932.
12. Kirkpatrick, H. J. R., and Murray, R. C.: Osteogenic fibroma of bone. A case, J. Bone Joint Surg. 37-B:606, 1955.
13. Lichtenstein, L.: Benign osteoblastoma. A category of osteoid- and bone-forming tumors other than classical osteoid-osteoma which may be mistaken for giant-cell tumor or osteogenic sarcoma, Cancer 9:1044, 1956.
14. Lichtenstein, L.: Bone tumors, ed. 2, St. Louis, 1959, The C. V. Mosby Co., pp. 97-108.
15. Lichtenstein, L.: Bone tumors, St. Louis, 1952, The C. V. Mosby Co., pp. 82-87.
16. Lichtenstein, L.: Medical progress. Pathology: Diseases of bone, N. Engl. J. Med. 255:427, 1956 (see Benign osteoblastoma, p. 428).
17. Lichtenstein, L., and Sawyer, W. R.: Benign osteoblastoma. Further observations and report of 20 additional cases, J. Bone Joint Surg. 46-A:755, 1964.
18. Mayer, L.: Malignant degeneration of so-called benign osteoblastoma, Bull. Hosp. Joint Dis. 28:4, 1967.
19. Mayer, L.: Benign (?) osteoblastoma. Letter to the editor, Bull. Hosp. Joint Dis. 29:236, 1968.
20. Pochaczevsky, R., Yen, Y. M., and Sherman, R. S.: The roentgen appearance of benign osteoblastoma, Radiology 75:429, 1960.
21. Rand, R. W., and Rand, C. W.: Intraspinal tumors of childhood, Springfield, Ill., 1960, Charles C Thomas, Publisher, pp. 330-339.
22. Rosensweig, J. Pintar, K., Mikail, M., and Mayman, A.: Benign osteoblastoma (giant osteoid osteoma). Report of an unusual rib tumour and review of the literature, Can. Med. Assoc. J. 89:1189, 1963.
23. Sanchis-Olmos, V., Torrelles, M. F., and Criado, M. F.: Osteoma Parostal de Clavicula, Acta Ortoped. Traumatol. Iberica 4(Fasc. 2°):471-486, 1956.
24. Schein, A. J.: Osteoblastoma of the scapula. A case report, J. Bone Joint Surg. 41-A:359, 1959.
25. Stewart, F. W.: Personal communication, Dec. 9, 1954.

Chapter 11

Nonosteogenic fibroma of bone (nonossifying fibroma, metaphyseal fibrous defect, fibrous cortical defect)

Our present views in regard to this relatively common, tumorlike lesion have developed in two phases. The first came in 1942 when Jaffe and I[9] separated the lesion from the jumble of giant-cell tumor variants, so-called (it had been called the healing, spindle-cell, or xanthic variant), and established that it had nothing in common with genuine giant-cell tumor of bone. It was also pointed out that some instances of the lesion had been called xanthoma and xanthogranuloma, mainly because its spindle connective tissue cells had taken up lipid in places and become converted to nests of foam cells. Incidentally, this aspect of the lesion, prominent though it may be in some instances (Fig. 11-7, *B*), appears to represent a secondary change. One encounters many specimens in which the presence of lipid cannot be demonstrated, even in serial sections stained with Sudan. At the time little was known of the natural history of the lesion and, inasmuch as some of the instances observed were good-sized fibrous growths within the medullary cavity, capable of substantial further enlargement under observation (Fig. 11-3, *A*, for example), the inference that we were dealing with a benign tumor seemed logical. This impression was reinforced by the cellularity of the constituent fibroblastic cells, which was impressive enough to cause some pathologists to interpret the lesion as low-grade fibrosarcoma, as well as giant-cell tumor (Fig. 11-7, *A*). This still happens occasionally, though much less often.

The second phase came some years later, when it was recognized that the condition appears with surprising frequency as an incidental finding; that some lesions, particularly the smaller subcortical or intracortical ones, may involute spontaneously; and that occasionally one encounters multiple foci in the same patient. Hatcher[8] was among the first to question whether the condition represented a genuine neoplasm and proposed the designation of metaphyseal fibrous defect, presumably resulting from some developmental aberration. He also stressed its association with concomitant epiphyseal disorders. Additional insight

122 Bone tumors

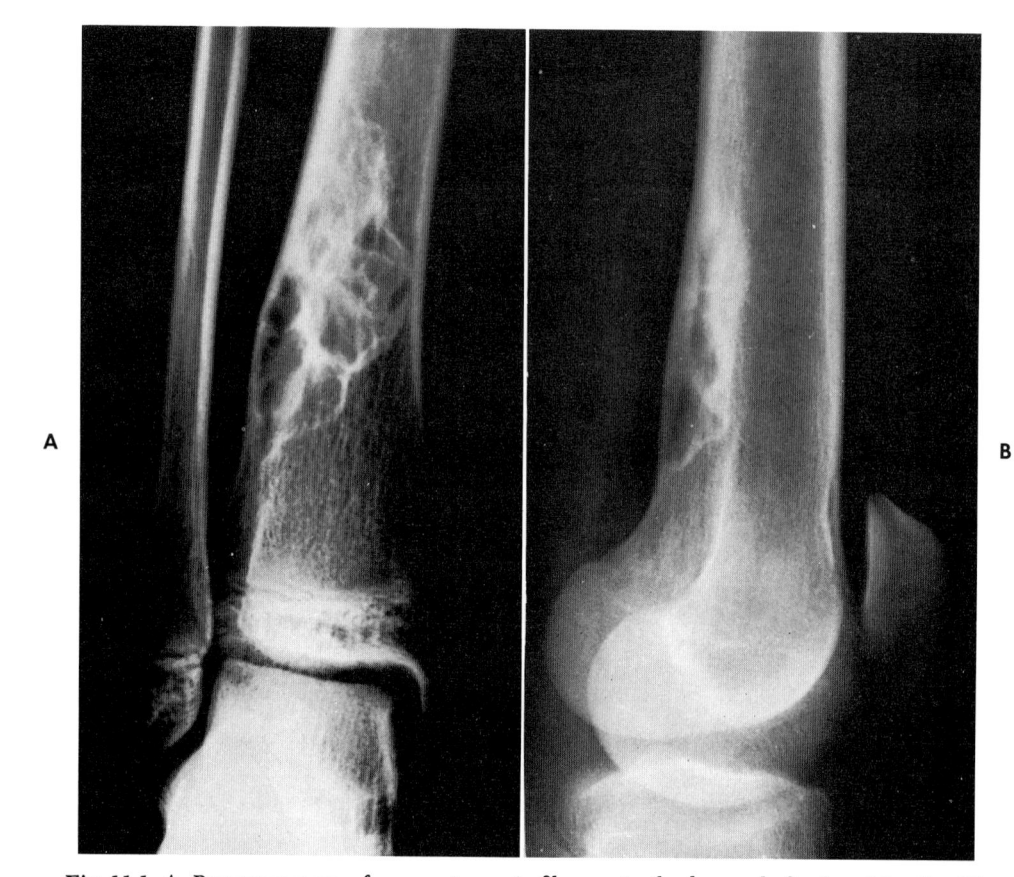

Fig. 11-1. A, Roentgenogram of a nonosteogenic fibroma in the lower shaft of a tibia of a 15-year-old boy, which was discovered following an injury to the ankle. The lesion is eccentrically situated, loculated, and sharply delimited internally by sclerotized bone. The overlying cortex is in part thinned and slightly bulging. This picture is so characteristic of the lesion as to leave little doubt as to its identity even before tissue examination. The tumor in this instance was thoroughly curetted and packed with bone chips. **B,** Another clinically silent lesion of nonosteogenic fibroma in the lower end of a femur, discovered on roentgen survey in a patient who also presented an osteogenic sarcoma in the opposite femur.

has also been gained from periodic mass roentgenographic surveys of the growing bones of young children (especially in the knee joint region). Whether the ephemeral small growth defects described by Sontag and Pyle[17] in the metaphyses of large limb bones, especially in the distal femoral metaphysis, are relevant is a moot point, although Jaffe apparently accepts them as such. The observations of Caffey[4] are more impressive. He has shown that "benign cortical defects," so-called, are common in children after the age of 2 years, that 90% of these occur in the femur, that about 50% are bilateral, and that they tend to come and go. In pathologic terms, he interprets them as segments or patches of localized fibrosis in the cortical walls. Jaffe's view is that occasionally an enlarging defect of this nature penetrates into the medullary cavity and acquires the character of nonossifying (or nonosteogenic) fibroma. This explanation has been

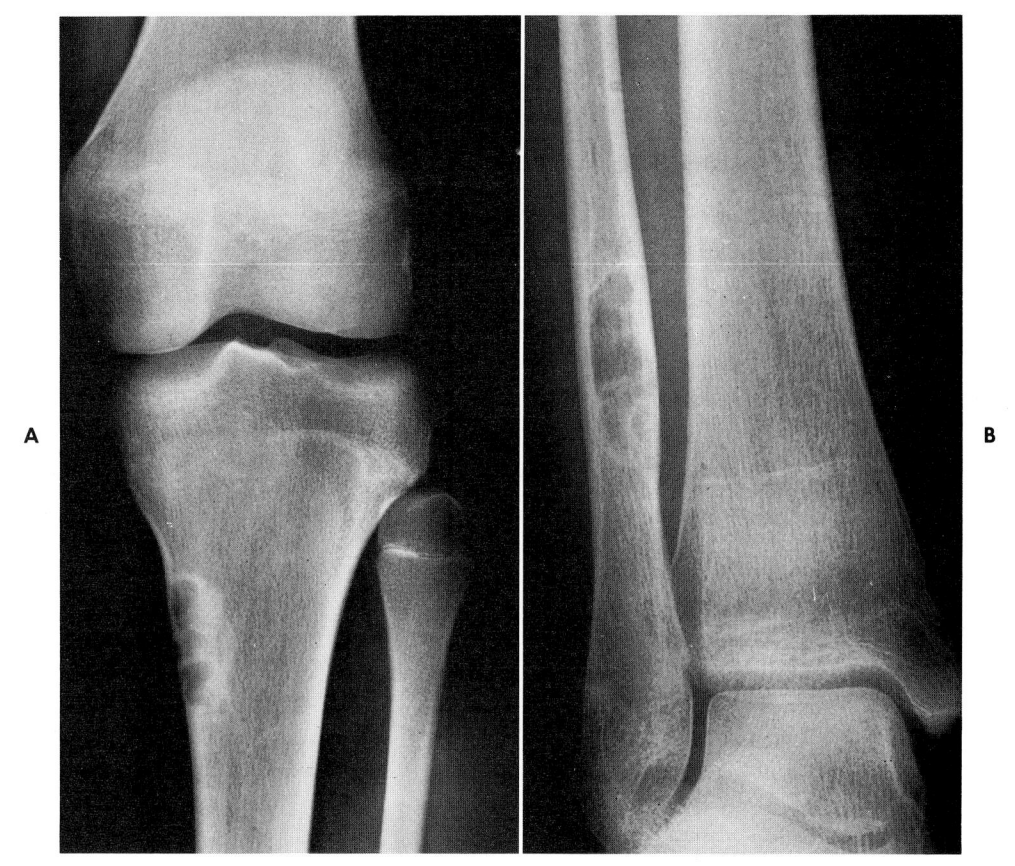

Fig. 11-2. **A**, Roentgenogram of a nonosteogenic fibroma in one of its more common sites. Note its subcortical position and its sharp delimitation by a zone of sclerotized bone. **B**, Another pertinent lesion in the lower shaft of a fibula. In a small limb bone like a fibula (or an ulna) the lesion may occupy the entire width of the affected bone, and its roentgen picture then becomes more equivocal and not readily distinguishable from that of a small bone cyst or a focus of fibrous dysplasia.

accepted by others.[13] All of the surgical material I have seen in recent years has come from subcortical or intramedullary lesions in patients in the second decade; therefore I have no basis for any independent judgment.

In any event, however one interprets the pathogenesis of this peculiar lesion, in its fully evolved state it presents a very distinctive roentgenographic and pathologic appearance that enables one to identify it readily. It is usually encountered in the shaft of a long bone, commonly a bone of the lower limb, not far from an epiphyseal cartilage plate. In a large limb bone, like the femur or tibia, the lesion tends characteristically to have an eccentric position, hugging the cortex, and to be sharply delimited internally by a sclerotized margin of bone. On the other hand, in a narrow tubular bone, such as the fibula or ulna, the lesion may come to occupy the full width of the shaft, in which case it may have to be differen-

124 Bone tumors

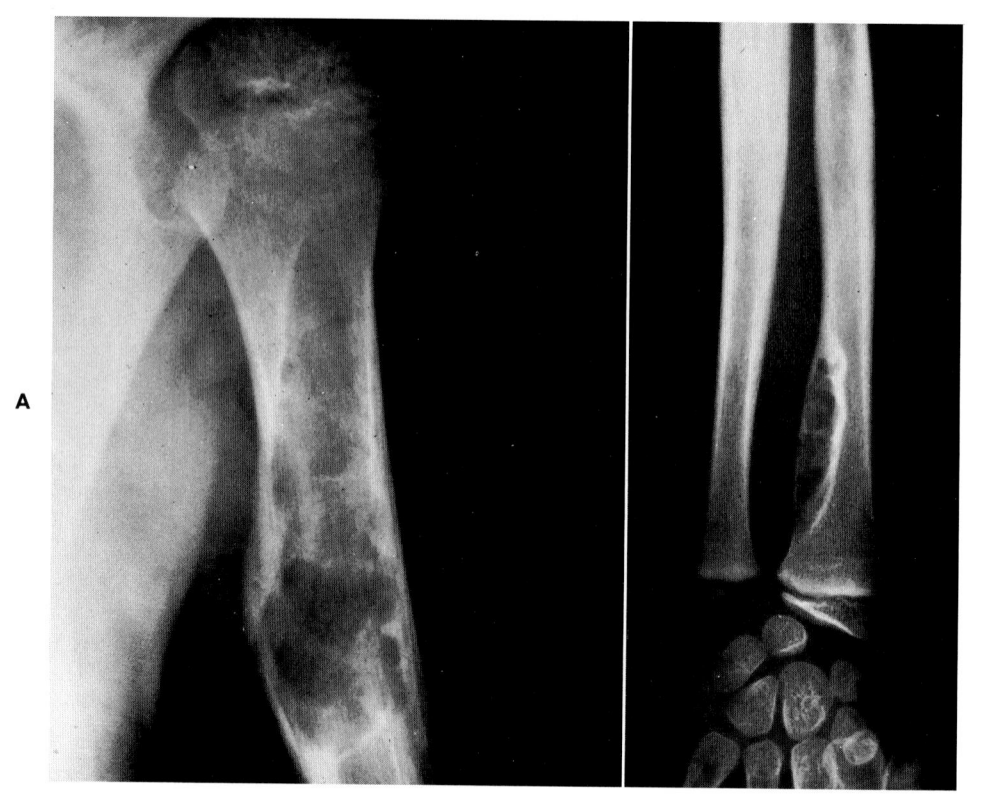

Fig. 11-3. A, Roentgenogram of a relatively large, nonosteogenic fibroma situated within the upper shaft of a humerus, an unusual location for it. The patient was a 6-year-old boy who had sustained a pathologic fracture in a fall some six weeks previously. The tumor tissue on curettement was found to be solid and yellowish in color. B, Another pertinent lesion situated beneath the cortex of the lower metaphysis of a radius in a child.

tiated roentgenographically from a bone cyst or a focus of fibrous dysplasia. In the gross, the lesion appears as a single focus or as a honeycomb of smaller contiguous foci of yellow or brown fibrous tissue, well demarcated by sclerotized bone. Its cytologic pattern is essentially that of whorled bundles of spindle-shaped connective tissue cells, among which occasional rather small and also spindly multinuclear giant cells may be interspersed. Within some lesions, though by no means all, smaller or larger collections of foam cells may also be observed in places.

With increasing recognition of the lesion by radiologists and orthopedic surgeons, not nearly as many are operated upon as formerly. When relevant material is referred to me for opinion now, it is usually because the examining pathologist considered the diagnosis of giant-cell tumor, because the picture was complicated by fracture and callus formation, or because multiple lesions were encountered. Pertaining to the effect of fracture, I have had occasion to see an unusual lesion in the upper tibia of an 11-year-old boy, in which, following a

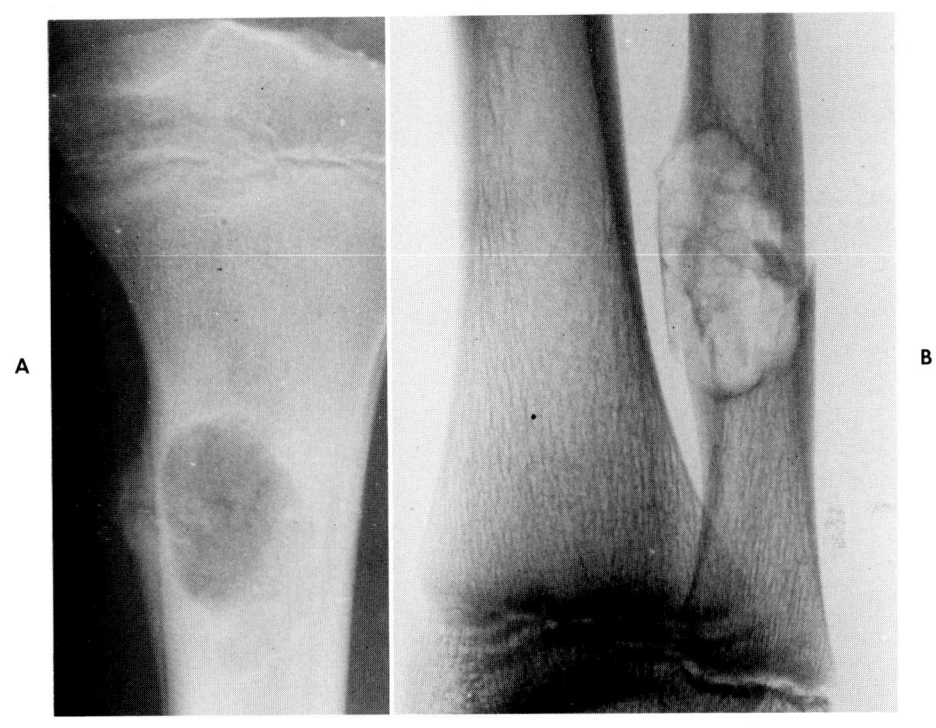

Fig. 11-4. A, Roentgenogram of a nonosteogenic fibroma in the upper metaphysis of a tibia of an 11-year-old boy, showing fracture and callus formation. The distal portion of the lesion showed evidence of spontaneous reconstruction. B, Another lesion in the lower fibula of a 12-year-old boy showing pathologic fracture.

fracture, the distal half ossified, but the proximal half continued to enlarge (Fig. 11-4, A). Among interesting cases showing multiple defects was one with as many as four (one in each lower femoral metaphysis, one in an upper tibia, and one in the continguous fibula); another with a large lesion in the lower tibial metaphysis and another smaller one in the upper shaft of the same bone; and two others in a fibula presenting two separate lesions. In one of the latter cases there was an interval of four years before the second defect came to clinical attention, and, interestingly enough, the initially presenting defect had reappeared despite previous surgery (Fig. 11-5).

Clinical features
Age and sex incidence and localization

The lesion is encountered notably in children and adolescents, although an occasional one, presumably of long standing, may be discovered incidentally on roentgen examination of a young adult. There does not appear to be any predilection for either sex. As for localization, the lesion is encountered regularly in long limb bones, as noted, and it is seldom observed elsewhere. I have seen tissue from a focus of nonossifying fibroma in an iliac bone adjacent to its sacral

126　Bone tumors

articulation, but this finding is unique in my experience (Fig. 11-5, *B*). As also indicated, the lower limb bones show particular predilection, specifically the tibia, femur, and fibula, although occasionally a bone of an upper limb, such as the ulna or humerus, may be the site of involvement. In any event, the lesion is usually found in the shaft, toward the upper or lower end of the bone, and extending, as a rule, within an inch or two of the adjacent epiphyseal plate.

Clinical complaints

There is nothing characteristic about the clinical history, nor is the latter particularly helpful in diagnosis, except insofar as it directs attention to the necessity for roentgen examination. In most instances the complaints are of brief duration, although this does not mean that the lesion was not of longer standing, developing slowly and insidiously before it was discovered. Many patients complain of

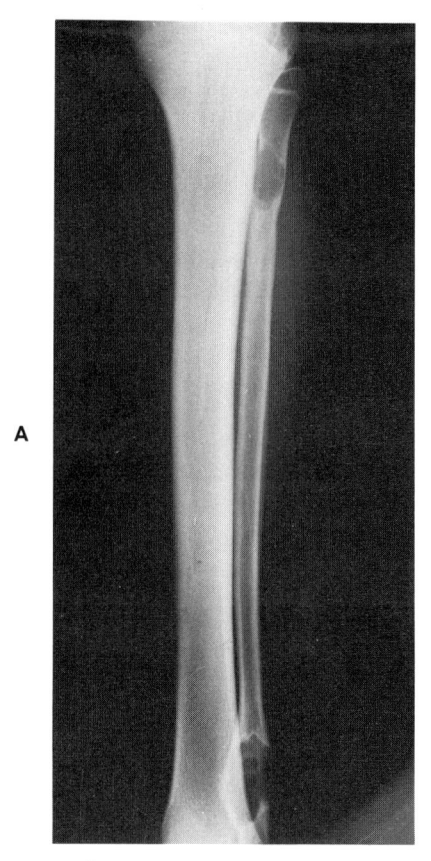

Fig. 11-5. A, Roentgenogram of an unusual instance in which two lesions of nonosteogenic fibroma developed in a fibula, one in the upper end and another in the lower end. The upper focus apparently healed after a fracture, only to reappear four years later, at which time a second focus in the other end of the bone was discovered. B, Roentgenogram of a nonosteogenic fibroma (proved by tissue examination) in a very unusual location—the iliac bone bordering on its sacral articulation. C, Roentgenogram of a comparatively large nonosteogenic fibroma in the distal femur, with a comminuted pathologic fracture of the cortex.

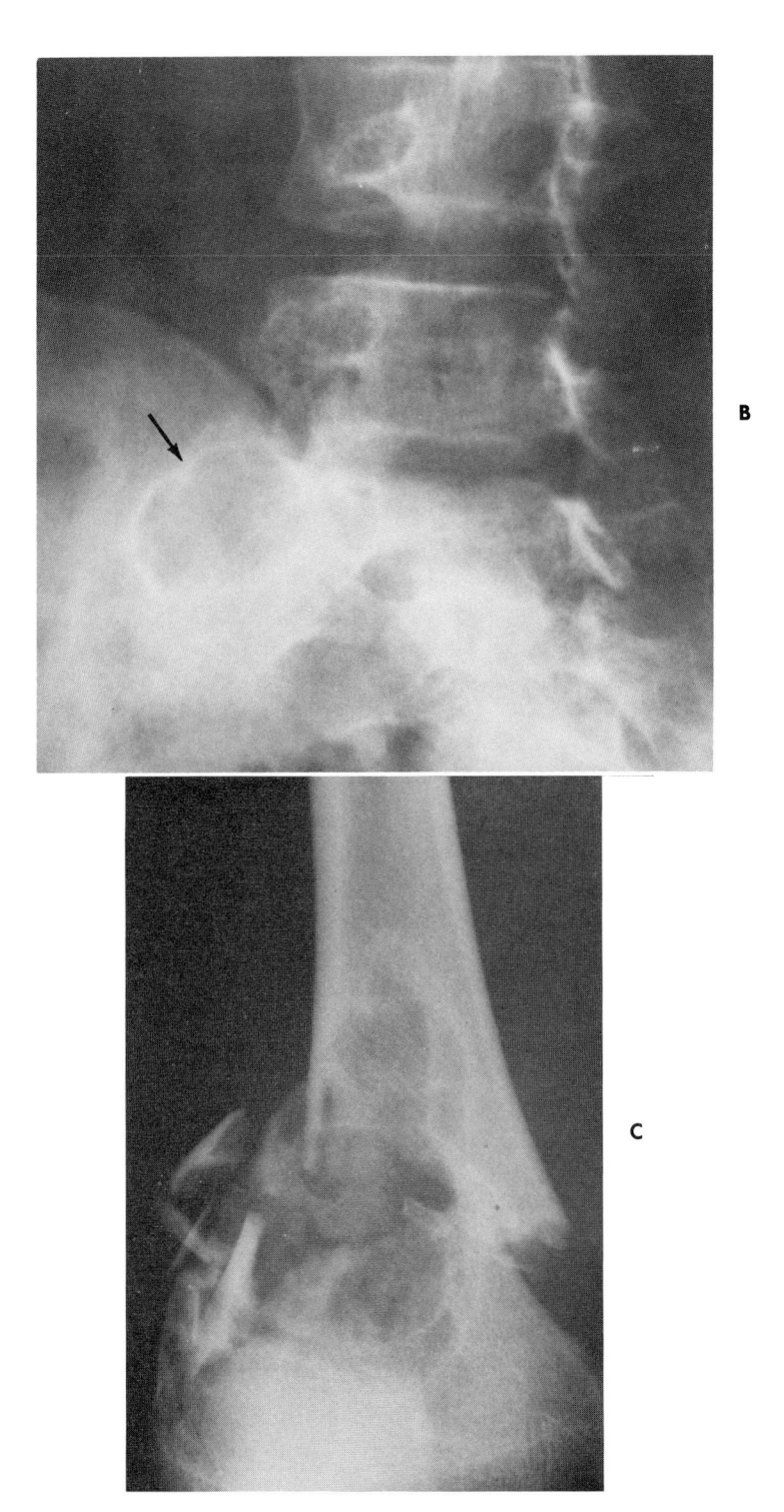

Fig. 11-5, cont'd. For legend see opposite page.

pain and swelling of an ankle, knee, or wrist and attribute their difficulty to some trauma, such as a sprain, kick, or fall, to the region in which the bone lesion was discovered. Others, while giving no history of trauma, likewise had pain and swelling of a joint as their chief complaint. Occasionally, pathologic fracture through the attenuated cortex overlying the lesion may be the first manifestation of its presence. In many instances, a clinically silent lesion may be discovered as an incidental finding on roentgen examination of the part for some other skeletal difficulty. Thus, I have observed several cases of osteogenic sarcoma of the lower femur, in which x-ray examination of the knee region also revealed the presence of an unsuspected nonosteogenic fibroma of the upper tibia.

Roentgenographic findings

Most instances of nonosteogenic fibroma present so distinctive a roentgenographic appearance as to be readily recognizable, if one is familiar with the picture. The usual location of the lesion in the upper or lower third of a long bone at some distance from the adjacent epiphyseal cartilage plate has already been emphasized. In a large limb bone, like the tibia or femur, the lesion is found characteristically to have an eccentric position abutting on the inner aspect of the cortex and to be sharply outlined internally by a sclerotized line. The lesion itself casts a rarefied shadow, which may appear loculated, owing to the presence of thin, dividing, bony partitions. The cortex delimiting the lesion peripherally is often thinned and sometimes slightly expanded, but its continuity is preserved, unless there has been a pathologic fracture (Fig. 11-5, C). As to size, the lesion may be rather small or as much as 6 cm. or more in greatest dimension, but, in any event, its long axis coincides with that of the bone in which it arises.

When the lesion develops in a slender limb bone, such as the fibula or ulna, it tends to occupy the entire width of the bone and to bring about some expansion and attenuation of the overlying cortex. Its appearance is otherwise essentially similar to that presented by lesions in large limb bones, but one cannot be certain without tissue examination that one is not dealing with a bone cyst or a solitary focus of fibrous dysplasia. Even when the lesion occupies a central position, its sharply defined and sclerotized outline should preclude any serious thought of giant-cell tumor of bone, as should also its metaphyseal or shaft location and its common occurrence in patients below the age of 20 years.

Pathologic features

Whether the lesion is eccentric in position and abutting on the cortex or whether it extends across the entire width of the shaft, it usually consists of several discrete but contiguous foci of gray-yellow or yellow-brown, firm, fibrous connective tissue. Each focus may be outlined in part by a thin shell of sclerotic bone, and some of the individual foci may also be separated from each other by bits of sclerotic spongiosa. As for the overlying cortex, this may show endosteal erosion and thinning in some places, and thickening in others. The periosteum

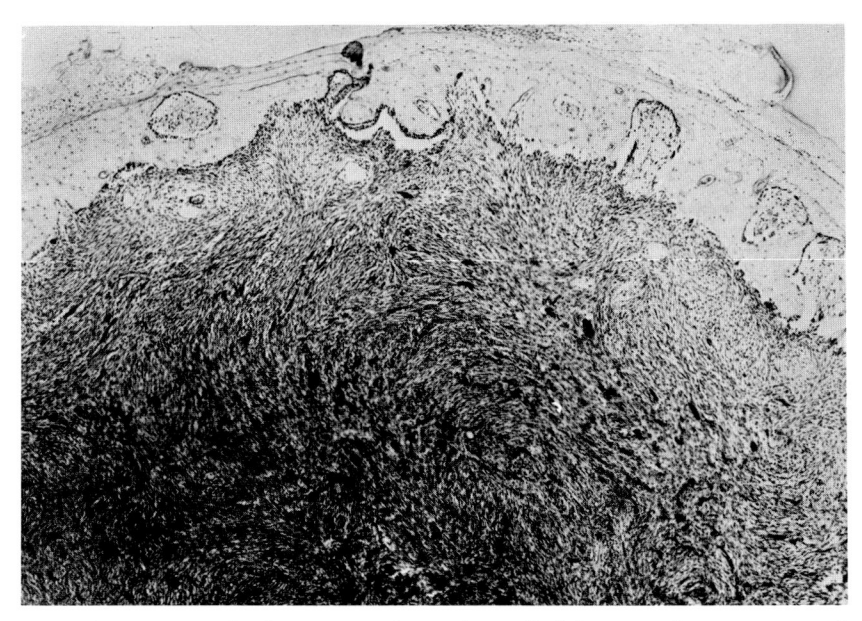

Fig. 11-6. Photomicrograph of a pertinent lesion (in a fibula). Its cytologic pattern is that of whorled, compact, small spindle-shaped connective tissue cells, interspersed among which are scattered, spindly multinuclear cells. The cortical bone has been attenuated and somewhat expanded. (×35.)

of the affected portion of the shaft is not particularly thickened, except at the site of a pathologic fracture.

On microscopic examination, as noted, the general pattern of the lesion is that of whorled bundles of connective tissue cells. However, the cellularity of the stroma varies from one lesion to another, or even from one focus to another within the same lesion. There is also some variation in regard to the vascularity of the lesion, the prominence of multinuclear giant cells within it, and its content of lipid, if any, in the form of collections of foam cells. In a distinctly brown lesion or focus, the connective tissue cells are spindle shaped and closely compacted, being interspersed with but little collagenous intercellular material. Many of the stromal cells are likely to contain granules of hemosiderin in their cytoplasm, and it is mainly this that accounts for the brownish color of the lesion as a whole, although some scattered capillary hemorrhages may also contribute to it. Irregularly dispersed among the stromal cells are small, often elongated multinuclear giant cells. These cells, sparse on the whole, may be more numerous and clustered together in some fields, especially about areas of recent capillary hemorrhage. The giant cells seem to be formed through fusion of the spindle-shaped stromal cells, and, like the latter, many of them contain granules of hemosiderin in their cytoplasm.

In a distinctly yellowish lesion or focus, nests of lipid-containing foam cells are seen, admixed with and encircled by the stromal tissue. The latter then con-

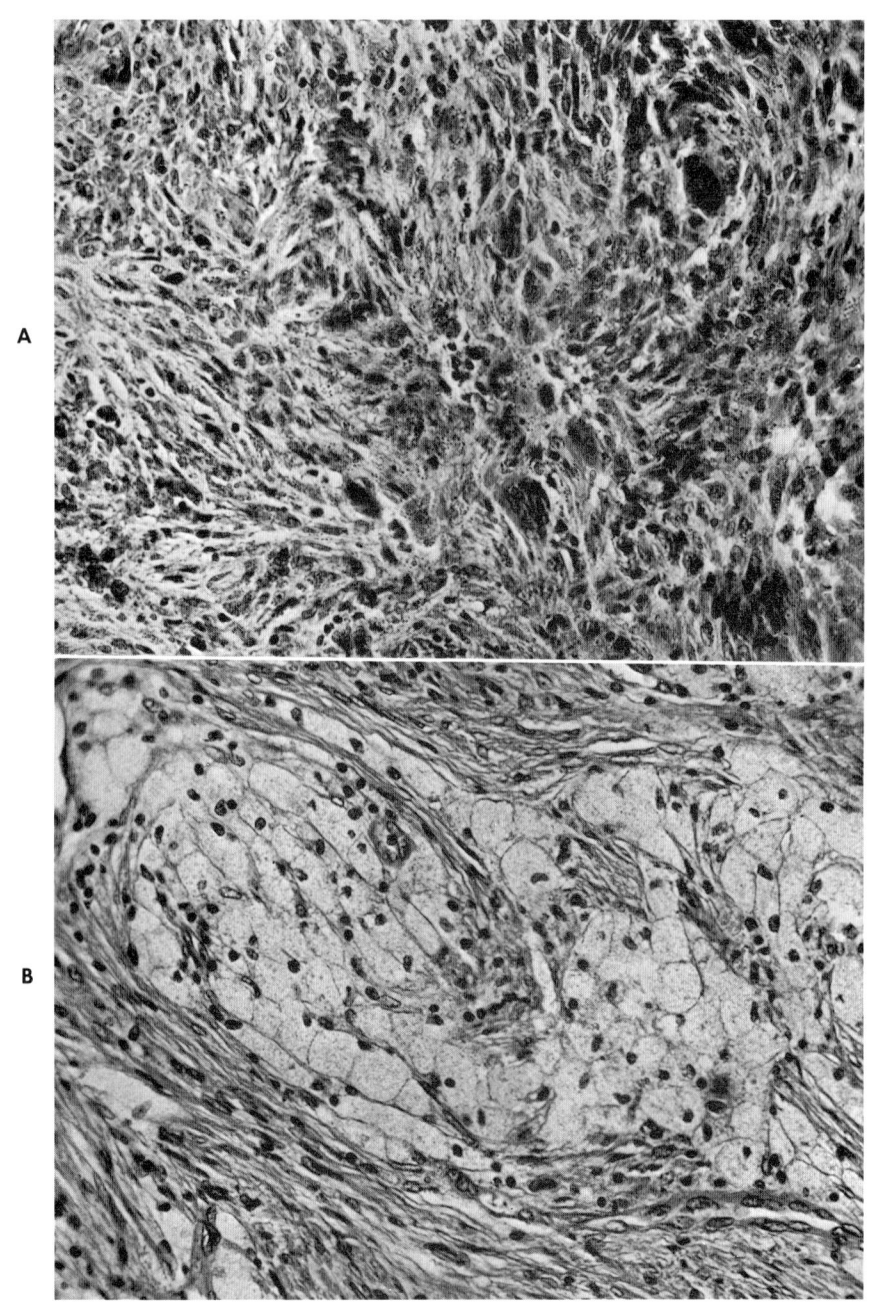

Fig. 11-7. **A,** Photomicrograph of a field of a nonosteogenic fibroma showing occasional small, compressed multinuclear cells within the connective tissue stroma. It is the presence of such multinuclear cells that may cause the lesion to be mistaken at times for giant-cell tumor. (×250.) **B,** Another field of a nonosteogenic fibroma in which the connective tissue cells have taken up lipid and been converted to foam cells. This feature is not a constant one and is observed only in certain lesions, some of which have been labeled in the past as "xanthoma" or "xanthogranuloma." (×250.) **C,** Photomicrograph of a desmoplastic fibroma of bone, for contrast with **A.** (×150.)

sists of rather collagenous, spindle-shaped connective tissue cells in winding thick strands or whorled bundles, honeycombed by the foam cells (Fig. 11-7, B). It can be shown that these lipid-containing cells arise through conversion of the spindle cells into lipophages, and that the lipids contained within the latter are, to a large extent, of the nature of cholesterol esters. On the whole, the more yellow the lesion or focus, the more lipophages it contains and the more collagenous the intervening stromal tissue appears; and furthermore, the less it shows of hemosiderin pigment in the stromal cells or of multinuclear giant cells among them. Why the disappearance of the hemosiderin pigment and giant cells should parallel the appearance of foam cells in the lesion we do not know, but the fact that it does so is clear from the findings in areas representing intermediary stages of yellow or brown pigmentation.

Thus, in an individual lesion, one may see fields in which the stromal connective tissue cells are rich in hemosiderin and interspersed with giant cells, and other fields in which pigment-bearing cells and giant cells are sparse or absent and foam cells are numerous. However, in about half of our cases, the entire lesion failed to show any lipid at all, although the latter was sought for in frozen sections of material stained for fat, and foam cells were looked for in paraffin sections prepared from many areas of each lesion. It seems clearly unjustifiable, therefore, to place undue emphasis upon the inconstant lipid component by designating the lesion a xanthoma or xanthofibroma of bone.

Furthermore, none of the lesions examined showed evidence of osteogenesis as a feature of their cytology, and the lack of bone formation within these lesions

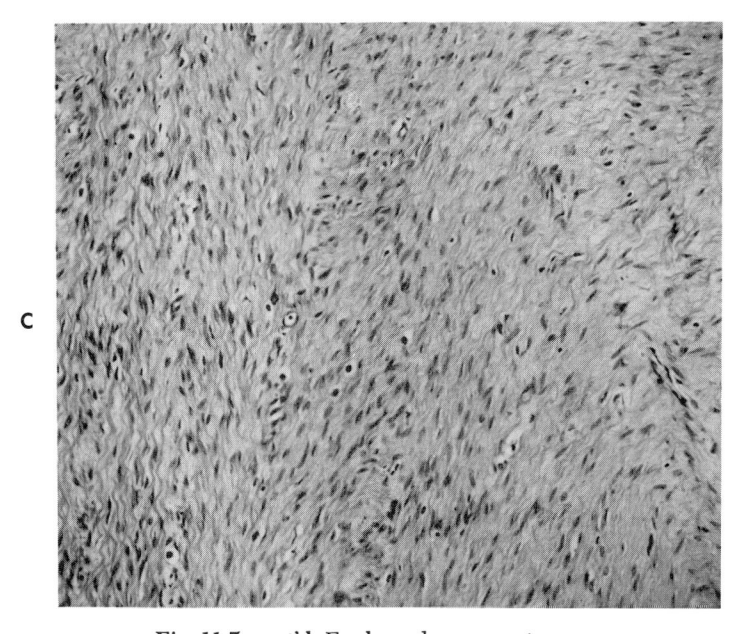

Fig. 11-7, cont'd. For legend see opposite page.

is a consistent and striking finding. It is true that individual foci may be walled off or delimited at their periphery by a narrow zone of bone. Also, where it abuts upon the cortex of the shaft, the lesion may provoke thickening of the cortex in places, just as in other places it may erode it. However, in either case, such bone formation represents a response of the neighboring tissue to the lesion and is not a feature of the lesion itself.

The lesion under discussion must be clearly differentiated from the tumor in bone that has been designated *desmoplastic fibroma* by Jaffe[10] and others.[15] The latter would seem to represent the conventional benign fibroblastic tumor analogous to fibroma elsewhere, although why it should develop so infrequently in bone is puzzling (Fig. 11-7, C). Some have interpreted the lesion as being analogous to (soft-tissue) fibromatosis, although I do not find this view convincing. Since Jaffe's brief account based on observation of some five cases, there have been a limited number of case reports, chief of which is that of Rabhan and Rosai[15] describing another ten instances. The lesion has been encountered mainly in children and young adults, and it may develop in the axial skeleton, as well as in limb bones, where it is more likely to be in the metaphysis than in the shaft. The tumor tissue in the gross is gray-white, firm, and rubbery and (microscopically) is composed of small fibroblasts, which tend to form abundant collagen, often in thick strands and bundles. Altogether, the gross and microscopic picture is quite different from that of nonossifying fibroma.

My own experience with this tumor is limited, although I would direct attention to two pitfalls that await the unwary pathologist. First, the presence of collagen bundles, per se, in a biopsy section of a fibroblastic tumor in bone does not indicate necessarily that it is benign—they may also be seen in fibrosarcoma (Fig. 17-8, C and D). Second, the cytologic differentiation between a desmoplastic fibroma and a slow-growing, well-differentiated fibrosarcoma can be tricky business. The fact that there was local recurrence after curettement in as many as one third of the reported cases of desmoplastic fibroma emphasizes this note of caution.

Treatment

The x-ray appearance of the lesion is so consistently distinctive that, in most cases, I now believe that biopsy or surgical removal is elective rather than mandatory. However, nonosteogenic fibroma of bone is readily amenable to treatment. The lesions discussed in this chapter were all treated surgically, the procedure in most cases being thorough curettement of the lesion. In several cases in which the lesion was in the fibula, subperiosteal resection of the affected portion of the bone was done. This seemed the easiest way of completely eradicating the focus of the disease in these particular cases, though, even in slender long bones, resection may not always be necessary. There were no local recurrences in any of the patients surgically treated. None of them received postoperative radiation therapy.

Whether the lesion would be amenable to radiation therapy alone (i.e., without surgical intervention), I cannot state from personal experience. Of course, without the histologic examination of tissue made possible by surgical intervention one could not be absolutely certain that the lesion being treated actually represented a nonosteogenic fibroma of bone. Furthermore, I am sufficiently impressed by recent observations on the prevalence of postirradiation sarcomas of bone to refrain from advocating x-ray therapy for benign tumors of bone that can be readily cured by conservative surgery.

Cognizance should be taken of a case report[2] of malignant transformation of a nonosteogenic fibroma of bone (to fibrosarcoma), the first of its kind that I am aware of. The details of the roentgen illustration were unclear. There was no follow-up, and I would have some reservation about accepting this case at its face value without reviewing the sections.

Summary

Whether one interprets this lesion as a benign fibroblastic tumor, at least in its advanced stage (nonosteogenic fibroma or nonossifying fibroma), or whether one conceives of it in all circumstances as a developmental or growth anomaly (metaphyseal fibrous defect, fibrous cortical defect), it is a relatively common entity with a distinctive roentgen and pathologic picture. Most of the patients are between the ages of 10 and 20, although an occasional one may be younger. There are no characteristic clinical manifestations, and, in fact, the lesion may be entirely asymptomatic, being discovered oftentimes on incidental roentgen examination or following a pathologic fracture. The usual site of the lesion is the shaft of a long tubular bone, most commonly of a lower limb, not far from the adjacent epiphyseal cartilage plate. The lesion tends to be of limited size and may not traverse the entire diameter of the affected bone, especially if the latter is a femur or tibia. Roentgenographically such a lesion presents as a sharply delimited, eccentric, somewhat loculated area of rarefaction, hugging and perhaps bulging out the cortex on one side. On the other hand, a lesion in a slender limb bone, such as a fibula or ulna, may appear as a multilocular area of rarefaction traversing the bone and even bulging it out on both sides.

On gross pathologic examination, the lesion is found usually to consist of several discrete but contiguous yellow-brown fibrous foci. The basic microscopic pattern is that of whorled bundles of spindle-shaped connective tissue cells loosely interspersed with small multinuclear giant cells, though, in some lesions areas containing foam cells may also be present.

In regard to treatment, thorough curettement or block resection of the affected area is all that is needed to effect a cure. In dealing with a lesion that is not giving rise to clinical difficulties and whose nature seems reasonably clear from its roentgen appearance, surgical removal is elective rather than mandatory. The lesion is entirely benign in my experience, and, if its connective tissue possesses any potentiality of aggressive growth or malignant change, I have never observed it, although there is a single case report on record of malignant transformation.

References

1. Bahls, G.: Uber ein solitäres Xanthoma im Knochen, Zentralbl f. Chir. **63**:1041, 1936.
2. Bhagwandeen, S.: Malignant transformation of a non-osteogenic fibroma of bone, J. Path. Bact. **92**:562, 1966.
3. Burman, M. S., and Sinberg, S. E.: Solitary xanthoma (lipoid granulomatosis) of bone, Arch. Surg. **37**:1017, 1938.
4. Caffey, J.: On fibrous defects in cortical walls of growing tubular bones, Adv. Pediatr. **7**:13, 1955.
5. Campbell, C. J., and Harkess, J.: Fibrous metaphyseal defect of bone, Surg. Gynecol. Obstet. **104**:329, 1957.
6. Compere, C. L., and Coleman, S. S.: Nonosteogenic fibroma of bone, Surg. Gynecol. Obstet. **105**:588, 1957.
7. Geschickter, C. F., and Copeland, M. M.: Tumors of bone, rev. ed., New York, 1936, American Journal of Cancer.
8. Hatcher, C. H.: The pathogenesis of localized fibrous lesions in the metaphyses of long bones, Ann. Surg. **122**:1016, 1945.
9. Jaffe, H. L., and Lichtenstein, L.: Nonosteogenic fibroma of bone, Am. J. Pathol. **18**:205, 1942.
10. Jaffe, H. L.: Tumors and tumorous conditions of the bones and joints, Philadelphia, 1958, Lea & Febiger, pp. 298-303.
11. Kolodny, A.: Bone sarcoma: the primary malignant tumors of bone and the giant cell tumor, Surg. Gynecol. Obstet. **44** (suppl. 1):1-214, 1927 (see Fig. 83, p. 186).
12. Maudsley, R. H., and Stansfeld, A. G.: Nonosteogenic fibroma of bone (fibrous metaphyseal defect), J. Bone Joint Surg. **38-B**:714, 1956.
13. Phelan, J. T.: Fibrous cortical defect and nonosseous fibroma of bone, Surg. Gynecol. Obstet. **119**:807, 1964.
14. Poinseti, I. V., and Friedman, B.: Evolution of metaphyseal fibrous defects, J. Bone Joint Surg. **31-A**:582, 1949.
15. Rabhan, W. N., and Rosai, J.: Desmoplastic fibroma. Report of 10 cases and review of the literature, J. Bone Joint Surg. **50-A**:487, 1968.
16. Schroeder, F.: Ein zentraler xanthomatöser Riesenzellentumor der Fibula Gleichzeitig ein Betirag zur Kenntnis der xanthomatösen Gewebsneubildungen, Arch. F. klin. Chir. **168**:118, 1931.
17. Sontag, L. W., and Pyle, S. I.: The appearance and nature of cyst-like areas in the distal femoral metaphyses of children, Am. J. Roentgenol. **46**:185, 1941.

Chapter 12

Giant-cell tumor of bone (osteoclastoma)

The subject of giant-cell tumor of bone is one that was in a state of confusion for a long time, not so much because genuine instances of it are difficult to recognize (quite the contrary), as because the diagnosis of giant-cell tumor was frequently applied indiscriminately to other bone lesions, mainly because they presented a scattering of multinuclear cells. It is true that noteworthy progress has been made since the rather chaotic situation prevailing some thirty years ago when no clear distinction was drawn between the brown tumors, so-called, of advanced hyperparathyroidism and the bona fide giant-cell tumors of surgical practice; when, collaterally, the neoplastic nature of giant-cell tumor of bone was open to question; when a wide variety of unrelated and generally less serious skeletal lesions were arbitrarily associated with giant-cell tumor in the guise of "variants"; and when, on the whole, no general appreciation of the seriousness of many giant-cell tumors of bone existed.

There are still a number of clinical problems, but these relate not so much to diagnosis as to the value of cytologic appraisal through grading, the choice of appropriate therapy especially for recurrent tumors, and prognosis generally.[32] In my opinion at least, no amount of enzymatic and ultramicroscopic analysis, interesting as this may be, is calculated to resolve these problems, and there is no easy substitute for continued painstaking clinical and pathologic correlation. A number of additional valuable surveys[12,16,34,38] in recent years have helped to provide some tentative guidelines, which will be discussed later, but much still remains to be done. The recent analysis of some 218 cases by Goldenberg, Campbell, and Bonfiglio[12] is an important step in the right direction.

Speaking as a pathologist, the more I see of giant-cell tumor material, the less I understand it in the sense that I become increasingly aware of subtle questions for which there are no ready answers. To indicate a number of such queries, why do certain lesions that are not neoplastic simulate giant-cell tumor histologically (Fig. 12-1, A), and what does one mean precisely by such terms as giant-cell reparative granuloma; why do some few giant-cell tumors develop in the shaft of a limb bone,[40,42] rather than at its epiphyseal end; why do occasional tumors otherwise resembling giant-cell tumor contain tracts of connective tissue in which cartilage or bone may be found, and how does one classify such tumors; why are the giant-cell tumors arising in Paget bone biologically different with respect to localization and relatively favorable behavior[12,15,39]; why do occasional giant-cell tumors that are not cytologically malignant nevertheless metastasize to the lungs,[12,26,37] and why are the pulmonary metastases of such tumors often limited or even indolent in their growth.[12]

In 1940, Jaffe, Portis, and I[24] attempted to define what should properly be

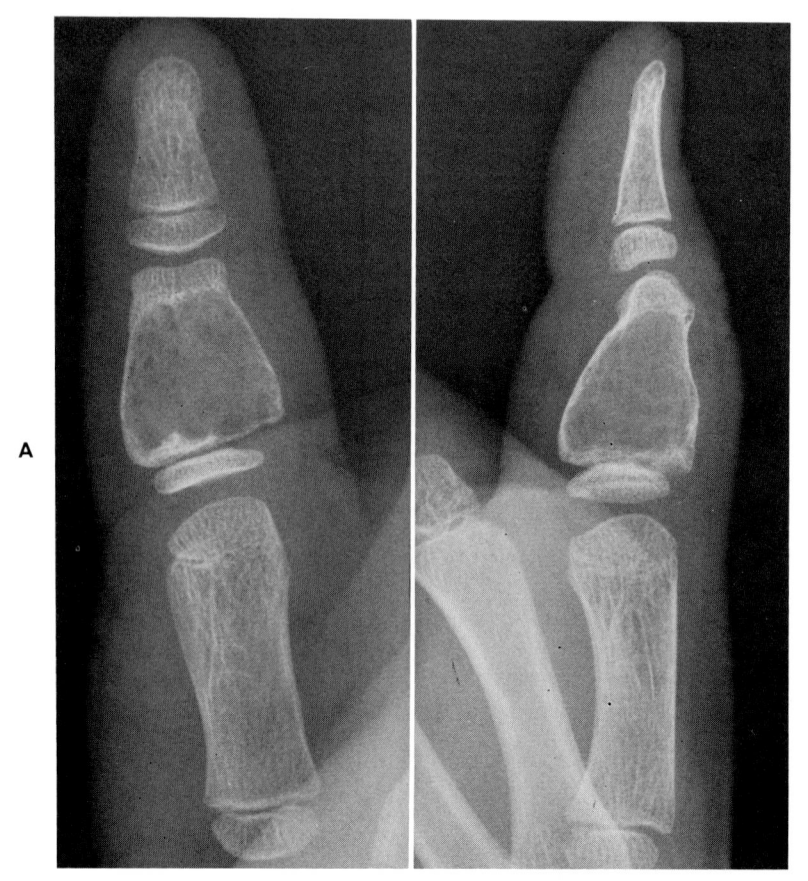

Fig. 12-1. **A**, Roentgenogram showing an expanded rarefied lesion in the metaphysis and shaft of a middle finger phalanx of a boy aged 9. It simulated giant-cell tumor cytologically and was considered to be that by the referring pathologist. Because of its location outside the epiphysis, as well as the age of the patient, I was inclined to interpret the lesion as an unusual giant-cell tumorlike reaction, possibly to hemorrhage in the bone. **B**, Roentgenogram of a giant-cell tumor developing in the upper end of a tibia. Treatment in this case consisted of thorough curettement. **C**, Roentgenogram of another representative giant-cell tumor situated in the lower end of a femur. Fracture occurred at the time of surgery, followed by some drainage and delayed healing. Six months later it was decided to use roentgen therapy, which proved efficacious (despite the popular admonition against combined treatment). At the follow-up five years later, the patient was well and doing heavy manual labor.

regarded as genuine giant-cell tumor, as a basis for more accurate diagnosis and rational therapy. In this survey, giant-cell tumor of bone was interpreted as a distinctive neoplasm arising apparently from the nonbone-forming, supporting connective tissue of the marrow, which could be readily identified on the basis of its cytologic details. Specifically, it was stated that the tumor was composed of a vascularized network of spindle-shaped or ovoid stromal cells, regularly and rather heavily interspersed with multinuclear cells (apparently syncytial stromal cells) as an integral part of the cytologic pattern. As an important corollary of this study, it became evident that genuine giant-cell tumor should be completely divorced from its spurious "variants" with which it had been and to some extent still is confused.

As a result of subsequent detailed investigation of the alleged variants of giant-cell tumor, there evolved a clearer concept of these lesions as distinct clinical and pathologic entities in their own right. Thus, the spindle-cell or healing or xanthic variant, so-called, was superseded by the rather common lesion now called nonosteogenic fibroma of bone (fibrous cortical defect). The "calcifying or chondromatous giant-cell tumor" described by Kolodny, Ewing, and Codman was

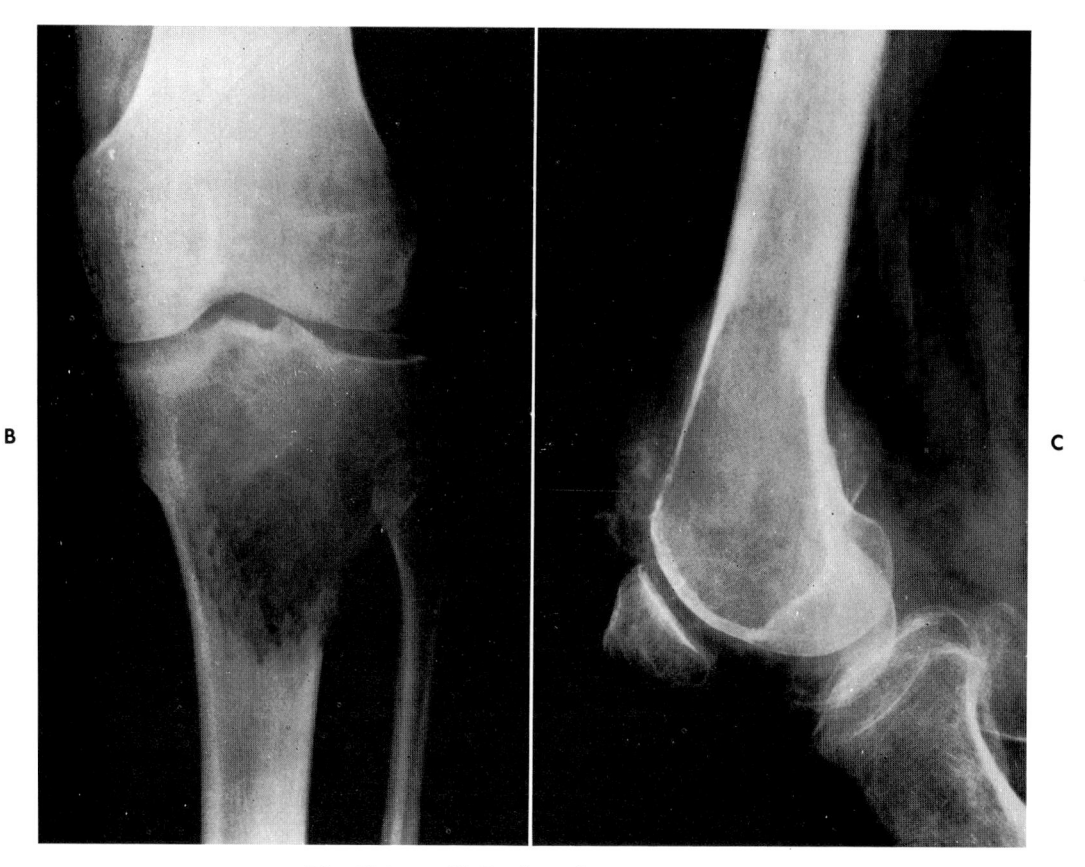

Fig. 12-1, cont'd. For legend see opposite page.

reinterpreted and designated benign chondroblastoma of bone[20,33] in the belief that it represents an independent benign tumor of cartilage-forming connective tissue derivation that is unrelated histogenetically to giant-cell tumor of bone. In another article dealing with solitary unicameral bone cyst,[23] it was pointed out that, while the lining tissue of a bone cyst might show appreciable giant-cell reaction in fields of blood extravasation, there was no sound basis for postulating any relationship between bone cyst and giant-cell tumor. Still another rather common pathologic entity frequently mistaken for giant-cell tumor and formerly referred to as "atypical, subperiosteal giant-cell tumor in unusual locations" has been clearly delineated under the designation of aneurysmal bone cyst.[28-30] As for the lesions that Ewing,[8] in his last classification of bone tumors (1939), referred to rather vaguely and paradoxically as "certain benign, circumscribed spindle-cell myxosarcomas with few or no giant cells, which run the usual course of giant-cell tumors," it is difficult to trace the reference but altogether conceivable that the lesions so designated represented instances of the distinctive neoplasm that Jaffe and I[21,31] have described under the head of chondromyxoid fibroma of bone. Continuing in the same vein, Jaffe[17] expressed the view that certain tumors in the jaw bones of adolescents, which simulate giant-cell tumor cytologically and yet have a uniformly favorable prognosis, may be merely a peculiar expression of reaction to hemorrhage; to convey this concept, he has proposed the name "giant-cell reparative granuloma." Bullock and Luck[1] have taken up this idea and have suggested that on occasion comparable changes may ensue in bones other than the maxilla and mandible ("giant-cell tumor-like lesions of bone"). In regard to so-called giant-cell tumors of synovial or tenosynovial tissues, there now seems to be general agreement that such lesions are wholly unrelated to giant-cell tumor of bone. They appear to represent peculiar hyperplastic granulomas rather than true neoplasms, and Jaffe, Sutro, and I[25] have described the condition as such under the head of pigmented villonodular synovitis, bursitis, and tenosynovitis. If one recognizes these distinctions, and they have more than academic import, then it becomes evident that genuine giant-cell tumor is not nearly as common or as miscellaneous a lesion as was formerly supposed. In fact, on a fair-sized orthopedic hospital service, one is not likely to encounter more than two or perhaps three cases a year, on the average.

Clinical features
Age and sex incidence

Genuine giant-cell tumor, in contrast to some of the alleged variant lesions, has its greatest incidence in adults between the ages of 20 and 40, although it is by no means uncommon in older patients. It may be noteworthy that I have observed a proved giant-cell tumor in the distal femur of a woman of 61 and another comparable tumor in a patient of 84. It is not so unusual as we once thought in patients under the age of 20, and the lower limit of the range of incidence should now be placed closer to 15 years of age. Of some 45 cases of giant-cell tumor seen in consultation in recent years, as many as 10 were in patients 14 to 20 years of age, although these were mainly well-developed girls whose bone age was relatively advanced. Incidence below the age of 14 has been noted, but this is comparatively rare.

In this same series, females outnumbered males almost two to one, but this observation may not be statistically significant.

Localization

The majority of giant-cell tumors develop in the lower end of the femur, the upper end of the tibia, and the lower end of the radius (in that order of fre-

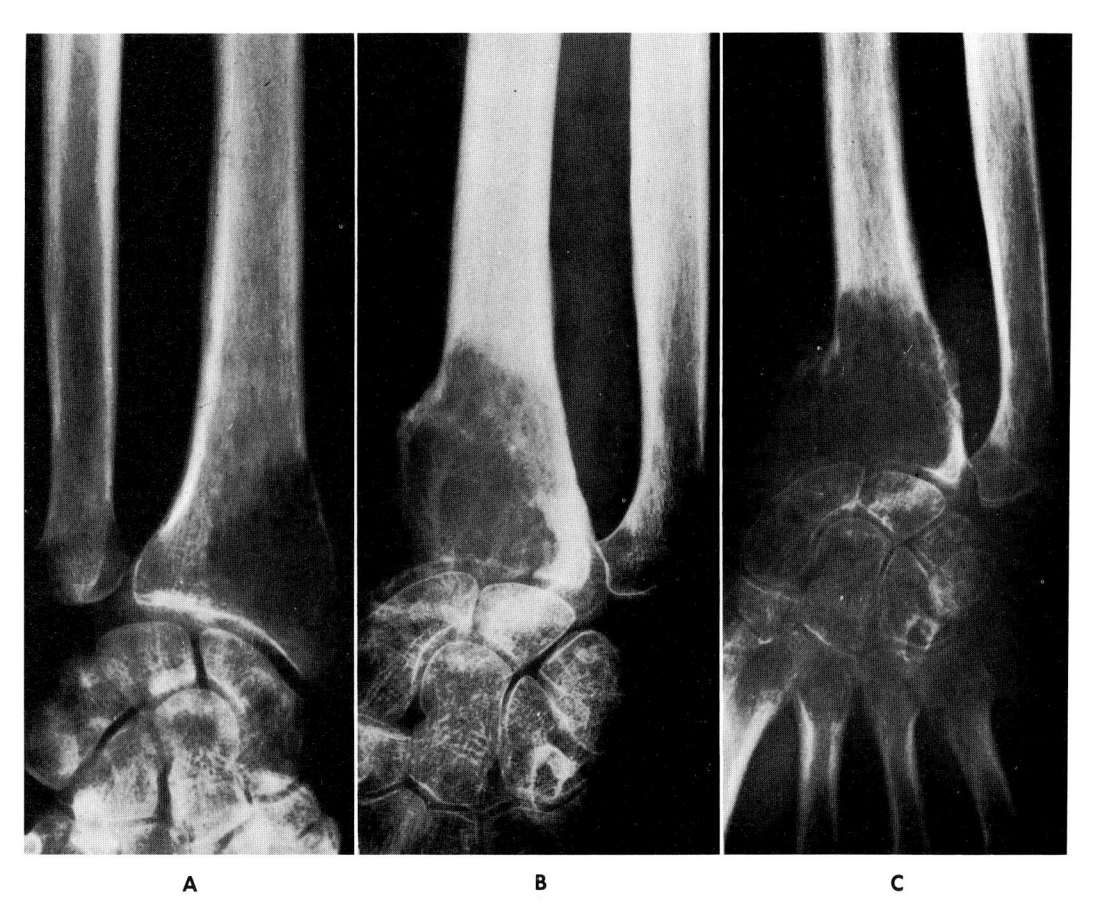

Fig. 12-2. A series of roentgenograms showing progression of a giant-cell tumor situated in the lower end of a radius, another frequent site of development. A, Initial film showing eccentric position of the tumor, its uniformly rarefied appearance, as well as thinning and slight expansion of the overlying cortex, which is still intact. B, The appearance of the tumor seven months later. C, Its appearance prior to surgical treatment (eleven months after the initial film). The tumor now occupies the entire width of the radius and has extended in places through the eroded cortex. The carpal bones show pronounced disuse atrophy. The importance of early diagnosis and prompt effective treatment cannot be too strongly emphasized.

quency). It has been reliably estimated by many observers that at least 60% of all giant-cell tumors develop in large limb bones. Occasional giant-cell tumors are observed also in jaw bones, in the upper end of the humerus, the upper femur, the upper end of the fibula, the lower end of the tibia, the patella, metacarpal heads, and even phalanges. In recent years I have observed material from one in the base of a metacarpal bone (of a thumb) and two in a finger phalanx; one of the latter metastasized to the lungs two years after amputation. In the same series, interestingly enough, there were as many as nine in the vertebral column, including the sarcum and coccyx (Fig. 12-3, A). Incidentally, these tumors in the spine and sacrum present a difficult problem in clinical management and may do poorly in spite of irradiation. I have observed relatively few instances in the innominate bone (Fig. 12-5) and have never encountered one in an ulna or a bone of the calvarium, although such tumors have been noted by others. Before

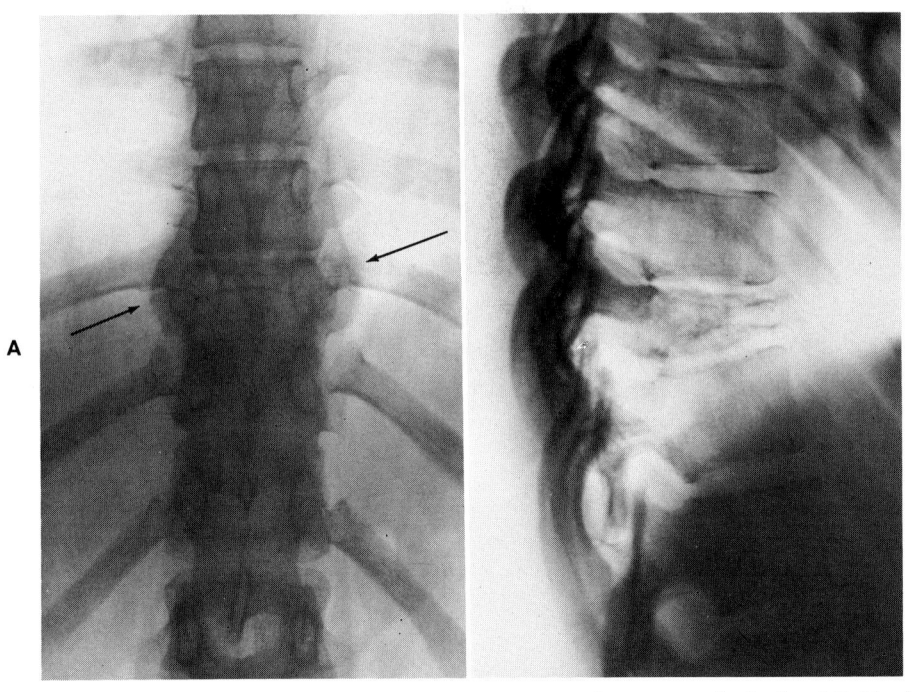

Fig. 12-3. **A,** Anteroposterior and lateral views of a giant-cell tumor in the body of D-10 of a young woman 20 years of age. The tumor subsequently induced paraplegia and continued to grow, producing a huge tumor occupying the right pleural cavity. Although it was not a sarcoma cytologically (Grade II), it behaved as such, and intensive irradiation (6,000 r) was ineffectual. (Courtesy Dr. T. Tajima, Niigata University Hospital, Japan.) **B,** Roentgenogram of a giant-cell tumor in the lower end of a femur of a 42-year-old man who had complained of pain, slight swelling, and limitation of motion for about four months. The tumor was thoroughly curetted (the wall of the cavity was not cauterized, nor were bone chips inserted). On microscopic examination this neoplasm was regarded as a giant-cell tumor, Grade II, that is, as one rather likely to prove aggressive and recur. **C,** Roentgenogram of the recurrent giant-cell tumor, nine months later. (See also Fig. 12-6.)

accepting ostensible giant-cell tumors in such unusual sites, one should require meticulous pathologic verification. Much of the old published statistical data, for example, the data cited in 1949 in an editorial in the *Journal of the American Medical Association*,[7] apparently culled from an article by Christensen,[5] give one a somewhat distorted impression of the incidence and localization of giant-cell tumor, particularly in the bones of the upper limb, the skull (exclusive of jaw bones), and the pelvis and vertebrae, where, as has been indicated elsewhere,[30] aneurysmal bone cyst is prone to develop. Cognizance should be taken, however, of the observation of Hutter and associates[15] that when *benign* giant-cell tumor complicates Paget's disease, as it may occasionally, it seems to show a predilection for the facial bones and the calvarium.

Mention should also be made of a few reported cases presenting more than one, or even several giant-cell tumors, in which the possibility of hyperparathyroidism was apparently excluded, but these are exceptional.

When a giant-cell tumor is situated in a long bone, it usually involves the end of the bone, and there are relatively few exceptions to this rule.[42] Willis[45] and

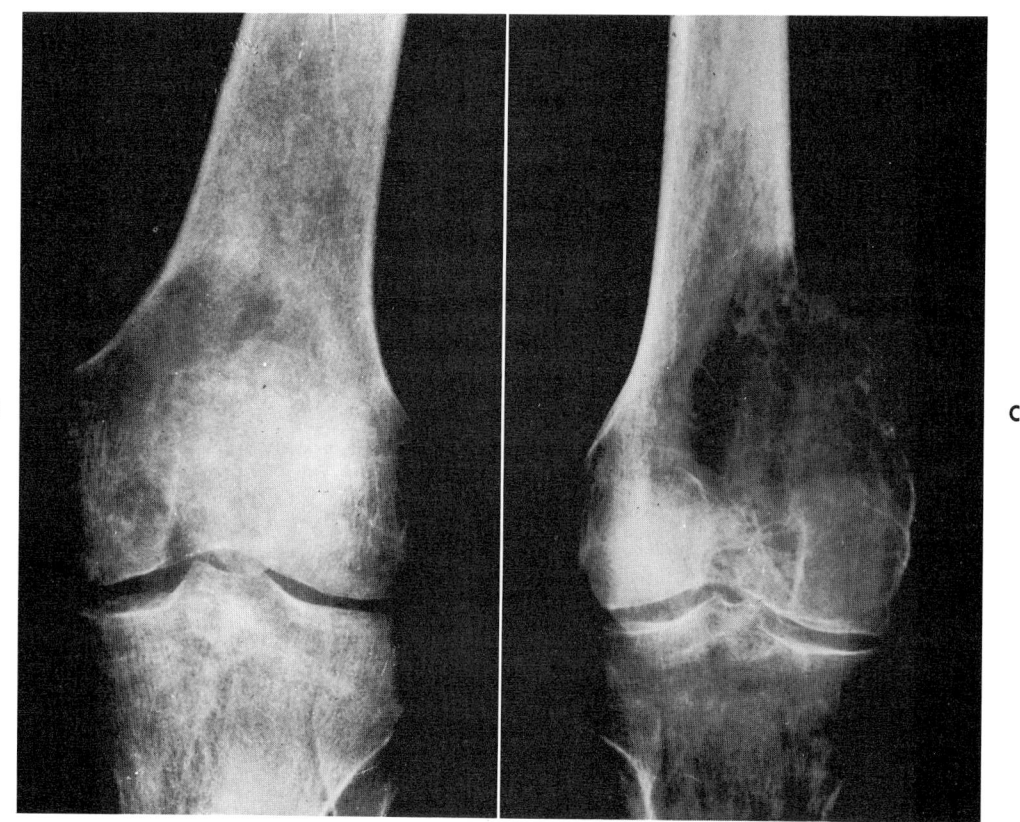

Fig. 12-3, cont'd. For legend see opposite page.

142   Bone tumors

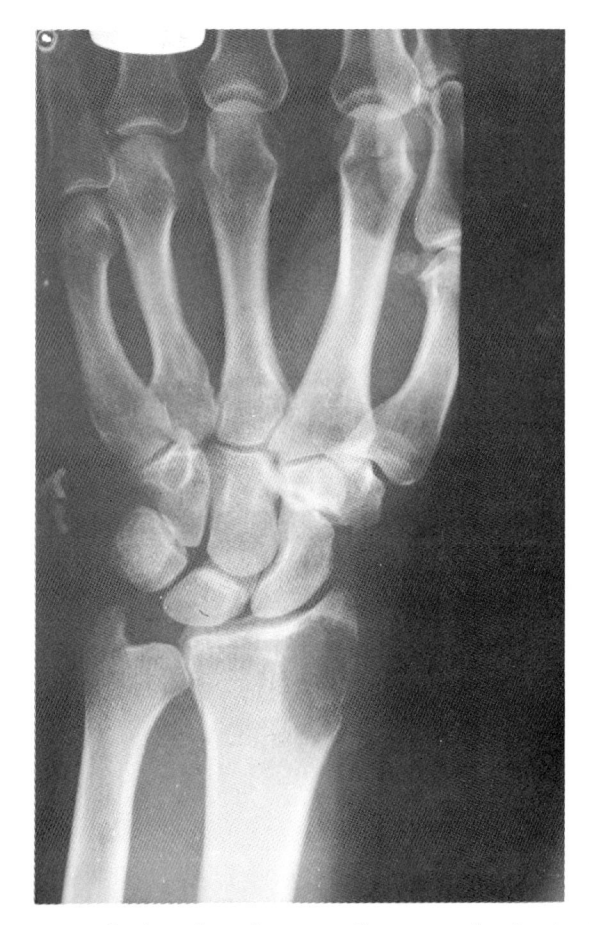

Fig. 12-4. Roentgenogram of relatively early giant-cell tumor in the distal radius of a 49-year-old man. Microscopic examination showed great cellularity, as well as muscle and vascular invasion, although there was no reason to anticipate this from the films.

some of his British colleagues were inclined to question the validity of this view, but it is my impression that they were not as critical as they might be in accepting as giant-cell tumors lesions that develop in the metaphyses of young patients. As noted, such lesions, in the great majority of cases, prove on close histologic scrutiny to be instances of other conditions, on the whole less serious than giant-cell tumor (nonosteogenic fibroma, bone cyst, chondromyxoid fibroma, etc.).

Clinical complaints

Like some other tumors of bone, giant-cell tumor develops insidiously and usually has attained appreciable size before its presence is recognized. Pain, slight swelling, limitation of motion of the neighboring joint, and tenderness on palpation are the complaints that are likely to direct attention to the lesion and point to the necessity for roentgenographic examination. Occasionally, infraction of the expanded and attenuated cortical bone overlying the tumor may provoke

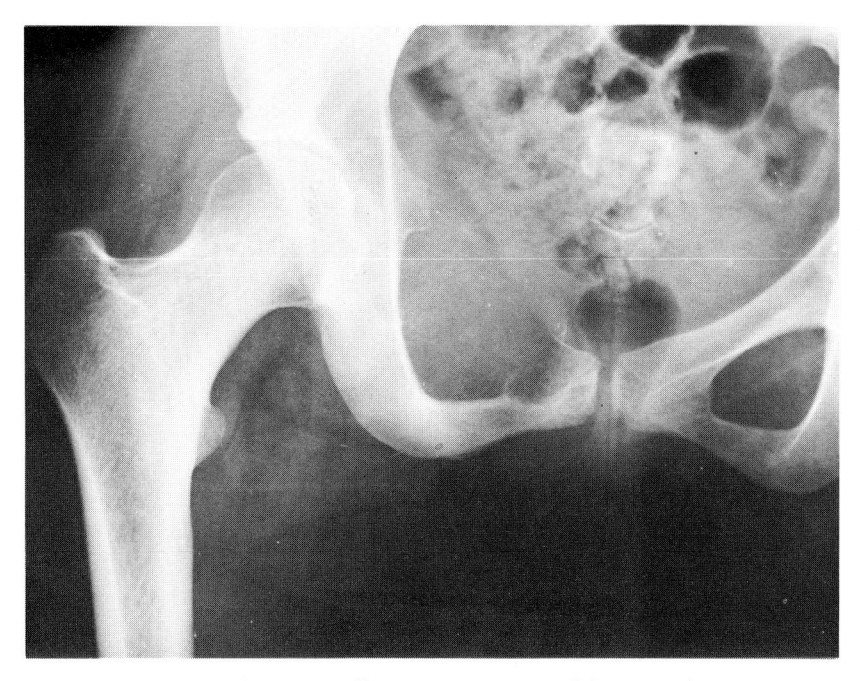

Fig. 12-5. Roentgenogram of a giant-cell tumor in an unusual location, the superior ramus of a pubis. The patient was an 18-year-old girl.

exacerbation of symptoms. Pronounced expansion and a sense of crackling of the cortical shell surrounding the lesion are manifestations of a far-advanced, neglected tumor that one does not see very often nowadays. In the case of some few giant-cell tumors, one may elicit a sense of pulsation reflecting great vascularity, but this finding, too, is rather unusual.

Roentgenographic appearance

It was formerly thought that giant-cell tumor of bone presented a characteristic multilocular cystlike appearance said to resemble an agglomeration of soap bubbles. As a matter of fact, this appearance is rather unusual for untreated giant-cell tumor and is much more likely to reflect the presence of lesions other than giant-cell tumor that grow more slowly, permitting the development of reactive grooves and spurs on the endosteal surface of the attenuated cortex overlying the lesion, e.g., hemangioma, nonosteogenic fibroma, fibrous dysplasia, and enchondroma.

Far more important diagnostically are the location of the area of rarefaction in the end of the bone and the thinning and expansion of the cortex, particularly on one side. Another significant point is the practical absence of periosteal new bone formation over the thinned and expanded cortex, not infrequently even where the latter has undergone pathologic fracture. However, in the last analysis, the latter features are not infallible either as roentgenographic guides to the correct diagnosis. Thus, a chondrosarcoma or a fibrosarcoma that has started in an epiphyseal end of a long bone may on occasion produce a roentgen picture closely simulating that of a giant-cell tumor. Further, we have seen cases in which a focus of myeloma did so. The recognition of a giant-cell tumor in sites other than a long tubular bone is likely to present a difficult problem in differentiation.

Altogether, then, despite the prevailing common opinion, there is *no* set of roentgenographic findings that can safely be regarded as typical of giant-cell tumor of bone. The necessity for reservation as to the diagnosis until a biopsy specimen has been studied is thus apparent. By the same token, the wisdom of the practice of instituting radiation therapy on the strength of a roentgen diagnosis alone, unverified by biopsy, is open to serious question.

Gross pathology

Inasmuch as most giant-cell tumors are treated, initially at least, by curettement or irradiation, it is only occasionally that one has the opportunity to study the gross specimen of an intact tumor, unmodified by treatment. Formerly, there was no lack of such material, since radical excision or amputation of the affected part was freely done as an initial (though late) procedure. Now, all that the pathologist usually sees of the lesion unmodified by treatment is a biopsy fragment or or a mass of curettings. If the lesion has been treated and has recurred, he may subsequently see the entire area involved, but by that time the gross appearance has been greatly modified by such influences as infection and hemorrhage, the effects of irradiation, and sometimes even spread of the tumor beyond the limits of the bone.

For information concerning the gross appearance of the natural lesion in its setting, the descriptions of Paget, Nélaton, and Gross are still of interest. However, these older descriptions usually relate to lesions that, through the very delay of treatment, had been allowed to attain large size, associated with the appearance of pronounced secondary changes. Consequently, these descriptions, with their emphasis on extensive necrosis, hemorrhage, cystic softening, and the formation of large blood spaces, though accurate as far as very advanced lesions are concerned, do not, on the whole, fit the gross picture of the giant-cell tumor as we see it, now that it is being treated more promptly. Schajowicz[38] in Buenos Aires has had as many as 35 segmental resections at his disposal, but our own surgeons are not yet ready to sacrifice a knee joint unless they have been forced by repeated recurrence or the threat of malignant change.

I have observed several intact resected tumors in the lower end of radius and two in the upper end of a fibula. The overall impression one obtains from such specimens is certainly that of a cellular neoplasm. As noted, the tumor involves the end of the bone and the adjacent metaphysis. In the affected area the bone outline is generally found expanded, at least in part. The distended area is usually delimited by a thin shell of bone, over which the periosteum is somewhat thickened. The thin bone shell represents newly formed bone that has replaced the resorbed original cortex. Whatever spongiosa there was originally where the tumor is present has also been resorbed. The tumor is often found to have extended to the articular cartilage in one place or another. If the bony end plate has been resorbed over any considerable area, the contour of this cartilage may no longer be entirely normal, but the cartilage is not likely to be found perforated by tumor tissue. Toward the shaft this tissue may extend into the major marrow cavity, though it is delimited from the marrow by a thin wall of fibrous tissue or bone.

As to the tumor itself, its gross appearance naturally depends to a considerable extent on the degree to which it has already undergone the secondary changes mentioned. Tumor tissue that has undergone but little modification is likely to be of a rather uniform dark red or red-brown color. Its more richly cellular areas, however, may be gray and of a fleshy consistency, though friable. In

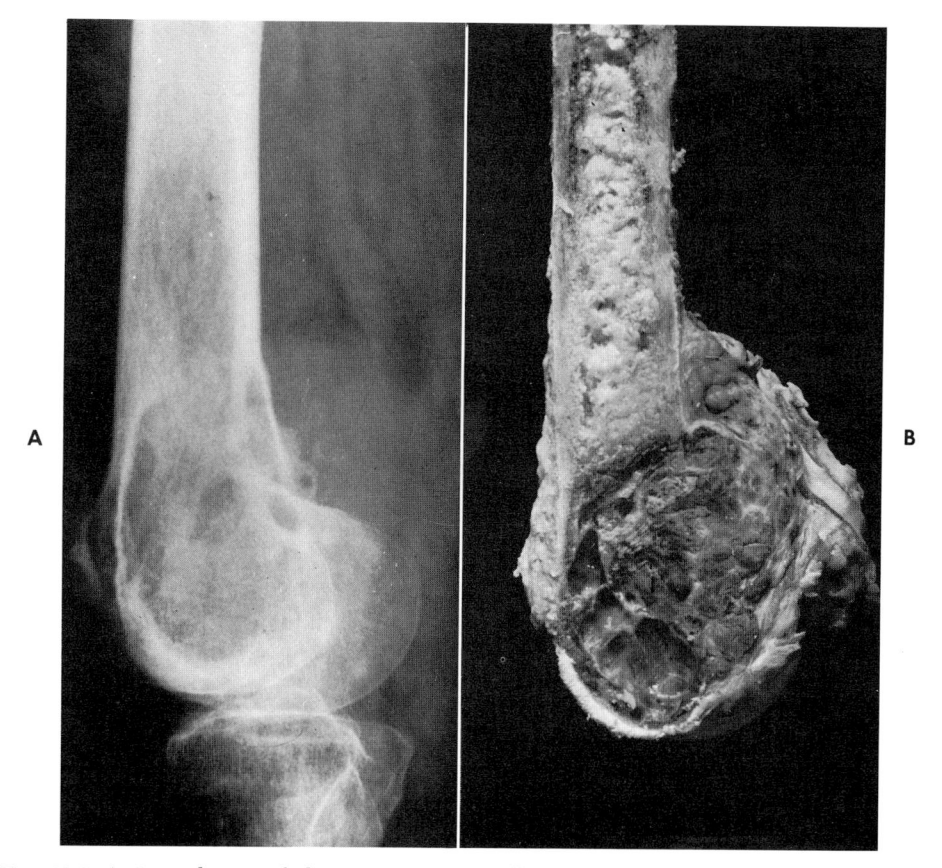

Fig. 12-6. **A**, Lateral view of the recurrent tumor illustrated in Fig. 12-3, **C**, showing extension into the contiguous soft parts posteriorly. Biopsy showed a cellular giant-cell tumor, Grade II, that, though invasive, was not yet frankly sarcomatous cytologically. **B**, Photograph of amputation specimen showing the aggressive recurrent giant-cell tumor illustrated in **A**. The cellular tumor tissue showed hemorrhage and cystic spaces in places (possibly reflecting previous curettement). Posteriorly, the neoplasm had broken through the cortex widely and invaded the adventitia of the popliteal vessels. At the follow-up after six years, this patient was ostensibly well and his chest was clear.

146   Bone tumors

fact, practically the entire lesion may present this appearance, especially if it is still small. In most specimens, however, the color and consistency are found altered by secondary changes that have occurred here and there throughout the tumor. The presence of hemorrhagic areas is evidenced in spots or blotches of bright red or blackish red and in greater softness of the tissue. Necrotic areas appear yellowish, amber, or orange and may even be found partly liquefied. It is after necrosis and hemorrhage have taken place in a giant-cell tumor that it may become partially cystic (Fig. 12-6, B).

The general description given represents the appearance of a lesion that has not yet broken its bounds. If it has been permitted to run its natural course after repeated pathologic fractures, the tumor may be found to have disrupted the periosteal cuff and perhaps grown along intermuscular septa. It may even have advanced into a neighboring bone, either by transgressing into the joint space or by extending through an interosseous membrane. These various consequences may also follow on recurrence after extensive curettement or on malignant transformation. They may appear whether or not there has been postoperative irradiation of the involved area and are especially likely to be found if an infection has

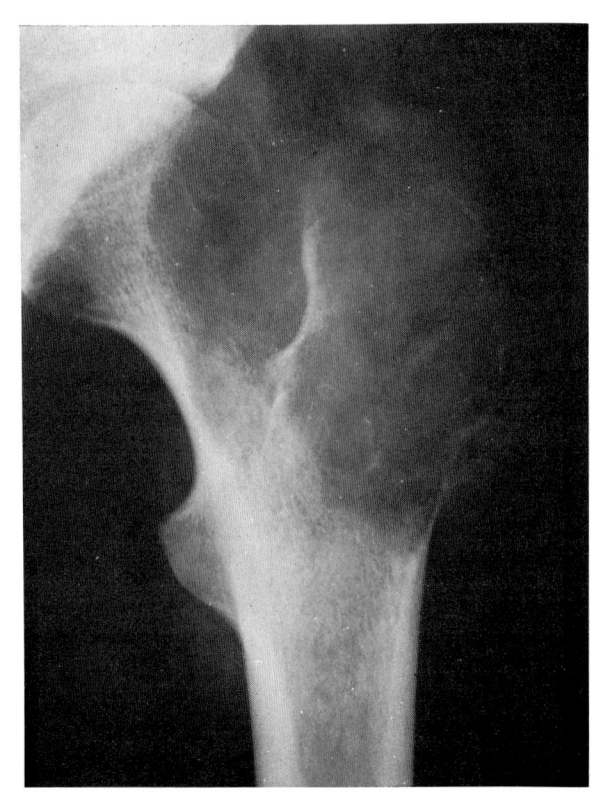

Fig. 12-7. Roentgenogram of an unusual giant-cell tumor that appears to have originated in the region of the greater trochanter.

Microscopic pathology

As indicated, a bona fide giant-cell tumor of bone is one of the easiest of neoplasms to identify. The cytologic details, however, may vary considerably from specimen to specimen and even within a given tumor. Nevertheless, a representative description can be made to serve for general histologic orientation and as the point of departure for discussion of the question of grading, which follows. The features characterizing the microscopic anatomy of any particular tumor stand out best in areas that have undergone few if any secondary changes. In these areas, as noted, the tumor consists of a moderately vascularized network of stromal cells and multinuclear giant cells meagerly interspersed with collagenous fibrils (Figs. 12-10 and 12-11).

The stromal cells are mononuclear and in general resemble young connective tissue cells. They are spindle shaped or ovoid in varying proportions. Correspondingly, the nucleus, which occupies much of the cell body, is longish or

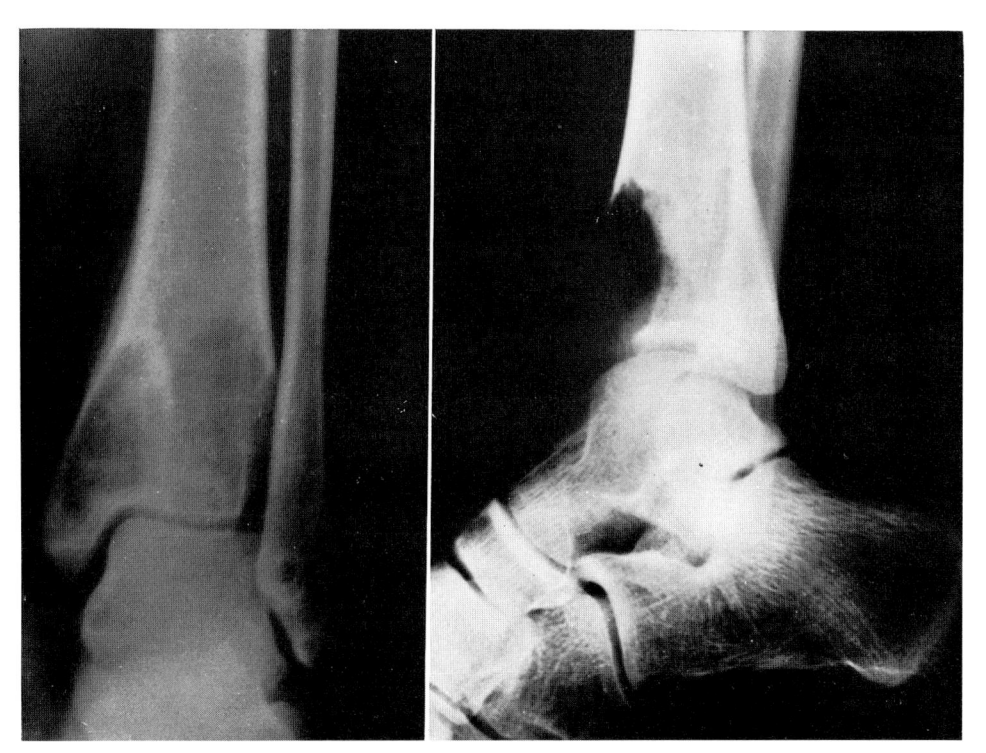

Fig. 12-8. Anteroposterior and lateral views of a giant-cell tumor in the distal tibia that was unusual with respect to location and the youthfulness of the patient (16 years of age). The clinical behavior of the tumor was aggressive, and this was reflected in its cytology (Grade II).

148   Bone tumors

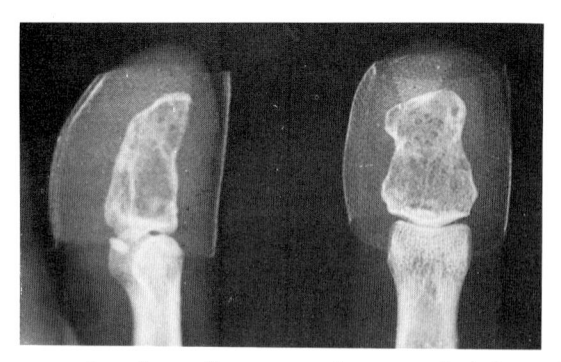

Fig. 12-9. Roentgenogram of a giant-cell tumor in the terminal phalanx of a thumb, a rare location for it. This tumor recurred wtihin a year after curettement. The surgeon elected to do a second curettement because he was loath to sacrifice the thumb, but is aware of the necessity for ablation in the event that the tumor recurs again.

roundish. It contains a moderate amount of chromatin and a more or less central nucleolus. The outlines of the individual stromal cells cannot always be traced completely, but it can almost regularly be seen that the cells have cytoplasmic processes. Occasional stromal cells may present evidence of mitotic division. The stromal cells of the tumor seem most plausibly explainable as arising through proliferation of the nonosteogenic supporting connective tissue of the marrow.

The multinuclear giant cells are found irregularly distributed between the stromal cells. In a given tumor they may be numerous or sparse, and their number may vary from part to part. They are generally from 30 to 60 microns in diameter, though sometimes they are 100 microns or even more. In a general way, the number of their nuclei increases with the diameter, and some of the cells may have many dozens. The nuclei tend to be agglomerated toward the middle of the cell. They are round or oval, and each has a nucleolus. On the whole, the nuclei of the giant cells are not much different from those of the ovoid stromal cells, and they may even be indistinguishable from them. The cytoplasm of the giant cells is usually considerable in amount and frequently granular and vacuolated. These cells, too, apparently have cytoplasmic processes, and some writers have shown that these processes anastomose with those of the stromal cells. The histologic facts favor the idea that the giant cells and the stromal cells have a common ancestry, if indeed the giant cells are not derived from the stromal cells by agglomeration or fusion. In any case, the giant cells should not be given the primal position in the genesis of the growth that has been assigned to them by many writers. This view finds support in recent electron microscopic studies of the ultrastructure and histogenesis of giant-cell tumor of bone.[14] Japanese investigators, particularly, have been interested in this question, and a sizable literature has accumulated. Doubtless, much of the confusion that exists in regard to the diagnosis and classification of the giant-cell tumor of bone and its supposed variants has resulted from undue emphasis on the giant cells. The enzyme studies carried out by Schajowicz[38] and others showed apparently that the giant cells

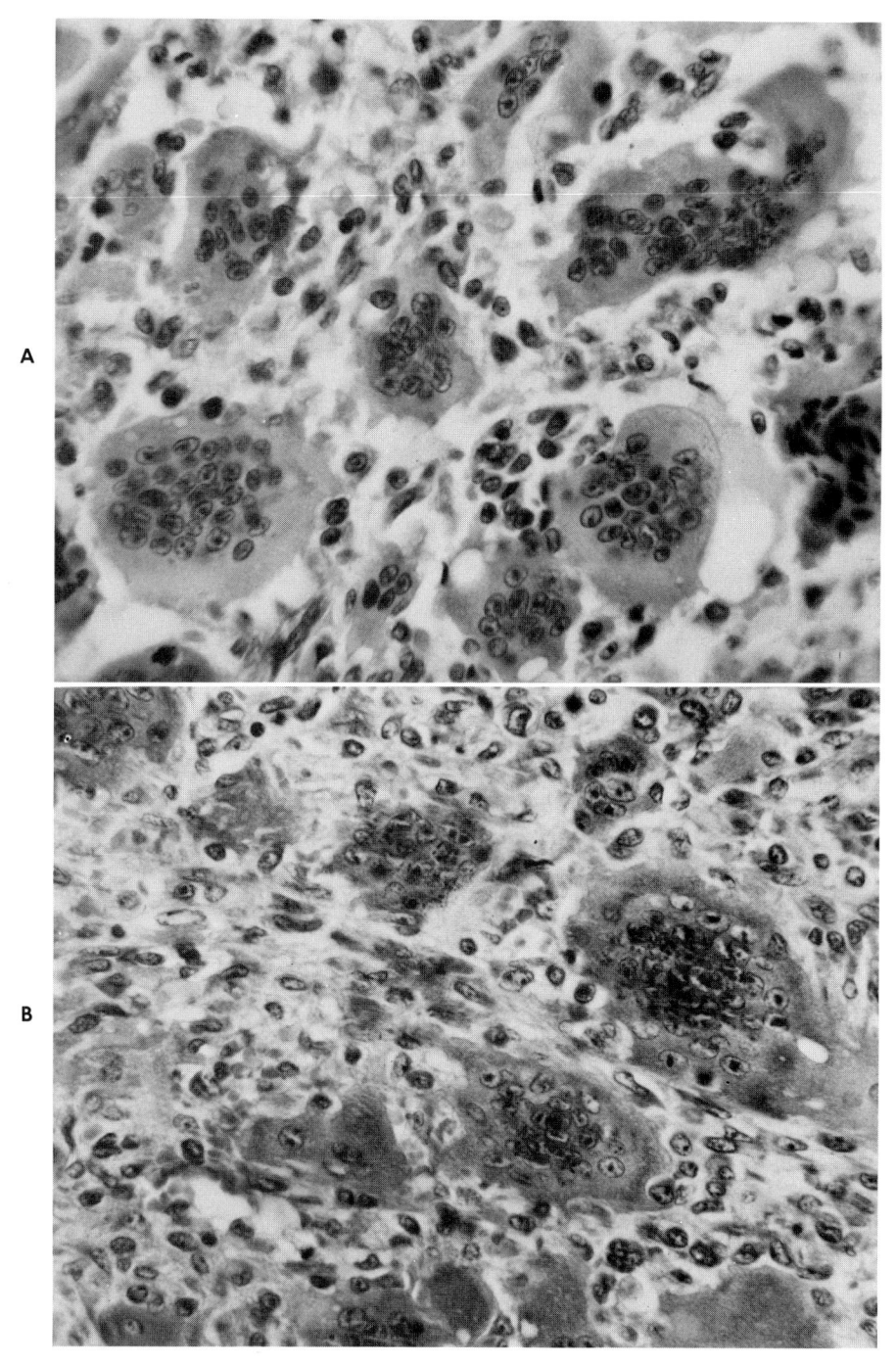

Fig. 12-10. A, Photomicrograph of a representative giant-cell tumor, Grade I, which is most likely to respond satisfactorily to treatment. (×420.) B, A more cellular giant-cell tumor of Grade II. This neoplasm developed in the head of a fibula (see Fig. 12-15) and recurred locally following resection. (×420.)

(but not the stromal cells) give reactions similar to those of osteoclasts, especially with reference to acid phosphatase activity and subcellular detail. Pathologically, however, the multinuclear cells of the giant-cell tumor, while resembling, also show definite differences from indubitable osteoclasts, such as one observes in connection with resorptive and reconstructive processes in a bone site.

The collagenous intercellular material in the giant-cell tumor is most abundant where the stromal cells are very spindly and loosely arranged. Where they are ovoid and closely packed, the collagenous material is sparse. In relatively unmodified tumor tissue, the blood vessels can be seen as small thin-walled channels lined by flattened cells. Some giant cells are usually seen in intimate relation with the vessel walls. Where there has been hemorrhage into the tumor, one finds large vascular sinuses, the walls of which are generally composed of stromal and giant cells. About such areas delicate trabeculae of osteoid may have been laid down. Trabeculae of osteoid and new bone are also observed, of course, within and around fields of organizing necrosis. In the vicinity of these regions some free and intracellular blood pigment is usually to be seen. Although it is generally reported that the giant-cell tumor of bone contains at least some lipoid-bearing phagocytes (foam cells), it is only in an occasional instance that they are significantly prominent.

Grading of giant-cell tumors

If one adheres to a strict definition of what should be regarded as giant-cell tumor and strips away all of the alleged variants, so-called, what is left constitutes a formidable neoplasm. The more I see of giant-cell tumors of bone, the more wholesome is my respect for them. Most of them in recent years have been aggressive or potentially aggressive tumors, although one must make allowance for the fact that the tumors that respond well to conservative treatment are not likely to be submitted for consultation. An appreciable number have manifested local recurrence after surgical extirpation, either in the surgical wound or in the operative field after resection. As notable cases among them, I may cite the appearance of a circumscribed tumor transplant (1) in the surgical wound some months after curettement of a giant-cell tumor in the upper tibia, (2) in proximity to an extensor-tendon sheath after curettement of a tumor in the head of a metacarpal, (3) as local recurrence in the soft parts after resection of the head of the fibula, and (4) in proximity to a bone graft inserted after resection of the lower end of the radius. In these circumstances, it is difficult and startling to realize that at one time there were those who maintained stoutly that giant-cell tumor did not represent a genuine neoplasm but a tissue reaction to trauma, hemorrhage, or chronic irritation. Altogether, it has become increasingly evident that, while giant-cell tumors are not necessarily "sarcomas," neither are they all "benign" as Bloodgood maintained. With respect to potential seriousness, they may run the whole gamut from one extreme to the other. There appears to be substantial agreement, among pathologists at least, that, while many giant-cell tumors are successfully treated by thorough curettement or irradiation, many are undoubtedly aggressive and prone to recur, and occasional ones behave like frank sarcomas, either when initially observed or, more often, after one or more local recurrences.[32] It is my impression as a working hypothesis that in a sizable group of proved giant-cell tumors at least one-half are likely to have a favorable outcome if properly treated by whatever method, at least one-third or more are likely to prove more aggressive and recur after treatment (and a considerable proportion of these may eventually come to amputation), while the remaining 10% to 15% more or less will be frankly malignant and prone to metastasize to the lungs. An occasional giant-cell tumor will be found to be malignant on initial tissue examination, but more often one has to reckon with malignant change incidental to one or more local recurrences. Empirical corroboration of this impression comes from the study by Thomson and Turner-Warwick[41] (among others) of some 34 giant-cell tumors, 18 of which recurred after local surgical or x-ray treatment, and 8 of these in turn eventually proved fatal from metastasis (2 of the sarcomas were associated with Paget's disease). The figures of Hutter and associates[15] at Memorial Hospital are somewhat more ominous; they found a recurrence rate of 62% and a malignancy rate as high as 30%. It is possible, however, that a greater number of more serious cases are referred to a cancer hospital for treatment. The experience at Massachusetts General Hospital, as analyzed recently by Mnaymneh and colleagues,[34] and that of Gilmer and associates at the Campbell Clinic in Memphis are more in line with our own. In Jaffe's material, too, the recurrence rate (after treatment by curettage) was estimated at 55% and the incidence of metastasis at about 15%. In the comparatively large series of 218 cases recently analyzed by Goldenberg, Campbell, and Bonfiglio,[12] the incidence of recurrence requiring secondary procedures was no more than 35%, and the fatality rate attributable to the tumor, less than 10%.

Along these lines, as a guide to therapy and with a view to forecasting prognosis within certain limits, we suggested as early as 1940 that giant-cell tumors be subdivided into three grades, designated numerically as I, II, and III, and showing, respectively, insignificant, moderate, and pronounced atypism of their stromal cells. The tumors of Grade III in this scheme are frankly malignant. The validity of this attempt at cytologic appraisal has become a controversial issue, which is really not too surprising. Willis[45] and Russell have contended that giant-cell tumors, which prove to be aggressive or eventually frankly malignant, may not be initially distinguishable from the benign ones. Similarly, Williams, Dahlin, and Ghormley[43] have not found the grading of giant-cell tumors helpful. Schajowicz[38] also remarked that grading of this neoplasm (at least of Grades I and II) has little value in his hands, although he went on to say that, "It is perhaps more common for the histologically aggressive tumor to grow more rapidly, to be more destructive, and to be more apt to recur." This is all we ever claimed actually.

It is quite true that a giant-cell tumor does not have to be frankly sarcomatous to be aggressive or capable of metastasizing, but neither does it look harmless cytologically. The point may be stressed here that some pathologists are prone

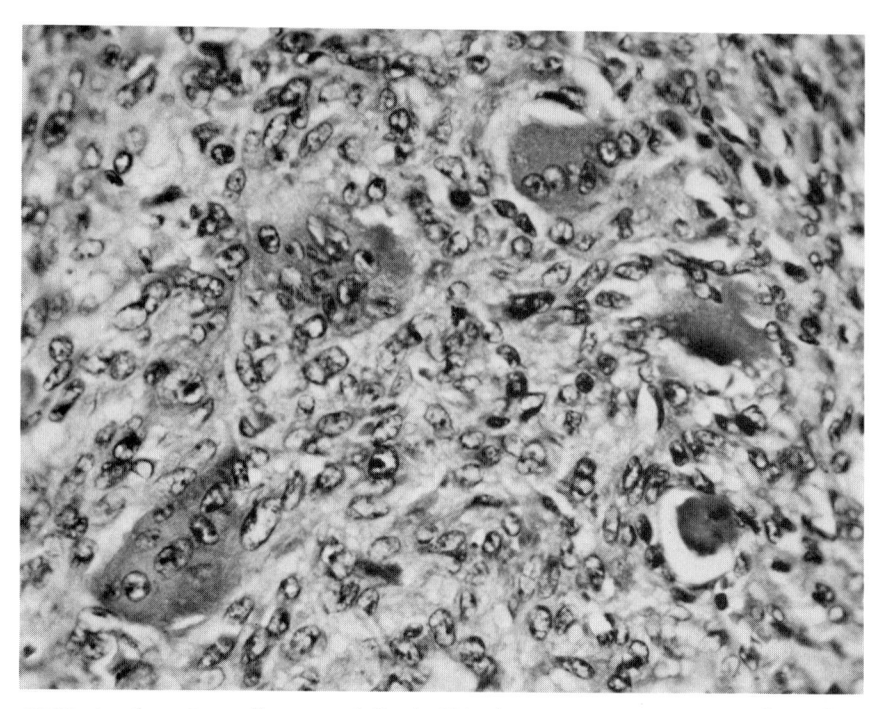

Fig. 12-11. Another giant-cell tumor of Grade II+ showing more ominous cytology than the neoplasms illustrated in Fig. 12-10, reflected in the swollen, pale appearance of its stromal-cell nuclei. The giant cells are sparse and contain relatively few nuclei that closely resemble those of the individual stromal cells. This neoplasm developed in the upper end of a tibia (see Fig. 12-16), and nine months after curettement, a small tumor node recurred in the surgical scar. (×420.)

to underrate the potential seriousness of giant-cell tumors. In this connection, I see not a few tumors in consultation, classed as Grade I by the examining pathologist, that are impressively cellular and show enough stromal cell abnormalities for me to class them as Grade II or II+. Generally speaking, I find rather consistently that the aggressive and malignant tumors are more cellular and show distinctly greater atypism of their stromal cells than the innocuous ones that respond well to conservative treatment (Figs. 12-11 to 12-13). I can only reiterate that, while no method of appraising potential aggressiveness from cytologic criteria is infallible, in my experience, the grading of giant-cell tumors has proved to be of practical value. Specifically, the giant-cell tumors that pursued an aggressive clinical course were, for the most part, tumors of Grade II or Grade II+ rather than Grade I initially, while those that eventually became frankly malignant (Grade III) likewise revealed a portent of this ominous tendency in previous tissue specimens. It should be stressed again that the examining pathologist must carefully scrutinize all the available tissue or a generous sample, if this is abundant, and pay close attention to detail, as will be indicated further on.

The usefulness of appraising giant-cell tumors as indicated has been sup-

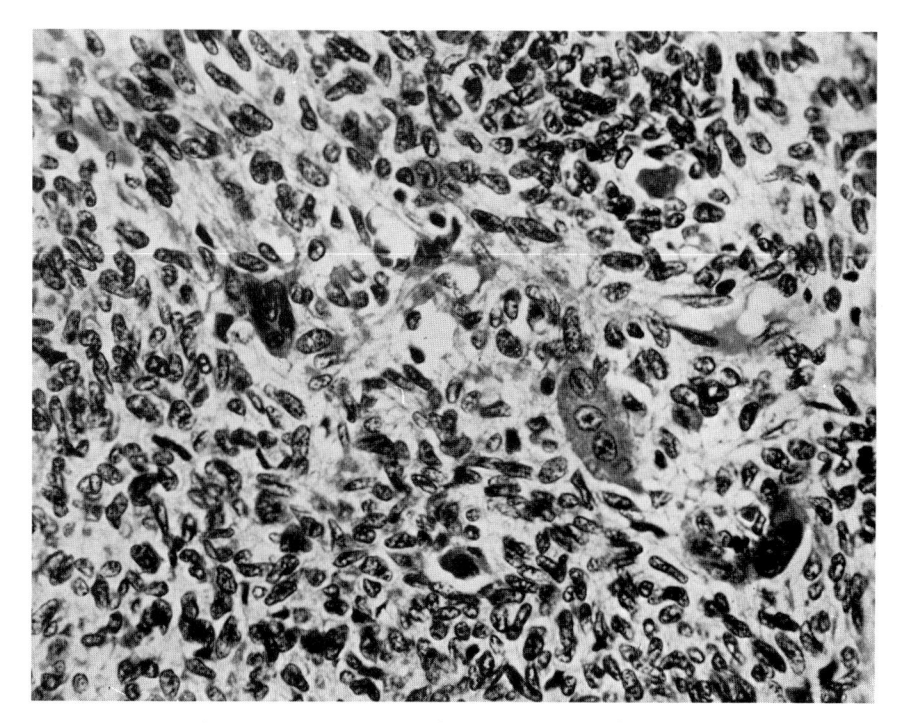

Fig. 12-12. A field of an aggressive giant-cell tumor (in the distal radius, invading the soft tissues) selected to show cellular tracts of plump spindle cells, reminiscent of early fibrosarcoma. Elsewhere, this tumor showed the classical cytology of a giant-cell tumor, Grade II+ (on a 1-to-3 scale). (×420.)

ported by the findings of Murphy and Ackerman,[35] who have subjected their material to close scrutiny. Similarly, the recent Massachusetts General Hospital survey[34] indicated a recurrence rate for Grade I tumors of 48% and for Grade II tumors, of 70%, as well as a significantly higher incidence of malignant change in the Grade II tumors. Gilmer and associates in Memphis also graded their giant-cell tumors numerically to indicate their aggressiveness or degree of malignancy, stating, "There is nothing esoteric about this system. It follows the conventional pattern of evaluating neoplasms on the basis of histologic features—specifically, cytologic atypicalities, extent of differentiation and mitotic activity. It is useful if the limitations are recognized: any may recur, and (occasionally) histologically benign tumors may behave in a malignant fashion."*

Continuing in the same vein, Hutter and associates[16] at Memorial Hospital qualified their giant-cell tumors histologically as being benign, borderline, or malignant, adding that "these designations are meaningful, prognostic, and subject to no greater fallibility than are any other microscopic diagnoses." I hold no

---

*From Gilmer, W. S., Jr., Higley, G. B., Jr., and Kilgore, W. E.: Atlas of bone tumors including tumorlike lesions, St. Louis, 1963, The C. V. Mosby Co.

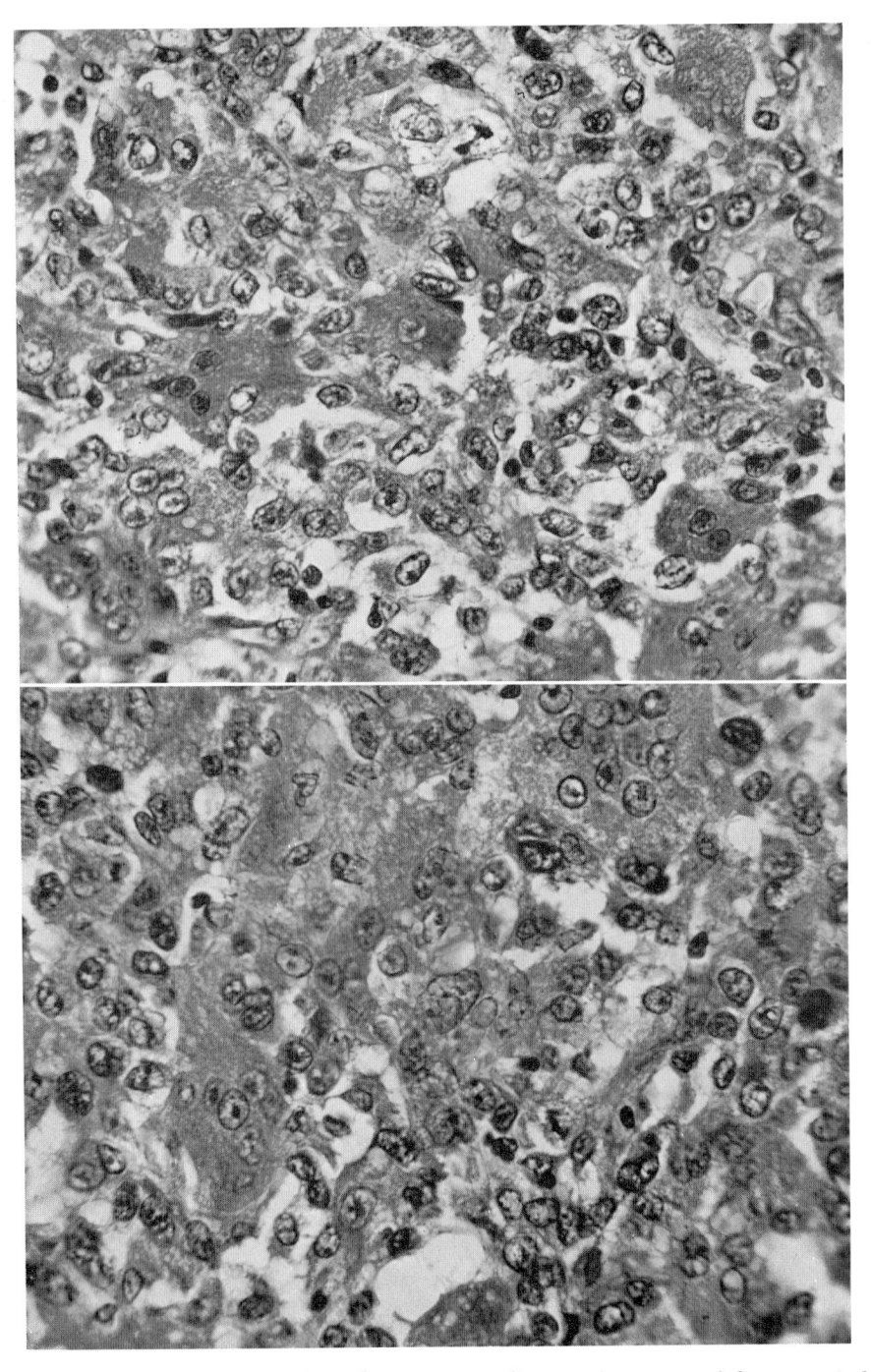

Fig. 12-13. Representative fields of a malignant giant-cell tumor (in a wing of the sacrum) that metastasized widely in spite of deep roentgen therapy. Although the architecture of giant-cell tumor is maintained, the stromal cells are compact and distinctly swollen and show significant hyperchromatism as well as an inordinate number of mitotic figures. Compare with Fig. 12-10, which was taken at the same magnification. (×420.) (Courtesy Professor Dorothy S. Russell, The London Hospital.)

brief particularly for numerical grading, and this appears to be a useful system of grading for any one who prefers it.

One argument that is sometimes used against the view that grading is of value relates to the phenomenon of the "benign" giant-cell tumor with pulmonary metastasis.[12,26,37] On the face of it, this appears to be a logical absurdity, and actually we seem to be dealing here with very occasional, biologically malignant giant-cell tumors that are not cytologically malignant. This is a disconcerting discrepancy that one observes in a good many other tumors—in itself, it seems to me, it does not negate the value of cytologic grading for most giant-cell tumors. For some peculiar reason, these metastasizing giant-cell tumors are prone to arise in the distal radius or in a hand bone, as well as in more common sites. With reference to the clinical course of such metastases, it is important to recognize, as has been noted by many observers, that solitary pulmonary metastases can often be cured by lobectomy and that even multiple tumor nodes in the lung fields may sometimes regress or disappear following irradiation or chemotherapy (Cytoxan), or even spontaneously. The long-term follow-ups in such cases, with survival ranging up to 20 years, are quite remarkable.

The tumors falling into the first group (Grade I), which seem to make up about half of any representative series of giant-cell tumors of bone, are those in which the cytologic features indicate the lowest degree of aggressiveness and, hence, a relatively favorable prognosis. The tumors delegated to the other two groups show successively more ominous cytologic features, those of Grade III being definitely malignant. In connection with grading, the details of the stromal cells should be closely scrutinized under high magnification, and one should judge the tumor by its most ominous-looking areas rather than by areas selected at random. It follows from this that, for a relatively safe judgment, more material is usually needed than is obtained in a needle or a punch biopsy specimen. In fact, when a mass of curettings is available, one should submit a considerable portion of it to cytologic study, using particularly the areas least modified by spontaneous secondary changes. Previous irradiation of the growth, too, is likely to be a confusing factor in the grading, since it may have induced fibrosis, hyalinization, and calcification as well as distortion and atypism of the stromal cells. Even though it has not been irradiated, a recurrent tumor that has become infected may also be somewhat difficult to grade, as it tends, on the whole, to look somewhat more ominous than it really it. Nevertheless, allowing for these modifying factors, one can usually still decide with reasonable plausibility on the grade to which a given tumor ought to be assigned.

To belong to Grade I, the lesion must show no appreciable atypism of its stromal cells. Though these cells are abundant, they are not densely compacted in a tumor of this grade. In the majority of cases they are predominantly spindle shaped, while in the remainder they are predominantly polygonal or ovoid. Whatever their shape (which does not seem to have any special significance), they are more or less uniform in size. Important also is the fact that one finds in a Grade I giant-cell tumor at most only an occasional stromal cell that has a hyperchromatic or abnormally large nucleus or perhaps two nuclei. A few of the stromal cells, to be sure, may exhibit nuclei in the process of mitotic division, but in any case the mitotic figures are not abnormal. The giant cells are numerous in most fields at least. Their nuclei vary in number, but each cell tends to have a good many of them, and they bear a close resemblance to the nuclei of the stromal cells (Fig. 12-10, A).

In regard to the prognosis for the tumors of Grade I, it is to be noted that recurrence can be expected in some instances, though not in the majority. Furthermore, in its recurrent state, particularly if it has recurred more than once, a Grade I tumor may finally come to exhibit characteristics that really put it in the next grade.

The tumors of Grade II constitute a somewhat varied group, ranging from those in which the stromal cells show only slight (though definite) atypism to those in which they are strikingly atypical though not yet sufficiently so to justify placing them in the category of the frankly malignant tumors. The stromal cells are abundant and closely compacted and may even show plainly an irregular whorled arrangement. In some cases they tend, on the whole, to be spindle shaped, though in some areas they may be plumper or ovoid, and an occasional cell may even appear anaplastic. At the other extreme there are cases in which the stromal cells are predominantly plump or ovoid, while their nuclei are large and swollen in proportion to the cell as a whole, often exhibiting atypism. Specifically, in the latter connection the nuclei may vary considerably in size, many of them may be hyperchromatic, and some of them may be multiple, two or three being present in a given cell. In these more ominous cases, in which the lesion may already be considered as potentially malignant, mitotic figures are rather frequently encountered, and some of the latter may appear abnormal (Figs. 12-10, B and 12-11). The giant cells are likely to be abundant in some or in many areas, though they may be sparse in others. Their nuclei may reveal atypism similar in a general way to that of the stromal cell nuclei and running more or less parallel to it. The compacted stroma may be found poorer in vascular channels than it is in the tumors of Grade I.

As to prognosis, it is to be noted that the tumors of Grade II tend strongly toward recurrence, and that some of them eventually undergo malignant transformation, although usually only after an interval of several years.

The tumors of Grade III constitute the small group of giant-cell tumors of bone that are frankly and obviously malignant, possessing a sarcomatous type of stroma and a capacity for metastasis. Their stromal cells are abundant and closely compacted and tend to present an irregular whorled arrangement. Their nuclei exhibit atypism almost uniformly and are likely to be unusually large and irregular. The giant cells tend to be dwarfed and to contain few nuclei, and the latter too, are likely to show atypism (Fig. 12-13).

Occasionally, one encounters a giant-cell tumor that is already frankly sarcomatous when tissue is first taken from it for study. More often, however, a malignant giant-cell tumor is one that originally belonged to Grade I or II but

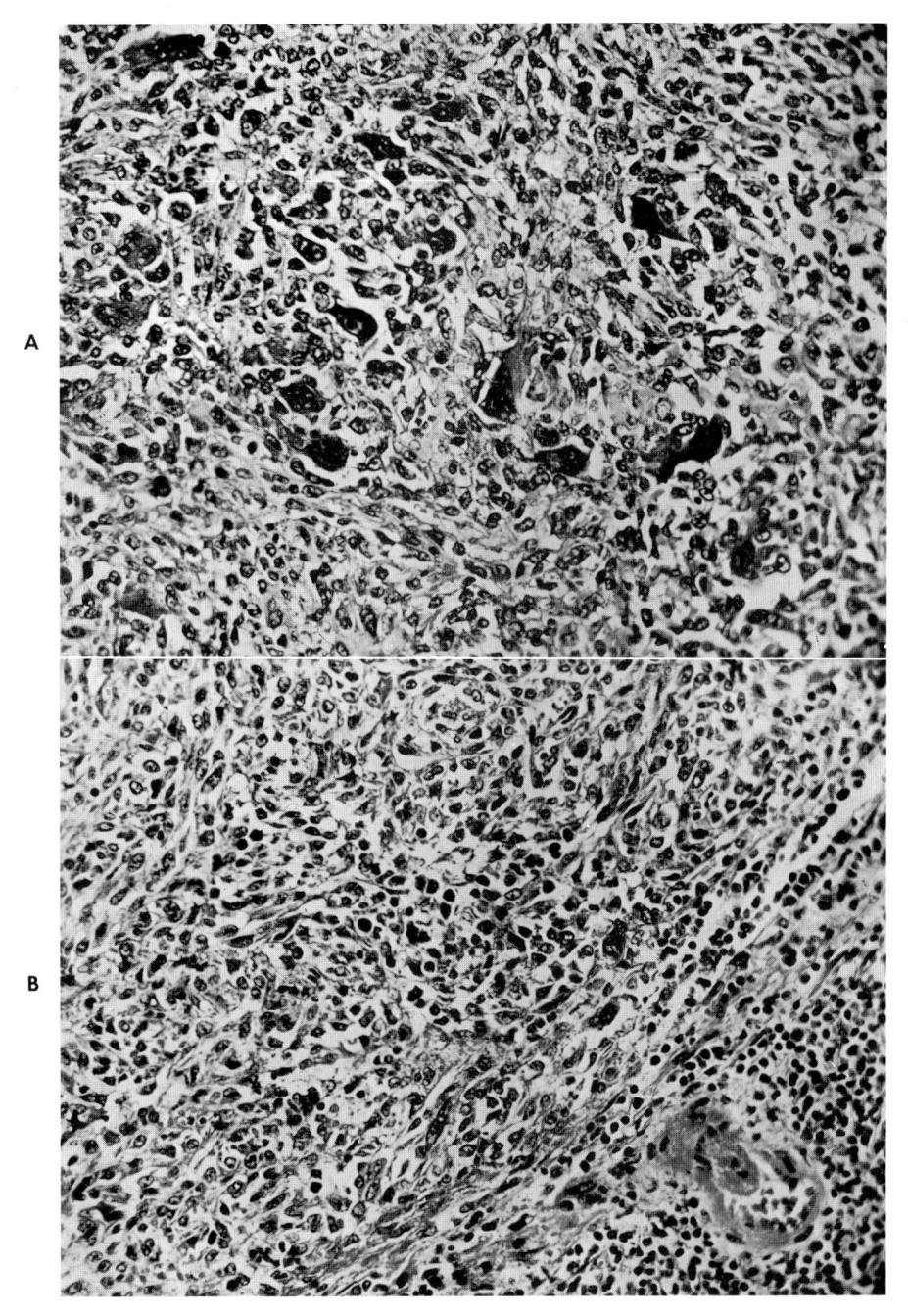

Fig. 12-14. **A,** Representative field of a pulmonary metastasis of the malignant giant-cell tumor illustrated in Fig. 12-13, showing a few dwarfed giant cells within a cellular spindle-cell stroma. (×20.) **B,** From a metastatic node in the spleen of the same case. From this pattern alone, one would hardly suspect that the primary neoplasm was a giant-cell tumor. (×220.)

that has become more and more aggressive in the course of years. Often the increased aggressiveness has followed on repeated curettage, infection, or irradiation, although it is possible that in these cases the malignant tendency of the growth was inherent in it from the beginning. Mention may be made here of a remarkable tumor interpreted as a malignant giant-cell tumor[3] that developed around a Moore (metallic) prosthesis some three years after its insertion, in an adult patient who had "phosphate diabetes" and osteomalacia. The tumors of Grade III metastasize sooner or later, particularly to the lungs. In their metastases, at least as I have observed, they do not show up as osteogenic sarcoma, if there has been no prior irradiation. In some instances, one can recognize the metastases as those of giant-cell tumor, although the giant cells may be scant and dwarfed; in others, they may look like undifferentiated fibrosarcoma (Fig. 12-14).

Problems in therapy

As indicated, biopsy should be resorted to before instituting treatment, irrespective of the method of treatment employed. If one is inclined to favor surgery, the diagnosis can be established by conservative but adequate surgical exposure (avoiding pathologic fracture of the attenuated cortex) and frozen section of a bit of representative tissue. There should be no difficulty on frozen section in identifying a giant-cell tumor and in ruling out a sarcoma, although the grading of the tumor may require good paraffin slides. At some clinics, aspiration biopsy is relied upon, but the interpretation of such specimens calls for a good deal of experience. The tumor may then be treated by excision, resection, or thorough curettement, depending upon its location and size. Whenever it is possible to excise or resect the tumor in toto, this should be the method selected as the most certain and quickest way to effect a cure. For large tumors in the upper femur and upper humerus, resection and prosthetic replacement may be considered (Fig. 12-15). Unfortunately, the majority of giant-cell tumors present as relatively large growths in the lower end of the femur or the upper end of the tibia, where resection would necessitate a major reconstruction, leading hopefully to arthrodesis without significant shortening. In some hospitals abroad,[38] this is undertaken as a routine procedure. In this country, thorough curettement is the initial procedure generally followed by those committed to surgery. It seems clear from

---

Fig. 12-15. A, Roentgenogram of a giant-cell tumor developing in the upper end of a fibula (its cytology is illustrated in Fig. 12-10, B). This patient was only 17 years of age—one of the occasional exceptions to the rule that giant-cell tumor is distinctly unusual below the age of 20 years. B, Roentgenogram of the resected upper end of the fibula showing the giant-cell tumor illustrated in A. Sections revealed that the neoplasm had extended through the expanded cortical shell in places into the contiguous muscle tissue. Within several months, local excision of recurrent tumor became necessary, but the patient remained well for the next three and one-half years. C, Roentgenogram of a giant-cell tumor in a young woman of 24; the tumor originated in the greater trochanter of the femur. It recurred five months after curettement and bone grafting; the upper femur was then resected and replaced by a prosthesis, D.

Giant-cell tumor of bone (osteoclastoma) 159

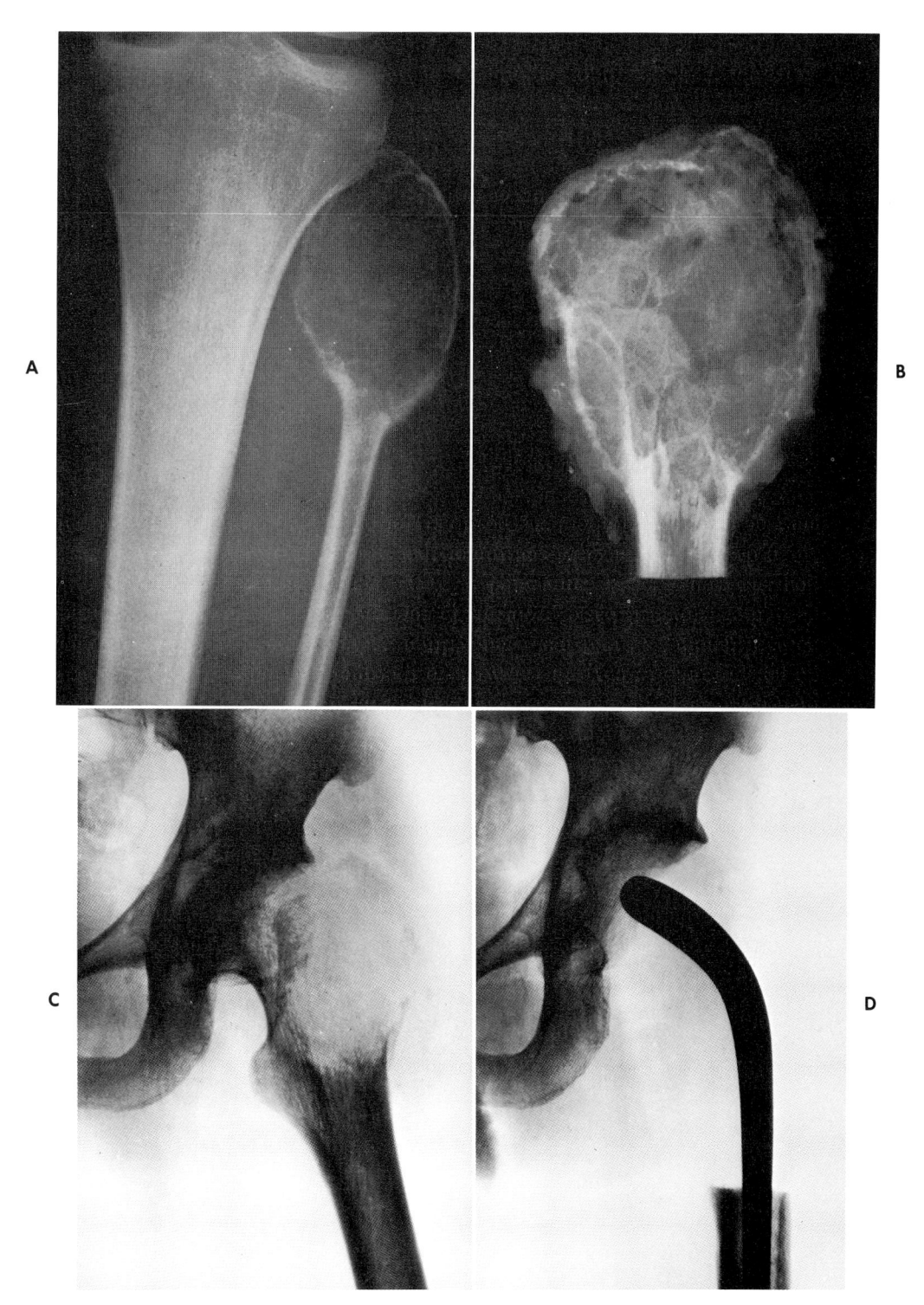

Fig. 12-15. For legend see opposite page.

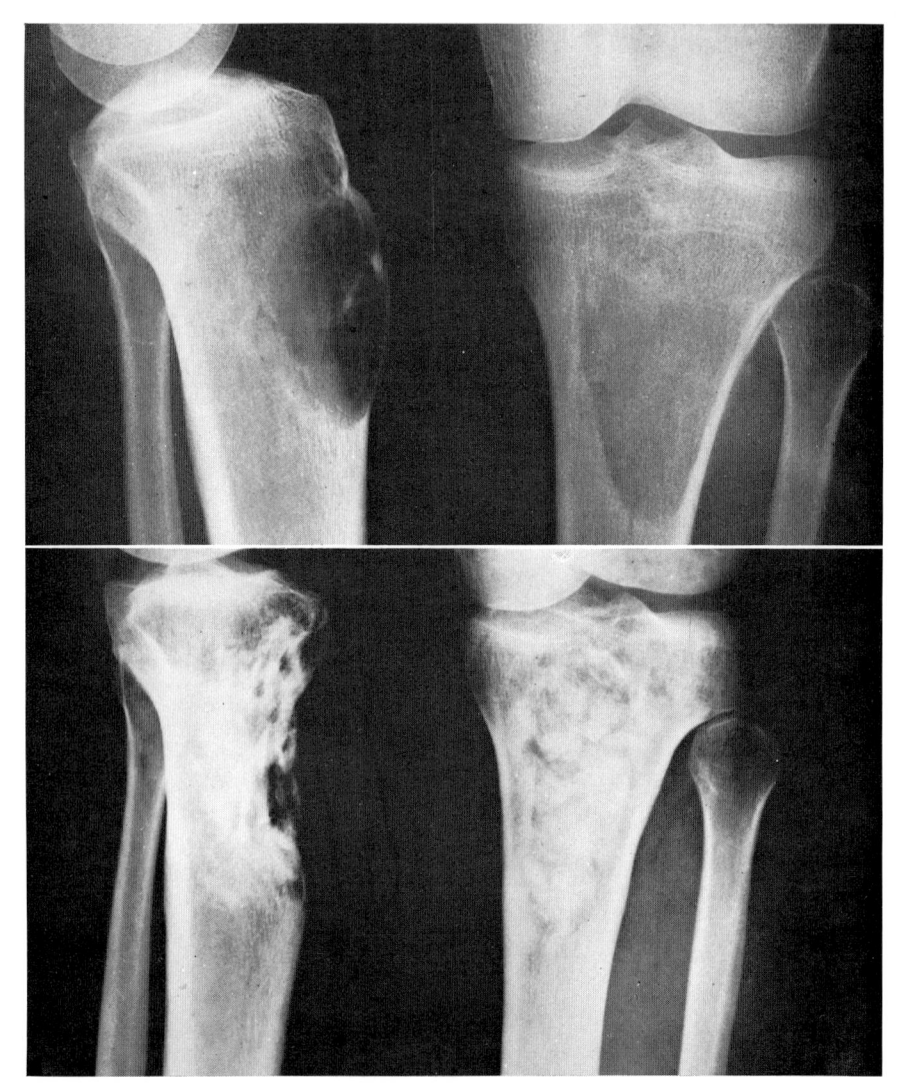

Fig. 12-16. Roentgenograms of another giant-cell tumor in the upper end of a tibia taken before and after thorough curettement and packing with bone chips. Complaints referable to the neoplasm had been noted for about one year. The cytology of this tumor is illustrated in Fig. 12-11. Although limited biopsy of the previously curetted area failed to reveal the presence of recurrent tumor, this case will bear close watching and may eventually come to amputation. About one year after surgery, a localized tumor node appeared in the subcutaneous tissue in the line of the surgical scar and was excised. Recurrence of giant-cell tumor in the upper tibia was noted three and one-half years after the initial curettement. It was decided to do a thorough curettement once again, and the patient has remained well to date.

the observations of Goldenberg, Campbell, and Bonfiglio[12] and others that the best results and the lowest recurrence rate are obtained by meticulous, *thorough* curettement and bone-grafting.

If one is committed to x-ray irradiation of giant-cell tumor by choice, then sufficient tissue for diagnosis can still be obtained by resorting to aspiration or drill biopsy, repeated if necessary in the event that the initial specimen is inadequate, or inconclusive. There seems to be good reason to hold empirically that x-ray irradiation per se is capable of effectively controlling a certain number of giant-cell tumors, particularly the less aggressive ones. To my knowledge, however, a well-controlled, altogether convincing, and sizable series of giant-cell tumors treated by roentgen therapy and followed for five to ten years has as yet to be presented.

One other important point needs to be stressed. If this modality is used in preference to surgery, the smallest tumor dose calculated to be effective should be used in view of the demonstrated hazard that some patients so treated may manifest the development of sarcoma in the lesion following a latent interval of five or more years after irradiation. I have personal knowledge of several cases in point in which sarcoma developed within an irradiated and ostensibly cured giant-cell tumor after a long latent interval, and indeed, I saw material from

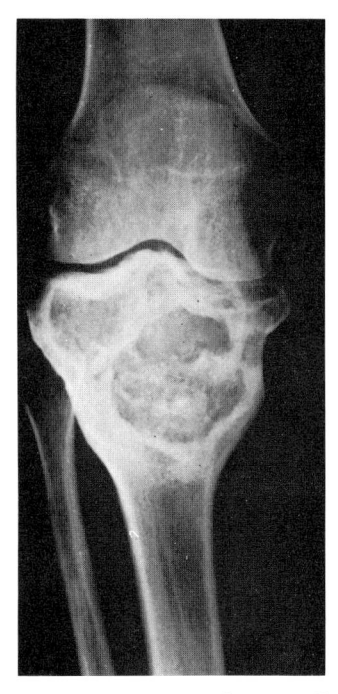

Fig. 12-17. Roentgenogram of a previously irradiated giant-cell tumor in the upper end of a tibia. It is noteworthy that biopsy performed seven years after treatment revealed the presence of residual giant-cell tumor tissue. This was distinctly modified by irradiation and impregnated by foam cells in places, but was still viable.

one recently in which an anaplastic fibrosarcoma developed thirty-four years after irradiation of a giant-cell tumor in the upper tibia (the details of irradiation were not available). Cahan and associates[2] reported several others in connection with a general survey of sarcoma in irradiated bone. Three additional instances in point were recorded also by Cruz, Coley, and Stewart.[6] In the series analyzed by Goldenberg, Campbell, and Bonfiglio,[12] postirradiation sarcoma developed in 3 of 46 patients (7%). In the Mayo Clinic material, as surveyed by Dahlin, sarcoma developed in as many as 7 of 36 patients so treated (19%), but perhaps the dosage was heavier. In any event, it is evident that giant-cell tumors cannot be irradiated with very large doses of x-ray with impunity.

The effective control of a giant-cell tumor that has already recurred locally following treatment, whether curettement or irradiation, raises still another set of problems that require some clarification. In the event that the initial therapy has been surgical, what is the likelihood that recurettement will effect a cure? According to Goldenberg,[*] some of these recurrences (usually within a two-year period) may reflect the fact that initial curettement was not complete, and thorough curettage and bone-grafting are therefore advocated. In the event that the recurrent tumor has broken through the cortex, resection and bone-grafting are recommended, and amputation is done only for unmistakably malignant tumors (Grade III), or for those that have become hopelessly infected or fractured. As for the use of supplementary irradiation, this seems to have lost favor, apparently because it is often ineffective and because of the hazard of postirradiation sarcoma.

In the event that the recurrent tumor has been initially treated by roentgen therapy in presumably adequate dosage, what is the likelihood that a second course of irradiation to the limit of tolerance will be any more effective? Insofar as the feasibility of supplementary surgery is concerned, one can readily appreciate the hazards of failure of tissue healing and of infection entailed in the curettement of irradiated tissues, but are these necessarily a deterrent in dealing with tumors that have received only moderate doses of x-ray, and, precisely, what is the limit of tolerance? If neither of these alternatives seems attractive, should one advocate surgical ablation for giant-cell tumors that have recurred in spite of what seemed to be adequate irradiation? As Coley[4] remarked, "There are few situations in the entire field of bone tumors which afford greater anxiety or which tax the judgment and intuition of the professional adviser more sorely than these cases of giant cell tumor which fail to yield to radiation therapy." I do not presume to have the answers to the questions raised, but I submit that, notwithstanding all that has been written on the subject of giant-cell tumor to date, there are still basic problems in therapy that require renewed consideration and cannot be circumvented by facile generalizations.

In dealing with a giant-cell tumor that has recurred a number of times, one must be circumspect about the possibility of frank malignant change and pulmo-

---

[*]Personal communication, Aug. 18, 1970.

nary metastasis. In particular, as Hutter and associates[16] emphasized, a recurrence after five years from first treatment should arouse great suspicion of malignant transformation. In reading the published case reports on malignant giant-cell tumors, one cannot fail to be impressed by the fact that in these cases amputation was resorted to much too late to be effective.

Summary

Giant-cell tumor of bone is a distinctive neoplasm arising apparently from the nonbone-forming, supporting connective tissue of the marrow, which can be readily identified on the basis of its cytologic details. The tumor is composed, cytologically, of a vascularized network of spindle-shaped or ovoid stromal cells, regularly and rather heavily interspersed with multinuclear cells (apparently syncytial stromal cells) as an integral part of the cytologic pattern. Giant-cell tumor, so conceived, is not nearly as common or as miscellaneous a lesion as has been supposed in the past. It must be clearly distinguished from the brown tumors, so-called, of advanced hyperparathyroidism, from most epulides, and from a variety of other less serious tumors of bone formerly associated with giant-cell tumor in the guise of "variants." Among the latter are such distinctive lesions as nonosteogenic fibroma, benign chondroblastoma, solitary unicameral bone cyst, aneurysmal bone cyst, and chondromyxoid fibroma of bone. They have little in common, clinically and anatomically, with genuine giant-cell tumor and little in common with each other except a uniformly favorable prognosis. If these distinctions are not clearly recognized, observations in regard to the efficacy of treatment by whatever method have but limited significance.

If one adheres to a strict definition of what should be regarded as giant-cell tumor and strips away all of the alleged variants, so-called, then what is left constitutes a formidable neoplasm to be reckoned with. With respect to potential seriousness, giant-cell tumors range the whole gamut from those that respond satisfactorily to well-conceived treatment, through those that are more aggressive and prone to recur locally, to those that may eventually become sarcomatous and metastasize. Along these lines, as a guide to therapy and with a view to forecasting prognosis within certain limits, it is suggested that giant-cell tumors be graded according to whether they show insignificant, moderate, or pronounced atypism of their stromal cells. In regard to therapy, I have surveyed some of the specific problems entailed in the treatment, by either surgery or irradiation, of a giant-cell tumor that is approached for the first time and of one that has already recurred after treatment.

From the clinical point of view, it is helpful in differential diagnosis to bear in mind that genuine giant-cell tumor is not likely to develop in patients under the age of 15 years. Also, despite the opinion once held, there is no such thing as a typical or characteristic roentgen picture of a giant-cell tumor. By the same token, the necessity for establishing accurate pathologic diagnosis before instituting treatment, whether surgery or irradiation, cannot be too strongly emphasized.

References

1. Bullock, W. K., and Luck, J. V.: Giant cell tumor-like lesions of bone, a preliminary report of a pathological entity, Calif. Med. 87:32, 1957.
2. Cahan, W. G., Woodard, H. Q., Higinbotham, N. L., Stewart, F. W., and Coley, B. L.: Sarcoma arising in irradiated bone. Report of eleven cases, Cancer 1:3, 1948.
3. Case Records of the Massachusetts General Hospital. Case 38-1965, N. Engl. J. Med. 273:494, 1965.
4. Coley, B. L.: Neoplasms of bone and related conditions. Their etiology, pathogenesis, diagnosis and treatment, New York, 1949, Paul B. Hoeber, Inc., p. 193.
5. Christensen, F. C.: Bone tumors. Analysis of one thousand cases with special reference of location, age and sex, Ann. Surg. 81:1074, 1925.
6. Cruz, M., Coley, B. L., and Stewart, F. W.: Postradiation bone sarcoma. Report of eleven cases, Cancer 10:72, 1957.
7. Editorial: Giant cell tumor of bone, J.A.M.A. 141:534, 1949.
8. Ewing, J.: A review of the classification of bone tumors, Surg. Gynecol. Obstet. 68:971, 1939.
9. Fennel, E. A.: Giant cell tumor: benign or malignant? Proc. Staff Meet. Clin., Honolulu 16:65, 1950.
10. Ferry, A. M.: Giant-cell tumors—surgery in the long bones, Clin. Orthop. 56:57, 1968.
11. Geschickter, C. F., Copeland, M. M., and Bloodgood, J. C.: Osteitis fibrosa and giant cell tumor, Arch. Surg. 19:169, 1929.
12. Goldenberg, R. R., Campbell, C. J., and Bonfiglio, M.: Giant-cell tumor of bone. An analysis of 218 cases, J. Bone Joint Surg. 52-A:619, 1970.
13. Haggart, G. E., and Hare, H. F.: Combined roentgen radiation and surgical treatment of large benign giant cell tumors of bone, Ann. Surg. 124:228, 1946.
14. Hanaoka, H., Friedman, B., and Mack, R. P.: Ultrastructure and histogenesis of giant-cell tumor of bone, Cancer 25:1408, 1970.
15. Hutter, R. V. P., Foote, F. W., Jr., Frazell, E. L., and Francis, K. C.: Giant cell tumors complicating Paget's disease of bone, Cancer 16:1044, 1963.
16. Hutter, R. V. P., Worcester, J. N., Jr., Francis, K. C., Foote, F. W., Jr., and Stewart, F. W.: Benign and malignant giant cell tumors of bone, Cancer 15:653, 1962.
17. Jaffe, H. L.: Giant-cell reparative granuloma, traumatic bone cyst, and fibrous (fibro-osseous) dysplasia of the jawbones, Oral Surg. 6:159, 1953.
18. Jaffe, H. L.: Giant-cell tumor (osteoclastoma) of bone: its pathologic delimitation and the inherent clinical implications, Ann. R. Coll. Surg. Engl. 13:343, 1953.
19. Jaffe, H. L.: Tumors of the skeletal system. Pathological aspects, Bull. N. Y. Acad. Med. 23:499, 1947.
20. Jaffe, H. L., and Lichtenstein, L.: Benign chondroblastoma of bone. A reinterpretation of the so-called calcifying or chondromatous giant cell tumor, Am. J. Pathol. 18:969, 1942.
21. Jaffe, H. L., and Lichtenstein, L.: Chondromyxoid fibroma of bone. A distinctive benign tumor likely to be mistaken for chondrosarcoma, Arch. Pathol. 45:541, 1948.
22. Jaffe, H. L., and Lichtenstein, L.: Non-osteogenic fibroma of bone, Am. J. Pathol. 18:205, 1942.
23. Jaffe, H. L., and Lichtenstein, L.: Solitary unicameral bone cyst. With emphasis on the roentgen picture, the pathologic appearance and the pathogenesis, Arch. Surg. 44:1004, 1942.
24. Jaffe, H. L., Lichtenstein, L., and Portis, R. B.: Giant cell tumor of bone. Its pathologic appearance, grading, supposed variants and treatment, Arch. Pathol. 30:993, 1940.
25. Jaffe, H. L., Lichtenstein, L., and Sutro, C. J.: Pigmented villonodular synovitis, bursitis and tenosynovitis, Arch. Pathol. 31:731, 1941.
26. Jewell, J. H., and Bush, L. F.: "Benign" giant-cell tumor of bone with a solitary pulmonary metastasis, J. Bone Joint Surg. 46-A:848, 1964.
27. Kraft, G. L., and Levinthal, D. H.: Acrylic prosthesis replacing lower end of the femur for benign giant-cell tumor, J. Bone Joint Surg. 36-A:368, 1954.
28. Lichtenstein, L.: Aneurysmal bone cyst. Further observations, Cancer 6:1228, 1953.
29. Lichtenstein, L.: Aneurysmal bone cyst. Observations on 50 cases, J. Bone Joint Surg. 39-A:873, 1957.
30. Lichtenstein, L.: Aneurysmal bone cyst. A pathological entity commonly mistaken for giant cell tumor and occasionally for hemangioma and osteogenic sarcoma, Cancer 3:279, 1950.
31. Lichtenstein, L.: Chondromyxoid fibroma of bone, Am. J. Pathol. 24:686, 1948.
32. Lichtenstein, L.: Giant cell tumor of bone. Current status of problems in diagnosis

and treatment, J. Bone Joint Surg. **33-A:** 143, 1951.
33. Lichtenstein, L., and Kaplan, L.: Benign chondroblastoma of bone. Unusual localization in femoral capital epiphysis, Cancer **2:**793, 1949.
34. Mnaymneh, W. A., Dudley, H. R., Jr., and Mnaymneh, L. G.: Giant-cell tumor of bone. An analysis and follow-up study of the 41 cases observed at the Massachusetts General Hospital between 1925 and 1961, J. Bone Joint Surg. **46-A:**63, 1964.
35. Murphy, W. R., and Ackerman, L. V.: Benign and malignant giant-cell tumors of bone; clinical-pathological evaluation of thirty-one cases, Cancer **9:**317, 1956.
36. Ores, R., Rosen, P., and Ortiz, J.: Localization of acid phosphatase activity in a giant cell tumor of bone, Arch. Pathol. **88:**54, 1969.
37. Pan, P., Dahlin, D. C., Lipscomb, P. R., and Bernatz, P. E.: "Benign" giant-cell tumors of the radius with pulmonary metastasis, Mayo Clinic Proc. **39:**344, 1964.
38. Schajowicz, F.: Giant-cell tumors of bone (osteoclastoma). A pathological and histochemical study, J. Bone Joint Surg. **43-A:** 1, 1961.
39. Schajowicz, F., and Slullitel, I.: Giant-cell tumor associated with Paget's disease of bone, J. Bone Joint Surg. **48-A:**1340, 1966.
40. Sherman, M., and Fabricius, R.: Giant-cell tumor in the metaphysis of a child, J. Bone Joint Surg. **43-A:**1225, 1961.
41. Thomson, A. D., and Turner-Warwick, R. T.: Skeletal sarcomata and giant-cell tumor, J. Bone Joint Surg. **37-B:**266, 1955.
42. Wilkerson, J. A., and Cracchiolo, A.: Giant-cell tumor of the tibial diaphysis, J. Bone Joint Surg. **51-A:**1205, 1969.
43. Williams, R. R., Dahlin, D. C., and Ghormley, R. K.: Giant-cell tumor of bone, Cancer **7:**764, 1954.
44. Willis, R. A.: Pathology of tumours, London, 1948, Butterworth & Co., Ltd. (see p. 684 and Fig. 329).
45. Willis, R. A.: The pathology of osteoclastoma or giant cell tumor of bone, J. Bone Joint Surg. **31-B:**236, 1949.

Chapter 13

Tumors of bone of vascular origin

Hemangioma, hemangioendothelioma, hemangiopericytoma (glomus), lymphangioma

Hemangioma

Although hemangioma in general represents a fairly common neoplasm, the occurrence of benign vascular tumors within bone is rather uncommon, at least in the sense of clinically or roentgenographically evident lesions constituting a surgical problem. Thus, Watson and McCarthy,[39] in reviewing a series of over 1,000 cases of vascular tumors of all types treated at Memorial Hospital, found only five that originated within bone. Of these, three were encountered within a lumbar vertebral body, one in a rib, and one in a mandible.

In 1962 Hartman and Stewart,[15] at the same hospital, reported on ten cases of hemangioendothelioma of bone, stressing the indolent course in many instances and cure by surgical extirpation. In four of these instances, one or more of the foot bones was involved; in three, the tibia (in one, there were multiple sites); in two, a bone of the skull; and in one, a rib. My own experience in recent years would indicate a somewhat greater incidence of hemangioma and hemangioendothelioma of bone than was once suspected. Since 1958, I have collected material submitted for consultation from as many as 27 cases (excluding those involving only the extraosseous soft parts), and these may be the subject of a detailed report later on. In nine instances there was involvement of two or more sites simultaneously, mainly in bones of the lower limb and especially in the knee region. The solitary lesions were encountered in the lower extremity, including the foot (eight); the upper extremity, including the hand (four); a frontal bone (one); a scapula (one); and the vertebral column (four). Two of the latter were unusual expanding lesions causing cord compression (Fig. 13-5).

The solitary localized tumors must be distinguished from the not too uncommon instances in which hemangioma formation in portions of one or more bones may be observed in association with comparable involvement of the contiguous soft parts (in a hypertrophied lower extremity, for example) as an integral part of a developmental anomaly of hemangiomatosis. These unusual expressions of hemangiomatosis may be manifested by involvement of the bones of one region, of an entire limb, or of a major part of the skeleton, tending to produce a striking degree of osteoporosis. For a valuable discussion of angiomatous lesions of the extremities, either congenital or becoming manifest during childhood, one may have recourse to the well-documented and superbly illustrated paper by Goidanich and Campanacci.[11] For consideration of instances of more widespread skeletal hemangiomatosis, the paper by Wallis, Asch, and Maisel[38] is useful. Cognizance must also be taken of comparable rare instances of lymphangiomatosis of bone, with or without associated involvement of the soft parts of the affected extremities.[12,27,28]

According to Sherman,[29] who surveyed some 60 cases of hemangioma of bone recorded in the literature, fully two-thirds were located in the skull or vertebral column, approximately one-fourth in the long bones, and the remainder in such sites as the innominate bones, the tarsal bones, and the scapula. The same author, in collaboration with Wilner,[30] has also published a comprehensive paper on the roentgen diagnosis of hemangioma of bone in general. A comprehensive discussion of hemangiomas of the skull, in particular, is to be found in a paper by Wyke[40] dealing with some 40 recorded cases. These developed most often in the

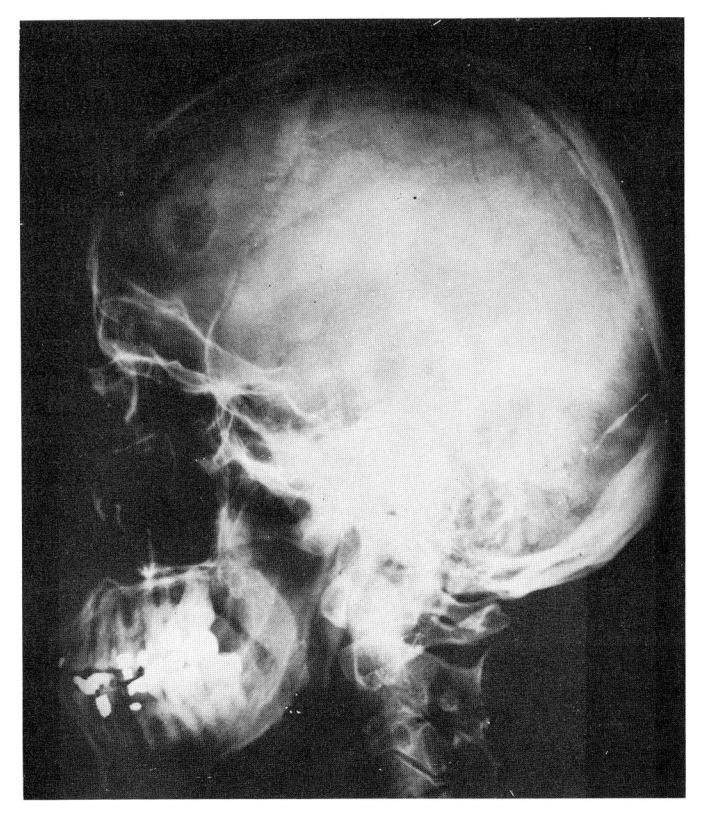

Fig. 13-1. Roentgenogram showing a small, circumscribed, lytic defect in the frontal bone of the calvarium, which proved to be a hemangioma (see Fig. 13-3).

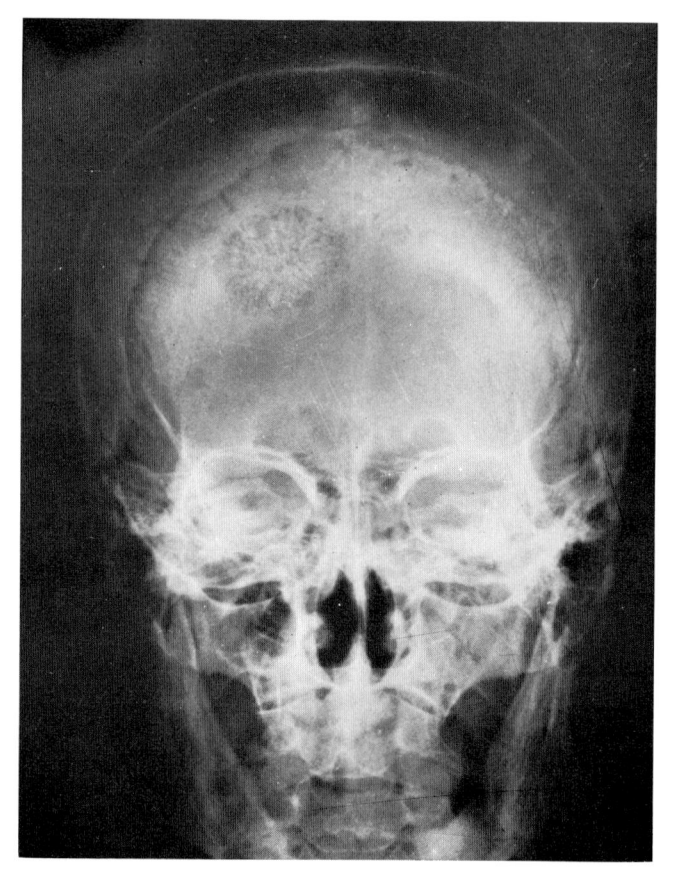

Fig. 13-2. Another hemangioma of a frontal bone showing the so-called "sunburst" effect that would lead one to suspect the diagnosis before surgery.

parietal and frontal bones and were encountered for the most part in adults past 30 years of age and especially in women. Roentgenographically, as Wyke and others[2] have pointed out, a hemangioma of the calvarium is likely to present as a circumscribed, round or oval, honeycombed area of rarefaction, tending to bulge the outer table. If the lesion is visualized in tangential views, another rather characteristic feature may be demonstrated, namely, the so-called "sun ray" appearance produced apparently by fine spicules of reactive new bone radiating from the center of the lesion (Fig. 13-2). It should be noted, however, by way of differential diagnosis that these striations do not all have a perpendicular orientation, such as one may observe when the calvarium reacts to the presence of an underlying eroding meningioma. On surgical exploration, a hemangioma of a calvarial bone presents as a hard, blue-domed lump lying beneath the intact pericranium. Histologically, its pattern may be either capillary or cavernous. In regard to prognosis, it is pertinent to note that in none of the cases surveyed by Wyke was there any indication of malignant change. Well-illustrated pathologic

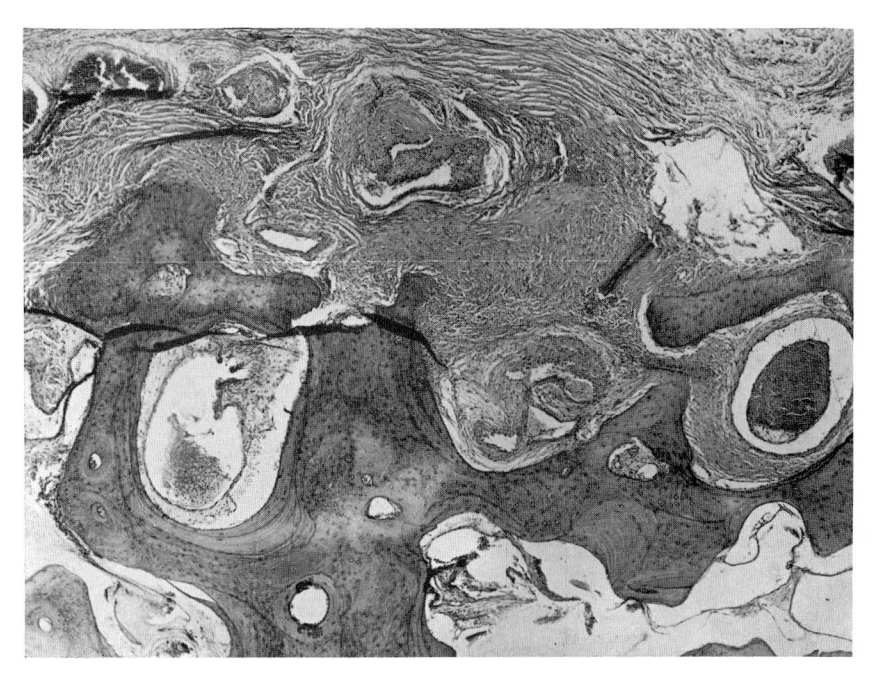

Fig. 13-3. Photomicrograph of the hemangioma (of a frontal bone) illustrated in Fig. 13-1. The overlying periosteal connective tissue is also permeated by numerous prominent blood vessels. (×35.)

data of value in regard to hemangiomas of the skull specifically may be found in a paper by Kleinsasser and Albrecht.[19]

Hemangiomas of vertebral bodies are said to be fairly common, and the anatomic studies of Töpfer[37] have been repeatedly cited to the effect that pertinent lesions in vertebrae held to represent hemangiomas were found in approximately 12% of over 2,000 subjects examined at autopsy. It is significant, however, that in none of these cases had the lesions in question provoked any clinical symptoms or been recognized roentgenographically. It is true that one occasionally encounters, as a fortuitous finding at autopsy, the presence of a circumscribed, roundish, bright red hemangioma-like focus within the spongiosa of a vertebral body, commonly a dorsal or a lumbar body. Such foci usually measure up to 1 to 2 cm. in greatest diameter and are found on microscopic examination to represent a congeries of closely approximated, thin-walled, dilated and engorged blood vessels, apparently venules and capillaries. They are not at all discernible roentgenographically, even in roentgenograms of specimens that afford great clarity of detail. Further, in sections of such lesions, one fails to observe any significant alteration of the surrounding bone. It has always seemed to me that such vascularized foci may reflect nothing more than localized venous stasis, and, as such, hardly represent hemangiomas in the sense of a neoplasm, any more than an esophageal varix or a plexus of dilated hemorrhoidal veins constitutes a tumor of blood vessels.

170 Bone tumors

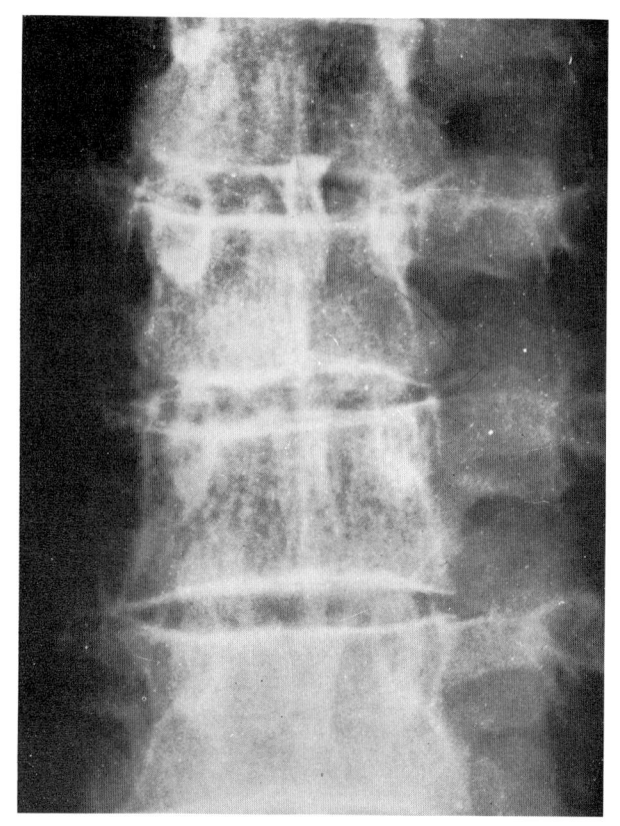

Fig. 13-4. Roentgenogram showing the vertical striated effect commonly held to be associated with hemangiomas of vertebral bodies.

In regard to clinically significant lesions reported as hemangiomas of the spine, it is relevant to point out that a certain number of them, at least, particularly those that have produced prominent expansion of the neural arch and perhaps part of the adjacent body of one or two contiguous vertebrae, may actually represent instances of aneurysmal bone cyst. In this connection, also, it perhaps needs to be emphasized that, in general, an unverified roentgen diagnosis of hemangioma of a vertebral body may not be too trustworthy. I recall a pertinent instance in which a peculiar, rarefied, and expanded lesion in a lumbar body was irradiated without prior needle biopsy on the premise that it represented a hemangioma, and it was not until two and one-half years later that it became quite evident that the lesion in question actually was an initially solitary focus of myeloma. It is not intended to convey the impression, however, that bona fide hemangiomas of vertebrae do not exist, but they are probably no more frequent there than they are in the calvarium. As Bucy and Capp[2] have emphasized, roentgenographically discernible hemangiomas of the spine are likely to present a distinctive, vertically striated appearance, and it is not unusual for them to in-

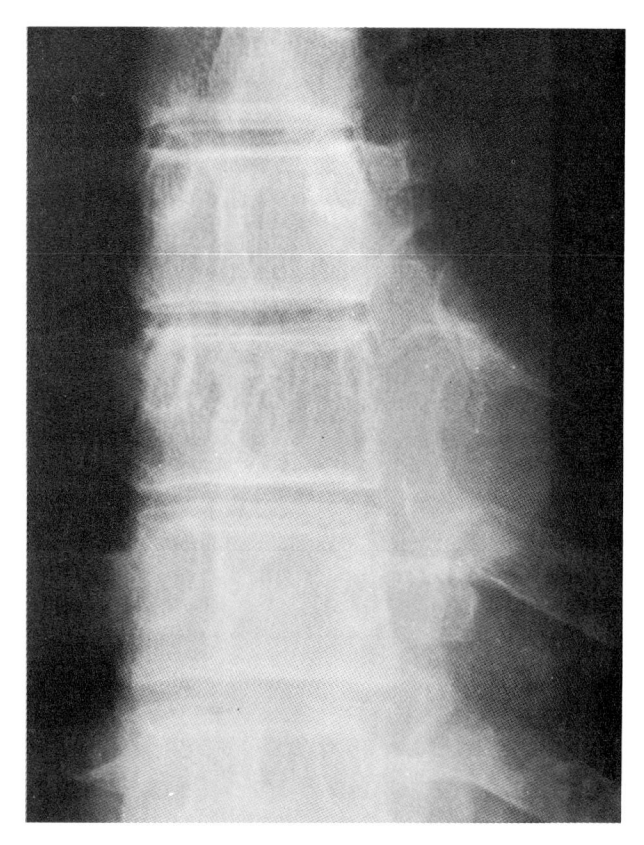

Fig. 13-5. Roentgenogram of an unusual expanded hemangioma in a tenth thoracic vertebra of a young man. Laminectomy was done for relief of cord compression, in the course of which a specimen was obtained for diagnosis; this showed a simple capillary hemangioma.

volve two or more contiguous bodies (Fig. 13-4). They may come to clinical attention because of symptoms of pressure on the spinal cord or its nerve roots (Fig. 13-5). For their effective control, it does not appear necessary to resort to hazardous laminectomy, and high-voltage roentgen therapy has been recommended by Watson and McCarthy[39] as the treatment of choice, affording complete relief of symptoms.

In a flat bone, such as a rib, a hemangioma may give rise to a symmetrical, fusiform expanded lesion presenting pronounced thinning of its distended cortex, without appreciable periosteal new bone reaction. The "sunburst" effect characterizing hemangioma in some other sites may be inconspicuous or entirely lacking, and one may observe instead a trabeculated or honeycombed pattern. A pertinent instance of this kind has been reported by Dorner and Marcy,[6] in which the expanded cortical shell at the site of rib involvement was found to contain soft reddish tumor tissue. The latter, on microscopic examination, was characterized by the presence of a meshwork of large, engorged, thin-walled blood vessels indicative of a cavernous hemangioma. A hemangioma in a foot bone may likewise present a pseudotrabeculated "soap bubble" appearance roentgenographically, and I have observed a pertinent instance in an os calcis, which was regarded as a probable giant-cell tumor prior to surgical exploration. This lesion was curetted and packed with bone chips and went on to uneventful healing (Fig. 13-7, A).

As for hemangiomas in long bones, the relatively few recorded instances indicate that here, also, hemangioma may give rise to fusiform or more localized expansion of the affected bone, often the end of the bone, as well as pronounced thinning of the overlying cortex, without necessarily provoking appreciable periosteal reaction. Roentgenographically, such lesions are likely to present a rather distinctive, coarsely loculated or honeycombed rarefied appearance that may

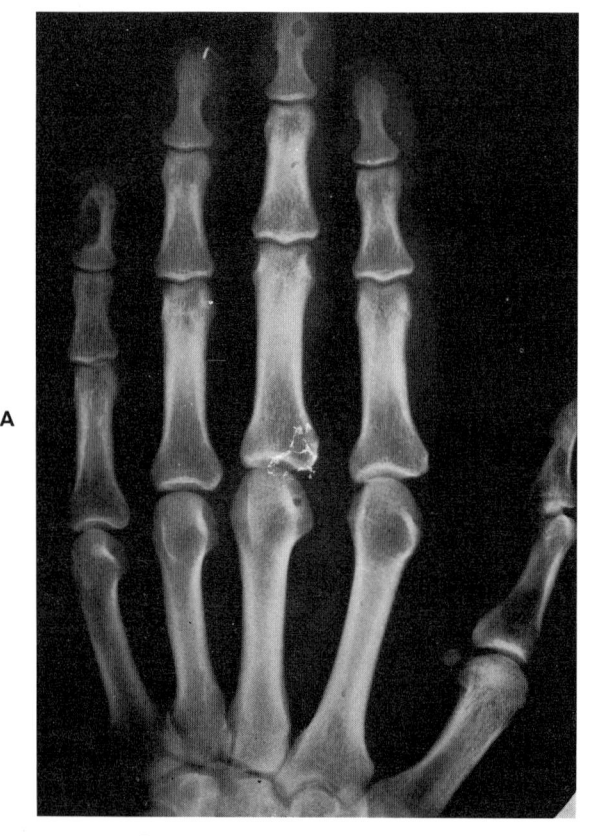

Fig. 13-6. A, Roentgenogram of a hand showing multiple, sharply punched-out, rarefied defects in the third and fifth fingers reflecting the presence of hemangioendotheliomas. (Biopsy material for microscopic examination was removed from the largest one in the distal phalanx of the fifth finger.) The patient also presented a small hemangioendothelioma in the subcutaneous tissue of the wrist. B, Roentgenogram of a hemangioma in the distal tibia, which expanded the bone and attenuated the cortex, without provoking appreciable periosteal new bone reaction. Its projection has a honeycombed appearance. C, Roentgenogram of a benign hemangioendothelioma in the region of the lesser trochanter of a femur in an adult, which provides no cue to its recognition as such.

suggest hemangioma, if one is alert to the possibility (Fig. 13-6, *B*). Some lesions in limb bones, however, may present as nondescript lucent defects, from which one would hardly suspect hemangioma (Fig. 13-6, *C*). Acceptable accounts of hemangiomas of limb bones (along with some others that seem clearly to deal with hemangioendotheliomas, though labeled hemangiomas) may be found in papers by Hitzrot,[17] Sherman,[29] Sherman and Wilner,[30] Thomas,[36] and Geschickter and Maseritz,[10] among others.

Malignant hemangioendothelioma

Malignant tumors of blood vessels are quite rare in general, and this is particularly true of those arising within bone. Furthermore, not all of the recorded tumors interpreted as malignant tumors of vascular origin are acceptable as such. It seems clear that some actually represent vascular neoplasms of other kinds, while the reports of some others are too vague or equivocal as to essential details to permit reliable classification. Altogether too few observers have resorted to silver staining to establish clearly the presence of atypical endothelia in relation to obscured vascular sheaths or the presence of free vascular anastomoses. In particular, it is pertinent to note that the tumors classified by Ewing in his

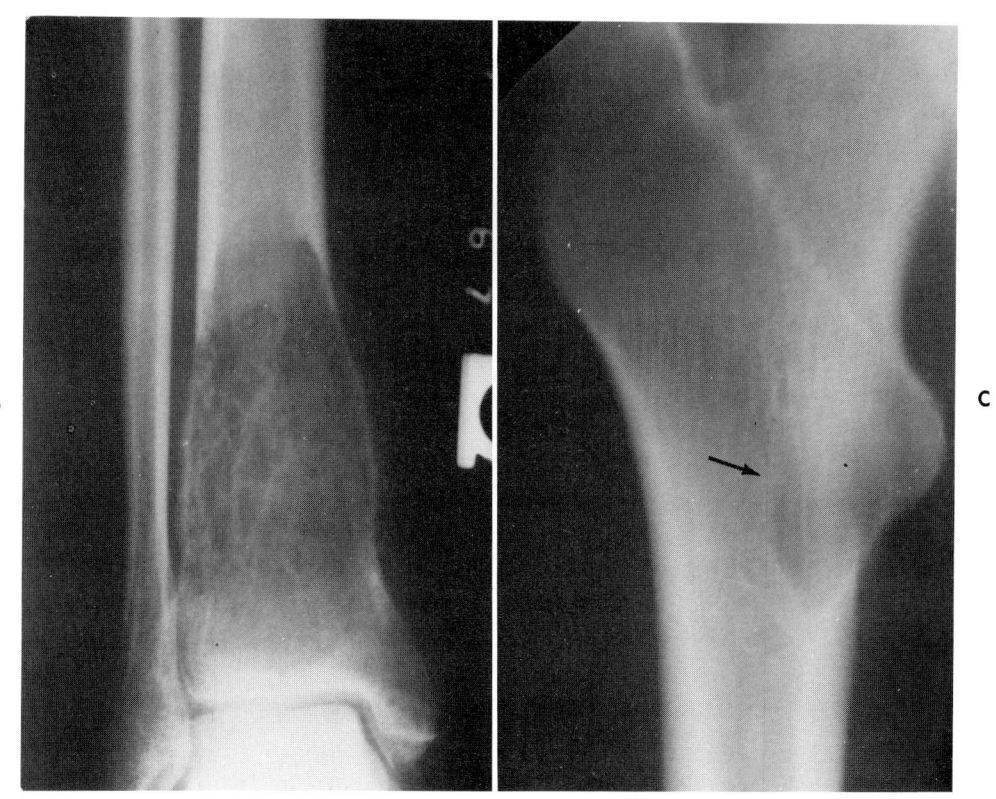

Fig. 13-6, cont'd. For legend see opposite page.

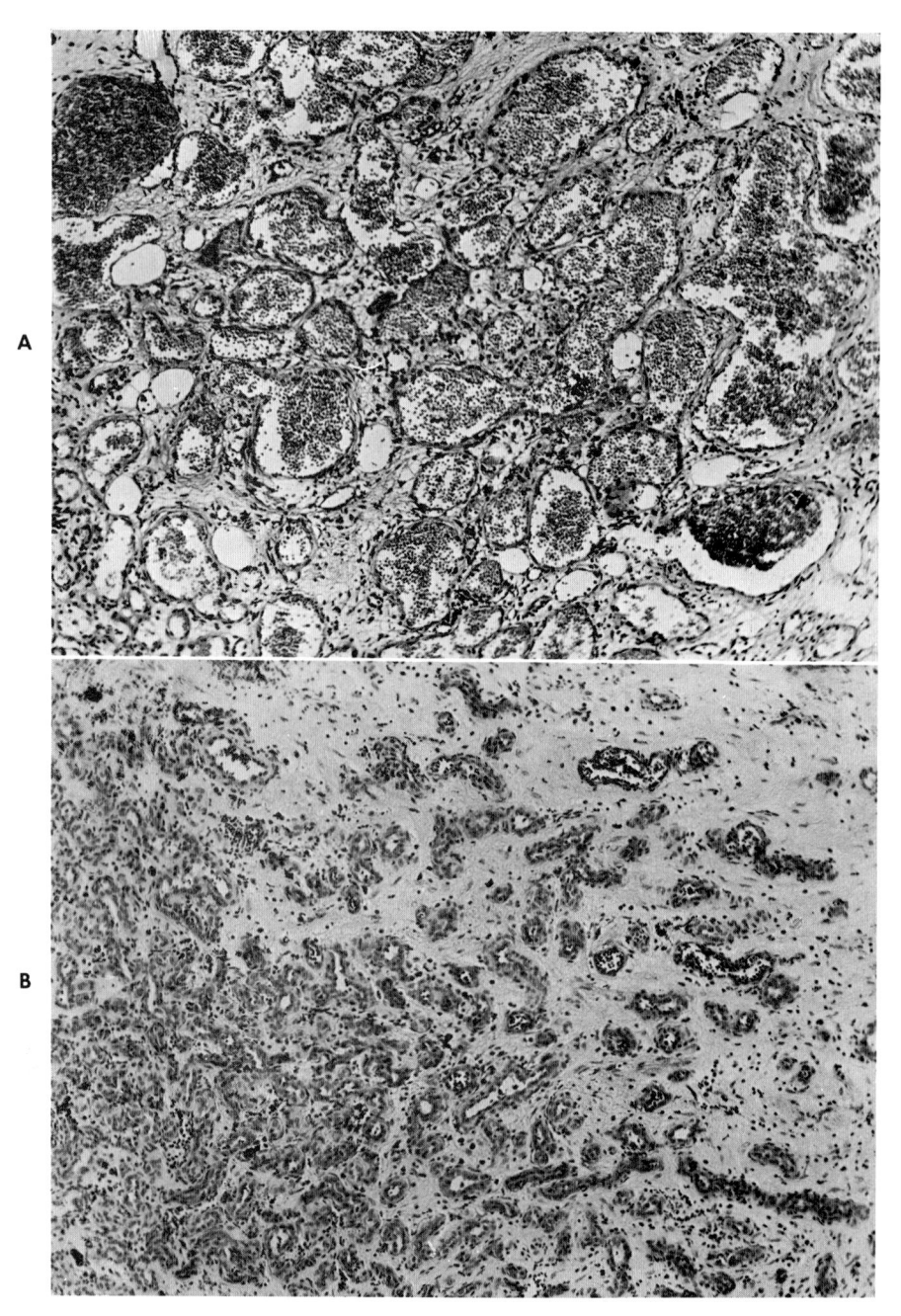

Fig. 13-7. **A**, Photomicrograph of a representative field of a capillary hemangioma that developed within a calcaneus and presented a well-circumscribed, pseudotrabeculated appearance roentgenographically. Thorough curettement of the lesion and packing of the defect with bone chips effected a clinical cure. **B**, Photomicrograph of hemangioendothelioma of an ischium. (×100.)

text as angioendotheliomas, and also reported as such by others,[22] have a striking resemblance to clear-cell renal carcinoma that, as is well known, may give rise to solitary skeletal metastasis, notably in the humerus. On the other hand, some of the cases reported as hemangioma of bone have obviously been underdiagnosed, as noted, and seem actually to represent instances of malignant hemangioendothelioma to judge by the illustrative photomicrographs. In regard to nomenclature, the use of such terms as angioblastoma and angiosarcoma, as well as telangiectatic sarcoma and malignant bone aneurysm, to denote obviously malignant tumors featuring blood vessel formation has further contributed to confusion. I am inclined to follow the suggestion of Stout that all the genuine malignant tumors of vascular origin, except for the aggressive or metastasizing hemangiopericytomas, be grouped under the single head of malignant hemangioendothelioma. As Stout has emphasized, these may be extremely malignant tumors that often have already extended by hematogenous spread before they are recognized. On the other hand, the experience of Hartman and Stewart,[15] previously cited, indicates that not a few hemangioendotheliomas of bone may pursue an indolent course with long survival after appropriate surgical therapy.

In the older literature one finds a number of well-documented cases of malignant hemangioendothelioma of bone recorded by Fienberg and Baehr,[9] Thomas,[36] Geschickter and Maseritz,[10] and Stout,[31] among others. The tumors cited were all malignant when first observed, and I have no knowledge of any hemangioendothelioma that developed through spontaneous malignant change in a benign hemangioma. The first-mentioned authors have reported a pertinent tumor arising in the tibia, which manifested its aggressiveness by extension to the popliteal artery. This patient survived for thirteen years after amputation without clinical evidence of tumor.[9] Hartman and Stewart[15] cited a comparable instance in which there was spread of tumor to the popliteal artery, as well as a lymph node in the vicinity, in spite of which the patient was well three years after treatment at last follow-up. Thomas,[36] in a survey of the relevant material of the Bone Sarcoma Registry, cited an instance of a recurrent malignant hemangioendothelioma (designated as "angiosarcoma"), involving a number of tarsal bones. Stout,[33] in a comprehensive discussion of some 18 collected cases of hemangioendothelioma in general, included two malignant neoplasms that originated in bone. The first of these, encountered in a 60-year-old woman, involved the lower ends of the tibia and fibula. Roentgenograms of the affected bones showed destruction, rarefaction, and widening, and at surgical exploration these were found to be filled with very vascular tissue, said to resemble sponge rubber in the gross. Roentgenograms taken three months later revealed further extension of tumor locally, as well as a suggestive area of involvement in the greater trochanter of the femur on the same side. The second pertinent tumor reported by Stout developed in a rib of a 20-year-old woman and metastasized widely, proving fatal within two or three years. On histologic examination this neoplasm showed, in some areas, vascular tubes lined by elongated cells; in other areas, rounded and heaped-up endothelia; and in still other areas, overproduction of tumor cells in solid masses, tending to obscure the vascular tubes. Gordon-Taylor and Wiles[13] have rendered a brief but interesting clinical account of a pulsating hemangioendothelioma of an iliac bone, over which a to-and-fro murmur was audible. It was elected to do a hindquarter amputation in this case. Pollak[26] reported an instance of a frankly malignant hemangioendothelioma of the sternum, which metastasized to the calvarium and a humerus, proving fatal shortly thereafter despite radical local resection and heavy x-ray irradiation. It is pertinent to note that in neither of the two foregoing cases were the roentgenograms sufficiently distinctive to suggest the diagnosis prior to surgical exploration. An extraordinary instance of hemangioendothelioma manifesting symmetrical involvement of both upper femora and progressive extension into the contiguous innominate bone has been reported by Hauser and Constant.[16] In this case, as in a number of others just cited, embarrassing hemorrhage from soft, friable, richly vascular tumor tissue was encountered at biopsy. It is noteworthy that this patient had survived for nine years without evident metastasis, even though the tumor in the interim had filled most of the pelvis.

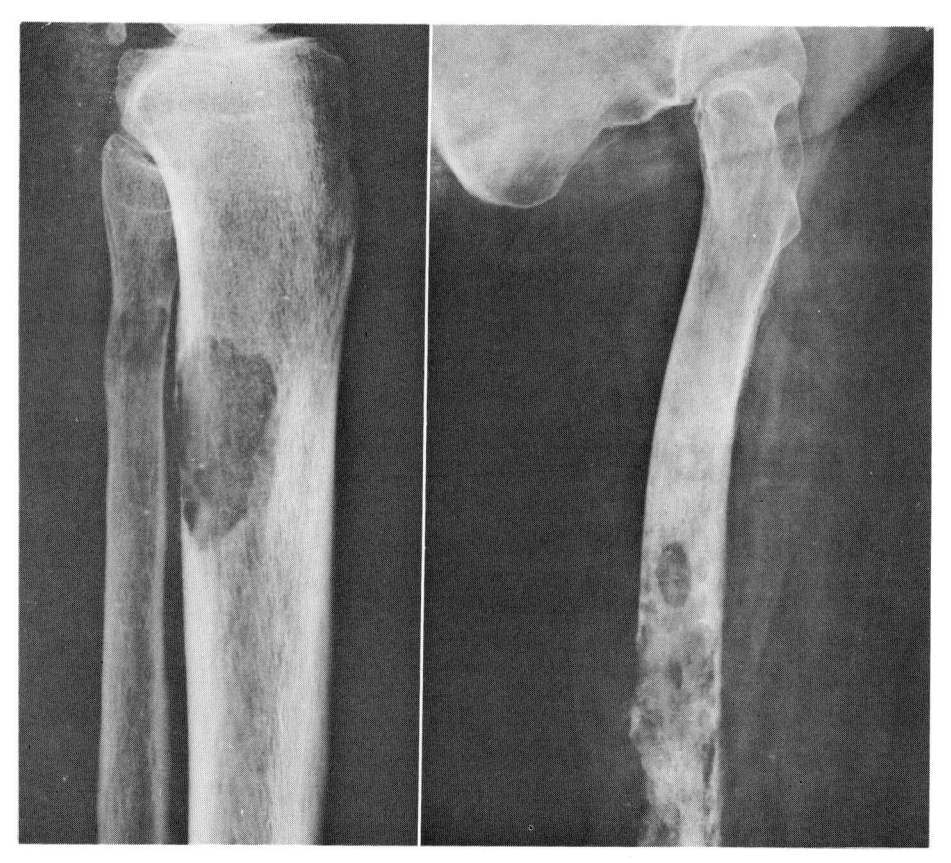

Fig. 13-8. Roentgenograms of a multicentric tumor in the femur, tibia, and upper fibula (ipsilateral) of an older woman, which proved on biopsy to be a malignant hemangioendothelioma.

I have also observed a number of frankly malignant hemangioendotheliomas in bone. One of these was in an iliac bone (in a 22-year-old young man), the roentgenograms of which were originally thought to suggest the presence of a chondrosarcoma. At exploration, the neoplasm was found to be composed of hemorrhagic, friable tumor tissue that was extending into the adjacent muscle. Sections showed that the tumor cells were freely invading blood vessels and flourishing as remarkable intravascular vasoformative tumor thrombi. Therefore, it was not surprising that metastasis to a rib was noted some months later, in spite of resection of the primary growth (Fig. 13-9, A). Another was in a humerus of a 38-year-old man and gave rise to pathologic fracture, still another was in a metacarpal bone, and one presented multiple foci in the femur, tibia, and fibula of the same lower extremity (Fig. 13-8). Still another was encountered in a lumbar vertebra of a young man of 20, and it had induced cord compression.

The two most recent malignant hemangioendotheliomas that were referred to me for opinion were both of unusual interest. One developed in a calcaneus at a site where, 25 years previously, a benign hemangioma had been irradiated (Fig. 13-9, B). The dosage employed was not known, nor were the original roentgenograms available. The surgeon elected to amputate the foot, and too little time has elapsed for any meaningful follow-up. The other malignant hemangioendothelioma developed in the distal femur around the end of an intramedullary Küntscher rod inserted fifteen years previously for a fracture of the femoral shaft (Fig. 13-9, C).

In summary, then, malignant hemangioendotheliomas of bone are comparatively rare neoplasms that are usually not identified clinically and roentgenographically prior to surgical exploration. Some may be so aggressive or so far advanced by the time they are recognized as to have a serious prognosis despite radical surgery. On the other hand, as Hartman and Stewart[15] have stressed, some may pursue an indolent course and be cured by surgical resection. In such tumors, even vascular invasion does not make fatal dissemination inevitable. Otis and his associates,[25] reporting more recently from the same institution, had reason to be less optimistic. They pointed out, incidentally, that in their experience multiple lesions had a more favorable prognosis than solitary ones. Altogether, the clinical behavior of malignant hemangioendotheliomas in bone would seem to be unpredictable, and we do not know enough about them as yet to make any dependable forecast from their cytology. It would also appear that perhaps too much reliance has been placed in the past upon the efficacy of irradiation, although this may provide satisfactory palliation.

Hemangiopericytoma (glomus)

The concept of the glomus tumor, along with its distinctive clinical and cytologic picture, has become increasingly familiar in recent years, but it is perhaps not generally known that the lesion may develop as a primary tumor within bone. Thus, Lattes and Bull[20] reported in 1948 an unusual instance of a glomus tumor that was completely encased within the terminal phalanx of a finger. Their

178   Bone tumors

patient was a 28-year-old woman who complained of sharp, stabbing, recurrent pain referable to the lesion for about four years. Roentgen examination revealed a localized, honeycombed area of rarefaction, suggesting an enchondroma or possibly a bone cyst. The overlying cortex was markedly attenuated, and the lesional tissue was soft and jellylike. This was curetted and a bone graft was inserted, resulting in complete relief of symptoms. The illustrative photomicrograph is quite consistent with the diagnosis of glomus tumor. In their search of the literature, the authors were able to find only one other comparable tumor, likewise situated within the terminal phalanx of a finger, which had been reported by Iglesias de la Torre, Gomez Camejo, and Palacios.[18] In this instance also, severe pain of four years' duration, radiating up the extremity and tending to paroxysmal exacerbations following slight trauma, was completely relieved by ablation of the affected phalanx.

Through the courtesy of Dr. M. Zeiler of Los Angeles, I have also observed material from a glomus tumor situated within a terminal phalanx of a finger. Its

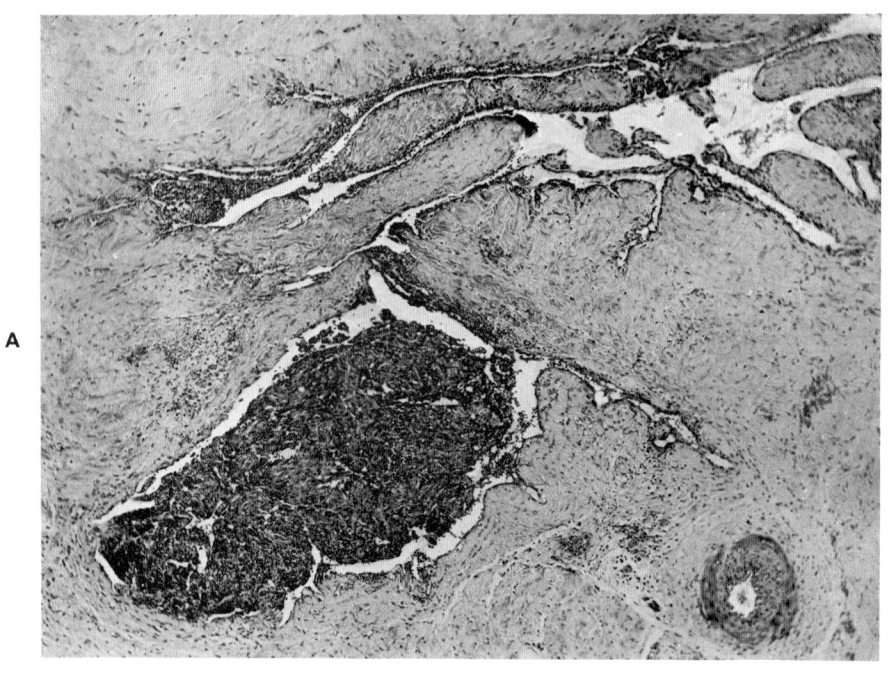

Fig. 13-9. A, Photomicrograph of a field of a malignant hemangioendothelioma showing an intravascular vasoformative tumor thrombus. This neoplasm developed in an iliac bone of a 22-year-old man and metastasized to a rib, despite local resection. (×65.) B, Tomogram of a cytologically malignant hemangioendothelioma in a calcaneus, which developed some twenty-five years after irradiation of a benign hemangioma at the same site. The details of dosage are not known. C, Roentgenogram of a tumor developing in the distal femur around the end of an intramedullary rod, some fifteen years after its insertion, which proved on biopsy to be a malignant hemangioendothelioma. (Courtesy Dr. S. J. Catanzaro, Fort Lauderdale, Fla.)

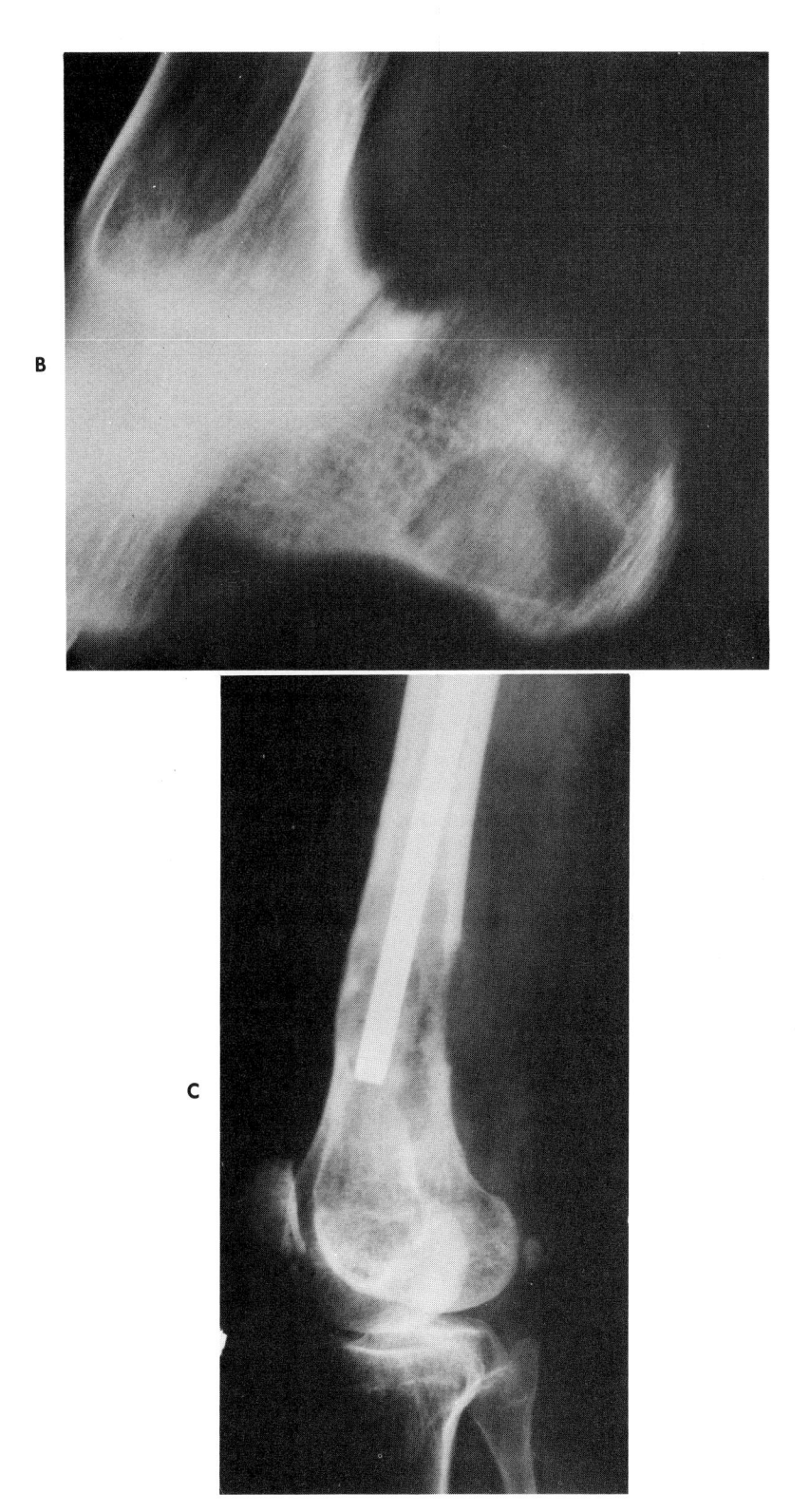

Fig. 13-9, cont'd. For legend see opposite page.

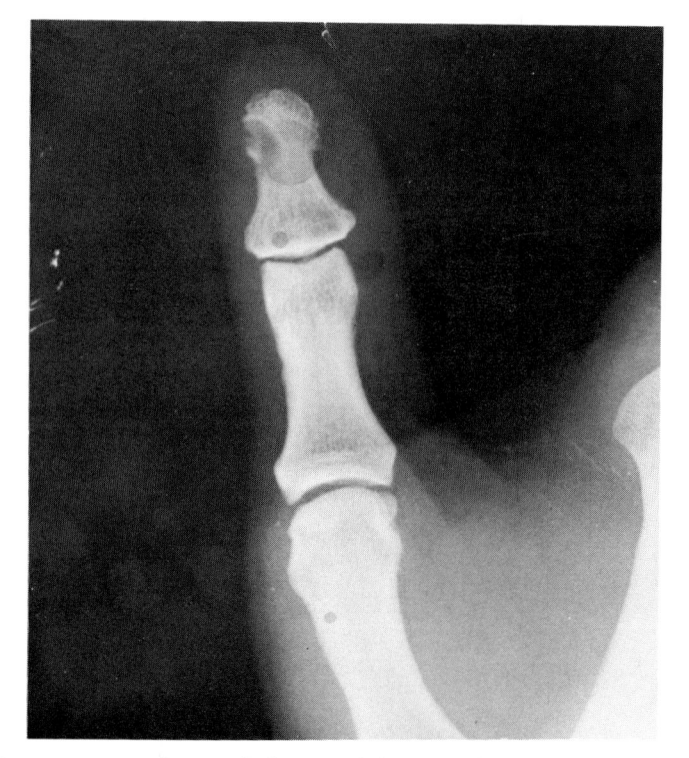

Fig. 13-10. Roentgenogram of an eroded terminal finger phalanx caused by a glomus tumor.

roentgen picture was not unlike that of an enchondroma, and the lesion had been only moderately painful. Subsequently, I had occasion to see another case in point, this one situated in the terminal phalanx of a thumb in a 37-year-old woman. The lesion had been tender for about five years, and the preoperative roentgen impression was that of a bone cyst. The tumor was described as mucoid in the gross, and it shelled out readily. Its microscopic picture closely resembled that illustrated in Fig. 13-11.

Hemangiopericytomas less differentiated than the glomus tumor may also arise within bone. They appear to be distinctly unusual, although it is entirely possible that some of them, at least, are not recognized by the examining pathologist. In a discussion by Stout[34] in 1956 covering 197 hemangiopericytomas in general, three were cited that involved bone, although no details were given of these cases specifically. Dahlin[5] illustrated one hemangiopericytoma in an expanded ramus of a mandible, but gave no further details. In 1960, Marcial-Rojas[23] reported, in the clavicle of an 83-year-old woman, a primary hemangiopericytoma that metastasized to the lungs. I have had occasion to observe a hemangiopericytoma in a rib (as a resected specimen). It appeared four years after removal of a meningeal tumor of comparable cytology. The slides of both tumors were reviewed by Dr. A. P. Stout and Dr. H. M. Zimmerman, who concurred in the diagnosis of hemangiopericytoma (Fig. 13-12).

Tumors of bone of vascular origin 181

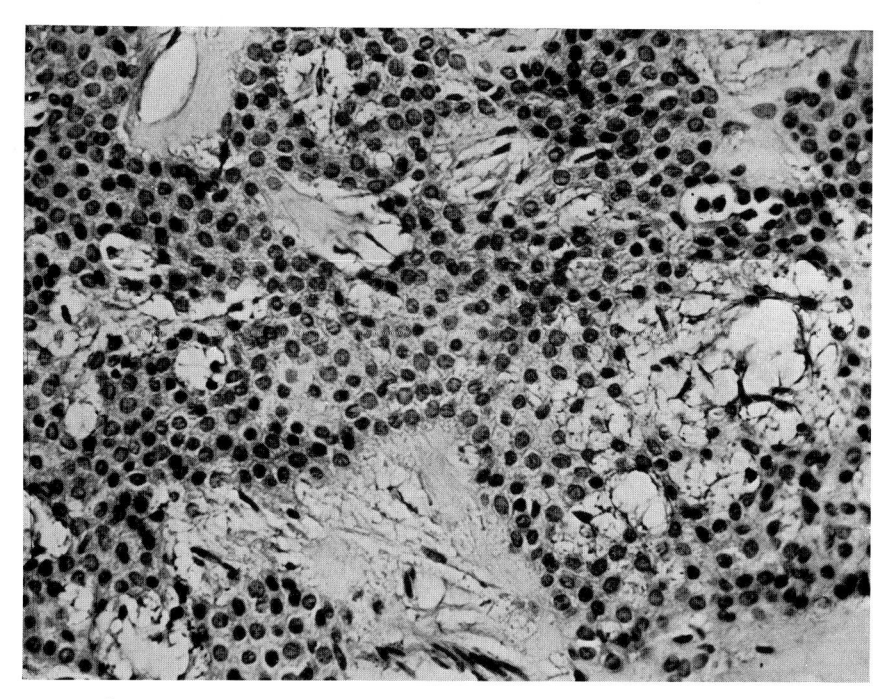

Fig. 13-11. Photomicrograph of a glomus tumor of a finger that eroded the terminal phalanx. (×250.)

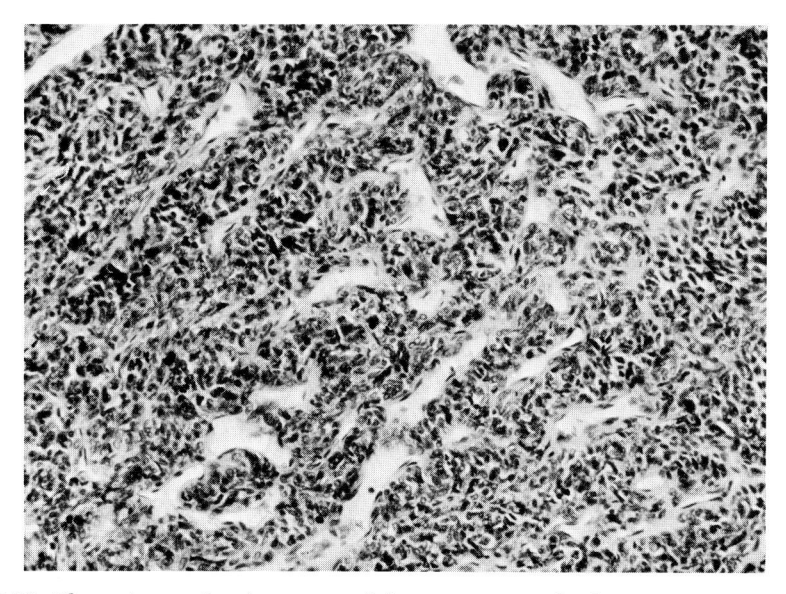

Fig. 13-12. Photomicrograph of an expanded tumor in a rib that was interpreted as a hemangiopericytoma. A meningeal neoplasm of comparable cytology had been removed four years previously. Drs. A. P. Stout and H. M. Zimmerman also saw the slides and concurred in our impression. (×160.)

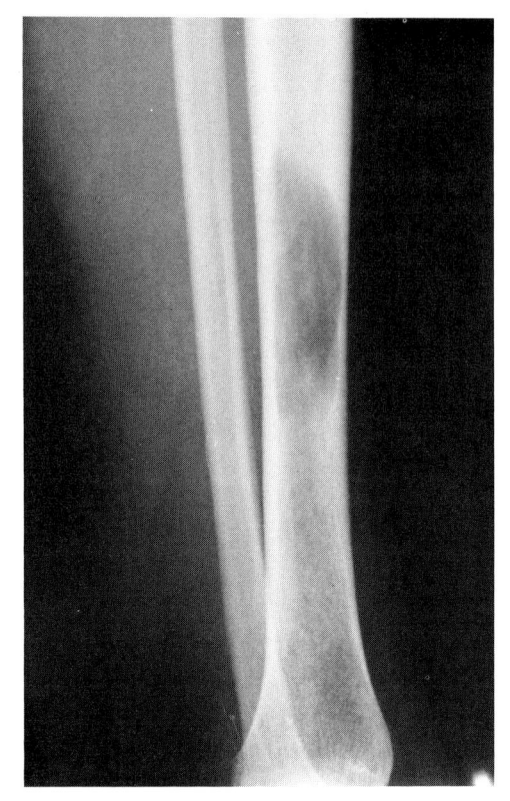

Fig. 13-13. Roentgenogram of a benign lesion in the shaft of a tibia, which on biopsy showed congeries of thin-walled vascular channels devoid of blood, and was interpreted, therefore, as a lymphangioma.

Lymphangioma

On rare occasions, one may encounter in bone a benign tumor of vascular origin in which the channels are completely devoid of blood, and which may logically be interpreted, therefore, as a lymphangioma.[27] I have observed only one such tumor, in the tibial shaft of an adult woman, which came to clinical notice after a pathologic fracture through the attenuated overlying cortex. Its roentgen picture (Fig. 13-13) was that of a nondescript, circumscribed, lucent defect.

More frequently encountered are instances of multiple lymphangiomas of bone (analogous to hemangiomatosis), as part of a congenital systemic disorder in which such extraskeletal manifestations as chylopericardium[12] or cystic hygromas of the neck and axilla[28] may also be present.

References

1. Bickel, W. H., and Broders, A. C.: Primary lymphangioma of the ilium; report of a case, J. Bone Joint Surg. 29:517, 1947.
2. Bucy, P., and Capp, C. S.: Primary hemangioma of bone with special reference to roentgenologic diagnosis, Am. J. Roentgenol. 23:1, 1930.
3. Bundens, W. D., Jr., and Brighton, C.

T.: Malignant hemangioendothelioma of bone, J. Bone Joint Surg. 47:762, 1965.
4. Campanacci, M., Cenni, F., and Giunti, A.: Angiectasie, Amartomi, E Neoplasmi Vascolari Dello Scheletro ("Angiomi", emangioendotelioma, emangiosarcoma), Chir. degli Organi Di Movimento 58 (Fasc. VI): 472, 1969.
5. Dahlin, D. C.: Bone tumors, Springfield, Ill., 1957, Charles C Thomas, Publisher (see p. 87).
6. Dorner, R. A., and Marcy, D. S.: Primary rib tumors. Survey of literature and a report of 7 additional cases, J. Thorac. Surg. 17:690, 1948.
7. Ewing, J.: Neoplastic diseases, ed. 4, Philadelphia, 1940, W. B. Saunders Co., p. 362.
8. Falkmer, S., and Tilling, G.: Primary lymphangioma of bone, Acta Orthop. Scand. (Fasc. 2) 25:99, 1956.
9. Fienberg, R., and Baehr, F. H.: Hemangioendothelioma of the tibia with metastasis to the popliteal artery, Arch. Pathol. 31: 811, 1941.
10. Geschickter, C. F., and Maseritz, I. H.: Primary hemangioma involving bones of the extremities, J. Bone Joint Surg. 20: 888, 1938.
11. Goidanich, I. F., and Campanacci, M.: Vascular hamartomata and infantile angioectatic osteohyperplasia of the extremities. A study of 94 cases, J. Bone Joint Surg. 44-A:815, 1962.
12. Goldstein, M. R., Benrchimol, A., Cornell, W., and Long, D. R.: Chylopericardium with multiple lymphangioma of bone, N. Engl. J. Med. 280:1034, 1969.
13. Gordon-Taylor, G., and Wiles, P.: Pulsating angio-endothelioma of the innominate bone treated by hindquarter amputation, J. Bone Joint Surg. 31-B:410, 1949.
14. Harris, R., and Prandoni, A. G.: Generalized primary lymphangiomas of bone; report of case associated with congenital lymphedema of forearm, Ann. Intern. Med. 33:1302, 1950.
15. Hartman, W. H., and Stewart, F. W.: Hemangioendothelioma of bone. Unusual tumor characterized by indolent course, Cancer 15:846, 1962.
16. Hauser, E. D. W., and Constant, G. A.: Skeletal hemangio-endothelioma. A case report, J. Bone Joint Surg. 30-A:517, 1948.
17. Hitzrot, J. M.: Hemangioma cavernosum of bone, Ann. Surg. 65:476, 1917.
18. Iglesias de la Torre, L., Gomez Camejo, M., and Palacios, G.: Considerationes clínicas, anatómicas, radiológicas y quirúrgicas del glomus tumoral de Masson; una observación, Cir. ortop. y traumatol., Habana 7:11, 1939.
19. Kleinsasser, O., and Albrecht, H.: Bei Hämangiome und Osteohämangiome der Schädelknocken, Langenbeck's Arch. ü Dtsch. Z. Chir. 285:115, 1957.
20. Lattes, R., and Bull, D. C.: A case of glomus tumor with primary involvement of bone, Ann. Surg. 127:187, 1948.
21. Lichtenstein, L.: Aneurysmal bone cyst. A pathological entity commonly mistaken for giant-cell tumor and occasionally for hemangioma and osteogenic sarcoma, Cancer 3:279, 1950.
22. Lutz, J. F., and Pusch, L. C.: Angio-endothelioma of bone, J.A.M.A. 113:1009, 1939.
23. Marcial-Rojas, R. A.: Primary hemangiopericytoma of bone. Review of the literature and report of the first case with metastases, Cancer 13:308, 1960.
24. Morgenstern, P., and Westing, S. W.: Malignant hemangio-endothelioma of bone. Fourteen-year follow-up in a case treated by radiation alone, Cancer 23:221, 1969.
25. Otis, J., Hutter, R. V. P., Foote, F. W., Jr., Marcove, R. C., and Stewart, F. W.: Hemangioendothelioma of bone, Surg. Gynecol. Obstet. 127:295, 1968.
26. Pollak, A.: Angiosarcoma of the sternum, Am. J. Surg. 77:522, 1949.
27. Schopfner, C. E., and Parker, A. R.: Lymphangioma of bone, Radiology 76:449, 1961.
28. Seckler, S. G., Rubin, H., and Rabinowitz, J. G.: Systemic cystic angiomatosis, Am. J. Med. 37:976, 1964.
29. Sherman, M. S.: Capillary hemangioma of bone, Arch. Pathol. 38:158, 1944.
30. Sherman, R. S., and Wilner, D.: The roentgen diagnosis of hemangioma of bone, Am. J. Roentgenol. 86:1146, 1961.
31. Stout, A. P.: Hemangio-endothelioma: A tumor of blood vessels featuring vascular endothelial cells, Ann. Surg. 118:445, 1943.
32. Stout, A. P.: Hemangiopericytoma. A study of 25 cases, Cancer 2:1027, 1949.
33. Stout, A. P.: Tumors of blood vessels, Texas State J. Med. 40:362, 1944.
34. Stout, A. P.: Tumors featuring pericytes; glomus tumor and hemangiopericytoma, Lab. Invest. 5:217, 1956.
35. Stout, A. P., and Murray, M. R.: Heman-

giopericytoma; a vascular tumor featuring Zimmerman's pericytes, Ann. Surg. **116**:26, 1942.
36. Thomas, A.: Vascular tumors of bone. A pathological and clinical study of twenty-seven cases, Surg. Gynecol. & Obstet. **74**:777, 1942.
37. Töpfer, D.: Ueber ein infiltrierend wachsendes Hämangiome der Haut und multiple Kapillarektasien der Haut und inneren Organe; zur Kenntnis der Wirbelangiome, Frankfurt. Ztschr. f. Path. **36**: 337, 1928.
38. Wallis, L. A., Asch, T., and Maisel, B. W.: Diffuse skeletal hemangiomatosis, Am. J. Med. **37**:545, 1964.
39. Watson, W. L., and McCarthy, W. D.: Blood and lymph vessel tumors. A report of 1056 cases, Surg. Gynecol. Obstet. **71**: 569, 1940.
40. Wyke, B. D.: Primary hemangioma of the skull: a rare cranial tumor, Am. J. Roentgenol. **61**:302, 1949.

Chapter 14

Tumors of nerve origin

Neurofibroma, ganglioneuroma, neurilemoma, malignant schwannoma

Inasmuch as bone as a structure is supplied by nerves, accompanying blood vessels for the most part, it is not surprising that one should occasionally encounter a neurofibroma or a neurilemoma (benign schwannian neoplasms), and rarely a malignant schwannoma arising within bone. In addition, one may observe comparable tumors, e.g., in Recklinghausen's neurofibromatosis, which appear to develop parosteally or within the periosteal connective tissue, and secondarily erode the cortex or even invade the medullary cavity of an affected bone.

Solitary neurofibromas within bone, comparable to those observed not infrequently in soft parts, are surprisingly rare, and one finds very little information in regard to them in the literature. I do not recall having observed more than one pertinent lesion, situated in a condyle of a humerus. It seems to be well established, however, that such tumors may occasionally develop in relation to bone as a manifestation of neurofibromatosis, though by no means as often as is generally assumed. As noted, they may develop subperiosteally and erode the underlying cortex, appearing roentgenographically as a blisterlike lesion between the eroded cortex and the elevated periosteum, whose inner surface may be delimited by a delicate shell of bone. Brooks and Lehman,[1] for example, have described a histologically proved, globular-shaped neurofibroma of this type, situated on the upper end of a tibia. Comparable instances in a number of sites have been recorded by Holt and Wright,[10] McCarroll,[13] and Hensley,[9] among others. It may be noted that I have observed a number of similar periosteal neurofibromas in patients without any apparent manifestations of Recklinghausen's disease (Figs. 14-1 and 14-2). Very occasionally also in neurofibromatosis, a neurofibroma may develop within the interior of a bone, and Uhlmann and Grossman[18] have reported what appears to be a tumor in point (in a 16-year-old girl, presenting a loculated, rarefied lesion in a mandible). Another pertinent instance in the case records of the Massachusetts General Hospital[2] is that of a comparatively large, slowly expanding neurofibroma in the right portion of the sacrum in a 54-year-old woman. The tumor had destroyed the first three segments.

There had been a five-year history of increasing involvement of the sacral nerve roots before the tumor was surgically extirpated.

Mention should also be made here of an apparently unique case of mature ganglioneuromas in multiple bone sites (a humerus, an ulna, a tibia, and a vertebral body) reported by Wilber and Woodcock.[19] In interpreting remarkable cases such as this, one must consider the possibility, as Goldman, Winterling, and Winterling[6] have suggested, that the ganglioneuromas may conceivably have resulted from the maturation of old neuroblastoma metastases.

As for the specific nerve sheath tumor (neurilemoma, neurinoma, schwannoma), it, too, is observed as a primary central bone tumor only on rare occasions, although precisely why this should be so is not altogether clear. Thus,

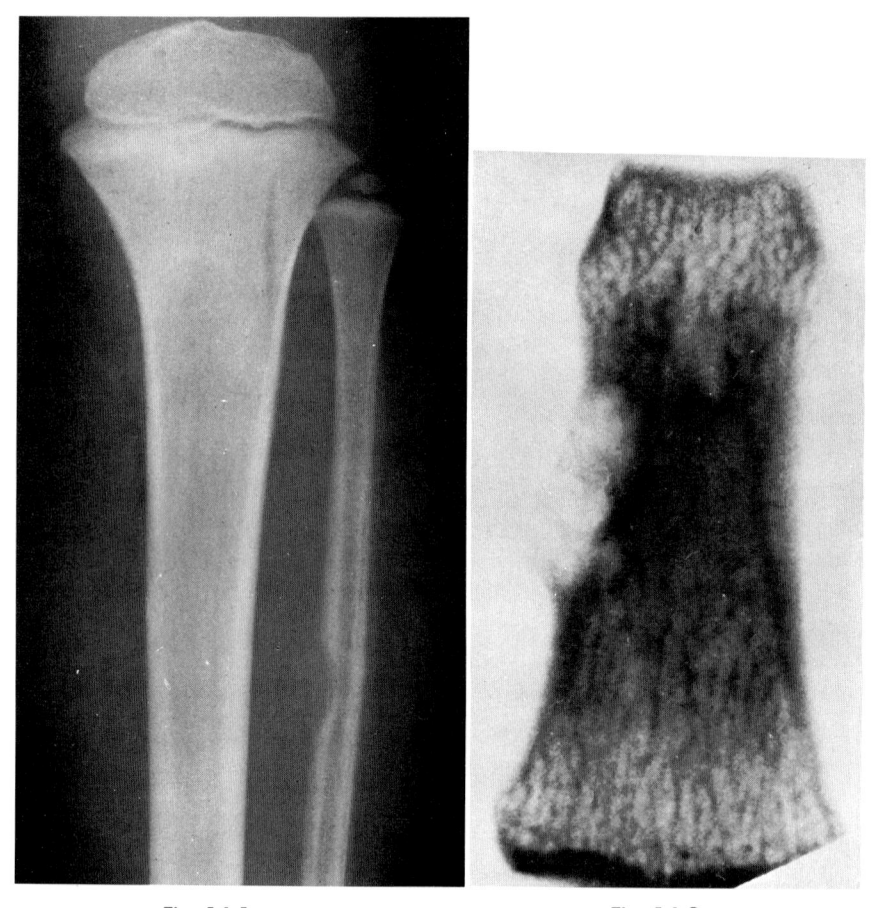

Fig. 14-1

Fig. 14-2

Fig. 14-1. Roentgenogram showing, in the shaft of a fibula, a defect caused by a neurofibroma arising apparently in the periosteum. The convex dome of this blisterlike lesion was more clearly outlined in the original x-ray film.

Fig. 14-2. Roentgenogram (enlarged from a Kodachrome reproduction) of another periosteal neurofibroma that eroded a phalanx of a finger (of a young woman). Local surgical excision afforded relief of pain.

Stout[16] in a survey of some 246 cases of peripheral nerve sheath tumors, including 52 of his own, did not mention a single instance in which the tumor was encountered in bone. There are, however, a few such cases reported in the literature, in none of which were any stigmas of generalized neurofibromatosis observed. The first of these, reported by Gross, Bailey, and Jacox,[7] deals with a neurilemoma of the shaft of a humerus in a 30-year-old woman who had been aware of an aching lump on her arm for about three years. Roentgenograms revealed a well-outlined, though rather nondescript, ovoid area of rarefaction, with some erosion also of the contiguous cortex and periosteal new bone apposition at the lower angle of the lesion. At exploration, a soft, fleshy, slightly fasciculated, ovoid, well-encapsulated tumor, about 2 by 1 by 1 cm., was found at the site indicated, apparently arising in the interior of the bone. Microscopically, the tumor presented a palisaded architecture, as seen commonly in neurilemomas of peripheral nerve sheaths, although the authors designated the tumor as a neurofibroma. Another case, reported by DeSanto and Burgess,[4] deals with a comparable tumor in the midshaft of an ulna of a 37-year-old man, who, interestingly enough, had sustained no fewer than five pathologic fractures over a period of eight years before the lesion was resected. It is interesting to note also that the tumor was not particularly painful. The initial x-ray examination showed a somewhat eccentric, hemispherical area of rarefaction, with localized expansion of its cortical contour. At surgery, it was noted that the tumor appeared to arise

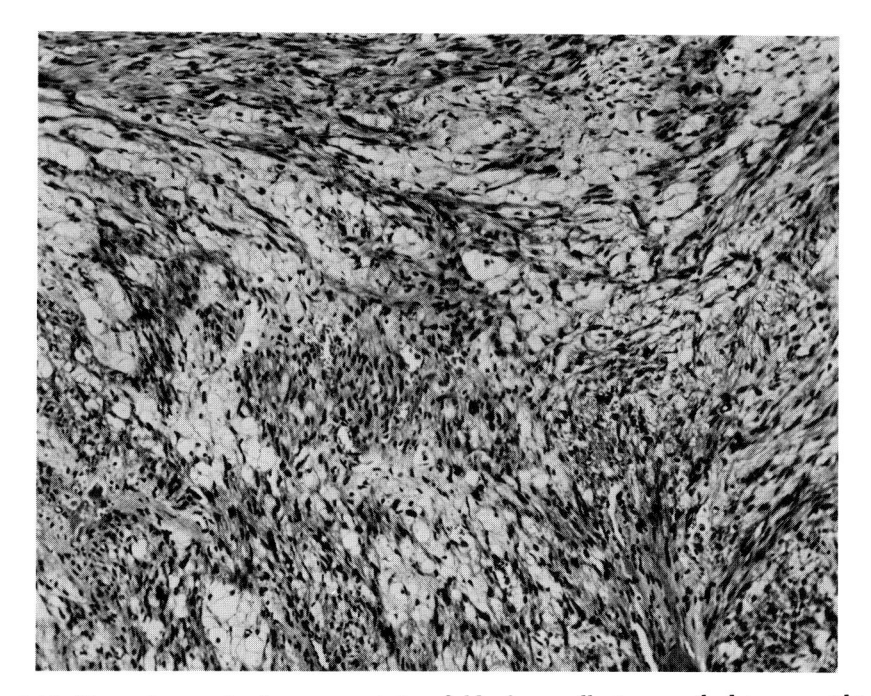

Fig. 14-3. Photomicrograph of a representative field of a small circumscribed tumor within a patella, which was interpreted as a neurilemoma. Such tumors are rarely encountered in bone, as noted.

from, and grow out of, the shaft of the ulna, and the illustrative photomicrographs leave no doubt that it was a typical neurilemoma. The same authors also described an unusual instance of a neurilemoma arising from the dorsal root of the fifth lumbar nerve and invading the right sacral wing secondarily, producing a large irregular defect in the first and second sacral segments. This tumor, though comparatively large for a neurilemoma (6 by 4 cm.), was circumscribed, and the authors emphasize that bone erosion is not per se indicative of malignancy. On the other hand, it is possible for such tumors to be malignant, and I recall a remarkable autopsy specimen of a spine, which showed erosion of a number of vertebral bodies by malignant schwannomas developing in a case of Recklinghausen's neurofibromatosis.

Apropos of neurilemoma of bone also, I have observed another pertinent instance of a small, circumscribed, surgically extirpated tumor developing within a patella, the whorled, palisaded histologic pattern of which was clearly that of a nerve sheath tumor (Fig. 14-3). Still another beautifully illustrated and well-documented case is that reported by Jones,[12] dealing with a neurilemoma of a metacarpal bone. The involved bone area was resected, and a graft was used for reconstruction, with a good functional result. A neurilemoma in a sacrum was illustrated by Jaffe,[11] and one in a mandible by Schroff.[15] In a survey of the Mayo Clinic material, Fawcett and Dahlin[5] found some seven instances in point, four of them in the mandible.

In regard to malignant schwannoma of bone, one of the few well-documented relevant accounts that I can find in the literature is that of Peers.[14] This deals with a tumor situated again in the midshaft of a long bone (an ulna) in a 55-year-old man. The tumor was labeled as a primary intramedullary neurogenic sarcoma (perineural fibroblastoma). The cytology of this tumor seems clearly to establish its schwannian character. Amputation was performed in the belief that it was malignant, and the follow-up did not extend beyond twenty months. Another comparable instance is that reported by Güthert[8] of a malignant neurinoma in the midshaft of a humerus of a 20-year-old man. The tumor was comparatively small but had extended through a cortical perforation into the contiguous soft parts, so that it was deemed necessary to amputate the affected limb. Many fields of the tumor were still clearly recognizable as neurinoma microscopically.

With respect to nomenclature and, in particular, to the use of the term "neurogenic sarcoma," it is relevant to cite the conviction of Stout[17] that this term is ill conceived and should be abandoned as confusing and obstructive. He maintains rather forcefully that tumors called neurogenic sarcomas (if they are not fibrosarcomas starting from fascial and other tissues outside the nerve and secondarily involving it) are actually malignant schwannomas and should be so designated. According to this view, there is no sound basis for the supposition that there is a special variety of nerve fibrosarcoma that can be designated a "neurogenic sarcoma."

The paucity in the literature of malignant schwannomas arising in bone is somewhat puzzling, although it is possible that such neoplasms go unrecognized for the most part, as Stout points out, through unfamiliarity with the remarkable versatility of schwannian cells. These cells by metaplasia are said to be capable of producing a wide variety of tissues (cartilage, bone, fat, striated muscle, etc.) not ordinarily thought of as being derived from them. Obviously, this consideration raises many subtle problems in differential diagnosis and, unfortunately, most pathologists do not have facilities for tissue culture studies at their disposal.

References

1. Brooks, B., and Lehman, E. P.: The bone changes in von Recklinghausen's neurofibromatosis, Surg. Gynecol. Obstet. 38:587, 1924.
2. Case Records of the Massachusetts General Hospital, Case 45102, N. Engl. J. Med. 260:496, 1959.
3. Dahlin, D. C.: Bone tumors, Springfield, Ill., 1957, Charles C Thomas, Publisher, p. 95.
4. DeSanto, D. A., and Burgess, E.: Primary and secondary neurilemmoma of bone, Surg. Gynecol. Obstet. 71:454, 1940.
5. Fawcett, K. J., and Dahlin, D. C.: Neurilemoma of bone, Am. J. Clin. Pathol. 47:759, 1967.
6. Goldman, R. L., Winterling, A. N., and Winterling, C. C.: Maturation of tumors of the sympathetic nervous system. Report of long-term survival in 2 patients, one with disseminated osseous metastases, and review of cases from the literature, Cancer 18:1510, 1965.
7. Gross, P., Bailey, F. R., and Jacox, H. W.: Primary intramedullary neurofibroma of the humerus, Arch. Pathol. 28:716, 1939.
8. Güthert, H.: Ein malignes Neurinom des Knochen, Zentralbl. Allg. Pathol. 88:185, 1952.
9. Hensley, C. D., Jr.: The rapid development of a "subperiosteal bone cyst" in multiple neurofibromatosis; a case report, J. Bone Joint Surg. 35-A:197, 1953.
10. Holt, J. F., and Wright, E. M.: The radiologic features of neurofibromatosis, Radiology 51:647, 1948.
11. Jaffe, H. L.: Tumors and tumors conditions of the bones and joints, Philadelphia, 1958, Lea & Febiger (see Fig. 73).
12. Jones, H. M.: Neurilemmoma of bone, Brit. J. Surg. 41:63, 1953.
13. McCarroll, H. R.: Clinical manifestations of congenital neurofibromatosis, J. Bone Joint Surg. 32-A:601-617, 626, 1950.
14. Peers, J. H.: Primary intramedullary neurogenic sarcoma of ulna, Am. J. Pathol. 10:811, 1934.
15. Schroff, J.: Solitary neurofibroma of the oral cavity (neurilemmoma, neurinoma), Am. J. Dent. 32:199, 1945.
16. Stout, A. P.: The peripheral manifestations of the specific nerve sheath tumor (neurilemoma), Am. J. Cancer 24:751, 1935.
17. Stout, A. P.: Tumors of the peripheral nervous system, J. Missouri Med. Assoc. 46:255, 1949.
18. Uhlmann, E., and Grossman, A.: Von Recklinghausen's neurofibromatosis with bone manifestations, Ann. Intern. Med. 14:225, 1940.
19. Wilber, M. C., and Woodcock, J. A.: Ganglioneuromata in bone. Report of a case, J. Bone Joint Surg. 39-A:1385, 1957.

Chapter 15

Chondrosarcoma of bone

The family of benign and malignant cartilage tumors is a large one and includes not only central and peripheral tumors in bone, but also those arising in the periosteum, in synovial joints and tendon sheaths, in the cartilage of the larynx, bronchi,[7] nose, etc., and in soft parts,[11,12] particularly in the hand and foot and rarely in the muscle or connective tissue of the lower extremity. This is not surprising, if one considers that phylogenetically the major part of the skeleton is preformed in cartilage and that the capacity for cartilage formation, as well as bone formation, appears to be inherent in all paraskeletal connective tissue. Each member of this large family has its own rules of biologic behavior that can only be ascertained empirically, and generalizations may have little validity. Thus the rules we laid down in 1943[21] for the recognition of early chondrosarcoma apply strictly to tumors *in* bone and particularly to central chondrosarcoma.

This chapter will deal specifically with the largest and most important group of malignant cartilage tumors of bone, and some of the others will be considered briefly in later chapters. Chondrosarcoma of bone may arise either in the interior of the medullary cavity (central) or through malignant growth of the cartilage cap of an osteochondroma (peripheral), usually in patients with hereditary multiple exostosis, and this distinction has important implications for therapy. Amputation is mandatory for a central chondrosarcoma, in a limb bone for example, whereas cure of a peripheral chondrosarcoma can often be achieved by adequate local excision, without sacrificing the affected part. The central chondrosarcomas may arise *de novo* or through malignant change in a preexisting enchondroma. The latter hazard is substantially greater in patients with skeletal enchondromatosis (Ollier's disease).

On rare occasions, a central chondrosarcoma may develop as an unfortunate sequel of therapeutic irradiation (as may osteosarcoma or fibrosarcoma).[6,14,27] I have observed a chondrosarcoma that developed in a lower rib of a girl of 11, some eight years after irradiation of the site of a Wilms' tumor. I have also had occasion to see material from a chondrosarcoma that appeared in a distal femur six years after irradiation of a Ewing's tumor[27] (see page 272 for further details). The development of chondrosarcoma in Paget bone has also been observed,[22] although this is distinctly unusual. It may also be noted here that chondrosarcoma of bone can be induced experimentally in rabbits by the intravenous administration of certain beryllium compounds, and such tumors can be transplanted successfully to the anterior chamber of the eye.[16]

The peripheral chondrosarcomas are composed uniformly of actively growing facets of mature hyaline cartilage. Most of the central chondrosarcomas are likewise composed of well-differentiated hyaline cartilage, but in some it is only partially differentiated or more myxoid, and in a few it is poorly differentiated or mesenchymal in character. These latter tumors, which may be designated as chondroid, have already been discussed in Chapter 8.

That the pathologic appraisal and appropriate therapy of cartilage tumors continue to give pathologists and clinicians cause for concern is evidenced by the fact that more than fifty chondrosarcomas of bone were submitted for opinion in recent years. (This is in addition to many benign and malignant cartilage tumors in skeletal soft parts.) As many as eight of these were in children or teen-agers, and these were mainly of poorly differentiated or primitive type, rather than the conventional ones composed of faceted hyaline cartilage. More than a few were in unusual sites, e.g., the lumbar spine and sacrum, the bones of the hand and foot, the nasal bones, or the skull bones. Some were submitted because delay in the pathologic recognition of chondrosarcoma had led to formidable problems in clinical management; others, because the pathologic indications of malignancy were borderline or subtle, rather than obvious; still others, particularly the poorly differentiated ones with myxoid fields, because they were confused with chondromyxoid fibroma.

The basic differences between chondrosarcoma and osteogenic sarcoma are now generally appreciated, and the insistence upon their clear separation is important clinically, insofar as treatment and prognosis are concerned. Chondrosarcoma ordinarily pursues a much slower course, not metastasizing to the lungs for years, while osteogenic sarcoma has often already metastasized by the time it is recognized (even though roentgenograms of the chest may still appear negative). The basic anatomic difference is that chondrosarcoma develops out of full-fledged cartilage (though not necessarily hyaline cartilage), while osteogenic sarcoma issues from more primitive tissue, developing out of bone-forming mesenchyme. Ordinarily, in an osteogenic sarcoma, most of the proliferating connective tissue, which may be quite anaplastic, becomes converted into neoplastic osteoid tissue and bone directly, though it usually also forms some neoplastic cartilage, which in turn tends to undergo rapid calcification and ossification. In an occasional osteogenic sarcoma, osteogenesis may even proceed predominantly via the cartilage stage, and cartilage may thus be a prominent feature in the histologic composition of the lesion. However, even in such an osteogenic sarcoma, if one does not limit one's scrutiny to a small field of the tumor, and particularly to the periphery of it, one will also see that in other places the basic proliferating connective tissue is merging directly into neoplastic osteoid tissue and bone. On the other hand, in a chondrosarcoma, though large areas of the hyaline matrix may have become myxomatous or even calcified and ossified, the basic proliferating tissue of the tumor is full-fledged cartilage. In contrast to osteogenic sarcoma, properly so-called, chondrosarcoma never shows neoplastic osteoid tissue and bone evolving directly from a sarcomatous stroma.

There was a tendency in the past[5,9,10,17,20] to underrate the potential seriousness of actively growing cartilage tumors until their aggressive clinical behavior could no longer be ignored or until their histologic picture (as seen in surgical specimens) had become crudely and obviously sarcomatous. At this stage, unfortunately, the chances for cure, even by drastic measures, may be sharply reduced. As we showed in 1943,[21] subtle but telltale histologic indications of malignant change are already present even in the early stage of the evolution of a chondrosarcoma of bone. They may have to be searched for, particularly in an early lesion, but in any case they can be recognized if adequate material is examined and proper significance attached to relatively inconspicuous cytologic abnormalities. Keiller,[18] in 1925, pointed out clearly the importance of attention to details regarding the cells (and particularly the cell nuclei) as a means of distinguishing between benign and malignant cartilage growths. Our own experience has taught us that a cartilage tumor is no longer to be regarded as benign if, when viable noncalcifying areas are examined, it shows, even in scattered fields: (1) many cells with plump nuclei, (2) more than an occasional cell with two such nuclei, and especially (3) giant cartilage cells with large single or multiple nuclei or with clumps of chromatin. The importance of making the correct diagnosis early resides in the relative amenability of chondrosarcomas in accessible sites to early radical surgical treatment. The criteria indicated have gained wide empirical acceptance, and their validity has been supported by the observations of O'Neal and Ackerman,[25] Dahlin, Barnes and Catto,[3] and others who have reviewed and analyzed their own hospital material.

For the examining pathologist, I would stress the following useful rule. Sample the tissue submitted generously (concentrating on areas that are viable and not heavily calcified or ossified), scan all the sections meticulously (using high magnification, as indicated), and judge the tumor by the worst-looking areas in it, since these are a portent of what the entire tumor will look like eventually. The finding of even occasional fields showing cartilage-cell nuclei of the type described above should suffice for a diagnosis of early chondrosarcoma. The absence of mitotic figures is of little importance. In recurrent tumors, these cytologic indications of atypical active growth will, of course, become more obvious. Late in the evolution of a chondrosarcoma, one may occasionally see spindle-cell fields as an expression of dedifferentiation.

Considerable interest has been evinced in the subject of chondrosarcoma in recent years, and for additional comment on its clinical and pathologic aspects, the reader may have recourse to the extensive case material published by Ackerman and Spjut,[1] Henderson and Dahlin,[15] and Barnes and Catto,[3] among others. The last paper is particularly recommended for its astute, objective comment, as well as its bibliography.

Clinical features
Age and sex incidence and localization

Most of the patients with chondrosarcoma have reached adult life, although some may be children or adolescents, as noted. The majority are between 30 and 60 years of age. The disorder appears to be somewhat more frequent in males.

The large limb bones (particularly the femur, the tibia, and the humerus), the scapula, the ribs, and the innominate bone are the most common sites. Malignant change in solitary enchondromas of bones of the hand and foot is not as unusual as was once thought, and in patients with skeletal enchondromatosis it is, of course, fairly common. I have seen at least half a dozen instances in recent years in which biopsy of a central cartilage tumor in one or another of the tubular bones of the hand and foot showed evidence of early malignant change by the usual pathologic criteria (Figs. 5-2 and 15-9, A). Other less common sites are the vertebral column, the nose, the maxilla, and the bones of the skull (particularly at the base, which is preformed in cartilage).

The cartilage tumors arising in the nose that I have seen in consultation (some five in number) have all been malignant and presented a formidable problem in treatment. The most recent one, for example, was a chondrosarcoma in a child of 3. It had spread to the maxilla, antrum, and orbital floor and would have required an extensive, mutilating resection for any attempt at cure.

The cartilage tumors arising at the base of the skull,[24] on the other hand, as I have encountered them, have been more slowly growing and circumscribed chondrosarcomas (of somewhat varied cytology), which at least permitted substantial partial removal affording relief of symptoms.

Clinical findings

In most of our cases the patients had already had a long but not dramatic history at the time of admission. This was true irrespective of the bone affected and of the central or peripheral origin of the chondrosarcoma. On the whole, the history tended to be longer in the cases of peripheral chondrosarcoma. Very short histories, associated with a rapidly fatal clinical course, are clearly exceptional. Thus, in a case of peripheral chondrosarcoma that evolved from a costal osteochondroma, the patient stated that for twelve years she had been aware of a painless mass that grew slowly to the size of an egg. In a case in which the chondrosarcoma (a huge one) developed from an osteochondroma of a tibia, the patient stated that for twenty-four years he had been conscious of a slowly enlarging but not disabling tumor mass in the upper part of the leg. In another case of peripheral chondrosarcoma of an innominate bone there was an eight-year history of a slowly progressive tumorous enlargement associated with scarcely any clinical difficulty.

While the histories in the cases of central chondrosarcoma tend to be somewhat shorter, it is not unusual in such cases for the history to date back several years. For instance, in one of the cases of central chondrosarcoma of a femur, the patient stated that he had had dull, aching, local pains at intervals for five years, with exacerbations from time to time. It was not until he accidentally palpated a mass along the lateral aspect of this femur that he sought medical care. On the other hand, in another case in which the chondrosarcoma was in a femur, the complaint was of only six months' standing. This patient gave a history of pain and functional disability in the region of the knee, worse at times, but never bad enough to confine him to bed. In one of the cases of central chondrosarcoma of an innominate bone, there was a five-year history of moderate and intermittent pain and disability in the region of the hip joint, associated with pains shooting down the entire leg.

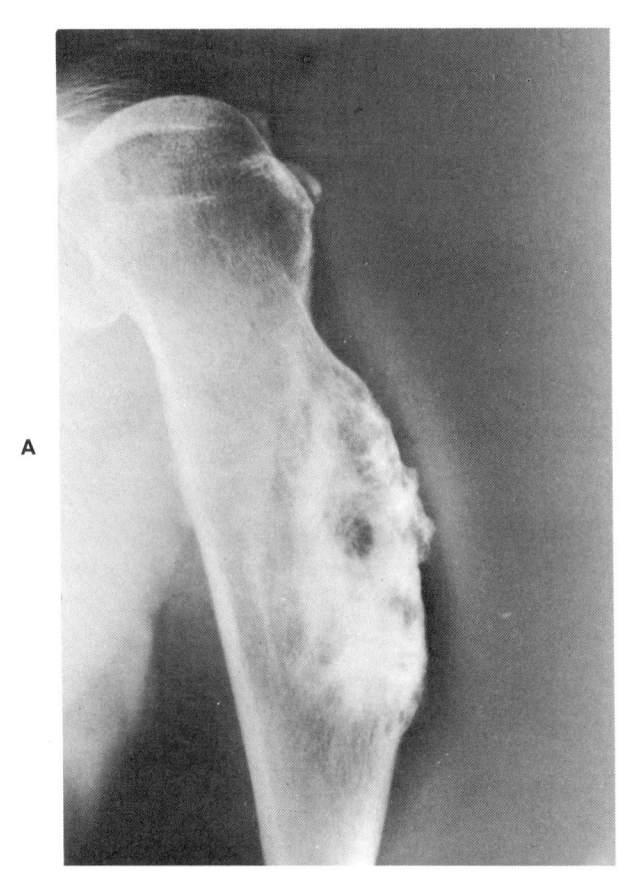

Fig. 15-1. **A**, Roentgenogram showing an unusual peripheral chondrosarcoma on the upper shaft of a humerus that developed through malignant change in the cartilage cap of a *solitary* osteocartilaginous exostosis. **B**, Roentgenogram of a peripheral chondrosarcoma growing out from an iliac bone. The vague outline of the tumor mass may give the observer a false impression of invasiveness and inoperability. **C**, Roentgenogram of a slice of the surgically extirpated neoplasm demonstrating that it is actually well circumscribed and that only the calcified areas are clearly discernible in the clinical x-ray film. **D**, Low-power photomicrograph of a peripheral field of the chondrosarcoma illustrated in **B** and **C**, showing focal calcification within facets of hyaline cartilage. Close scrutiny of many high-power fields is usually necessary to demonstrate significant atypism of cartilage-cell nuclei. (See also Fig. 15-2, *C*.)

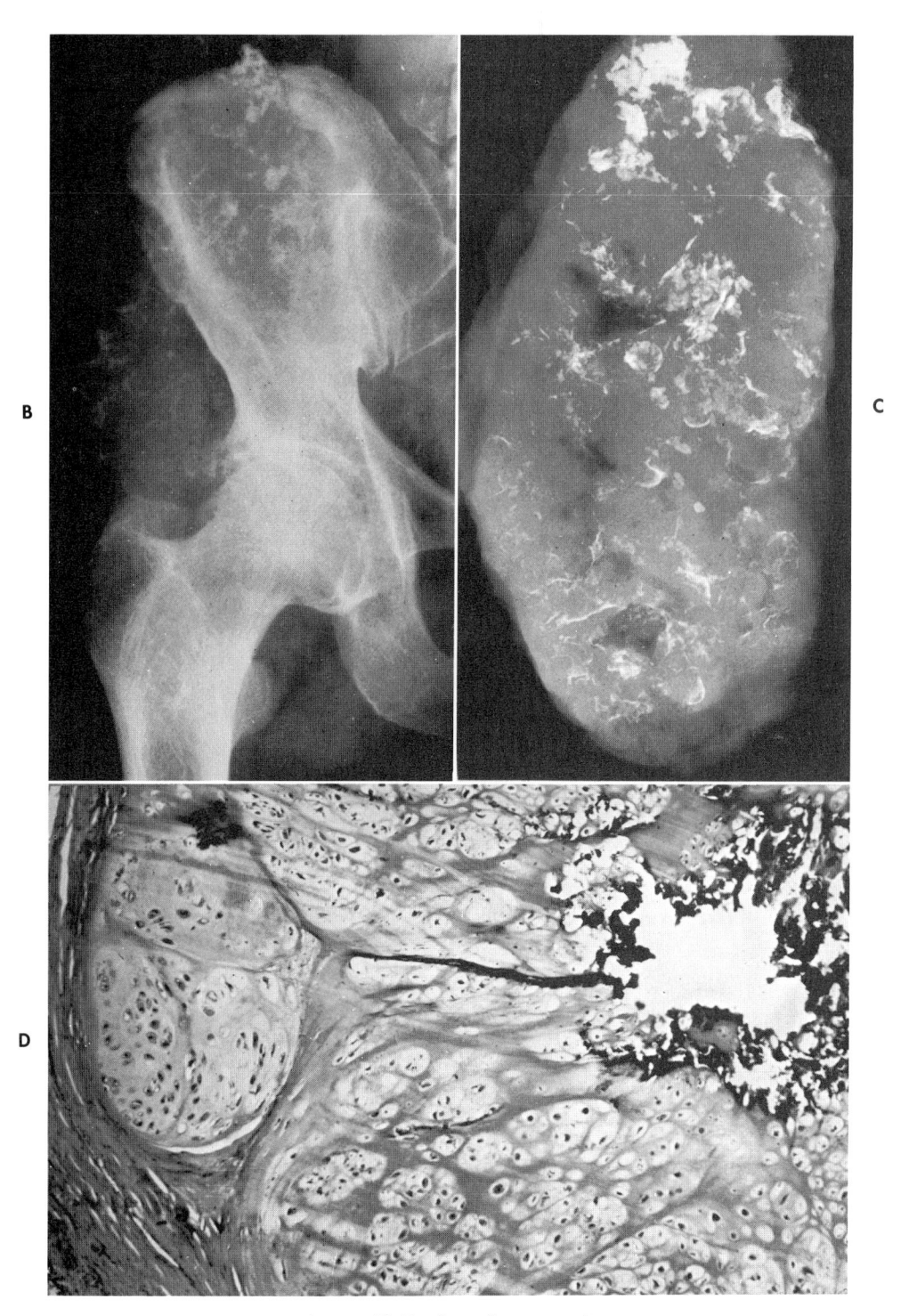

Fig. 15-1, cont'd. For legend see opposite page.

Physical examination in most instances revealed some enlargement of the area affected. The enlarged part was firm or bone hard, usually not very tender, and the overlying skin was never red or warm. When the area involved was near a joint, the latter was likely to be found somewhat swollen and its motion somewhat restricted.

Significance of trauma

Although one must be critical of the role of trauma in the development of bone tumors in general, in dealing with chondrosarcoma specifically I have been impressed by the frequency with which an injury was followed, after a reasonable interval, by malignant change. This is only an impression, however, and is not susceptible to statistical proof.

Roentgenographic findings

The roentgenographic findings may go far toward confirming the suspicion, perhaps already aroused by the history and physical findings, that one is dealing with a chondrosarcoma. Certainly, a long bone presenting an irregularly mottled and calcified shadow in its interior and a fuzzy area of localized destruction of the cortex should make one suspect tumor of this type. This suspicion is all the more justified if, where the cortex is undergoing destruction, it is somewhat thickened in part or throughout and is overlaid by tissue casting an abnormal shadow.

In the absence of mottling and calcification as a clue to the cartilaginous nature of a central bone lesion, it may not be clear at all that a given malignant tumor in a long bone is a chondrosarcoma.

The peripheral chondrosarcomas are, on the whole, not difficult to single out. A benign osteochondroma, whether small or large, presents roentgenographically a more or less uniform texture and a well-defined peripheral outline, beyond which there are no abnormal shadows. In contrast, an osteochondroma that has undergone transformation into a chondrosarcoma presents a dense, blotchy appearance over a considerable area, usually associated with the presence of more ragged, irregular radiopaque streaks extending away from the main part of the lesion. It is the older part of the tumor, particularly, that is prone to manifest heavy calcification and ossification.

Central chondrosarcoma

As noted, a chondrosarcoma within the interior of an affected bone may develop as a primary malignancy or, secondarily, through insidious malignant change in a preexisting enchondroma, which may be of long standing. Primary chondrosarcoma is encountered commonly, in the innominate bone, for example. Malignant change in an enchondroma is observed more often in large limb bones, notably the femur, upper tibia, and humerus, than in the peripheral small bones of the hand and foot. The onset of pain in a patient with an old enchondroma and the demonstration of cortical perforation roentgenographically may be indi-

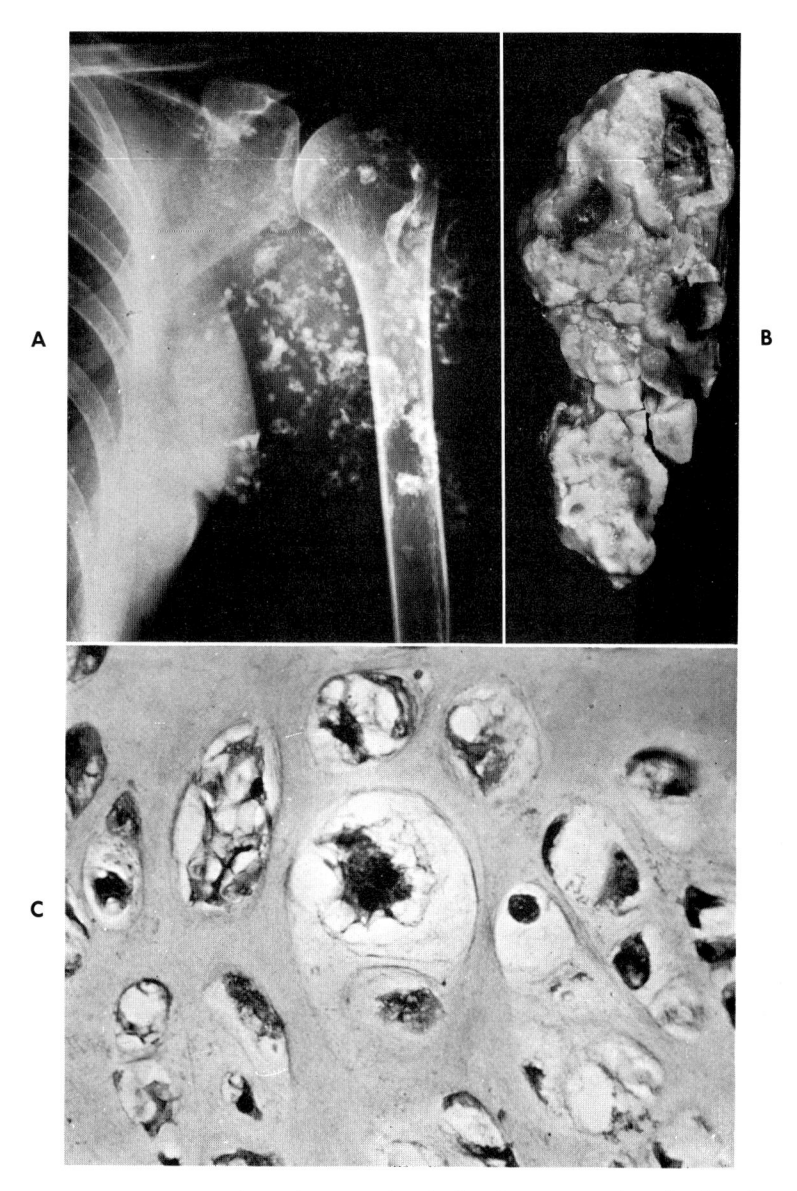

Fig. 15-2. **A**, Roentgenogram of another peripheral chondrosarcoma that developed originally from the cartilage cap of an osteochondroma on the upper shaft of the humerus. This represents a third recurrence of the chondrosarcoma after surgical removal over a period of about ten years. Despite the ominous impression created by the roentgenogram, it was possible to extirpate the neoplasm completely without resorting to radical resection. **B**, Photograph (appreciably reduced) of a representative slice of the peripheral chondrosarcoma illustrated in **A**. The tumor is composed of facets of whitish hyaline cartilage showing focal areas of softening, as well as calcification. **C**, Photomicrograph of a field showing a cartilage cell with two plump nuclei. (×250.)

cations of early malignant changes. In patients with skeletal enchondromatosis (Ollier's disease) the hazard of malignant change in one or more enchondromas is always present, and any rapid tumorous enlargement must be viewed with suspicion.

Peripheral chondrosarcoma

As indicated, chondrosarcoma may also develop through malignant change in the cartilage cap of an osteochondroma. In dealing with a solitary osteochondroma, whatever its location may be, this complication is very unusual, and its incidence has been estimated at something less than 1% (Fig. 15-1, A). In patients with hereditary multiple exostosis, however, the incidence of malignant

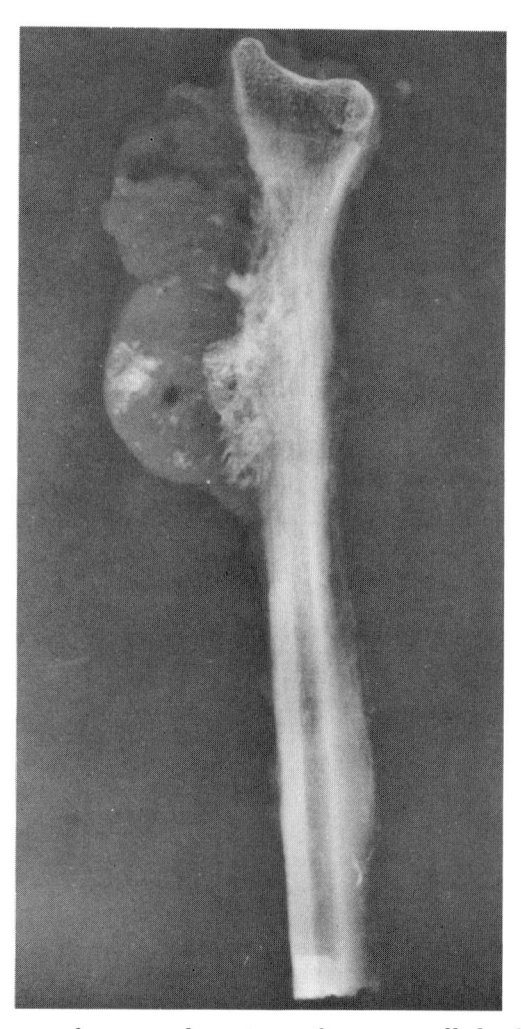

Fig. 15-3. Roentgenogram of a resected specimen of an upper fibula showing a peripheral chondrosarcoma. The radiopaque foci reflect calcification and secondary ossification of tumor cartilage.

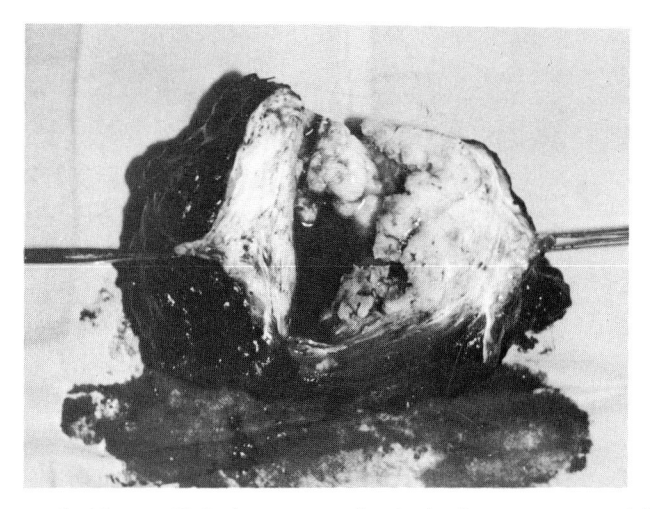

Fig. 15-4. Photograph (from a Kodachrome reproduction) of a recurrent peripheral chondrosarcoma of a scapula.

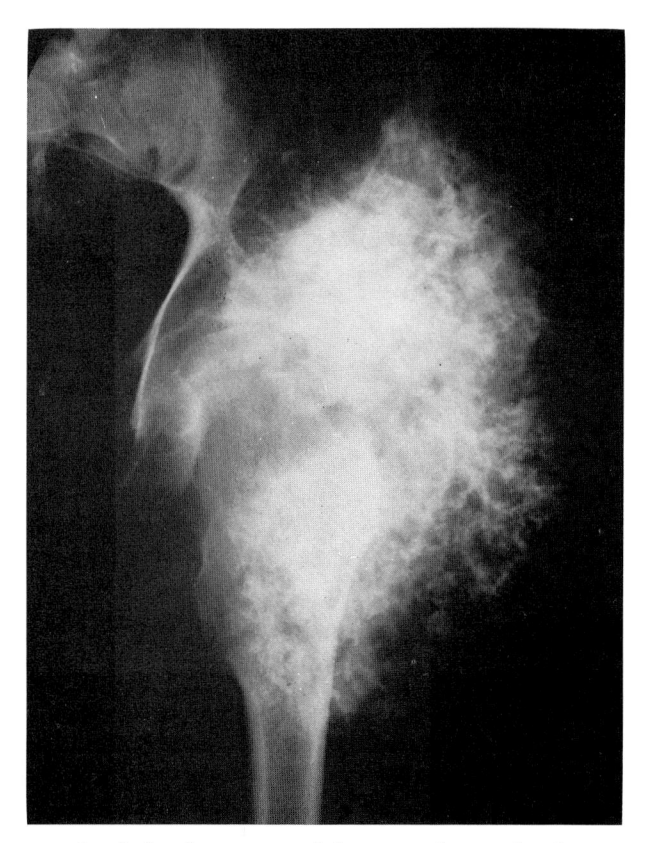

Fig. 15-5. Large peripheral chondrosarcoma of the upper femur, developing in a 28-year-old man who had shown multiple exostoses since childhood. The tumor had been enlarging steadily for some five years, and, when extirpated, was found to measure as much as 30 cm. in its greatest dimension.

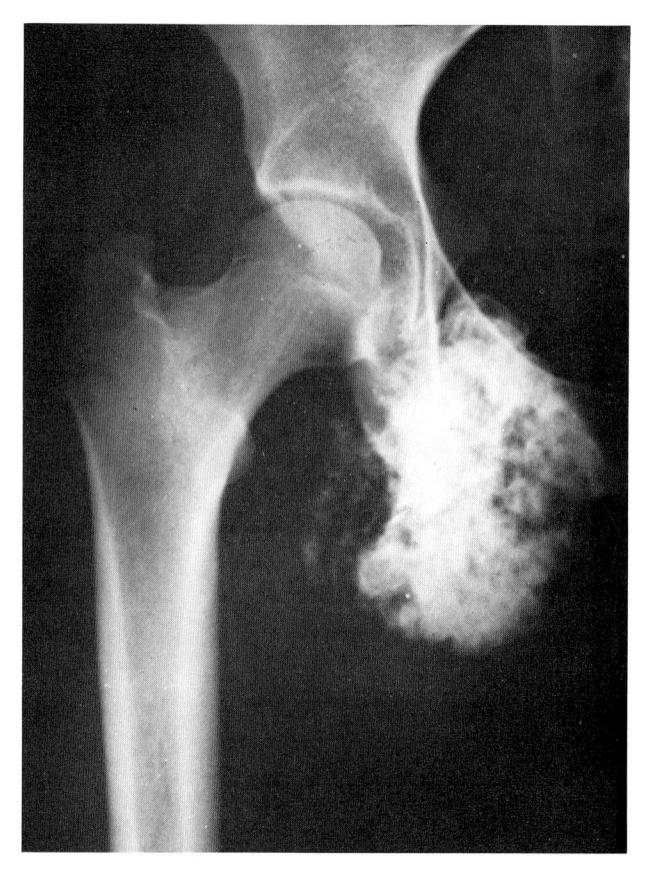

Fig. 15-6. Early chondrosarcoma arising in the right ischium of a 26-year-old woman. The tumor had been gradually enlarging for about one year, and the patient sought treatment mainly because it interfered with sitting. Such tumors, if they are not extirpated while still operable, tend to enlarge steadily over a period of years and may eventually attain huge size.

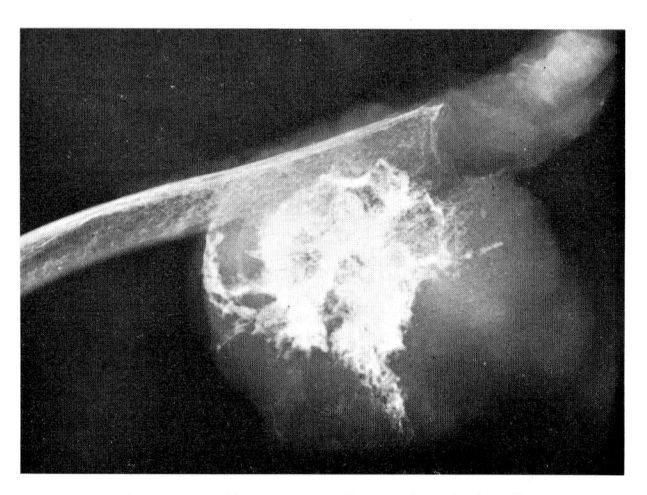

Fig. 15-7. Roentgenogram of a surgically extirpated peripheral chondrosarcoma protruding from the inner aspect of a rib. Only the older, central portion of the tumor is heavily calcified. This neoplasm developed insidiously and was discovered by chance in a chest film taken because the patient had developed pneumothorax following an injury. The pleura was not yet invaded by tumor, and the prospect for cure in this instance is good.

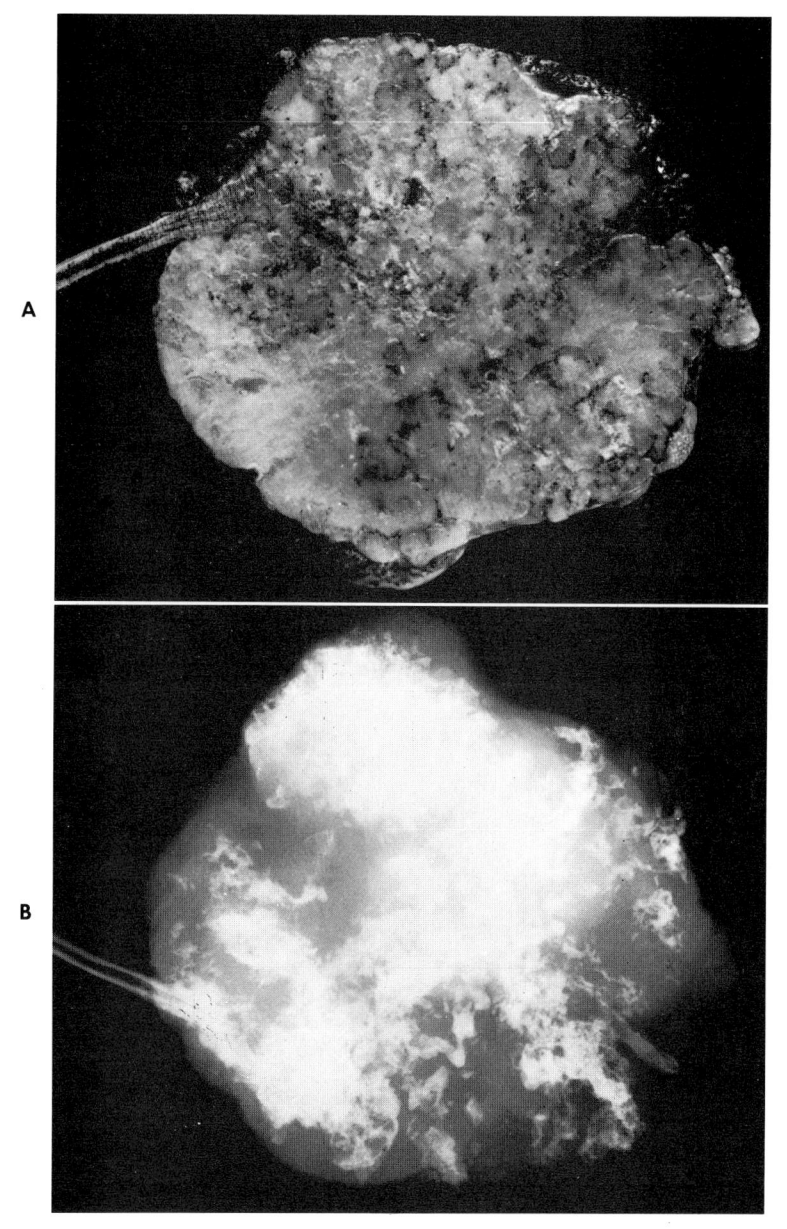

Fig. 15-8. A, Photograph (reduced to one-half natural size) of another surgically extirpated chondrosarcoma of a rib, which had been slowly enlarging in the chest wall for several years. It is not possible to trace the evolution of a chondrosarcoma that is so far advanced. (Compare with tumor illustrated in Fig. 15-7.) B, Roentgenogram of the chondrosarcoma illustrated in A, emphasizing the presence of foci of heavy calcification and ossification throughout the neoplasm. At the follow-up four years after resection, this patient was well and apparently free of tumor.

202   Bone tumors

changes is very appreciable (possibly about 20% or more), especially if one follows them well into adult life.

Such peripheral chondrosarcomas may attain rather large size by the time they are operated upon. The roentgen picture (Figs. 15-1, B, 15-2, and 15-5) may create a false impression of invasiveness and inoperability, if one is not familiar with it (only the areas that are calcified or ossified stand out sharply). Actually, however bulky a peripheral chondrosarcoma may be, it is found on surgical exploration to be a discrete, circumscribed mass, and cure can be obtained by adequate local excision, provided (1) that the tumor is cleared peripherally (blunt dissection should be avoided) and (2) that the bone at its site of attachment is resected. Even if the tumor recurs, it does so locally, and such tumors

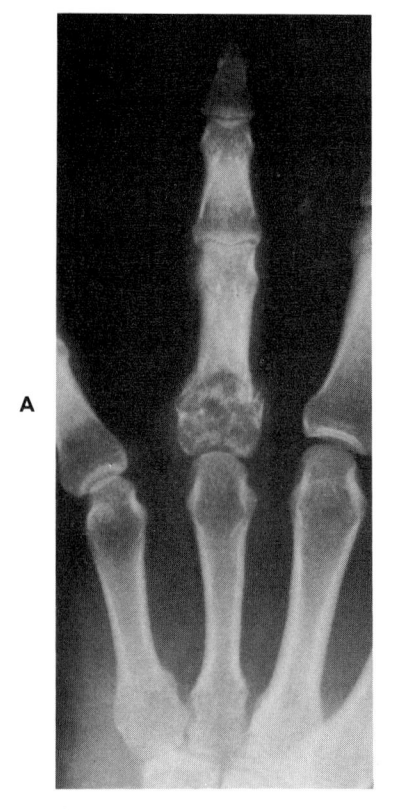

Fig. 15-9. A, Roentgenogram of a central cartilage tumor in the proximal end of the proximal phalanx of a fourth finger of a man of 31. Biopsy showed evidence of early chondrosarcoma by the usual pathologic criteria, and ray amputation was advised. It would appear that malignant change in solitary enchondromas of bones of the hand and foot is not as unusual as was once thought. B, Roentgenogram of a rarefied, tumorlike lesion in the upper shaft and intertrochanteric region of a femur with a pathologic fracture through it, which proved to be a chondrosarcoma. From this initial x-ray film alone one could hardly venture any more definitive opinion than that of a malignant neoplasm. C, Roentgenogram of the same chondrosarcoma, now heavily calcified and ossified, taken seven years later. The patient had declined the recommendation of disarticulation (which would probably have effected a cure), and he eventually developed pulmonary metastases.

may recur repeatedly over a period of years, without showing any tendency to distant metastasis (Fig. 15-2).

The sarcomatous nature of a tumor of comparatively large size is likely to be obvious. In dealing with smaller peripheral tumors (Fig. 15-7), the most important single pathologic observation is measurement of the width of the cartilage cap. If this exceeds 1 cm. (and if the patient is an adult), then the cartilage has been actively growing and, as such, represents chondrosarcoma. In selecting blocks for microscopic examination, the pathologist should concentrate on well-preserved peripheral fields showing little calcification or ossification, but, even in these, there may be so much degeneration or necrobiosis that he may have to scan many fields for cartilage-cell nuclear changes indicative of malignancy (Figs. 15-1, *D* and 15-2, *C*).

Extension and metastasis

An occasional central chondrosarcoma may metastasize early, seeding the lungs. I can recall two such tumors in the calcaneus, for example, which metastasized within a year after amputation of the foot (Fig. 15-11). This is the excep-

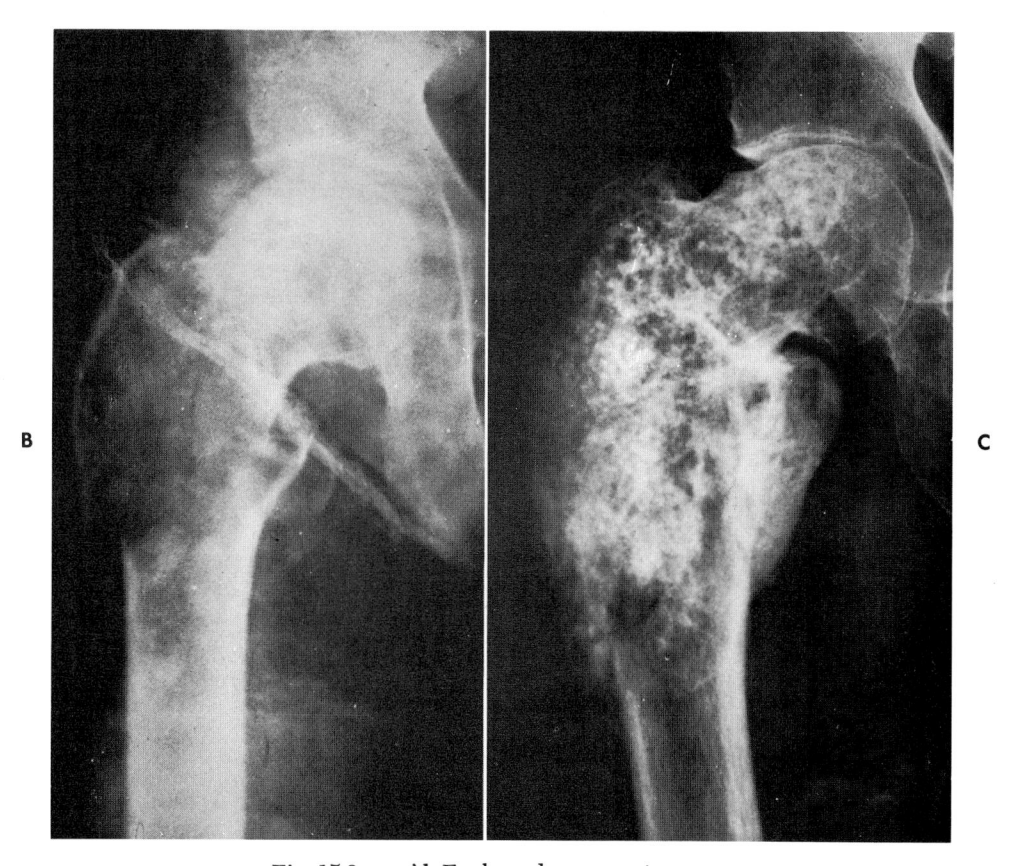

Fig. 15-9, cont'd. For legend see opposite page.

204 *Bone tumors*

tion, fortunately, rather than the rule. Most chondrosarcomas are likely to remain locally invasive for some time, even after an unsuccessful attempt at surgical removal, so that, under favorable auspices, the cure rate for tumors in accessible sites is substantially higher than it is for osteogenic sarcoma. By the same token, inoperable chondrosarcomas in the pelvic region may eventually attain tremendous size before causing the death of the patient from a variety of complications incidental to local spread.

When an advanced chondrosarcoma finally does become aggressive, it tends to break into the regional venous channels, and, by intravascular growth and extension, without necessarily adhering very much to the vessel walls, may reach

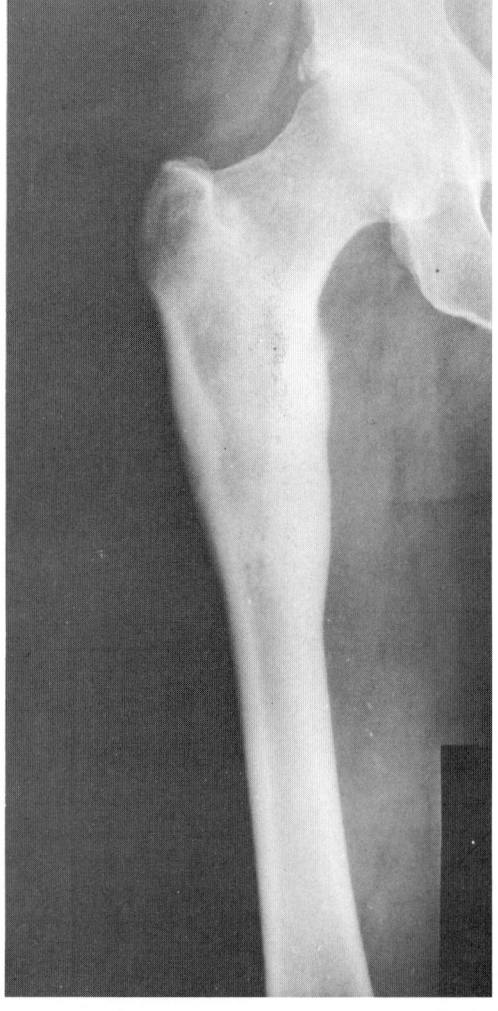

Fig. 15-10. Roentgenogram of a chondrosarcoma in the upper shaft of the femur in an adult which developed sufficiently slowly to permit marked cortical thickening.

the heart and lungs. Though it is ordinarily years before this occurs, in an occasional case the disorder runs its course so rapidly that the patient is dead within some months after the original tumor in the bone is first noted. The presence of severe respiratory and cardiac difficulties for a time before death in a patient with chondrosarcoma may well be a clinical indication that cordlike intravascular growth and extension of the tumor to the heart and lungs has taken place.

A remarkable example of such neoplastic extension is the case described by Ernst[8] of a chondrosarcoma involving the lower part of the vertebral column. In this case there were tumor plugs in both the renal and the suprarenal veins, the left internal spermatic vein, the azygos vein, the inferior vena cava, the right auricle, and the branches of the right and left pulmonary arteries, and still the pulmonary parenchyma was free from metastases. Kósa[19] described a femoral chondrosarcoma with neoplastic extension to the ipsilateral femoral and iliac veins, the inferior vena cava, the right heart, and both branches of the pulmonary artery, even to the capillaries, again without the occurrence of any parenchymal metastases, even in the lungs.

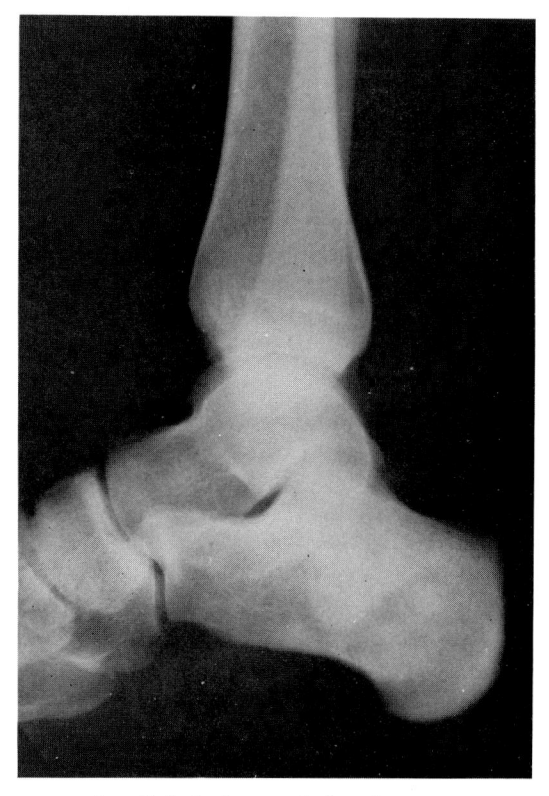

Fig. 15-11. Roentgenogram of an ill-defined, irregularly sclerosing tumor in the calcaneus of an adolescent girl. This tumor proved, on microscopic examination, to be a chondrosarcoma. The radiopaque areas reflect secondary ossification of tumor cartilage. Pulmonary metastases appeared within one year of amputation of the foot.

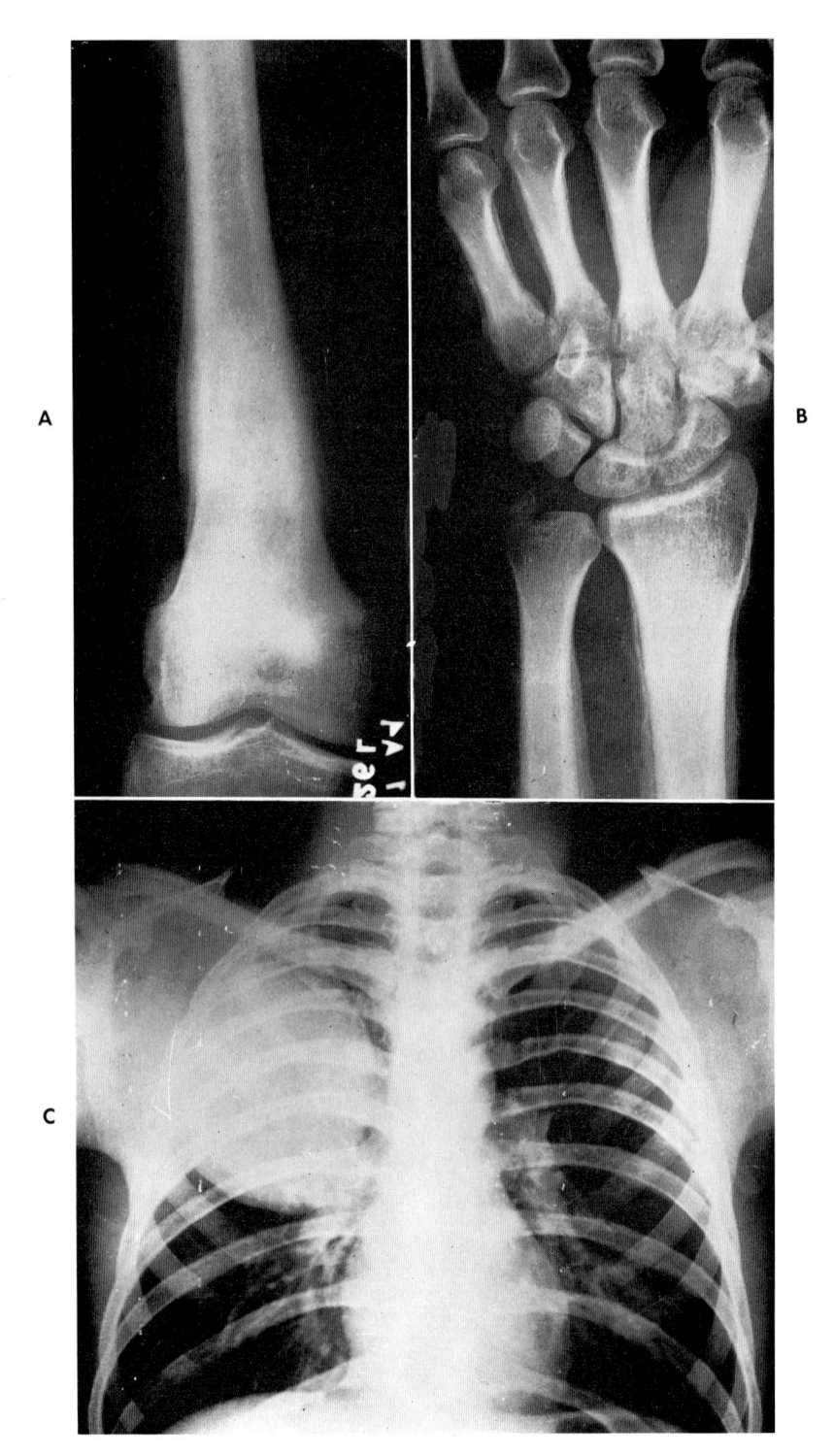

Fig. 15-12. **A**, Roentgenogram of another central chondrosarcoma in the lower shaft of a femur that has provoked lamellated ("onionpeel") deposition of periosteal new bone. **B**, Roentgenogram of the same patient showing periosteal new bone apposition on the metacarpal and forearm bones as an expression of pulmonary hypertrophic osteoarthropathy. **C**, Roentgenogram showing a large, solitary (slowly enlarging) metastasis in the right lung, responsible for the changes illustrated in **B**.

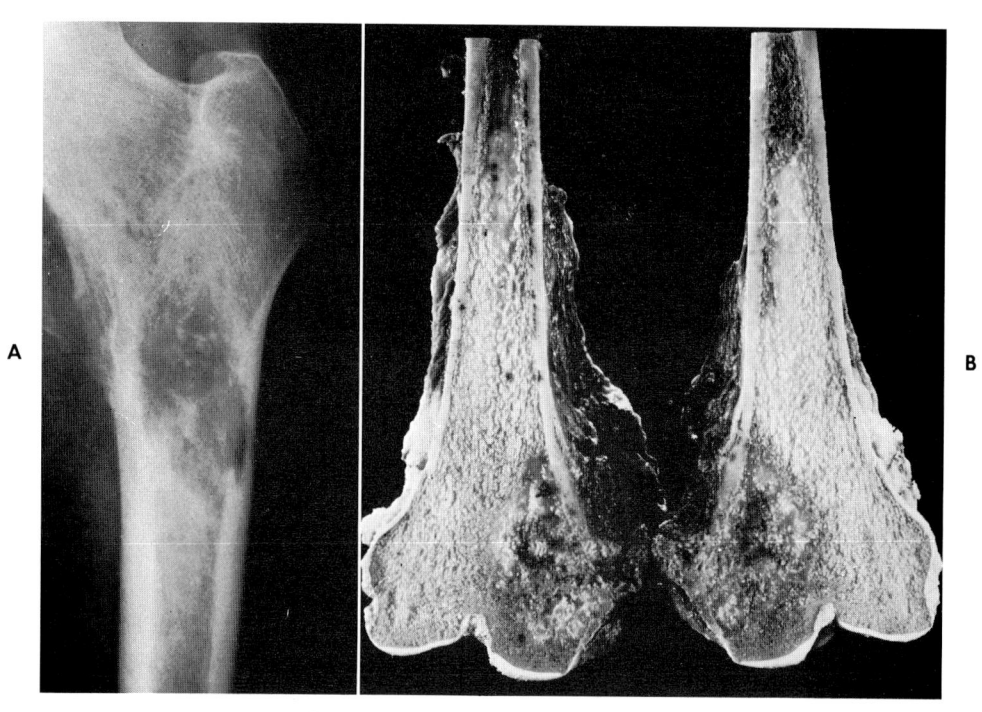

Fig. 15-13. **A,** Central chondrosarcoma of the upper femur in an older adult. This chondrosarcoma caused partial destruction and avulsion of the lesser trochanter. The presence of light calcific stippling of the central portion of the tumor affords the only clue to its recognition. **B,** Photograph (reduced) of the two halves of a lower femur amputated for chondrosarcoma in the medial condyle. Though still comparatively small, the tumor had already penetrated the cortex. The subperiosteal hematoma resulted from biopsy, performed several days previously.

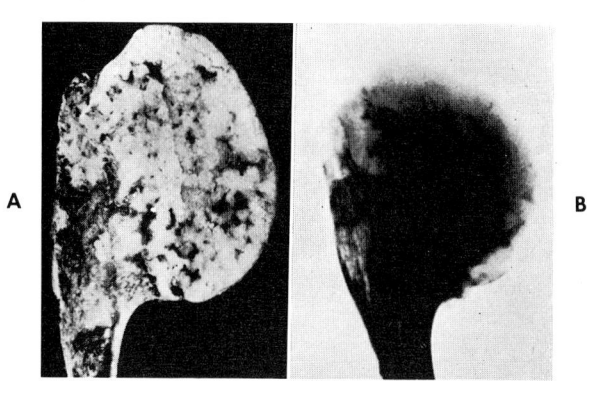

Fig. 15-14. **A,** Photograph (reduced) of a chondrosarcoma developing in the resected distal end of an ulna of a 19-year-old young man with skeletal enchondromatosis limited to the bones of the right hand and forearm (Ollier's disease). The protruding tumor mass measured 6 by 5 by 5 cm. and was continuous with tumor cartilage in the interior of the ulna. **B,** Roentgenogram of the specimen illustrated in **A.** The radiopaque central area reflects ossification of neoplastic cartilage.

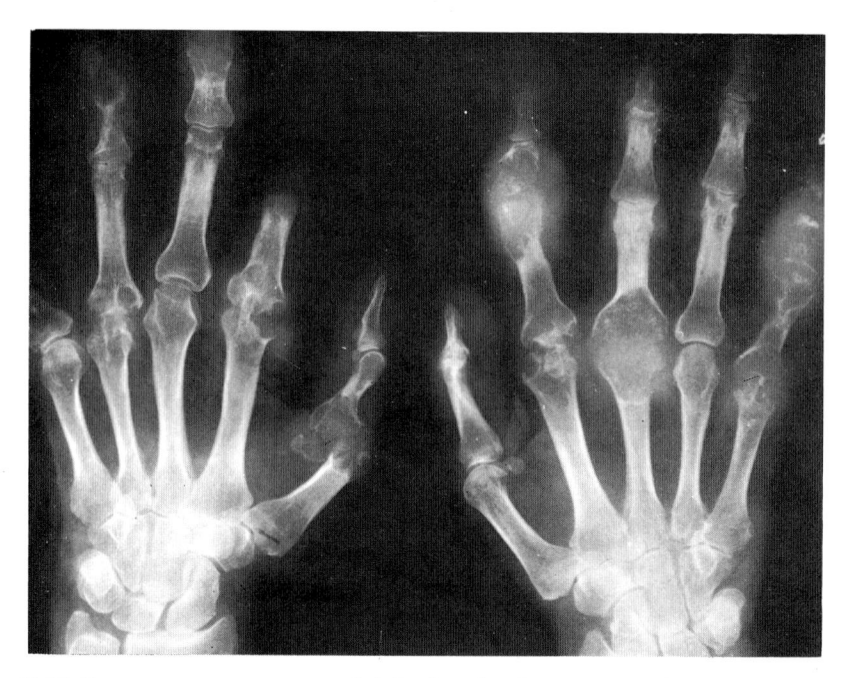

Fig. 15-15. Roentgenogram in a case of skeletal enchondromatosis involving both hands (Ollier's disease). Biopsy showed early malignant change in the metacarpal bone of the right thumb (shown on the left).

In other cases, while extending into the large venous channels, the tumor also gives rise to parenchymal metastases, at least in the lungs. In the case described by Weber[29] there were metastases not only in the lungs but also in the liver (around tumor-plugged branches of the portal vein); in the case reported by Warren,[28] however, the metastases were limited to the lungs. Actually, metastases elsewhere than in the lungs are uncommon in connection with chondrosarcomas. The possibility of lymphatic spread also exists, and extension of the tumor to lymph nodes, especially regional, has occasionally been reported. I have observed extension of chondrosarcoma to the femoral lymph nodes in a hemipelvectomy specimen (the primary tumor was a large one in the upper femur and had spread extensively into the adjacent soft tissues). However, it is to be recognized that small secondary nodules of tumor not far from the primary mass might easily be wrongly interpreted as representing lymph nodes that have undergone complete replacement by tumor.

Treatment

In principle, the only form of therapy that offers any prospect of cure in chondrosarcoma is adequate surgery. Roentgen irradiation, even in heavy dosage, has only limited effectiveness and should be reserved for the palliation of advanced inoperable tumors (without any great expectation of benefit). The use of radioactive sulfur preparations is still experimental,[13] and results are too incon-

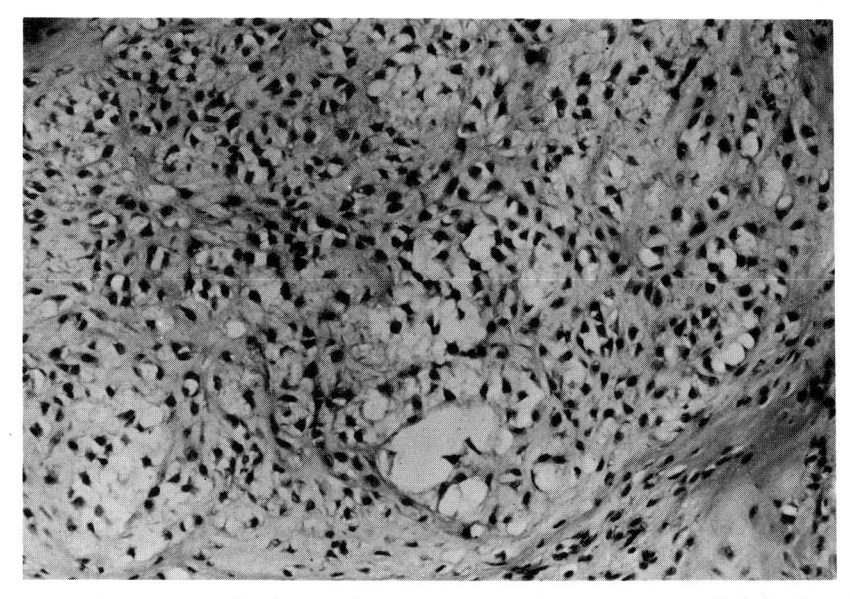

Fig. 15-16. Photomicrograph of a cartilage tumor in a finger in a case of skeletal enchondromatosis (Ollier's disease), which manifested recent active growth and malignant change. Note the relative cellularity and widespread nuclear enlargement and hyperchromatism. (×160.)

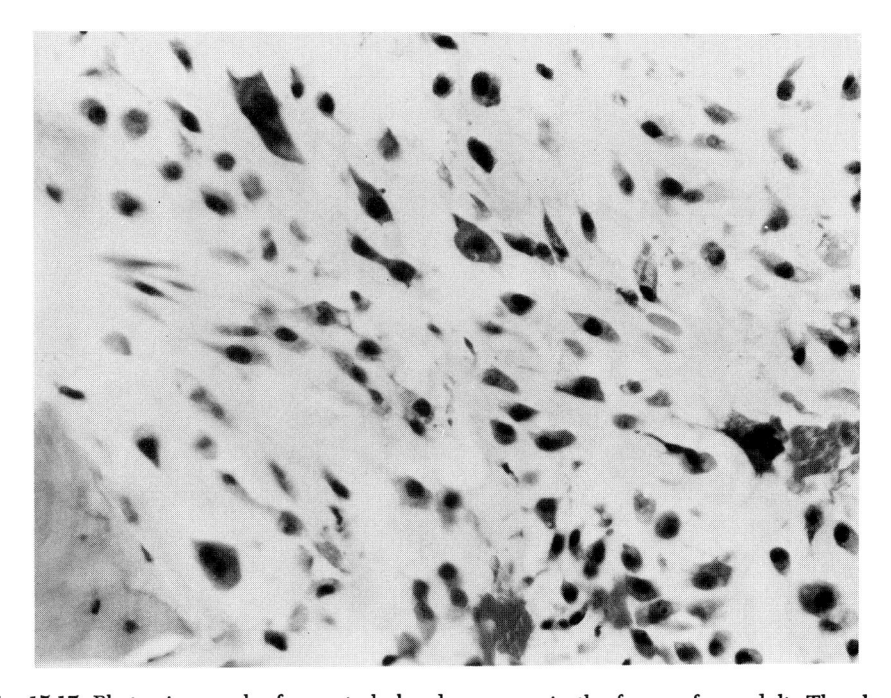

Fig. 15-17. Photomicrograph of a central chondrosarcoma in the femur of an adult. The chondrosarcoma had been present for some time before diagnosis. Note the plumpness and hyperchromatism of the nuclei generally, as well as the presence of scattered tumor cells with multiple large nuclei. (×300.)

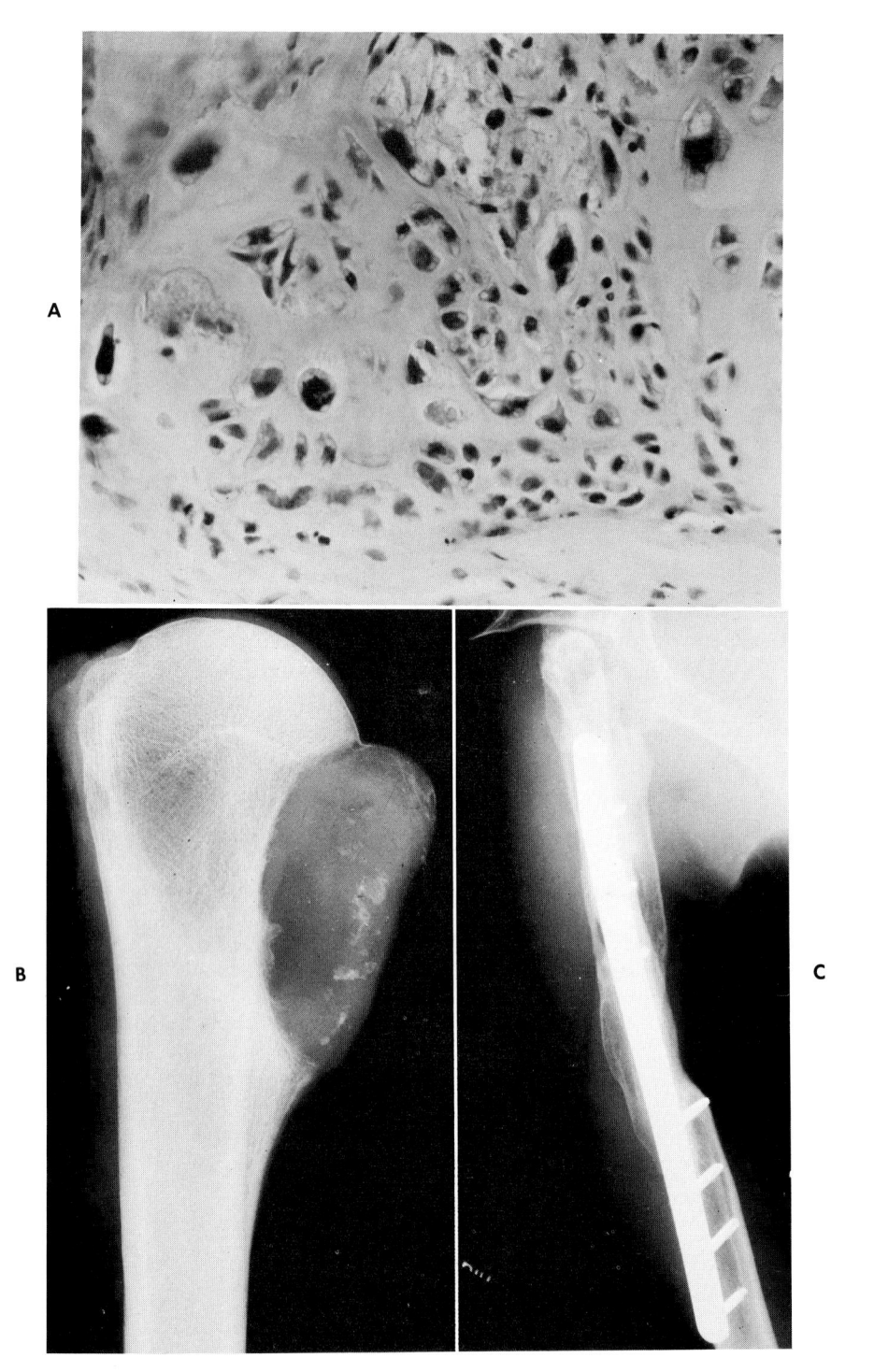

Fig. 15-18. A, Photomicrograph of a chondrosarcoma in the pubic bone showing the presence of numerous tumor cells with distinctly enlarged, hyperchromatic nuclei. The finding of even an occasional field such as this suffices for a diagnosis of malignancy. (×300.) **B,** Roentgenogram of an unusual, eccentrically placed, localized chondrosarcoma, for which it was possible to do a successful resection, followed by a fibula transplant for reconstruction, **C.** Resection and bone grafting may also be feasible for an occasional, early localized chondrosarcoma in the distal femur, such as the chondrosarcoma illustrated in **D.**

Chondrosarcoma of bone 211

clusive to warrant clinical application, except by way of investigational chemotherapy. As with so many other drugs, bone marrow depression appears to be a limiting factor. It is noteworthy, however, that Boström and his associates,[4] at the Karolinska Institute in Stockholm, were able to achieve remarkable palliation over a two-year period in a case of chondrosarcoma with pulmonary and skeletal metastases by the use of ^{35}S-sulfate. The usual deleterious systemic effects of high dosage were circumvented by intra-arterial and intravenous injection of the isotope.

The surgical management of peripheral chondrosarcomas by adequate local excision has already been discussed. In dealing with *central* chondrosarcomas in surgically accessible sites, one occasionally encounters early tumors that have not yet extended through the cortex, for which resection and reconstruction may be considered, e.g., in the humeral head, upper femur, or an iliac wing (Figs. 5-6 and 15-18). These are special situations, however. For most central tumors, treatment has to be radical, and the wider the margin of clearance, the better. The initial approach may well be the only opportunity to effect a cure, and once a

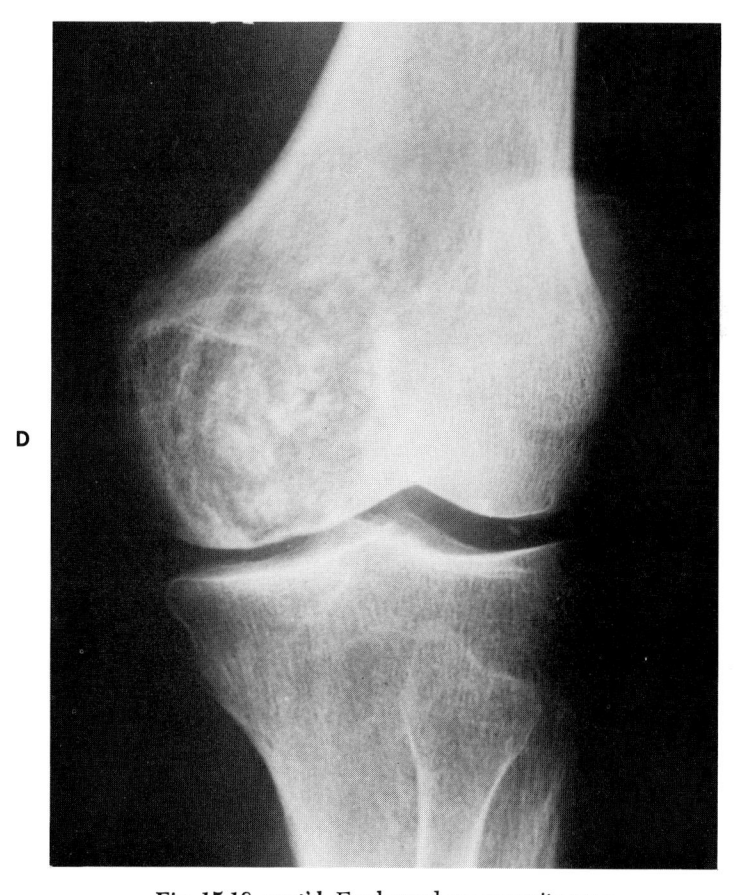

Fig. 15-18, cont'd. For legend see opposite page.

chondrosarcoma begins to spread, you may never be able to control it. For chondrosarcoma in the lower femur, for example, the level of amputation should be well above the proximal limit of the tumor (this does not imply disarticulation necessarily). For tumors higher up in the thigh or groin or in the iliac bone, hindquarter amputation may be feasible, and it is noteworthy that over 90% of the five-year survivors after this procedure are patients who had chondrosarcoma.

Summary

Chondrosarcoma should be regarded as a neoplasm distinct from osteogenic sarcoma of bone. The former develops out of full-fledged cartilage, while the latter issues from more primitive tissue, developing out of bone-forming mesenchyme. Some chondrosarcomas do show large areas in which the intercellular matrix of the tumor cartilage has become heavily calcified or ossified, and in some osteogenic sarcomas, tumor cartilage in considerable amounts may be formed in the course of osteogenesis from the primitive mesenchyme. However, in a chondrosarcoma, in contrast to osteogenic sarcoma, one never sees tumorous osteoid tissue and bone that is evolving out of a sarcomatous stroma directly, such as one always sees somewhere in an osteogenic sarcoma, no matter how much cartilage it contains.

In comparison with osteogenic sarcoma, chondrosarcoma is definitely less common, appears at a later age (on the average), runs a much slower course, and, especially if given radical surgical treatment at an early stage, has a much better prognosis, since the tumor has usually not yet metastasized at the time of initial surgical intervention. Even when the tumor is inadequately extirpated, it tends to recur locally one or more times before extending to the tributary veins or to the lungs.

A chondrosarcoma that begins its development within the interior of a bone may be denoted as a central chondrosarcoma, and one that begins in the cartilaginous cap of an osteochondroma may be denoted as a peripheral chondrosarcoma. It is in the peripheral chondrosarcomas and in the central ones that have clearly evolved from benign enchondromas that one finds, at least in the earlier stages of evolution of the lesion, heavy calcification or ossification of large parts of the intercellular matrix of the tumor cartilage. In other chondrosarcomas the neoplastic tissue is likely to consist, in the main, of compacted islands of cartilage with hyaline matrix, though, if the chondrosarcoma is very bulky, one may also see areas in which the cartilage is softer and myxomatous and perhaps even necrotic.

The histologic picture of any particular tumor does not have to be crudely and obviously sarcomatous to indicate chondrosarcoma. Even in the early stages of the evolution of a chondrosarcoma, one will find, at least in scattered fields, if adequate material is examined, subtle but telltale evidences of cytologic atypism of the cartilage cells that will betray the malignant character of the lesion. A cartilage tumor in bone should no longer be regarded as benign if, when viable and not heavily calcified areas are examined, it shows, even in scattered fields:

(1) many cells with plump nuclei, (2) more than an occasional cell with two such nuclei, and especially (3) any giant cartilage cells with large single or multiple nuclei or with clumps of chromatin. By observing these criteria, the tendency to "underdiagnosis" of chondrosarcoma in an early stage of malignancy can be overcome. In a more fully evolved chondrosarcoma these indications will be relatively easy to find if one recognizes their diagnostic importance, and in a fully developed chondrosarcoma, of course, the histologic picture may even be obviously sarcomatous.

From a clinical point of view, it may be emphasized that evidence of cortical perforation and the onset of pain in a cartilage growth that has previously been dormant is likely to be an ominous sign pointing to early malignant change and the necessity for biopsy and appropriate surgical therapy. If a chondrosarcoma is recognized early and is widely cleared at the first operation, the chances of obtaining a cure are fairly good and, in any event, very much better than with osteogenic sarcoma.

References

1. Ackerman, L. V., and Spjut, H. J.: Tumors of bone and cartilage, Washington, D. C., 1962, Armed Forces Institute of Pathology.
2. Anderson, C. E., Ludourieg, J., Ehring, E. J., and Horowitz, B.: Ultrastructure and clinical composition of chondrosarcoma, J. Bone Joint Surg. 45-A:753, 1963.
3. Barnes, R., and Catto, M.: Chondrosarcoma of bone, J. Bone Joint Surg. 48-B: 729, 1966.
4. Boström, H., Edgren, B., Friberg, U., Larsson, K. S., Nilsonne, U., Wengle, B., and Wester, P. O.: Case of chondrosarcoma with pulmonary and skeletal metastases after hemipelvectomy, successfully treated with 35 S-sulfate, Acta Orthop. Scand. 39:549, 1968.
5. Castrén, H.: Zur Kenntnis der metastasenbildenden Chondrome, Acta Soc. med. fenn. duodecim. (s.B.) 15:1, 1931.
6. Cohen, J., and D'Angio, G. J.: Unusual bone tumors after roentgen therapy in children. Two case reports, Am. J. Roentgenol. 86:502, 1961.
7. Daniels, A. C., Conner, G. H., and Straus, F. H.: Primary chondrosarcoma of the tracheobronchial tree, Arch. Pathol. 84: 615, 1967.
8. Ernst, P.: Ungewöhnliche Verbreitung einer Knorpelgeschwulst in der Blutbahn, Beitr. pathol. Anat. 28:255, 1900.
9. Ewing, J.: Neoplastic diseases, ed. 4, Philadelphia, 1940, W. B. Saunders Co., p. 207.
10. Flörcken, H.: Ein selten grosses Chondrom der Lendengegend und seine Behandlung, Z. Krebsforsch. 35:354, 1932.
11. Goldenberg, R. R., Cohen, P., and Steinlauf, P.: Chondrosarcoma of the extraskeletal soft tissues, J. Bone Joint Surg. 49-A:1487, 1967.
12. Goldman, R. L.: Mesenchymal chondrosarcoma, a rare malignant chondroid tumor usually primary in bone. Report of a case arising in extraskeletal soft tissue, Cancer 20:1494, 1967.
13. Gottschalk, K. F., Alport, L. K., and Albert, R. E.: The use of large amounts of radioactive sulfur in patients with advanced chondrosarcomas, Cancer Res. 19: 1070, 1959.
14. Hatcher, C. H.: Development of sarcoma in bones subjected to roentgen or radium irradiation, J. Bone Joint Surg. 27:179, 1945.
15. Henderson, E. D., and Dahlin, D. C.: Chondrosarcoma of bone. A study of 288 cases, J. Bone Joint Surg. 45-A:1450, 1963.
16. Higgins, G. M., Levy, B. M., and Yollick, B. L.: A transplantable beryllium-induced chondrosarcoma of rabbits, J. Bone Joint Surg. 46-A:789, 1964.
17. Kaufman, E.: Lehrbuch der speziellen pathologischen Anatomie, eds. 7 and 8, Berlin, 1922, W. de Gruyter & Co., pp. 1 and 941.
18. Keiller, V. H.: Cartilaginous tumors of bone, Surg. Gynecol. Obstet. 40:510, 1925.
19. Kósa, M.: Chondroblastom in der venösen Blutbahn, Virchows Arch. 272:166, 1929.

20. Le Conte, R. G., Lee, W. E., and Belk, W. P.: Enchondroma of the femur with repeated recurrences and ultimate death; report of case, Arch. Surg. 11:93, 1925.
21. Lichtenstein, L., and Jaffe, H. L.: Chondrosarcoma of bone, Am. J. Pathol. 19:553, 1943.
22. Lichtenstein, L.: Diseases of bone and joints, St. Louis, 1970, The C. V. Mosby Co., pp. 131-132.
23. Makrycostas, K.: Zur Histologie des bösartigen embryonalen Enchondroms, Virchows Arch. 282:737, 1931.
24. Minagi, H., and Newton, T. H.: Cartilaginous tumors of the base of skull, Am. J. Roentgenol. 105:308, 1969.
25. O'Neal, L. W., and Ackerman, L. V.: Chondrosarcoma of bone, Cancer 5:551, 1952.
26. Phemister, D. B.: Chondrosarcoma of bone, Surg. Gynecol. Obstet. 50:216, 1930.
27. Sirsat, M. V.: Some uncommon tumors in childhood, Indian J. Child Health, Jan., 1961, pp. 7-11.
28. Warren, S.: Chondrosarcoma with intravascular growth and tumor emboli to lungs, Am. J. Pathol. 7:161, 1931.
29. Weber, O.: Zur Geschichte des Enchondroms namentlich in Bezug auf dessen hereditäres Vorkommen und secundäre Verbreitung in innern Organen durch Embolie, Virchows Arch. 35:501, 1866.

Chapter 16

Osteogenic sarcoma of bone

Osteogenic sarcoma is probably the most frequently encountered primary malignant tumor of bone, with the possible exception of multiple myeloma (many instances of which go unrecognized clinically or are mistaken for skeletal carcinomatosis). The differentiation of osteogenic sarcoma from chondrosarcoma of bone has already been considered in connection with the latter tumor (Chapter 15). To reiterate, chondrosarcoma develops from full-fledged, clearly differentiated cartilage, while osteogenic sarcoma takes origin apparently from more primitive bone-forming mesenchyme. Ordinarily, in an osteogenic sarcoma, the proliferating connective tissue, which often is quite anaplastic, gives rise to tumor osteoid and bone directly, though it may also form some tumor cartilage, which in turn tends to undergo rapid osseous transformation. It is true that in an occasional osteogenic sarcoma, bone formation may proceed prominently via an intermediate cartilage stage, and tumor cartilage may thus be a conspicuous feature of its cytology. However, even in such an osteogenic sarcoma, if the observer does not limit his scrutiny to a small field of the tumor, and particularly to the periphery of it, he will readily perceive that in other places the basic connective tissue is directly forming neoplastic osteoid tissue and bone. With few exceptions, it should be possible to make a clear pathologic distinction between chondrosarcoma and osteogenic sarcoma, and, by the same token, there seems to be little justification for retaining such equivocal hybrid designations as chondro-osteosarcoma or osteochondrosarcoma.

Clinically, also, there are significant differences between chondrosarcoma and osteogenic sarcoma. Thus, osteogenic sarcoma is more frequent, occurs, on the whole, at an earlier age (with the exception of the occasional instances complicating Paget's disease), pursues a more rapid course, metastasizes to the lungs relatively early, and hence is more serious, even when amputation is resorted to as soon as the condition is recognized. By comparison, chondrosarcoma, as a rule, has a distinctly more favorable prognosis, provided that the neoplasm is in a surgically accessible site, is not underdiagnosed through failure to recognize subtle histologic criteria of early malignant change, and is widely cleared surgically at the initial operation. The practical importance of distinguishing between chondrosarcoma and osteogenic sarcoma is thus evident.

Fibrosarcoma of bone, also, should be clearly distinguished from osteogenic sarcoma, and I am in full accord with those who depart from the classification of the Bone Sarcoma Registry in recommending that central fibrosarcoma be removed from the category of osteogenic sarcoma and considered as an independent neoplasm. The nature and behavior of such neoplasms, and they are by no means rare, will be considered later (Chapter 17). Essentially, they represent malignant fibroblastic tumors that arise in the interior of the affected bone, and that, on thorough histologic sampling, fail to show any indication that the tumor cells are actually forming tumor osteoid and bone. Like chondrosarcoma, fibrosarcoma of bone in most instances also carries a better prognosis than does osteogenic sarcoma and can be cured by radical surgery, if the tumor has not already metastasized to the lungs.

In the revised classification of bone tumors of the American College of Surgeons Registry (1939), one finds outlined still other subdivisions of the "osteogenic series," so-called, such as medullary and subperiosteal, telangiectatic, and sclerosing, but I feel that retaining these is not particularly helpful, and that this makes the subject unnecessarily confusing. By the time their presence is recognized, virtually all osteogenic sarcomas are found to involve the medullary cavity and to have extended through the cortex beneath the elevated periosteum or even beyond it, into the adjacent muscle tissue. Also, some osteogenic sarcomas are more richly vascular than others, and some display more abundant new bone formation than others, to be sure, but such distinctions are of little practical importance. To state the issue bluntly, a given neoplasm of bone is either an osteogenic sarcoma or it is not, and if it is one, its prognosis is serious, whether it is richly vascular or only moderately so, whether it forms abundant tumor bone (sclerosing) or relatively little (osteolytic). Incidentally, it was found that about one quarter of the osteogenic sarcomas in our material showed relatively little ossification, another quarter a moderate degree of ossification, and about one half rather heavy ossification, obviously reflected roentgenographically.

A good deal of interest has been evinced in regard to this neoplasm in recent years, and an appreciable number of interesting and significant papers have appeared; these have been included in the references. They have dealt mainly with surveys of sizable groups of cases emphasizing treatment and prognosis, with tumors in special or unusual sites, with Paget's sarcoma, and with parosteal bone-forming tumors. Reference to these contributions will be made in due course.

That the prompt recognition and effective treatment of osteogenic sarcoma still present certain problems at times for both surgeon and pathologist is evidenced by my relevant consultation material in recent years. Some instances were treated initially as osteomyelitis; in some, the diagnosis was masked for a time by pathologic fracture; in several, the malignant nature of the lesion was not recognized at surgery, so that curettement was the initial procedure; and in more than a few, the pathologist thought he was dealing with some other neoplasm, such as malignant giant-cell tumor, benign osteoblastoma, chondromyxoid fibroma, or chondrosarcoma. To be sure, in most instances consultation was sought because the surgeon or the pathologist or both wanted a corroborative opinion on record before radical surgery was undertaken.

An occasional telangiectatic osteosarcoma may masquerade as an aneurysmal bone cyst, so that close attention must be directed to the character of the cells lining its pools of blood. It is my impression that the tumors in man and dogs that have been provisionally interpreted as "malignant aneurysmal bone cyst"[20] appear actually to be telangiectatic osteogenic sarcomas.

Clinical features
Age and sex incidence

The tumor appears to develop more often in males than in females. Its greatest incidence is in the age group between 10 and 25 years, and its next smaller peak of incidence is in older adults with Paget's disease. However, osteogenic sarcoma is by no means rare in patients in their thirties or forties, who show no evidence of Paget's disease.

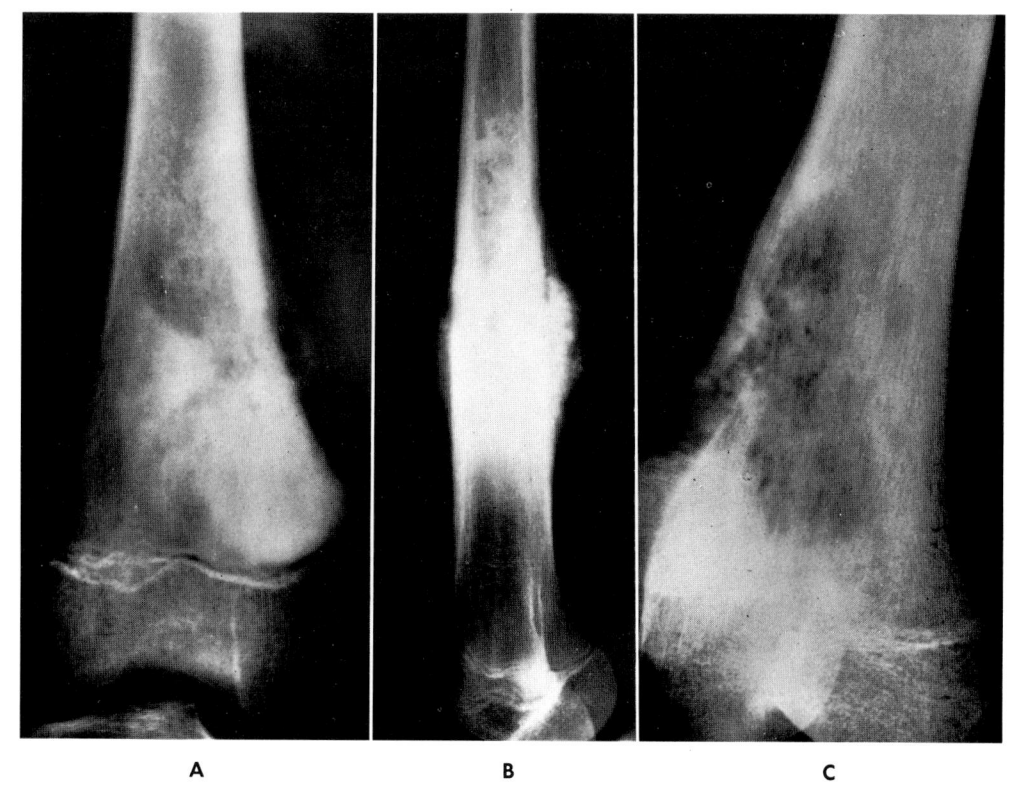

Fig. 16-1. A-C, Representative roentgenograms of several osteogenic sarcomas developing in the lower femur. The sclerosing tumor illustrated in **B** is situated in the shaft rather than at the end of the bone. The osteogenic sarcoma illustrated in **C** is noteworthy in that it shows "onionpeel" lamellation of periosteal new bone rather than the more usual perpendicular striation.

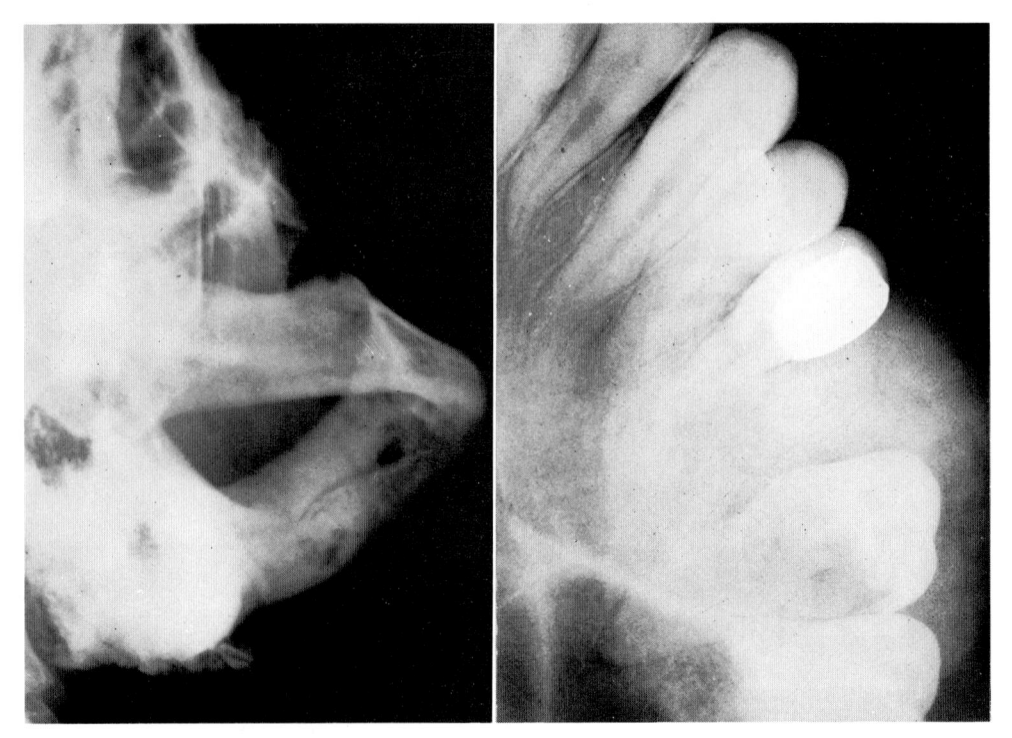

Fig. 16-2. Representative roentgenograms of two sclerosing osteogenic sarcomas developing in the mandible.

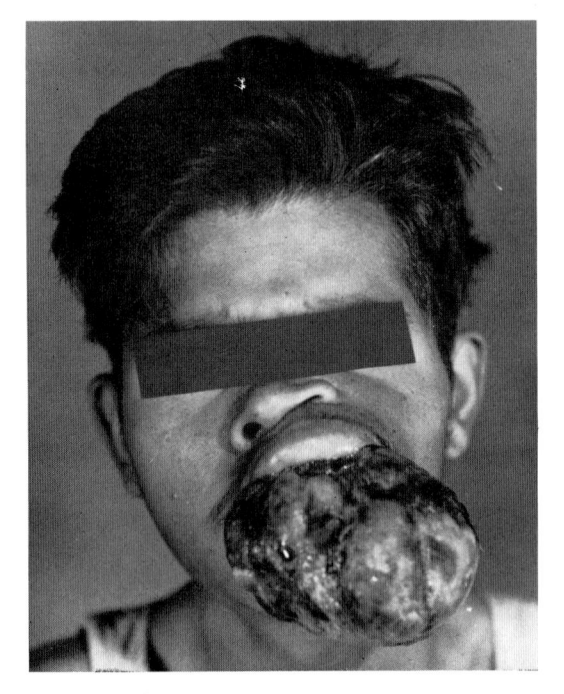

Fig. 16-3. A rapidly growing, neglected osteogenic sarcoma arising in the maxilla of a 17-year-old Indian boy. The tumor was already far advanced when he sought treatment, although he had been aware of it for only two and one-half months. (Courtesy Dr. M. V. Sirsat, Tata Memorial Hospital, Bombay, India.)

Location

The commonest sites of occurrence are the lower end of the femur, the upper end of the tibia, and the upper end of the humerus, in the order indicated. In my own material, about 90% of the tumors were encountered in long limb bones, over 70% in the femur or tibia, and about one-half in the lower femur or upper tibia. Occasionally, an osteogenic sarcoma may be encountered in the upper end of the fibula, in the iliac bone, in the vertebral column, or in a jaw bone, and rarely in other sites, such as a scapula, a clavicle, or a finger phalanx (Fig. 16-13, B and C). In a long bone, it is usually the end of the shaft and part of the adjacent epiphyseal area that are involved, but occasionally the tumor may develop more toward the midshaft region (Fig. 16-1, B).

Clinical picture

As with most tumors of bone, pain and swelling of the affected part are the usual presenting complaints. In patients (especially children) with rapidly growing sarcomas (e.g., in the lower femur), appreciable weight loss and moderately severe secondary anemia may also be observed, and under these circumstances pathologic fracture is not uncommon. In such instances in which the tumor eventually attains a very considerable size if allowed to follow its natural course, the affected limb becomes obviously swollen and its surface veins conspicuously dilated.

The interval between the onset of symptoms and the recognition of the neoplasm may vary from just a few weeks to six months or more. That the tumor develops insidiously is evidenced by the fact that it may be as large and far advanced in a patient presenting a history of only a few weeks' duration as in a patient who has been aware of a growth for many months before seeking medical advice.

Blood chemical findings as an aid in diagnosis

There are no significant changes in the serum calcium or phosphorus levels in cases of osteogenic sarcoma. However, as one might expect, the serum alkaline phosphatase value (which in general reflects a tendency to new bone formation) is significantly increased up to 20 or more Bodansky units in many instances, though by no means all. In such instances, there is a trend to decline to a more nearly normal level following removal of the primary tumor by ablation and to return to the initially high level or even beyond it when the presence of pulmonary metastases becomes evident.

Roentgenographic appearance

The ease with which an osteogenic sarcoma may be recognized roentgenographically in any particular instance depends largely upon how clear the indications are of cortical perforation and subperiosteal extension (as an expression of malignancy) and upon how evident the tendency to new bone formation within the neoplasm happens to be (as an indication of its osteogenic character).

In approximately half the cases of any sizable series of osteogenic sarcomas (the highly sclerosing tumors particularly), both of these features will be so obvious that even a relatively inexperienced observer will have no difficulty in properly interpreting them. It should be emphasized, however, that if one necessarily expects to find conspicuous perpendicular striations of new bone within the subperiosteal tumor cuff—a sign upon which undue emphasis has been placed—one is likely to miss a considerable number of osteogenic sarcomas. Moreover, this perpendicularly striated pattern of periosteal new bone formation is not specific for osteogenic sarcoma. I have observed it, on occasion, in cases of metastatic carcinoma, of advanced Ewing's sarcoma, and even of tuberculosis of the shaft of a long bone, so that one must consider the picture as a whole in relation to the relevant clinical facts before reaching a conclusion. An important corollary of this observation is that one is never justified in recommending ablation without confirmation by biopsy, however certain one may be of the accuracy of the roentgen diagnosis.

In approximately another one third of the cases of osteogenic sarcoma, the features just described will be apparent, though perhaps not obvious, and the examiner may have to scrutinize the films closely to discern them. In another smaller group of cases, these features may be scarcely evident, and I have observed proved instances of osteogenic sarcoma (essentially osteolytic in nature) that defy recognition roentgenographically even on the part of a skillful observer. In such instances, although one may entertain a suspicion of osteolytic osteogenic sarcoma, the diagnosis must rest essentially upon the biopsy findings.

Pathologic features

By the time one has an opportunity to examine a specimen amputated for osteogenic sarcoma, one finds, as a rule, that, while the bulk of the neoplasm is present within the medullary cavity of the affected bone area, the tumor has already extended through the cortex beneath the raised periosteum, where it forms a cuff extending around part of the circumference of the bone. Further, an osteogenic sarcoma that is far advanced may already have broken through this periosteal barrier and invaded the contiguous muscle tissue. From the examination of many such relevant specimens, one gains the distinct impression that osteogenic sarcoma originates within the interior of the affected bone area, though it readily penetrates the cortex to spread beneath the overlying periosteum. In the course of its extension, it may leave the affected cortical area substantially intact, apparently because the latter is permeated by tumor too rapidly to allow for appreciable resorption or for gradual expansion, such as one observes with chondrosarcoma on occasion.

The central portion of the tumor is the most heavily ossified, although the extent of ossification, as noted, varies from specimen to specimen. At one extreme, there are essentially osteolytic tumors that require roentgen examination of serial slices of the specimen for the clear demonstration of occasional rather small, densely mottled foci of new bone formation. These osteolytic tumors are rather likely to show appreciable necrosis, cystic softening, hemorrhage, and telangiectasis as conspicuous secondary features of their pathologic anatomy. At the other extreme, as is well known, there are highly sclerosing tumors that are so hard as to be substantially eburnated. On the other hand, the peripheral (subperiosteal) cuff of tumor is likely to be comparatively cellular, soft, and whitish in appearance, although it, too, usually displays prominent striae or more delicate and irregularly dispersed streaks of tumor bone within it.

The most cellular and least differentiated portion of an osteogenic sarcoma is usually represented by its advancing core within the medullary cavity. This conical plug of tumor tissue, which often measures several centimeters in length, may fail to exhibit any demonstrable evidence of ossification, even on roentgen examination, a factor that must be considered in determining the optimum level of amputation. An occasional specimen may show skip extension of tumor within the medullary cavity, and this possibility must also be borne in mind. In regard

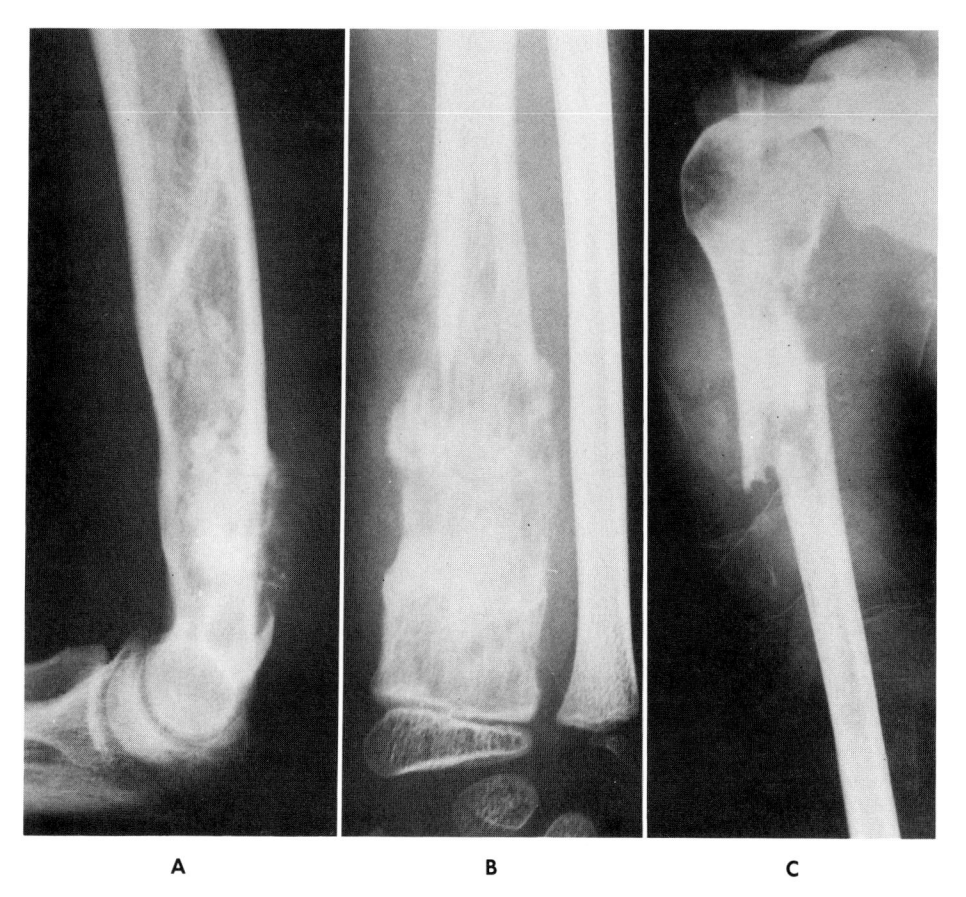

Fig. 16-4. A, Roentgenogram of a sclerosing osteogenic sarcoma in an unusual location, the lower end of a humerus. There is a healed fracture at the upper limit of the tumor. B, Another unusual osteogenic sarcoma developing in the lower metaphysis and shaft of a radius in a child. C, A sclerosing osteogenic sarcoma in the upper shaft of a humerus showing a pathologic fracture.

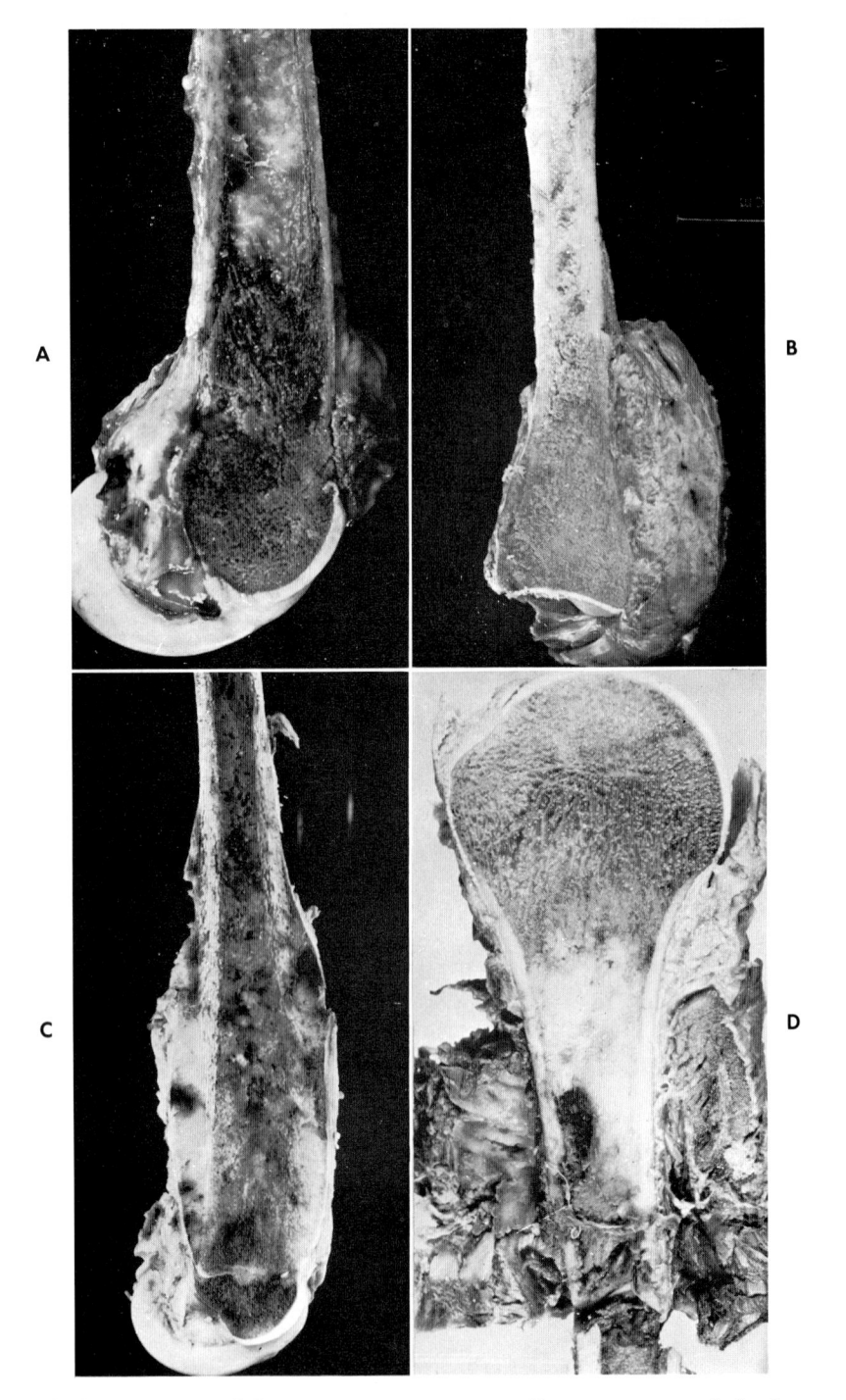

Fig. 16-5. A-D, A group of four amputation specimens illustrating some of the features of the gross pathologic anatomy of osteogenic sarcoma referred to in the text. The tumor shown in **B** is unusual as to location (lower end of a tibia) and presented an equivocal x-ray picture clinically. The tumor shown in **D** developed so insidiously that a pathologic fracture was its first manifestation. Despite the brief clinical history, there were already tumor nodules within the deltoid muscle.

Osteogenic sarcoma of bone 223

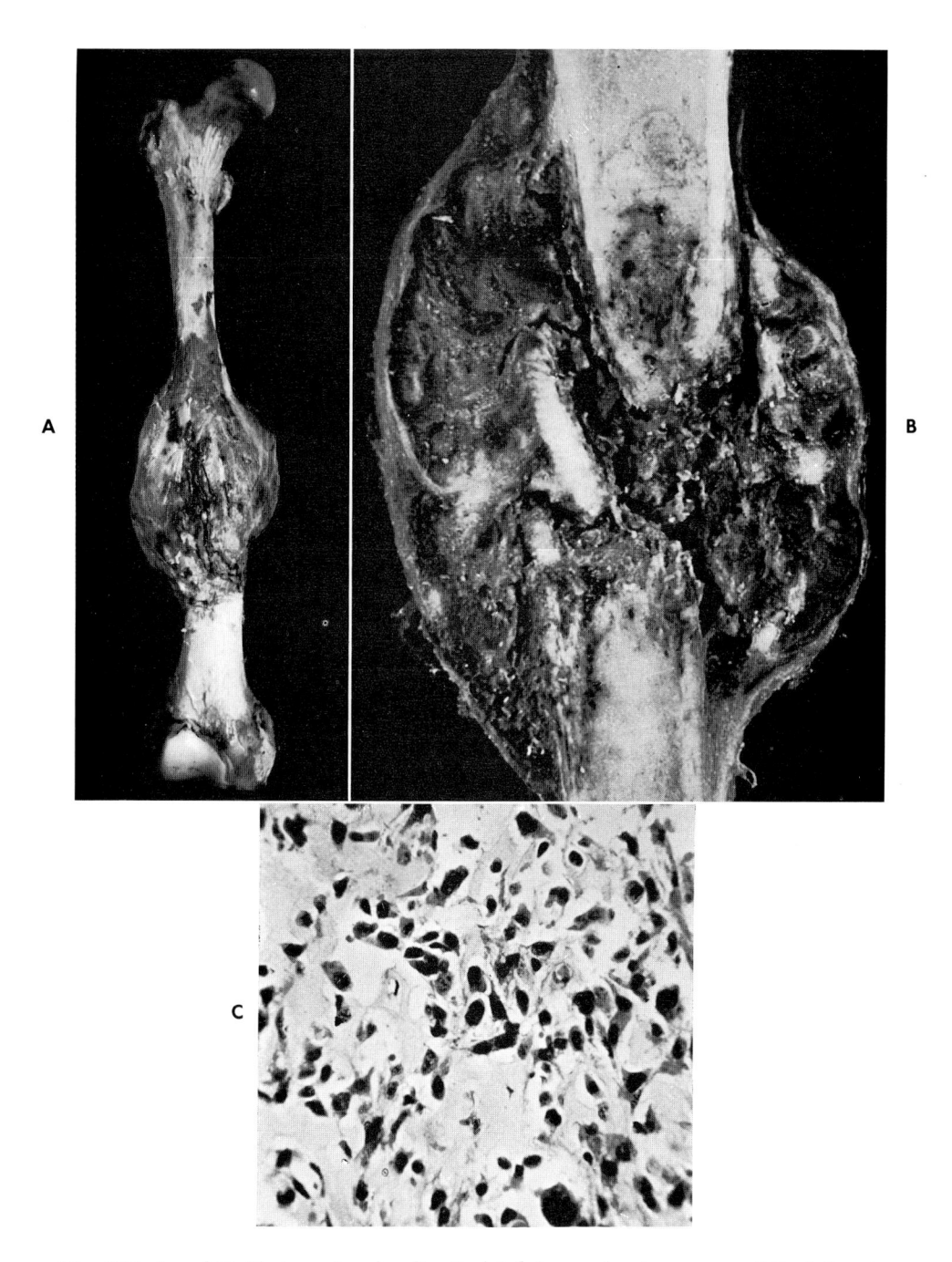

Fig. 16-6. **A** and **B**, Photographs of a disarticulated femur showing an essentially lytic osteogenic sarcoma in its midshaft. The osteogenic sarcoma has destroyed the continuity of the bone and has extended beneath the raised periosteum. The patient was not aware of the neoplasm until he sustained a pathologic fracture about one month before surgery was performed. **C**, A representative field of the osteogenic sarcoma illustrated in **A** and **B**, showing the formation of osteoid matrix by the malignant tumor cells.

to extension toward the end of the affected bone, it should be noted that a tumor developing in the metaphyseal region of a long bone, e.g., the lower end of a femur, tends to involve also part of the adjacent bone end (the epiphyseal area, if fusion has not yet taken place). While this may not be evident in a single random frontal or sagittal section of the specimen, it can usually be demonstrated on serial section. Where the tumor extends beneath the articular cartilage, the latter acts as an effective barrier. However, an osteogenic sarcoma may readily involve a neighboring joint through invasion of the capsule at the site of its attachment to the affected bone area, in which case one is likely to encounter blood-tinged synovial fluid.

The histologic pattern of osteogenic sarcomas is so variable that no two specimens are exactly alike. In any event, whatever this pattern may be in any particular instance, the essential criteria for the diagnosis of osteogenic sarcoma are (1) the presence of a frankly sarcomatous stroma and (2) the direct formation of tumor osteoid and bone by this malignant connective tissue. As noted, one may observe, in addition, more or less prominent fields of malignant tumor cartilage undergoing calcification and osseous transformation, but this should not alter one's impression of osteogenic sarcoma. In any given tumor, the con-

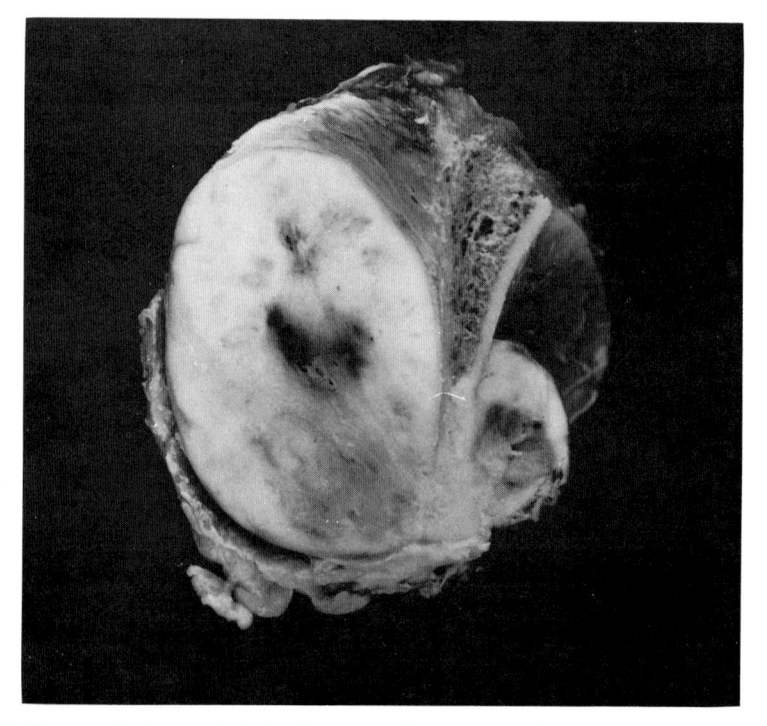

Fig. 16-7. Photograph (natural size) of a resected specimen of an osteogenic sarcoma in the wing of an iliac bone. The tumor extended into attached muscle on both sides. The encapsulation of sarcomas can be very deceptive, and an attempt at clearance by so slender a margin is not to be recommended.

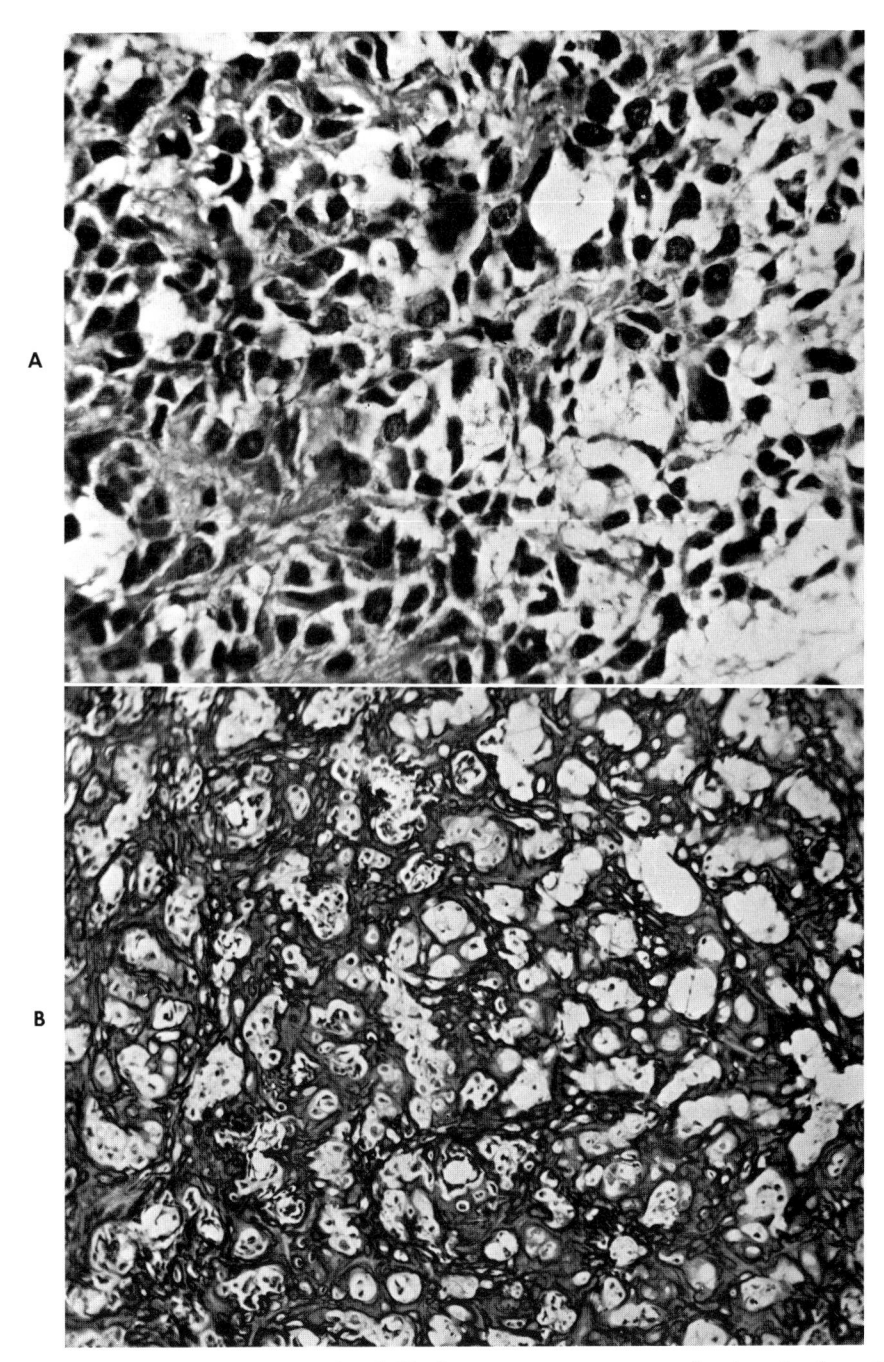

Fig. 16-8. A, Photomicrograph of a field of an osteogenic sarcoma showing the formation of intercellular osteoid matrix by a frankly sarcomatous cellular stroma. (×400.) B, A representative field of a sclerosing osteogenic sarcoma showing interlacing streamers of collagen that have undergone calcification and osteoid conversion. (×100.)

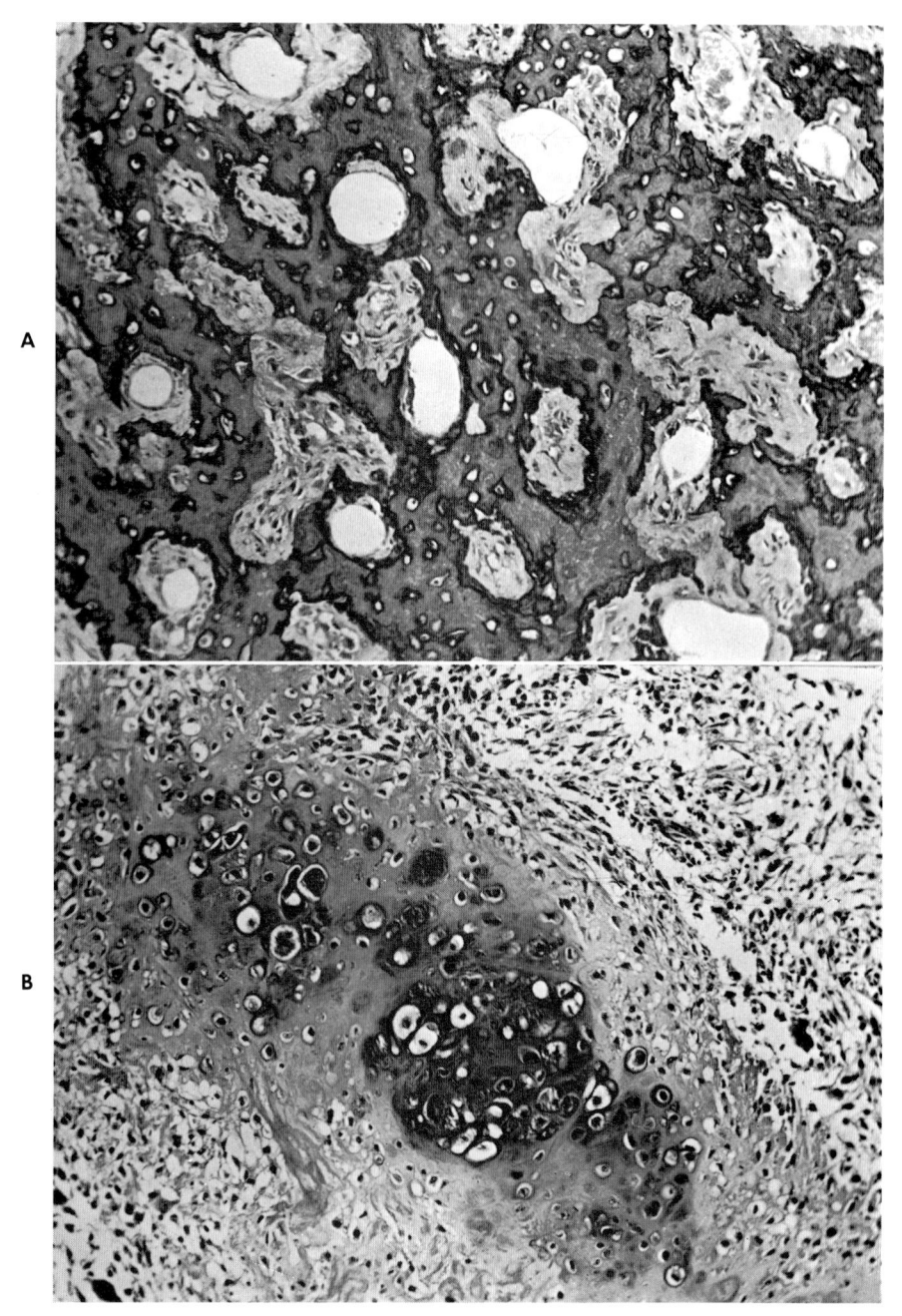

Fig. 16-9. A, Photomicrograph showing formation of tumor bone within a sclerosing osteogenic sarcoma. **B,** A field from another osteogenic sarcoma showing the formation of neoplastic cartilage. This may be a prominent feature in some pertinent tumors and an inconspicuous feature in others. (×110.)

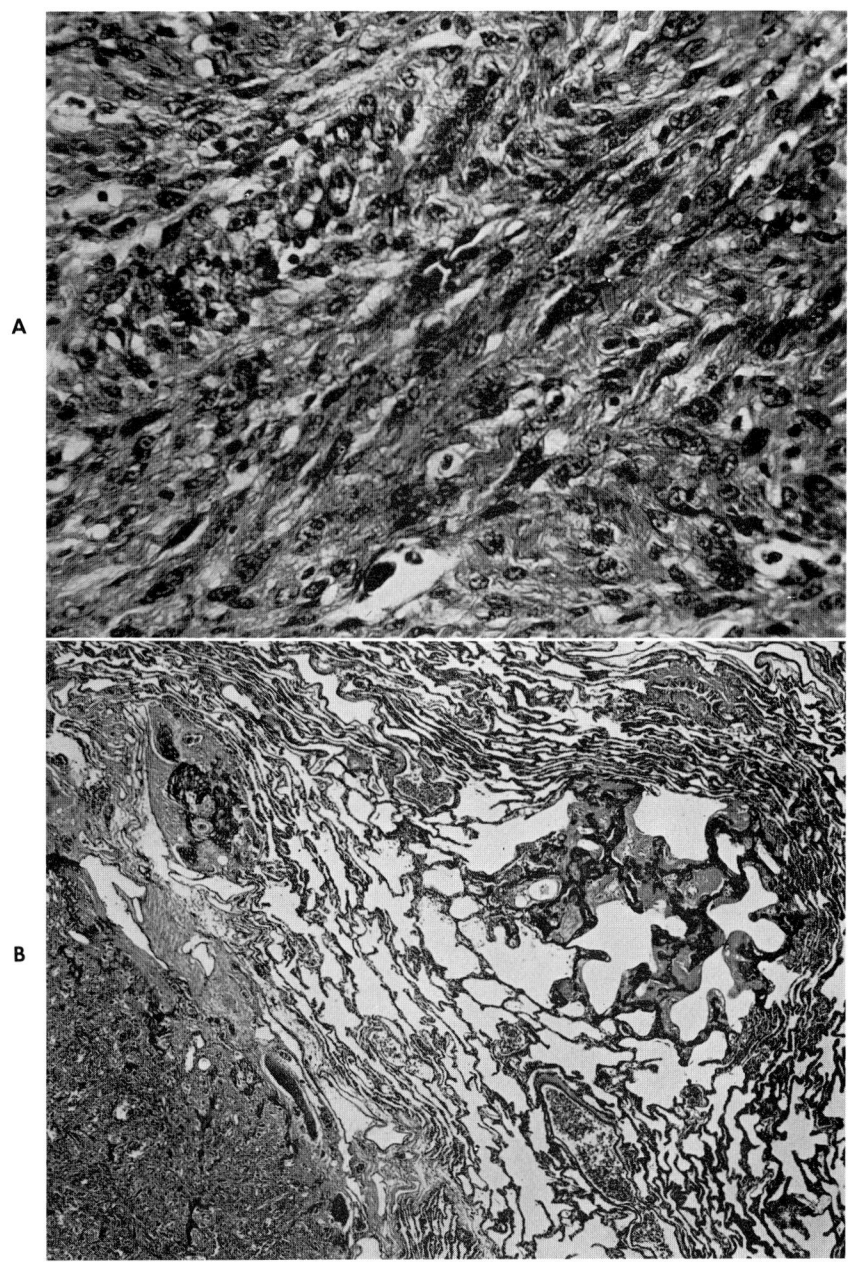

Fig. 16-10. **A,** A field from the periphery of an osteogenic sarcoma that, if viewed in a limited biopsy specimen without due consideration of the character of the neoplasm as a whole, might lead to a false impression of fibrosarcoma. **B,** Photomicrograph showing that in the pulmonary metastases of an osteogenic sarcoma one also observes neoplastic bone formation.

nective tissue stroma may be composed predominantly of large, atypical spindle-shaped cells or may be distinctly anaplastic and present a polymorphous cellular pattern, replete with tumor giant cells. Irregularly dispersed within this sarcomatous stroma, one observes fields in which osteoid and osseous transformation is in active progress. This may be preceded by collagenization of the intercellular matrix, often in the form of crisscrossing streamers, which, in turn, undergo osteoid conversion and focal calcification. The tumor cells that become enveloped in this intercellular matrix usually appear smaller, more rounded, and less ominous than those of the neighboring sarcomatous stroma, which has not as yet undergone collagenization and ossification.

If the neoplasm is one in which relatively little tumor osteoid and bone are laid down, the original spongy bone undergoes substantial resorption and dissolution. On the other hand, if the sarcoma is one that displays extensive osteogenesis, one observes in the highly sclerotized areas within the interior of the affected bone area that the deposits of tumor osteoid and bone have been built around the original spongy bone framework as a scaffold or have freely extended between the spongy trabeculae, with consequent obliteration of the marrow spaces. In such sclerosing tumors, the heavily ossified areas of tumor tissue outside of the cortex also show the intermingling of actively ossifying tumor tissue with reactive, nontumorous, periosteal new bone.

Metastasis in osteogenic sarcoma occurs almost exclusively by hematogenous spread and extension to regional lymph nodes, although it has been noted, appears to be of infrequent occurrence. On rare occasions, large arteries may be invaded and occluded by direct extension of tumor.[46] Pulmonary metastases are consistently found at autopsy. Judging by serial roentgenograms, these may start out as discrete multiple foci (usually also ossified), which, as they enlarge, tend to coalesce, so that ultimately one is likely to find a bulky solid tumor mass within the mediastinum, and/or one or another of the lungs. On occasion, one may observe late metastases in one or more of the other bones. According to Lowbeer,[25] if roentgen skeletal survey is used for detection and all the bones are examined at autopsy, late metastases in them may be found in "up to 15% of cases." Visceral metastases aside from those in the lungs are unusual. In this terminal stage also, cachexia, decubitus ulcers, flexion contractures, and secondary anemia, reflected anatomically in hemosiderosis of the reticulum-bearing organs, are common findings.

Sarcoma complicating Paget's disease

It is a well-known observation that sarcoma of bone develops with significant frequency in patients with Paget's disease. McKenna and associates,[28] in a comprehensive review of the Memorial Hospital material, recently reported 33 osteogenic sarcomas arising in Paget bone and surveyed an additional 137 well-documented cases in point collected from the English literature. Among other recent articles on this subject are those of Schatzki and Dudley,[39] Poretta, Dahlin, and Janes,[31] Freydinger, Duhig, and McDonald,[12] and Price and Goldie.[34]

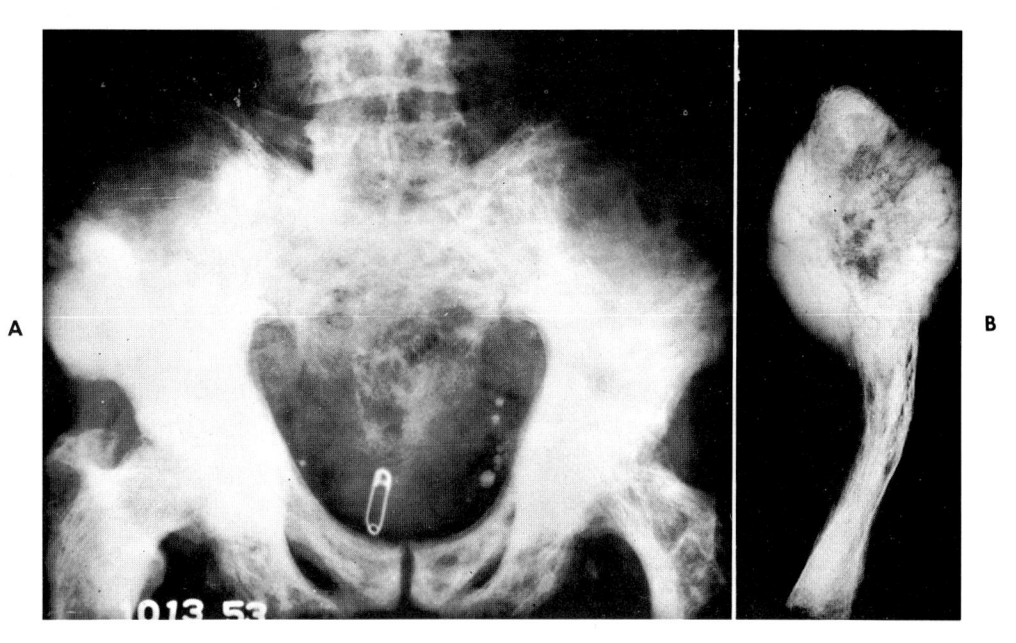

Fig. 16-11. A, Roentgenogram showing multicentric foci of sclerosing osteogenic sarcoma in the right iliac bone of an older man with advanced Paget's disease. The patient succumbed shortly after attempted resection. B, Roentgenogram of a sagittal section of one of the tumors in the ilium, which also shows coarse trabecular alteration indicative of Paget's disease.

This complication is usually observed in patients with fairly extensive Paget's disease of long standing, but it may occur in monostotic Paget's disease. Commonly, it is some one bone that manifests malignant change through the roentgenographic appearance of an ominous rarefied defect that had not been noted previously. However, it is not at all unusual to observe the development of two or more sarcomas, more or less simultaneously, within bones transformed by Paget's disease, e.g., in the calvarium, and in one or more of the large limb bones, particularly the femur, tibia, and humerus.

When bone sarcoma supervenes in the course of Paget's disease, it frequently is of the nature of an osteogenic sarcoma. It is perhaps not generally appreciated, however, that the sarcoma need not necessarily be osteogenic. In fact, it is not unusual under these circumstances to find, on pathologic examination, that the neoplasm in question represents a fibrosarcoma or a sarcoma whose stroma is so anaplastic and replete with tumor giant cells as to simulate a malignant giant-cell tumor. Whether the latter tumor should actually be regarded as a malignant giant-cell tumor of bone, as Russell has contended, is debatable, however. It is pertinent to note that the development of chondrosarcoma in Paget bone has also been observed, although this appears to be distinctly unusual.

The question is often raised as to the precise incidence of sarcoma complicating Paget's disease, and it is rather difficult to answer satisfactorily because of the necessarily limited experience of any one observer and the inaccuracies inherent in pooled material culled from the literature. Moreover, as Schmorl demonstrated, most cases of Paget's disease show limited skeletal involvement and go unrecognized clinically, the changes being confined to portions of the sacrum or to one or a few lumbar vertebral bodies. If one includes all lesions of Paget's disease of whatever nature, then the estimate of malignant change may well be less than 1%. However, if one considers only cases of more or less extensive, advanced Paget's disease, the usually cited estimate of approximately 10% to 15% seems plausible. The prognosis in such cases is distinctly bad, and I have no personal knowledge of a single instance of five-year survival. At the time our bone sarcoma cases were surveyed, there were seven instances of Paget's sarcoma among them, and follow-up observations showed that all had terminated fatally within six months of the time of initial observation. There are occasional survivors after radical surgery,[6,34] to be sure, but, as McKenna and associates[28] emphasized, the reported cures that stand up under close scrutiny can be counted on your hands.

Osteogenic sarcoma developing in multicentric foci

Brief mention should be made of certain rare but undoubted instances of osteogenic sarcomatosis, in which many or even innumerable tumors develop apparently simultaneously throughout the skeleton. An extraordinary case in point is that reported by Silverman,[41] which I saw at autopsy. Literally hundreds of separate tumors of the nature of osteogenic sarcoma, many of them still quite small, were found developing within all parts of the skeleton examined. Through the courtesy of Dr. E. LeMoncheck, of Los Angeles, I have observed another proved comparable instance in a 15-year-old boy, who presented many foci of sclerosing osteogenic sarcoma in the calvarium, vertebral column, and long bones, and whose lung fields were "snowballed" by radiopaque metastases. Dr. G. L. Kraft, also of Los Angeles, has called my attention to still another similar case of osteogenic sarcoma apparently developing in multicentric foci (Figs. 16-12 and 16-13). Through the courtesy of Dr. B. W. Drompp, of Lincoln, Nebraska, I have observed material from an extraordinary case[7] in which the development of an osteogenic sarcoma in a phalanx of a finger was followed some three years later by the appearance of a second osteogenic sarcoma in a phalanx of a finger of the opposite hand (Fig. 16-13, *B* and *C*). Continuing, Dr. Roy I. Peck, of Philadelphia, collected a sizable group of cases exhibiting multicentric osteogenic sarcoma (as yet unpublished to my knowledge). Also worth citing here is a case of multifocal osteogenic sarcoma reported by Price and Truscott,[33] in which tumor growth was relatively slow and had not given rise to pulmonary metastasis. In their paper these authors mention a few additional relevant case reports in the literature. Altogether, it would appear that osteogenic sarcoma developing in multicentric foci is by no means a rarity, as Lowbeer has emphasized.

In none of the instances cited had there been any exposure to radium, mesothorium, or other radioactive substances as a predisposing factor.[8,27] It is note-

Osteogenic sarcoma of bone   231

worthy that Evans and associates, following up the pioneer study of Martland,[27] have observed a 10% incidence to date of osteogenic sarcoma in persons with symptomatic radium poisoning. These tumors were distributed in random fashion throughout the skeleton, in contrast to spontaneous osteogenic sarcoma. Other complications of radium poisoning were dental abnormalities, spontaneous fractures through areas of necrosis and osteitis, osteomyelitis (of the jaw bones particularly), and, in a few instances, carcinoma of the paranasal sinuses or mastoid. These investigators point out that radium and mesothorium are deposited in

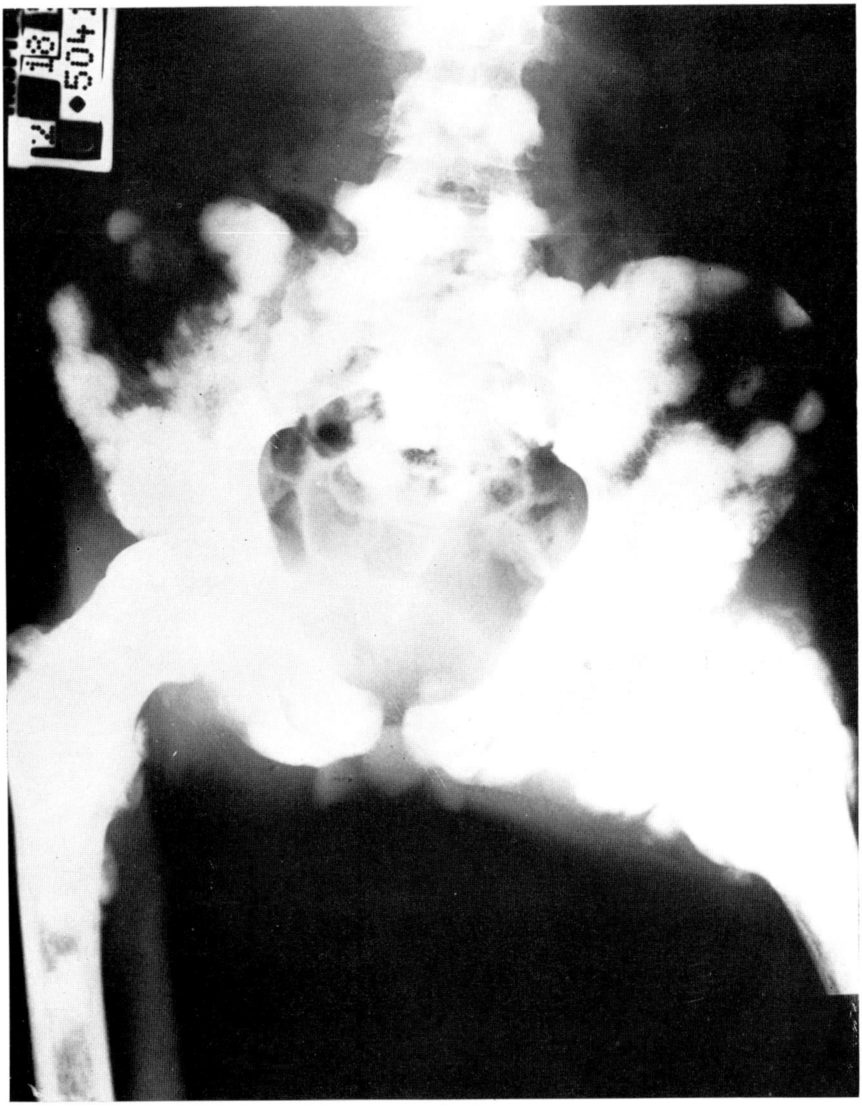

Fig. 16-12. Roentgenogram of an unusual multicentric osteogenic sarcoma. (Courtesy Dr. G. L. Kraft, Los Angeles, Calif.)

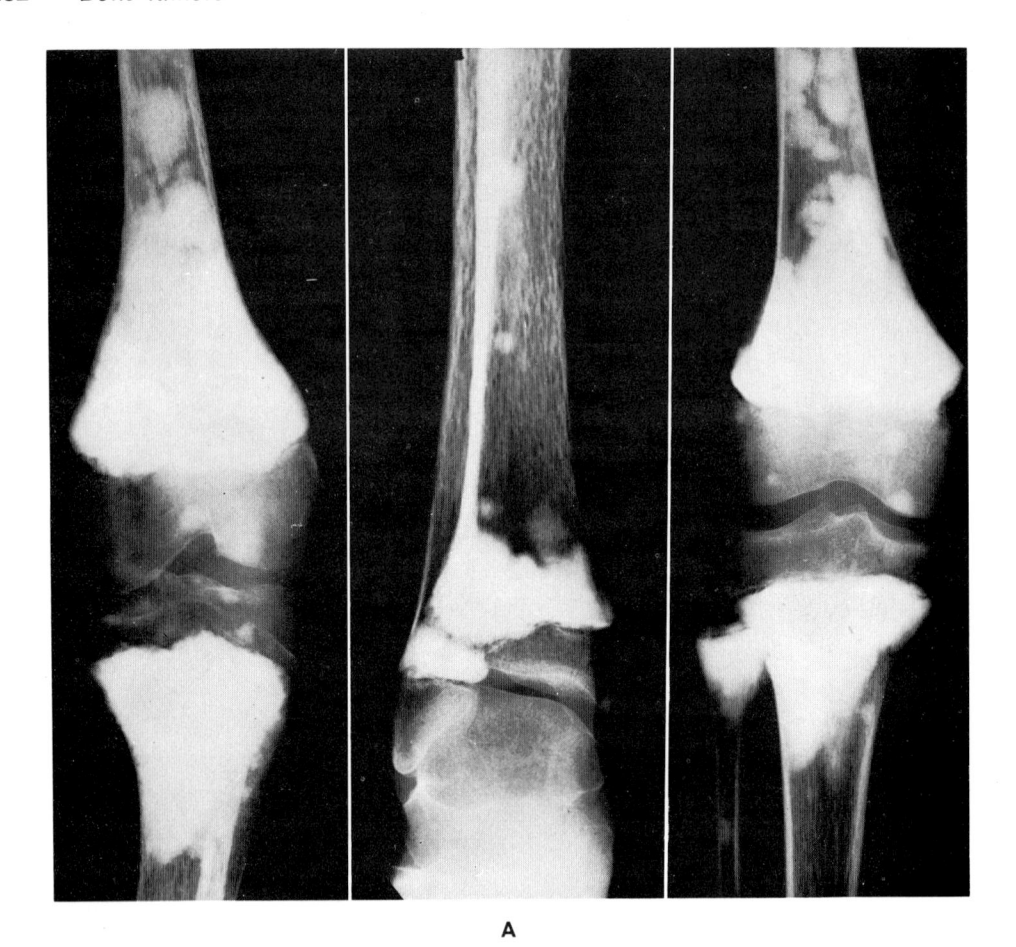

Fig. 16-13. A, Additional roentgenograms from the case illustrated in Fig. 16-12, showing numerous discrete foci of sclerosing osteogenic sarcoma, some of them still quite small, in the limb bones of both lower extremities. **B,** Roentgenogram of a sclerosing osteosarcoma in a proximal finger phalanx. **C,** Another comparable tumor that developed three years later in the opposite hand.

bone in an irregular pattern, with hot spots that contain a hundred times the concentration of radioactivity found in adjacent areas of bone. In the light of this information, one may have some concern about the long-term effects of radioactive fallout in certain parts of the world, especially that of the bone-seeking radioactive materials, such as plutonium or strontium 90. It may be added that osteogenic sarcoma has been induced experimentally by radium (in rats), by exposure to plutonium (in rats), and to radiostrontium (in mice), and even by embedding certain irritant plastics beneath the fascia of the anterior abdominal wall of rodents.

Cognizance must also be taken of the development of osteogenic sarcoma following therapeutic irradiation after a latent interval that may be as short as three years or as long as twenty to thirty years, or more. To the growing list of

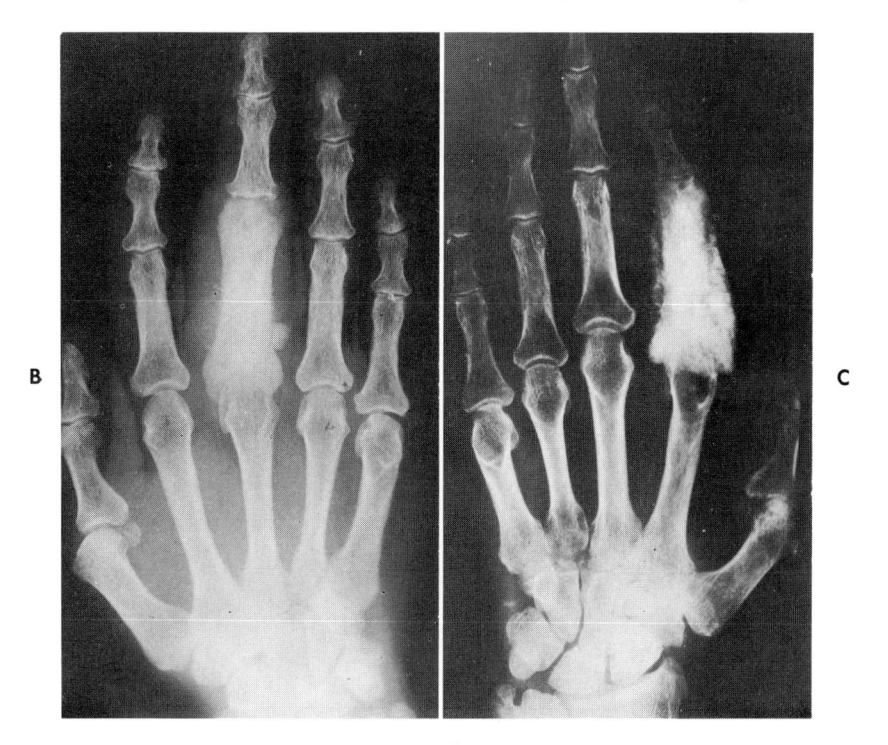

Fig. 16-13, cont'd. For legend see opposite page.

such cases in the literature, I may add mention of several noteworthy instances at this time: one in which osteogenic sarcoma of a lower rib appeared twenty years after irradiation of a Wilms' tumor, another in which a focus of extraskeletal osteogenic sarcoma appeared in the skin and subcutis of the cheek some thirty years after x-ray irradiation of the affected site (the dosage employed is not known), and still another in which osteogenic sarcoma developed in a frontal bone twenty-five years after irradiation for retinoblastoma. Similarly, Block has reported a case in which a pelvic osteogenic sarcoma appeared fourteen years after radiation therapy for carcinoma of the cervix. Dahlin and Coventry[6] cited several comparable instances, as well as three others in which osteosarcoma developed in the scapula after irradiation for carcinoma of the breast.

Treatment and prognosis

As is well known, central or intramedullary osteogenic sarcoma (as distinct from parosteal osteogenic sarcoma) has had an appallingly high mortality rate, in spite of prompt conventional radical surgery. This is particularly true of tumors in children and in older adults with Paget's sarcoma, but not too many of the others are successfully treated beyond a few years. Even when ablation or radical resection is resorted to as soon as the diagnosis is established, the prognosis is nevertheless serious, and my own experience leads me to believe that the five-year

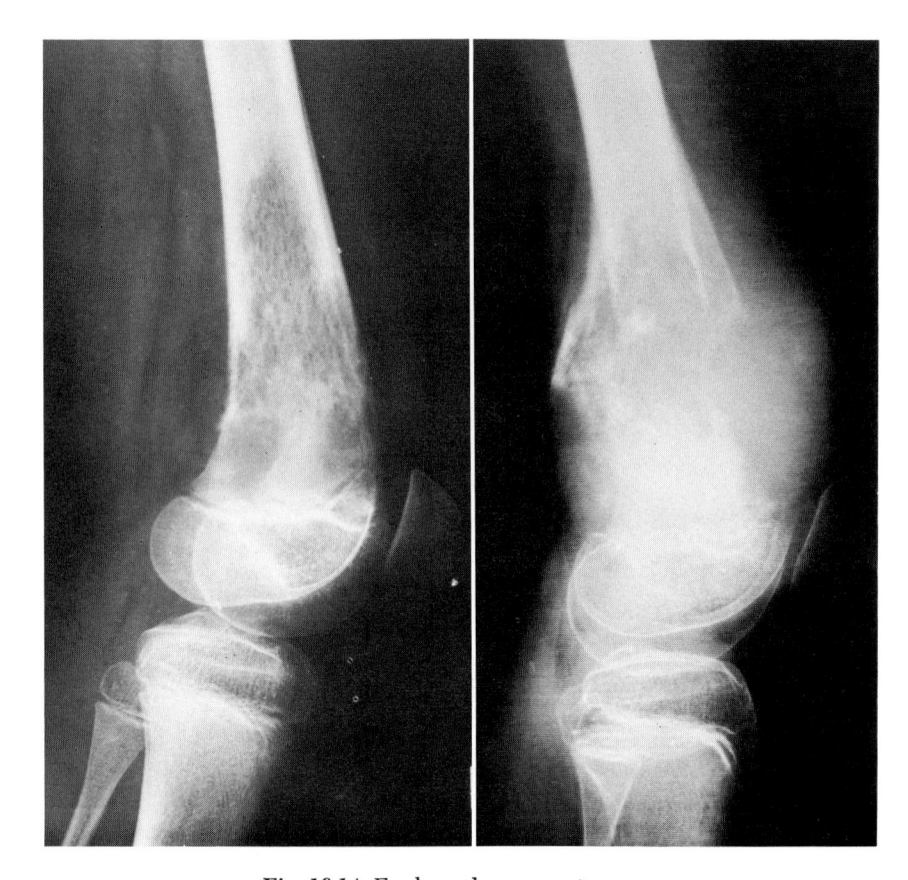

Fig. 16-14. For legend see opposite page.

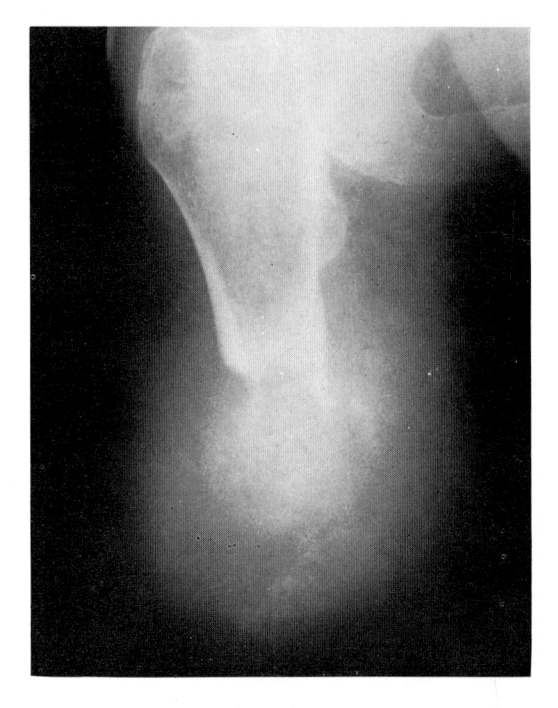

Fig. 16-15. For legend see opposite page.

Osteogenic sarcoma of bone 235

survival rate is probably no higher than 10%. This impression appears to be essentially in accord with that of many other observers: Jaffe[21] reported not much above 5%; Luck,[26] 10% or less; Hatcher,[18] about 5%; Gilmer, Higley, and Kilgore,[14] no more than 10%; and Weinfeld and Dudley,[47] 13%. Coventry and Dahlin[5,6] are not quite so pessimistic and claim an overall survival rate of 19% at five years and of 15% at ten years, but they include among their osteogenic sarcomas some tumors that others might designate as fibrosarcoma or chondrosarcoma. Similarly,

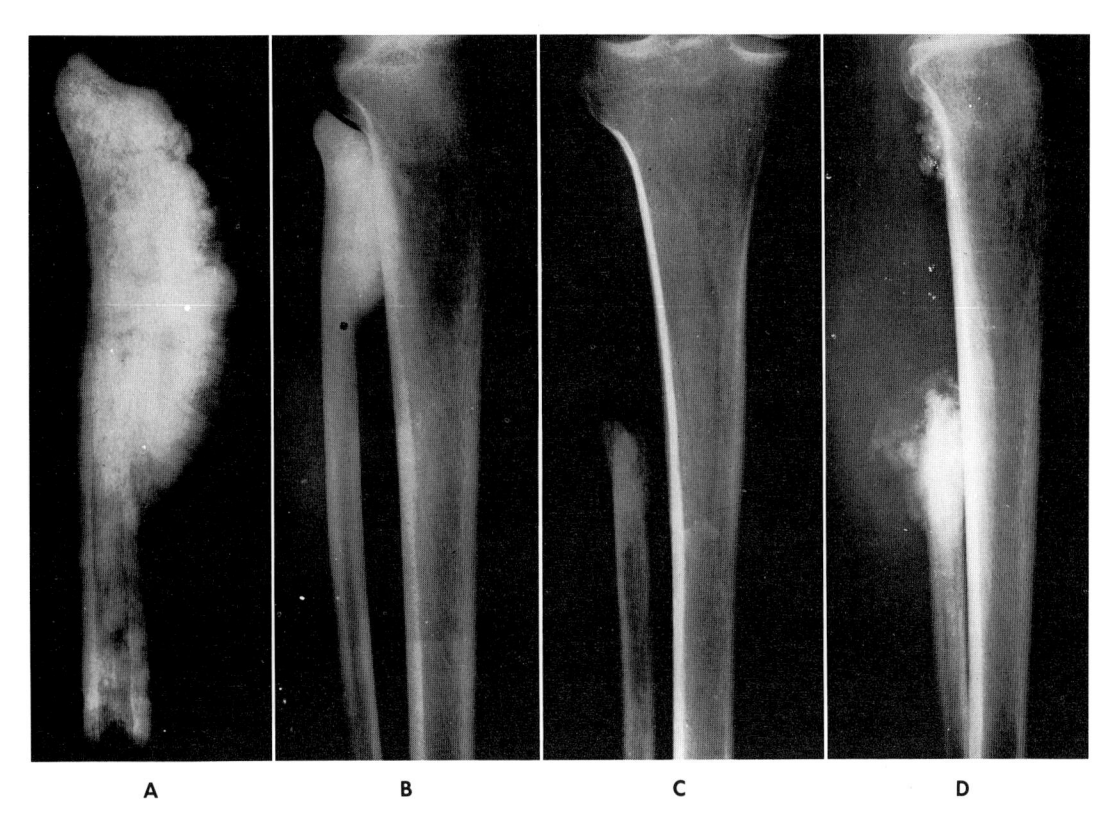

A B C D

Fig. 16-16. Roentgenograms demonstrating the futility of local resection for osteogenic sarcoma, except as a palliative measure. (The patient in this instance refused amputation.) **A,** Roentgenogram of resected specimen. **B,** The initial film showing a sclerosing osteogenic sarcoma in the upper end of a fibula. **C,** Film taken nine months after resection showing recurrence in the stump of the fibula. **D,** Film taken fifteen months postoperatively showing recurrent tumor at the upper as well as the lower end of the excision. Pulmonary metastases were already evident at this time.

Fig. 16-14. Roentgenograms of an osteogenic sarcoma in the distal femur, showing dramatic advance in only seven weeks. (Courtesy Prof. V. Barbera of the University of Bari, Italy.)

Fig. 16-15. Roentgenogram showing recurrence of osteogenic sarcoma in an amputation stump. This complication is not observed with sufficient frequency to justify routine disarticulation at the hip for tumors in the lower femur.

236 Bone tumors

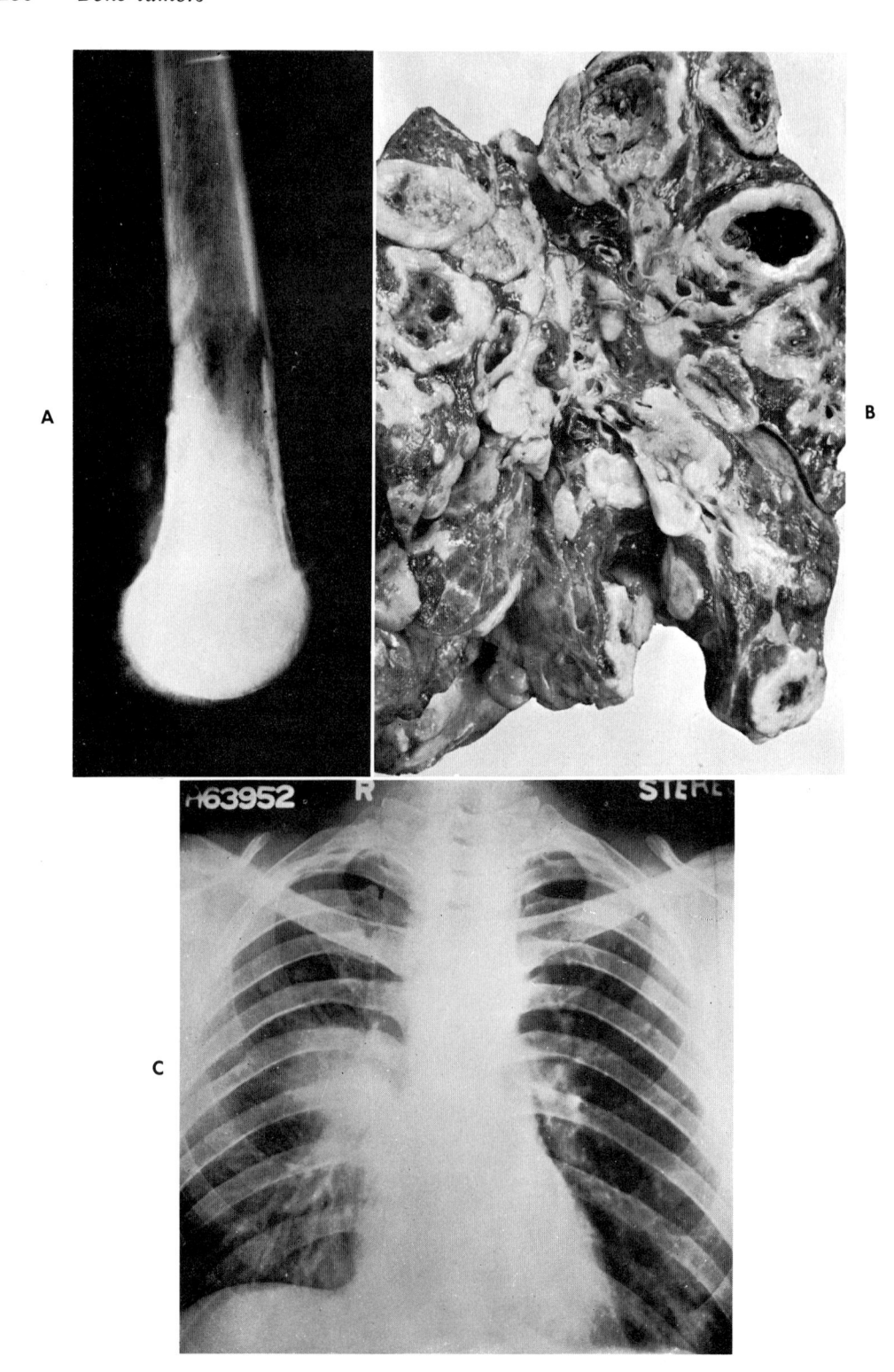

Fig. 16-17. For legend see opposite page.

Price[32] in Britain cites an overall five-year survival rate of 17% and Lindbom, Söderberg, and Spjut[24] in Stockholm, 18.5%.

It is true that there are older surveys reported in the literature, in which the estimated five-year survival rate was 20% or 30%, or even higher. However, there is good reason to infer that these more optimistic impressions are based upon the inclusion in the reported case material of lesions other than osteogenic sarcoma and, specifically, of nonmalignant bone-forming lesions mistaken for osteogenic sarcoma (fibrous dysplasia of bone, myositis ossificans, periosteal ossification, etc.), as well as of neoplasms less serious than osteogenic sarcoma proper (fibrosarcoma and chondrosarcoma particularly). In this same connection, it is pertinent to comment upon the much-discussed paper by Ferguson[10] who, after surveying the cases diagnosed as osteogenic sarcoma in the Bone Sarcoma Registry, came to the rather curious conclusion that the clinical results in patients operated upon after a delay of six months or more were significantly better than in those operated upon promptly. Here again, one is forced to suspect that the recorded impressions in regard to diagnosis in the Registry stand in need of critical review, and that the cases which terminated fatally in spite of prompt surgery were apparently genuine osteogenic sarcomas, whereas many of those in which delay of six months or more was feasible may well have represented other lesions less serious than osteogenic sarcoma. This view is supported by the finding of Budd and MacDonald[2] that of some 118 five-year cures of osteogenic sarcoma, so-called, in the files of the Bone Sarcoma Registry, no more than 14 (12%) were actually bone-producing sarcomas, whereas 93 (almost 80%) appeared to represent instances of either chondrosarcoma or fibrosarcoma.

The discouraging outlook in dealing with osteogenic sarcoma does not appear to be attributable to any significant delay in its clinical recognition. What seems more probable, unfortunately, is that many patients with osteogenic sarcoma already have pulmonary seeding by the time they present themselves for treatment, even though their chest films appears negative. It frequently takes several or many months for these metastases to attain sufficient size and radiopacity for their discernment, and it is apparently only in an occasional instance that pulmonary metastasis fails to develop early or, having developed, is followed by regression of the tumor transplants (Figs. 16-17 and 16-18). Pulmonary spread usually ensues without apparent involvement of large intermediate veins, although in one of the cases in our hospital files a large tumor thrombus was found in the inferior vena cava (at necropsy) in proximity to an osteogenic sarcoma that had extended well beyond the confines of the iliac bone of origin.

Fig. 16-17. A, Roentgenogram of an amputation specimen showing a sclerosing osteogenic sarcoma in the lower end of a femur. B, Photograph showing massive pulmonary metastasis as observed at autopsy less than a year later. Some of the tumor foci have undergone cystic softening. C, Roentgenogram in another comparable instance showing relatively early pulmonary metastasis.

238 Bone tumors

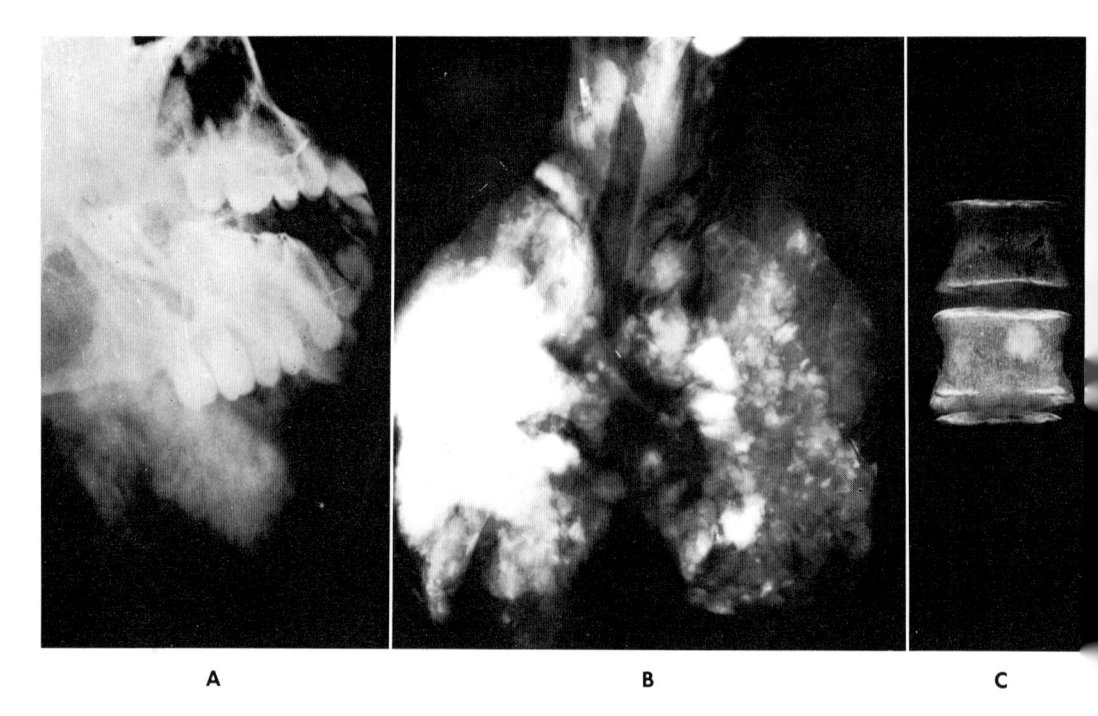

A B C

Fig. 16-18. **A**, Roentgenogram showing local recurrence of osteogenic sarcoma following resection of the mandible. **B**, Roentgenogram of the lungs in this case showing extensive metastatic foci of sclerosing osteogenic sarcoma, as observed at autopsy some months later. **C**, A focus of osteogenic sarcoma encountered within a lumbar vertebral body in this case. (Additional small tumor foci were also observed in the body of the sternum and in one of the ribs examined.)

It has been stated (by Jaffe and Dahlin) that osteogenic sarcomas in the tibia have a significantly better prognosis than do those in the femur. Similarly, Kragh, Dahlin, and Erich,[23] in a survey of 44 osteogenic sarcomas of the jaws and facial bones, stated that the survival rate at five years was as high as 25% or more. The reasons for this disparity in prognosis are not at all apparent. Another unpredictable variable is that of the immunologic response or resistance of the patient to his tumor. Sherman and Irani[40] have stressed this factor in reporting two cases of unexpected long survival (in patients 18 and 5 years of age, respectively) after delayed amputation for advanced, aggressive tumors. The same consideration arises when one attempts to explain the occasional cures by secondary lobectomy for solitary pulmonary metastases, or the sustained disappearance of pulmonary metastases after palliative irradiation (Francis and associates[11]). It may well be that when delicate specific immunologic tools become available for therapy, we shall witness many more such "miracles," and I am convinced that hope for the future lies in this direction. It may be noteworthy[29] here that recent immunofluorescent studies of antibodies to osteosarcoma in the sera of patients and their close relatives and associates, as well as tissue culture studies, have opened up the possibility at least of an oncogenic viral etiology. This could conceivably afford an explanation for the occasional reports of the familial incidence of osteosarcoma.

In principle, amputation should be performed proximal to the bone involved, rather than through it, since recurrent osteogenic sarcoma in an amputation stump is sometimes observed (Fig. 16-15). However, in dealing with osteogenic sarcoma in the lower end of the femur, by far the commonest site of localization, there is little empirical evidence to indicate that disarticulation at the hip is more effective than mid-thigh or high-thigh amputation.

In situations in which radical surgery is contemplated, it is important to emphasize again, self-evident as this may seem, that one should always insist upon confirmation of the clinical and roentgen impression of osteosarcoma by biopsy, however clear the diagnosis may seem. It is by no means rare for cases of exuberant callus[22] (due to whatever cause), active myositis ossificans, self-limited periosteal ossification, or metastatic carcinoma to be mistaken clinically and even pathologically for osteogenic sarcoma. This problem of differential diagnosis will be dealt with in a later chapter. The hazard of the spread of tumor by biopsy has probably been exaggerated. It is usually not necessary to incise the tumor widely or to enter the medullary cavity in order to obtain a satisfactory specimen. If prompt surgery is planned, and the pathologist has confidence in his frozen section diagnosis of sarcoma (of the lower femur or the upper tibia, for example), ablation can be carried out at the time of biopsy between two tourniquets previously applied. For tumors in the upper femur and for some in the innominate bone, hindquarter amputation may be indicated, as may interscapulothoracic amputation for osteosarcoma in the upper end of the humerus. Spread to regional lymph nodes appears to be a rarity and ordinarily is of little concern.

As indicated, however, radical surgery per se has distinct limitations in view of the tendency of osteosarcoma to spread to the lungs relatively early. In the previous edition of this book, I suggested supplementing radical surgery by irradiation of both lung fields through multiple ports as an experimental therapeutic procedure, in the hope of destroying microscopic tumor emboli, or at least reducing the spread to one or two metastatic sites that might be dealt with by lobectomy. In our present medicolegal climate, this suggestion has received only a very limited and inconclusive trial, if only for the reason that physicians are reluctant or unwilling to incur the possible risk of postirradiation pulmonary fibrosis.

Another approach to the use of supplementary irradiation is being widely tested, however—presurgical irradiation of the tumor itself, in the hope or expectation presumably of advantageously enhancing the patient's immune response to his tumor before the latter is extirpated. The expectation engendered by this regimen, which was quite popular for a time,[17] has apparently waned. Those who still advocate it[30] claim only that it may forestall radical surgery in patients in whom pulmonary metastasis has already developed (but has not yet shown up in roentgenograms).

Ossifying parosteal sarcoma (juxtacortical osteogenic sarcoma, parosteal osteogenic sarcoma, parosteal "osteoma")

Considerable interest has been evinced in this unusual category of neoplasms since the publication of the papers by Geschickter and Copeland,[13] Dwinnell, Dahlin, and Ghormley,[9] Scaglietti and Calandriello,[37] and van der Heul and von Ronnen,[45] among others. That they are by no means rare is evidenced by the fact that the last-named authors were able to collect as many as sixty-four well-documented cases from the literature, in addition to sixteen of their own from the Dutch Registry. These neoplasms develop apparently through slow but progressive proliferation of bone-forming (and also cartilage-forming) periosteal and/or parosteal connective tissue, and present as smaller or larger hard masses on the surface of limb bones, rather than in their interior. However, with increasing size, they may in time extend into the underlying cortex and eventually penetrate the medullary cavity. The distal femur particularly is a site of predilection, though occasionally the tibia, the humerus, the ulna, or some other long bone may be affected (Fig. 16-19). For a discussion of the roentgenographic recognition and differentiation of parosteal sarcomas, the reader may refer to the paper by Stevens, Pugh, and Dahlin.[43] To be sure, not all parosteal growths (on the lower femur posteriorly, for example) develop into sarcomas (Fig. A-5), and, for this reason, I cannot condone the practice of performing radical surgery on a presumptive clinical diagnosis, without confirmation by an adequate biopsy. However, the natural history of many of them indicates that they are potentially malignant, although the clinical course may be measured in years rather than months, and that they are capable of pulmonary metastasis eventually.

Much valuable, practical information based on long-term follow-up may be found in the paper by Scaglietti and Calandriello.[38] They point out that local excision of the lesion initially is nearly always followed by recurrence after a varying interval, and they therefore recommend block resection (with bone grafting) if this will encompass the entire lesion. When this is not possible or when recurrence has taken place, they advocate radical surgery, as do other observers who have studied the problem. Surgery had been refused by several of their patients, and the tumors were observed to attain huge size over a period of seven or eight years; in two such instances belated radical surgery did not forestall pulmonary metastasis. The necessity for adequate treatment without unduly prolonged temporizing is thus underscored. Under favorable clinical auspices the cure rate may be as high as 70% or more, in striking contrast to that of conventional intramedullary osteogenic sarcoma, with which the condition seems to have little in common.

The task of the pathologist in appraising the seriousness of a lesion in question from tissue sections alone may be quite difficult, particularly if the lesion is an early one, and he should always have the benefit of an adequate history and of the x-ray films for orientation. It is incumbent upon him to sample thoroughly all the tissue submitted and, particularly, to scrutinize the fields of

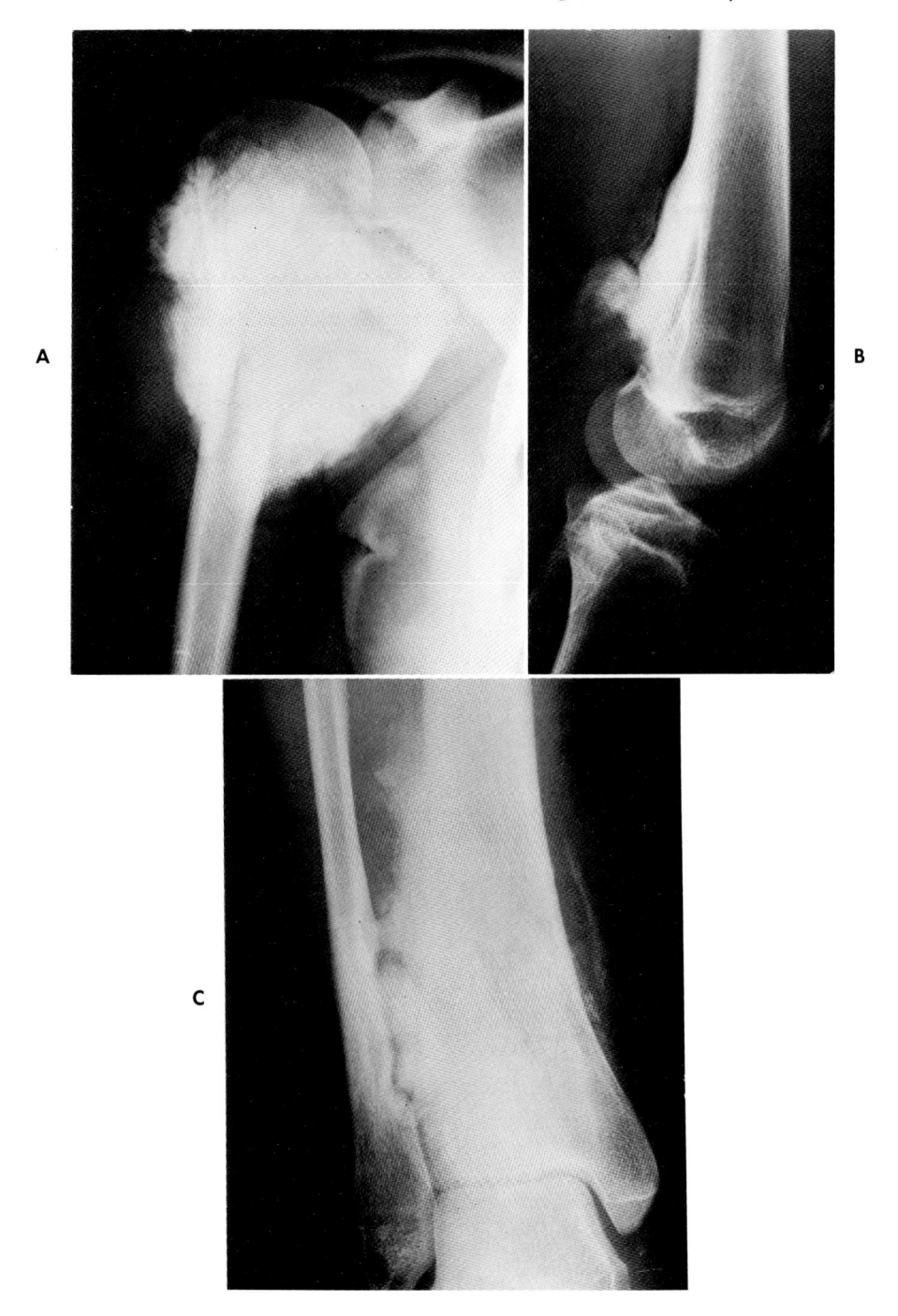

Fig. 16-19. A, Roentgenogram of a parosteal osteogenic sarcoma surrounding the upper humerus. This tumor was unusual in that it metastasized relatively early (within two years of the time it was recognized). B, Roentgenogram of a parosteal osteogenic sarcoma developing around the distal femur posteriorly in a girl of 12. This tumor recurred after an attempt at local excision. C, Another, more extensive, parosteal osteosarcoma developing around the distal tibia.

connective tissue closely for focal areas in which the spindle cells are more compact and have plump hyperchromatic or otherwise atypical nuclei. I might add that some of the published photomicrographs do not convincingly show sarcomatous change, by the usual standards at least, and I do believe that this area needs further clarification. The surgeon can help by sampling multiple (separately labeled) areas for biopsy, including one or two from the depth of the lesion, close to the periosteum and cortex where the proliferating connective tissue is likely to show its greatest activity.

References

1. Barry, H. C.: Sarcoma in Paget's disease of bone in Australia, J. Bone Joint Surg. 43-A:1122, 1961.
2. Budd, J. W., and MacDonald, I.: Osteogenic sarcoma. A modified nomenclature and a review of 118 five-year cures, Surg. Gynecol. Obstet. 77:413, 1943.
3. Coley, B. L., and Harold, C. C., Jr.: An analysis of 59 cases of osteogenic sarcoma with survival for five years or more, J. Bone Joint Surg. 32:307, 1950.
4. Cones, D. M. T.: An unusual bone tumor complicating Paget's disease, J. Bone Joint Surg. 35-B:101, 1953.
5. Coventry, M. B., and Dahlin, D. C.: Osteogenic sarcoma, J. Bone Joint Surg. 39-A:741, 1957.
6. Dahlin, D. C., and Coventry, M. B.: Osteogenic sarcoma—a study of six hundred cases, J. Bone Joint Surg. 49-A:101, 1967.
7. Drompp, B. W.: Bilateral osteosarcoma in the phalanges of the hand, J. Bone Joint Surg. 43-A:199, 1961.
8. Dunlap, C. E., Aub, J. C., Evans, R. D., and Harris, R. S.: Transplantable osteogenic sarcomas induced in rats by feeding radium, Am. J. Pathol. 20:1, 1944.
9. Dwinnell, L. A., Dahlin, D. C., and Ghormley, R. K.: Parosteal (juxtacortical) osteogenic sarcoma, J. Bone Joint Surg. 36-A:732, 1954.
10. Ferguson, A. B.: Treatment of osteogenic sarcoma, J. Bone Joint Surg. 22:916, 1940.
11. Francis, K. C., Hutter, R. V. P., Phillips, R. K., Eyerly, R. C., and Schechter, L.: Osteogenic sarcoma. Sustained disappearance of pulmonary metastases after only palliative irradiation, N. Engl. J. Med. 266:694, 1962.
12. Freydinger, J. E., Duhig, J. T., and McDonald, L. W.: Sarcoma complicating Paget's disease of bone, Arch. Pathol. 75:496, 1963.
13. Geschickter, C. F., and Copeland, M. M.: Parosteal osteoma of bone: a new entity, Ann. Surg. 133:790, 1951.
14. Gilmer, W. S., Higley, G. B., Jr., and Kilgore, W. E.: Atlas of bone tumors, St. Louis, 1963, The C. V. Mosby Co.
15. Goldenberg, R. R.: Eight-year survival of osteogenic sarcoma of tibia with pulmonary metastasis; case report, Bull. Hosp. Joint Dis. 15:67, 1954.
16. Goldenberg, R. R.: The skeleton in Paget's disease, Bull. Hosp. Joint Dis. 12:229, 1952.
17. Green, W. T.: Recent experiences with treatment of osteogenic sarcomata, J. Bone Joint Surg. 40-A:1437, 1958.
18. Hatcher, C. H.: J. Bone Joint Surg. 39-A:758, 1957 (discussion of paper by Coventry and Dahlin).
19. Horie, K., Makita, M., and Sato, K.: Experimental osteogenic sarcoma: histogenesis for osteogenic sarcoma, Gann 51:399, 1960.
20. Jacobson, S. A.: Malignant aneurysmal bone cyst, Bull. Pathol., July-Aug., 1969, p. 240; Malignant aneurysmal bone cyst: a new tumor of man and animals, Am. J. Pathol. 55:28(a), 1969.
21. Jaffe, H. L.: Tumors and tumorous conditions of the bones and joints, Philadelphia, 1958, Lea & Febiger.
22. Kahn, L. B., Wood, F. W., and Ackerman, L. V.: Fracture callus associated with benign and malignant bone lesions and mimicking osteosarcoma, Am. J. Clin. Pathol. 52:14, 1969.
23. Kragh, L. V., Dahlin, D. C., and Erich, J. B.: Osteogenic sarcoma of the jaws and facial bones, Am. J. Surg. 96:496, 1958.
24. Lindbom, A., Söderberg, G., and Spjut, H. J.: Osteosarcoma. A review of 96 cases, Acta Radiol. (Stockholm) 56:1, 1961.
25. Lowbeer, L.: Multifocal osteosarcomatosis, a rare entity, Bull. Pathol., March, 1968, p. 52.
26. Luck, J. B.: J. Bone Joint Surg. 39-A:757, 1957 (discussion of paper by Coventry and Dahlin).

27. Martland, H. S.: Occurrence of malignancy in radioactive persons; a general review of data gathered in the study of the radium dial painters. With special reference to the occurrence of osteogenic sarcoma and the inter-relationship of certain blood diseases, Am. J. Cancer 15:2435, 1931.
28. McKenna, R. J., Schwinn, C. P., Soong, K. Y., and Higinbotham, N. L.: Osteogenic sarcoma arising in Paget's disease, Cancer 17:42, 1964.
29. Morton, D. L., Malmgren, R. A., Hall, W. T., and Schidlovsky, G.: Immunologic and virus studies with human sarcoma, Surgery 66:152, 1969.
30. Phillips, T. L., and Sheline, G. E.: Radiation therapy of malignant bone tumors, Radiology 92:1537, 1969.
31. Poretta, C. A., Dahlin, D. C., and Janes, J. M.: Sarcoma in Paget's disease of bone, J. Bone Joint Surg. 39-A:1314, 1957.
32. Price, C. H. G.: Osteogenic sarcoma. An analysis of survival and its relationship to histological grading and structure, J. Bone Joint Surg. 43-B:300, 1961.
33. Price, C. H. G., and Truscott, E. D.: Multifocal osteogenic sarcoma. Report of a case, J. Bone Joint Surg. 39-B:524, 1957.
34. Price, C. H. G., and Goldie, W.: Paget's sarcoma of bone—a study of eighty cases from the Bristol and Leeds Bone Tumour Registries, J. Bone Joint Surg. 51-B:205, 1969.
35. Robbins, R.: Familial osteosarcoma. Fifth reported occurrence, J.A.M.A. 202:1055, 1967.
36. Russell, D. S.: Malignant osteoclastoma and the association of malignant osteoclastoma with Paget's osteitis deformans, J. Bone Joint Surg. 31-B:281, 1949.
37. Scaglietti, O., and Calandriello, B.: Il Sarcoma Parostale Ossificante, Arch. Putti 6:9, 1955.
38. Scaglietti, O., and Calandriello, B.: Ossifying parosteal sarcoma, J. Bone Joint Surg. 44-A:635, 1962.
39. Schatzki, S. C., and Dudley, H. R., Jr.: Bone sarcoma complicating Paget's disease. A report of three cases with bone survival, Cancer 14:517, 1961.
40. Sherman, M., and Irani, R. N.: Osteogenic sarcoma. Two cases of unexpectedly long survival, J. Bone Joint Surg. 44-A:461, 1962.
41. Silverman, G.: Multiple osteogenic sarcoma, Arch. Pathol. 21:88, 1936.
42. Sirsat, M. V.: Osteogenic sarcoma of the maxilla, Indian J. Med. Sci. 9:537, 1955.
43. Stevens, G. M., Pugh, D. G., and Dahlin, D. C.: Roentgenographic recognition and differentiation of parosteal osteogenic sarcoma, Am. J. Roentgenol. 78:1, 1957.
44. Tapp, E.: Osteogenic sarcoma in rabbits following subperiosteal implantation of beryllium, Arch. Pathol. 88:89, 1969.
45. Van der Heul, R. O., and von Ronnen, J. R.: Juxtacortical osteosarcoma—diagnosis, differential diagnosis, treatment and an analysis of eighty cases, J. Bone Joint Surg. 49-A:415, 1967.
46. Van Way, C. W., III, and Lawler, M. R.: Osteogenic sarcomatous emboli to the femoral arteries, Am. J. Surg. 117:745, 1969.
47. Weinfeld, M. S., and Dudley, H. R., Jr.: Osteogenic sarcoma. A follow-up study of the 94 cases observed at the Massachusetts General Hospital from 1920 to 1960, J. Bone Joint Surg. 44-A:269, 1962.

Chapter 17

Fibrosarcoma of bone

Fibrosarcoma of bone may be defined as a primary malignant fibroblastic tumor that, upon thorough histologic sampling, fails to exhibit any tendency to form tumor osteoid and bone, either in its local growth or in its metastases. As early as 1943, Budd and MacDonald[1] advocated the separation of (central) fibrosarcoma from osteogenic sarcoma proper ("osteosarcoma") as a distinctly less serious neoplasm, pointing out that such tumors accounted for 31% of the five-year cures of so-called osteogenic sarcoma filed in the Bone Sarcoma Registry. Phemister[11] also supported the concept of fibrosarcoma as a distinctive neoplasm of bone, emphasizing that it is much more frequently primary in the medullary region than in the periosteum and that the tumor tissue does not form bone, although periosteal new bone may be laid down as a result of cortical perforation and pathologic fracture.

Fibrosarcoma of bone occurs distinctly less frequently than osteogenic sarcoma or chondrosarcoma. As indicated, it starts its development within the interior of the affected bone, usually a large limb bone, but, like other intramedullary malignant neoplasms, it tends eventually to penetrate the overlying cortex and extend into the contiguous periosteum and muscle. When it does so, it must be distinguished from the occasional fibrosarcoma that arises parosteally and invades the interior of the contiguous bone secondarily by direct extension. These basic concepts, once controversial, have been amply supported by the investigations of McLeod, Dahlin, and Ivins[9] and of Gilmer and MacEwen,[5] among others.[4,6,7]

The femur and tibia are by far the most common sites, and only occasionally is the humerus or some other long limb bone involved. Occurrence of fibrosarcoma elsewhere is distinctly unusual in my experience. Of the last twenty-five instances observed, fully two-thirds developed in the femur or tibia, in shaft locations as well as the ends of these bones. Only three were not in a long limb bone (a cuboid, a finger, and an iliac bone). While most of these patients were adults whose ages ranged from 30 to 70 years, it is noteworthy that four were comparatively young (11, 17, 20, and 21 years of age). This experience is essentially in accord with that of other observers.[5,9] The presenting clinical complaints, as in most bone tumors, were pain and swelling, and their duration varied

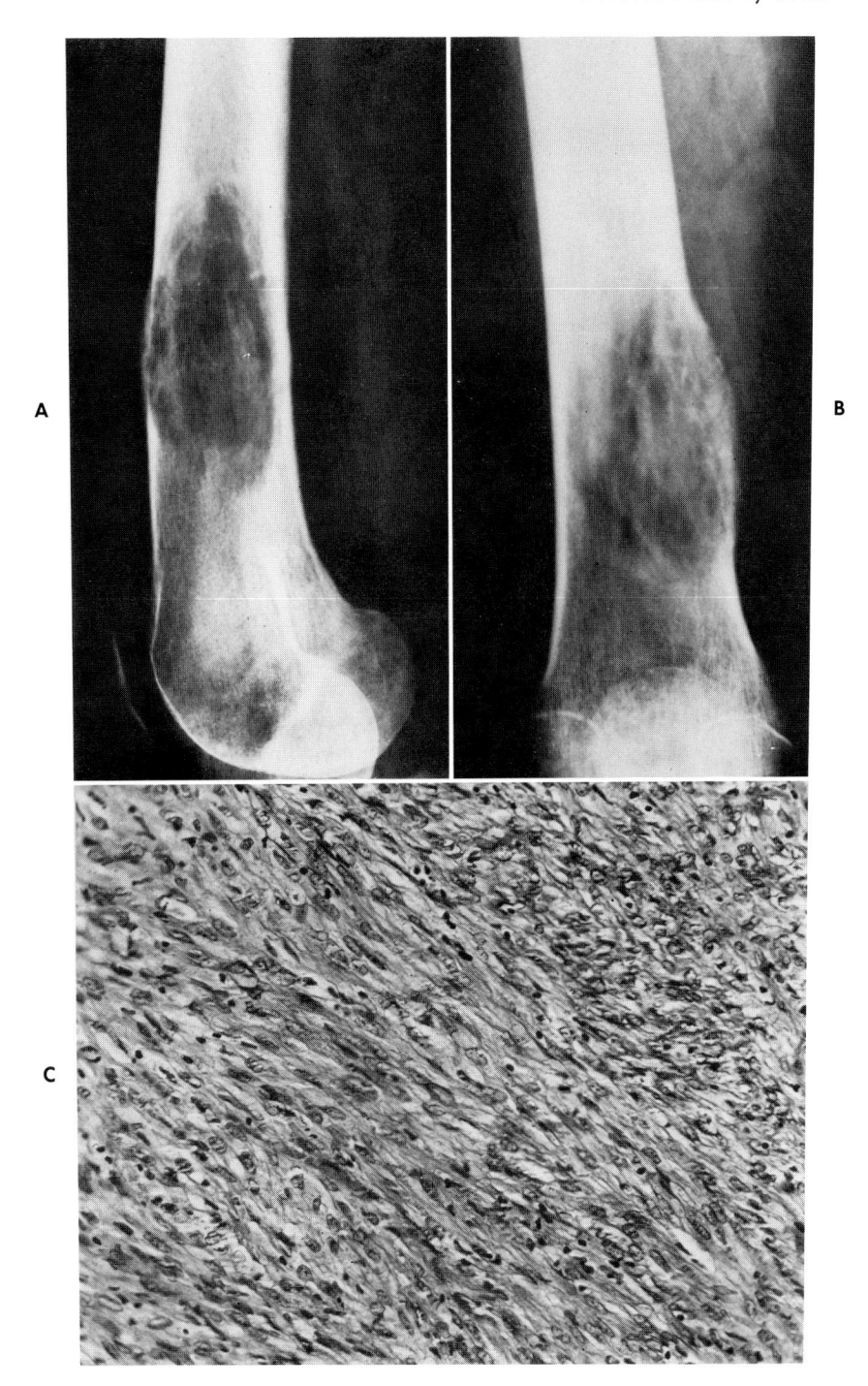

Fig. 17-1. A and B, Roentgenograms of a primary malignant neoplasm in the lower shaft of the femur of an older adult, which on biopsy proved to be a fibrosarcoma. Amputation was carried out promptly. From the x-ray study alone, one might suspect the presence of a primary sarcoma, though not necessarily fibrosarcoma. C, Photomicrograph of the fibrosarcoma illustrated in A and B, as observed in the biopsy specimen. (×200.)

246 Bone tumors

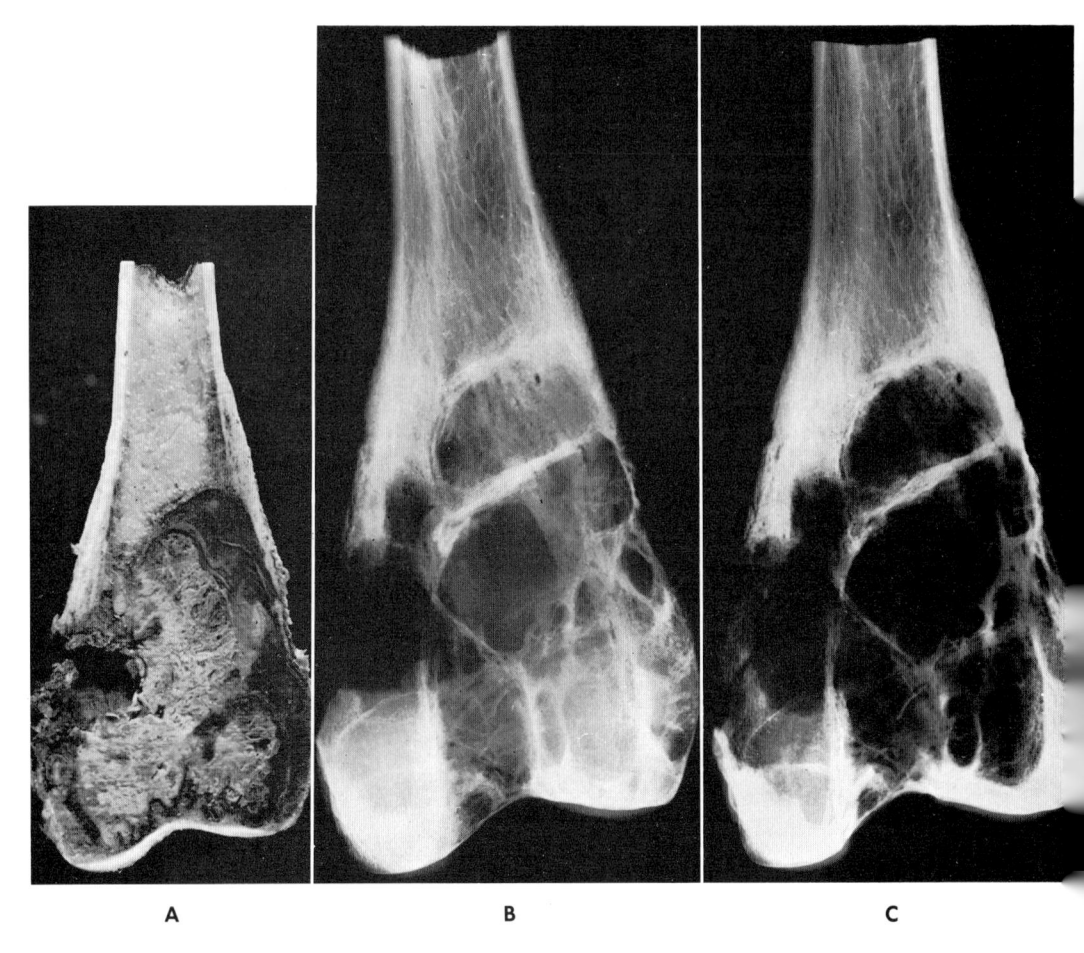

A   B   C

Fig. 17-2. **A**, Photograph of a central fibrosarcoma in the lower end of the femur of an adult. The cortical defect represents the biopsy site. The neoplastic tissue showed extensive old hemorrhage and necrosis. This tumor developed relatively slowly over a period of several years and then took on a spurt of growth, reflected in its cytologic picture (Fig. 17-6, *A*). Nowhere in any of the numerous fields examined was there evidence of tumor osteoid or new bone formation. **B**, X-ray film of the amputation specimen shown in **A**. **C**, X-ray film of the same specimen taken after all of the tumor tissue had been carefully scooped out, leaving only the surrounding bony shell. This demonstrates convincingly that the trabeculated pattern observed in **B** reflects endosteal reaction to the slowly expanding tumor.

considerably from a few months to several or many years. In several instances pathologic fracture was the initial manifestation.

It seems to be unusual for a roentgen diagnosis of fibrosarcoma to be made before biopsy. The picture is rather nondescript and essentially that of an ill-defined rarefaction. The rule of thumb that I follow is this: if a lesion suggests a primary malignant bone tumor, but not any one in particular, then think of fibrosarcoma as a possibility, especially if the lesion is in the femur or tibia of an adult.

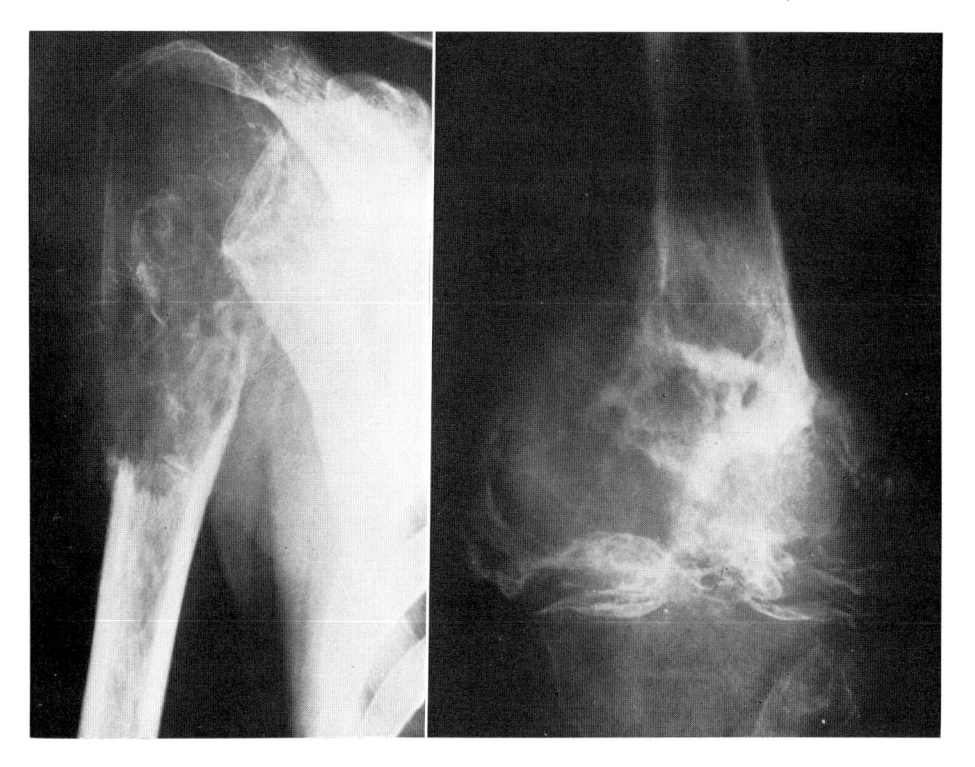

Fig. 17-3   Fig. 17-4

Fig. 17-3. Roentgenogram of a large lytic lesion in the upper end of the humerus of a 31-year-old man. The cortical and intramedullary dissolution (not evident in previous x-ray films) proved to be due to the presence of a fibrosarcoma. The circumstances pertaining to the case strongly suggested that this tumor may well have developed within an old solitary unicameral bone cyst.

Fig. 17-4. Roentgenogram showing an advanced, destructive tumor in the lower end of a femur, which proved to be fibrosarcoma. This site had been irradiated some years previously for another condition (total dosage is not known). The subsequent clinical course was featured by amputation after considerable delay, recurrence in the stump, and eventual spread to other bones and soft parts.

The consultation material in my files indicates that often pathologists, too, may have difficulty in making a diagnosis of fibrosarcoma from examination of a biopsy specimen. Of the last eighteen instances in point, there were as many as nine in which the examining pathologist missed the diagnosis of fibrosarcoma initially and considered instead the possibility of fibrous dysplasia, nonossifying fibroma, desmoplastic fibroma, or some other benign lesion. This may reflect lack of clinical orientation and failure to look at the x-ray films, the fact that some fibrosarcomas are well differentiated, and also the limitations of random sampling. With reference to the latter point particularly, it may be emphasized that desmoplastic reaction in a biopsy field does not mean necessarily that the tumor as a whole is well differentiated; it may be richly cellular and ominous in other areas (Fig. 17-8, *C* and *D*). Whatever the reason may be, failure to establish a diag-

248 Bone tumors

nosis of fibrosarcoma promptly, leading to curettement of a tumor initially or to long delay in its recognition, is cause for concern.

Some predisposing or contributory causes for the development of fibrosarcoma of bone may be considered briefly here. It is well known, for example, that sarcoma developing in Paget bone may sometimes be of the nature of fibrosarcoma (Fig. 17-6, *B*). Similarly, some of the malignant neoplasms developing as an untoward sequel of therapeutic irradiation may take the form of fibrosarcoma. Malignant change in giant-cell tumor of bone, with or without previous irradiation, may give rise to tumors resembling fibrosarcoma (Fig. 12-14, *B*), and, in a sense, malignant giant-cell tumor may be regarded as a special kind of fibrosarcoma. In the survey of the Mayo Clinic material by McLeod, Dahlin, and

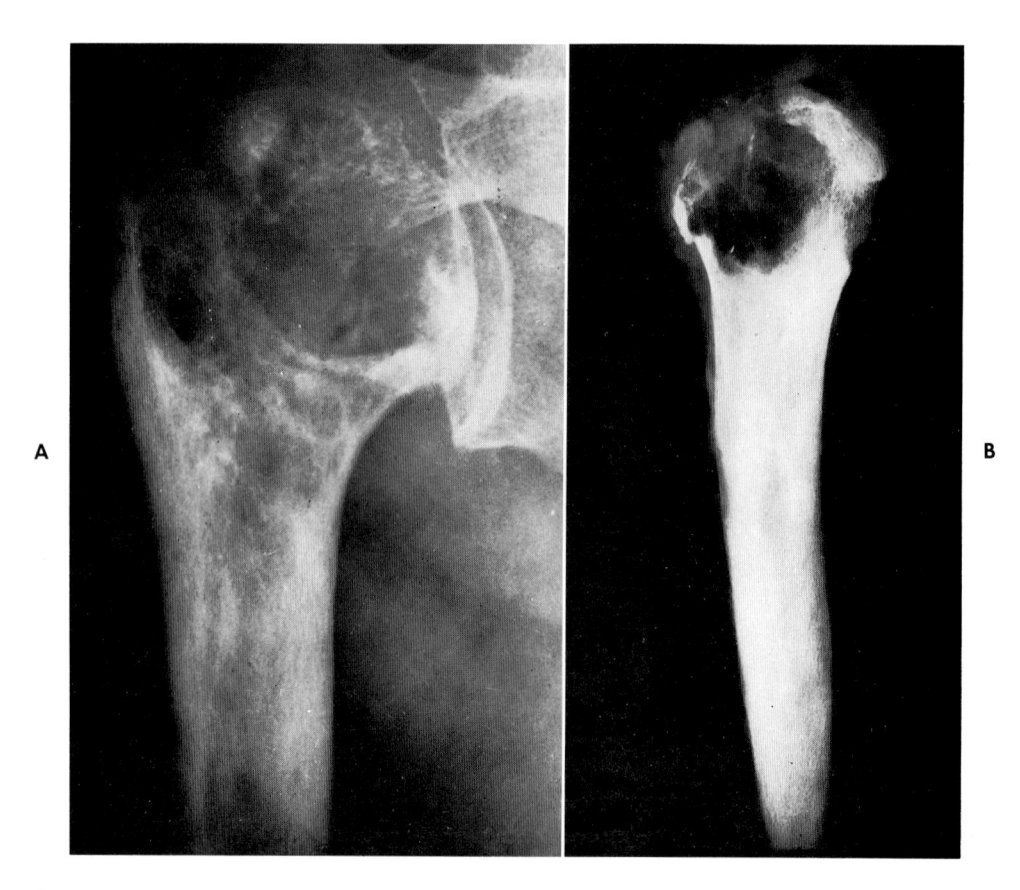

Fig. 17-5. **A**, Roentgenogram of a primary malignant neoplasm in the upper end of the humerus of an older woman, which proved on biopsy to represent a fibrosarcoma (Fig. 17-6, *B*). Despite ablation, this patient developed metastases within a few months. Examination of the cortical bone in the head and upper shaft of the humerus revealed the presence of Paget's disease. **B**, Roentgenogram of the amputation specimen (reduced) showing the lytic tumor defect and perforation of the cortex (this developed after the film shown in **A** was taken), as well as changes in the humerus incidental to Paget's disease (these changes, of course, were more clearly seen in the original roentgenogram).

Fibrosarcoma of bone 249

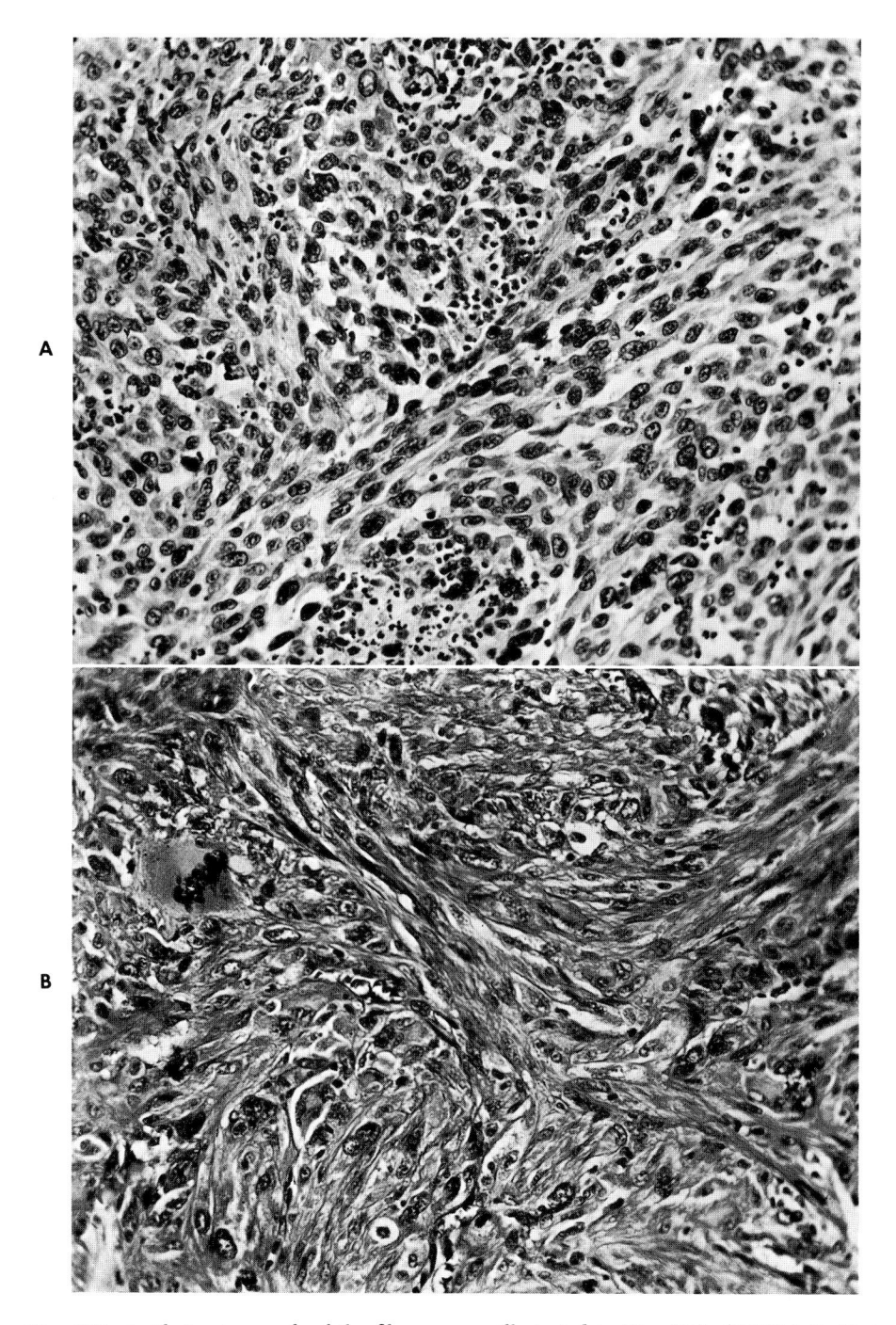

Fig. 17-6. A, Photomicrograph of the fibrosarcoma illustrated in Fig. 17-2. (×220.) B, Photomicrograph of the fibrosarcoma complicating Paget's disease of the humerus illustrated in Fig. 17-5. The anaplasia and formation of tumor giant cells are features commonly associated with Paget's sarcoma. (×200.)

250   Bone tumors

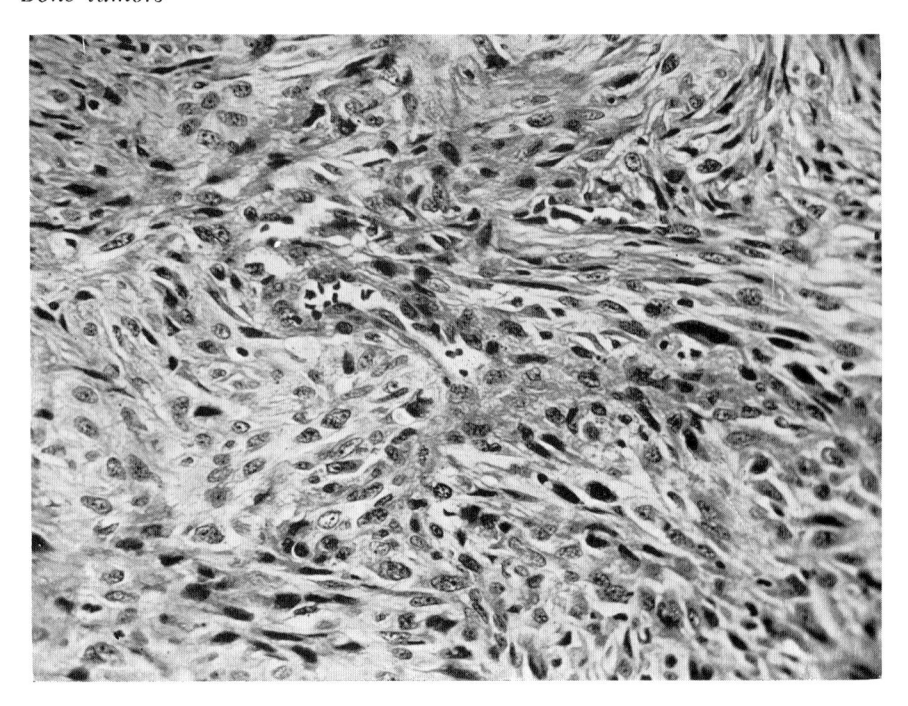

Fig. 17-7. Photomicrograph showing a representative field of a postirradiation fibrosarcoma developing in the upper humerus of a child and necessitating disarticulation. This site had been heavily irradiated some years previously (without prior biopsy) on the premise that a giant-cell tumor was present. Actually, review of the x-ray films indicated that the lesion initially was, in all probability, a solitary unicameral bone cyst. (×220.)

Ivins,[9] as many as ten out of fifty instances of fibrosarcoma in general were of this nature. Continuing, fibrosarcoma may on rare occasions develop in association with lesions of fibrous dysplasia. There is reason to believe also that once in a great while fibrosarcoma may develop out of the lining tissue of a previously treated bone cyst (Fig. 17-3). Finally, osteomyelitis of long standing may be a predisposing factor. Morris and Lucas[10] reported a case of fibrosarcoma arising within a draining osteomyelitic sinus of forty-one years' duration, and they cited several additional similar instances in the literature.

As has been emphasized by other investigators also,[5,8,9] fibrosarcomas in bone show wide variation in growth potential and aggressiveness, and this is usually, though not invariably, reflected in their cytologic appearance. At one extreme, there are highly malignant fibroblastic neoplasms that, by virtue of their rapid and aggressive growth, their ominous cytology (reflected in moderate anaplasia, cell irregularity, and rather numerous mitotic figures), and their tendency to early pulmonary metastasis, behave not unlike osteogenic sarcomas, though failing to exhibit any tendency whatever to form tumor osteoid and bone, even upon the most searching histologic examination of entire amputation specimens. At most, one observes scattered small focal areas of hyalinization and calcification, just as one may in fibroblastic meningiomas, for example. There are still

Fibrosarcoma of bone 251

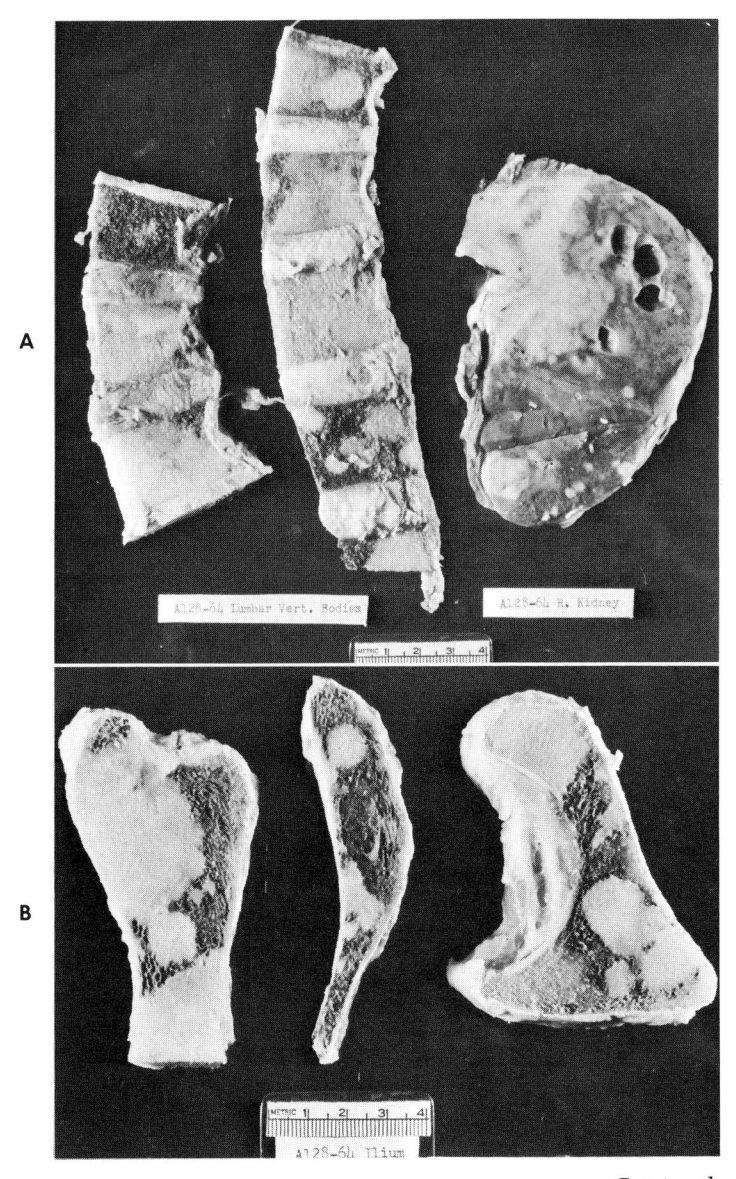

Continued.

Fig. 17-8. **A** and **B**, Photographs showing widespread dissemination at autopsy of a fibrosarcoma that arose in the proximal femur of a 65-year-old man. There was no indication of Paget's disease. This was a desmoplastic fibrosarcoma microscopically, and its cytology is illustrated in **C** and **D**. **C**, Low-power photomicrograph of the fibrosarcoma illustrated in **A** and **B**, showing its desmoplastic character. This specimen from the original tumor in the femur was obtained by needle biopsy. (×64.) **D**, Photomicrograph of another tumor focus in bone from the case of fibrosarcoma illustrated in **A**, **B**, and **C**. The stroma here is succulent and more obviously malignant than that shown in **C**. (×300.)

252 Bone tumors

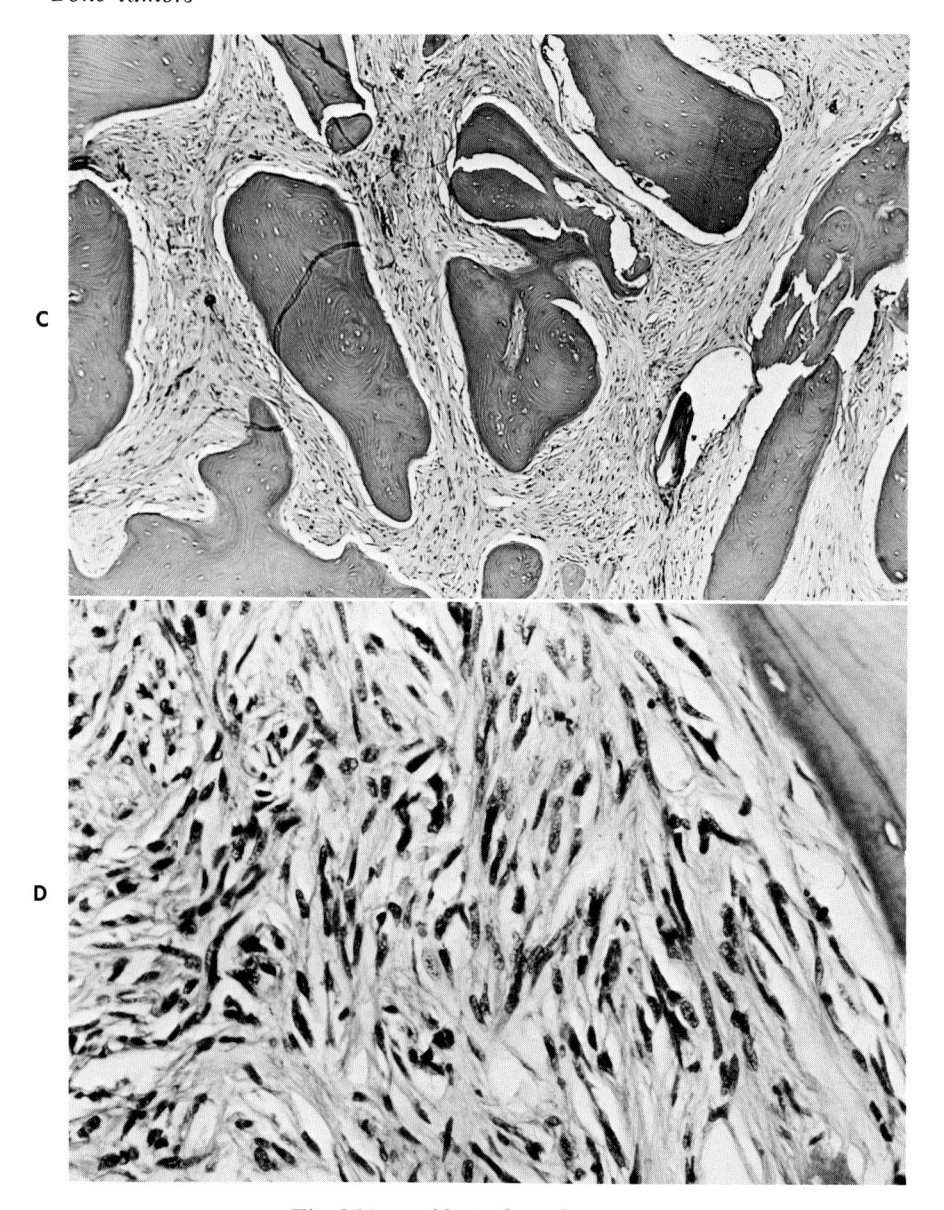

C

D

Fig. 17-8, cont'd. For legend see p. 251.

some who believe that such neoplasms should be regarded as osteogenic sarcomas that have not manifested their osteogenic potentiality, but this concept hardly seems to make good sense as a practical working hypothesis. In my opinion, a neoplasm should be appraised in the light of what it does and what it actually looks like, rather than by any preconceived notion in regard to what it might do under other circumstances. In dealing clinically with such neoplasms, the outlook is serious in spite of prompt radical surgery, and one must be guarded in the matter of prognosis.

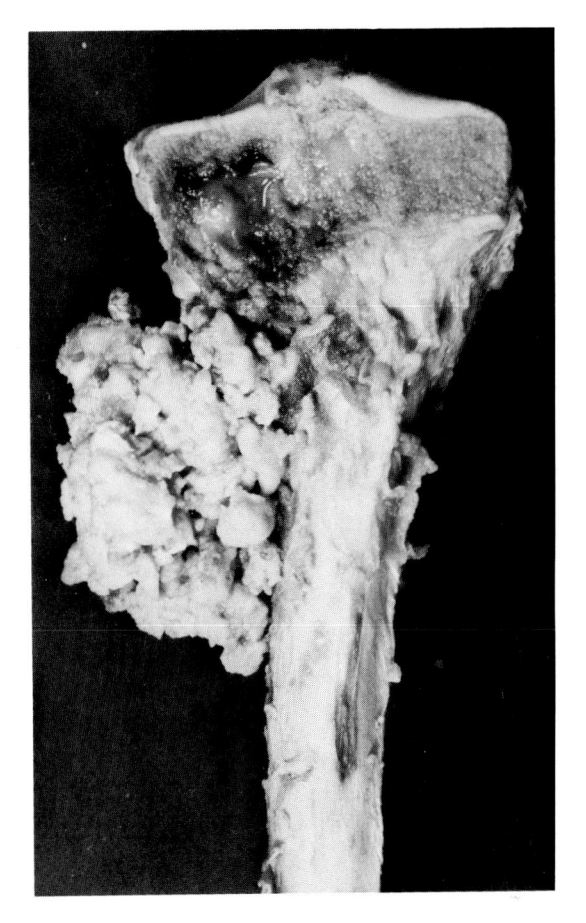

Fig. 17-9. Amputation specimen (from a woman of 55) showing a fibrosarcoma originating in the upper end of a tibia, which has perforated the cortex and extended into the contiguous soft tissues.

In the middle ground, there are other less serious fibrosarcomas that develop more slowly, although they may eventually penetrate the cortex of the affected bone. At the other extreme of the entire range, there are occasional tumors whose cytology makes a diagnosis of fibrosarcoma mandatory by the usual criteria, but that are nevertheless surprisingly indolent in their growth. In fact, such neoplasms may show relatively little progress in clinical and roentgenographic observations over a period of several years or more. I have knowledge of a tumor in point, situated in the midshaft of the tibia of an older adult, which did not manifest appreciable activity until ten years after its presence was recognized (review of the original biopsy specimen clearly showed fibrosarcoma). It should be emphasized, however, that even these favorable central fibrosarcomas are not to be regarded too lightly, since they may at any time take on a spurt of growth and become aggressive.

These differences in clinical behavior and cytologic appearance among fibrosarcomas of bone led Gilmer and MacEwen[5] and also McLeod, Dahlin, and Ivins[9] to grade them numerically as a guide to therapy and prognosis. Along similar lines, Jaffe[8] divides them into two general groups, the well-differentiated and the poorly differentiated fibrosarcomas, emphasizing that among the latter there are some that may be frankly anaplastic and of very serious import. Still another rich source of case study material is to be found in the Italian literature in a comprehensive article by Goidanich and Venturi.[6] The recent survey of Eyre-Brook and Price,[4] of Bristol, England makes available another valuable collection for comparative study.

Treatment and prognosis

When a diagnosis of central or intramedullary fibrosarcoma of bone is firmly established, radical surgery is indicated as a rule, if this is feasible and if roentgenograms of the chest are still negative (Fig. 17-9). The only exception one might consider applies to an early, well-differentiated tumor that is still confined by the cortex and hence considered suitable for block excision and reconstruction. Even in this special situation there should be an end to temporizing at the first indication of local recurrence. Spread to regional lymph nodes appears to be very unusual and not a matter of real concern. Radiation therapy is not calculated to be effective, any more than it is effective against osteosarcoma or chondrosarcoma, although it may have some palliative value.[3,4]

In the matter of prognosis, the biologic behavior of the individual tumor, as indicated by its clinical course and expressed pathologically in its relative cellularity, growth activity, degree of differentiation, anaplasia, etc. (whether this be indicated by words or numbers), has a distinct bearing on the outcome. Considered altogether as a group, the five-year survival rate, according to Gilmer and MacEwen,[5] is not nearly so good as that of soft tissue fibrosarcomas, but appreciably better than that of osteosarcoma. More specifically, the overall cure rate after radical surgery in their twenty-two cases was only 26%. The estimate of McLeod, Dahlin, and Ivins,[9] based on somewhat more extensive material, is comparable. The inference to be drawn from their experience would seem to be that for any fibrosarcoma of bone that is not slowly growing and well differentiated the prognosis should be guarded, at least for the first two years of follow-up.

Multicentric fibrosarcomas of bone

In the discussion of osteogenic sarcoma it was pointed out that in certain rare instances multiple tumors may develop apparently independently and more or less simultaneously over the entire skeleton. It would appear from the extraordinary case reported by Steiner[12] that, similarly, multicentric tumors of the nature of fibrosarcoma may develop within the skeleton as well as the visceral soft parts, as an expression of a peculiar generalized fibrosarcomatosis (unrelated to either Paget's disease or Recklinghausen's neurofibromatosis). The point is of greater academic interest than of practical moment, however, and for further details the reader is referred to the original paper.

References

1. Budd, J. W., and MacDonald, I.: Osteogenic sarcoma. A modified nomenclature and a review of 118 five-year cures, Surg. Gynecol. Obstet. 77:413, 1943.
2. Cunningham, M. P., and Arlen, M.: Medullary fibrosarcoma of bone, Cancer 21: 31, 1968.
3. Dahlin, D. C., and Ivins, J. C.: Fibrosarcoma of bone. A study of 114 cases, Cancer 23:35, 1969.
4. Eyre-Brook, A. L., and Price, C. H. G.: Fibrosarcoma of bone. Review of fifty consecutive cases from the Bristol Bone Tumor Registry, J. Bone Joint Surg. 51-B:20, 1969.
5. Gilmer, W. S., Jr., and MacEwen, G. D.: Central (medullary) fibrosarcoma of bone, J. Bone Joint Surg. 40-A:121, 1958.
6. Goidanich, I. F., and Venturi, R.: I Fibrosarcomi Primitivi Dello Scheletro, Chir. d. org. di movimento (Fasc. 1) 46:1, 1958.
7. Jaffe, H. L.: Tumors of the skeletal system: pathological aspects, Bull. N. Y. Acad. Med. 23:497, 1947 (see pp. 503-504).
8. Jaffe, H. L.: Tumors and tumorous conditions of the bones and joints, Philadelphia, 1958, Lea & Febiger, pp. 304-313.
9. McLeod, J. J., Dahlin, D. C., and Ivins, J. C.: Fibrosarcoma of bone, Am. J. Surg. 94: 431, 1957.
10. Morris, J. M., and Lucas, D. B.: Fibrosarcoma within a sinus tract of chronic draining osteomyelitis, J. Bone Joint Surg. 46-A: 853, 1964.
11. Phemister, D. B.: Cancer of bone and joint, J.A.M.A. 136:545, 1948.
12. Steiner, P. E.: Multiple diffuse fibrosarcoma of bone, Am. J. Pathol. 20:877, 1944.

Chapter 18

Ewing's sarcoma

There is now general agreement among pathologists and clinicians in regard to the existence of Ewing's sarcoma of bone as a rather primitive, multicentric primary malignant tumor of bone, however one interprets its histogenesis. It is a relatively uncommon neoplasm affecting mainly children, adolescents, and young adults. With few exceptions it spreads (in spite of successful local treatment) to many other bones and, eventually, to the lungs. Cytologically, as Jaffe and I[22] as well as other investigators have shown, it is composed of compact, strikingly uniform cells with indistinct borders and fairly large, prominent, round or ovoid nuclei containing scattered chromatin (which gives them a relatively dark, often smoky appearance). As such, Ewing's sarcoma of bone is different from other marrow tumors, particularly reticulum-cell sarcoma, and distinguishable from certain metastatic neoplasms in bone, which may on occasion mimic it cytologically, notably neuroblastoma and undifferentiated round-cell carcinoma. More specifically, there are valid and useful pathologic as well as clinical grounds for making a clear distinction between Ewing's tumor and primary reticulum-cell sarcoma of bone marrow. Nor is the point an academic one—for the individual patient, it means a difference between a survival rate of 5% (or less) and one of approximately 50%. The fact that this distinction may not be easy in actual practice, when one is dealing with meager biopsy specimens showing extensive degeneration or necrosis, does not negate the general principle.

For twenty years or more following publication of Ewing's original pertinent papers (under the titles of "Diffuse Endothelioma of Bone"[8] and "Endothelial Myeloma of Bone"[9]), the subject was one of the most controversial in the field of bone tumors. Much of the confusion resulted from undue reliance upon certain clinical features that proved not to be specific and from faulty pathologic delineation (based largely upon run-of-the-mill biopsy material), let alone a theory of histogenesis that did not meet with wide acceptance. As a consequence, as Willis cogently pointed out, the diagnosis was often applied uncritically to instances of other tumors.

It is my impression that there is still too great a tendency on the part of some pathologists to base an unequivocal diagnosis of Ewing's sarcoma upon technically poor or inadequate biopsy preparations. As noted, positive identification

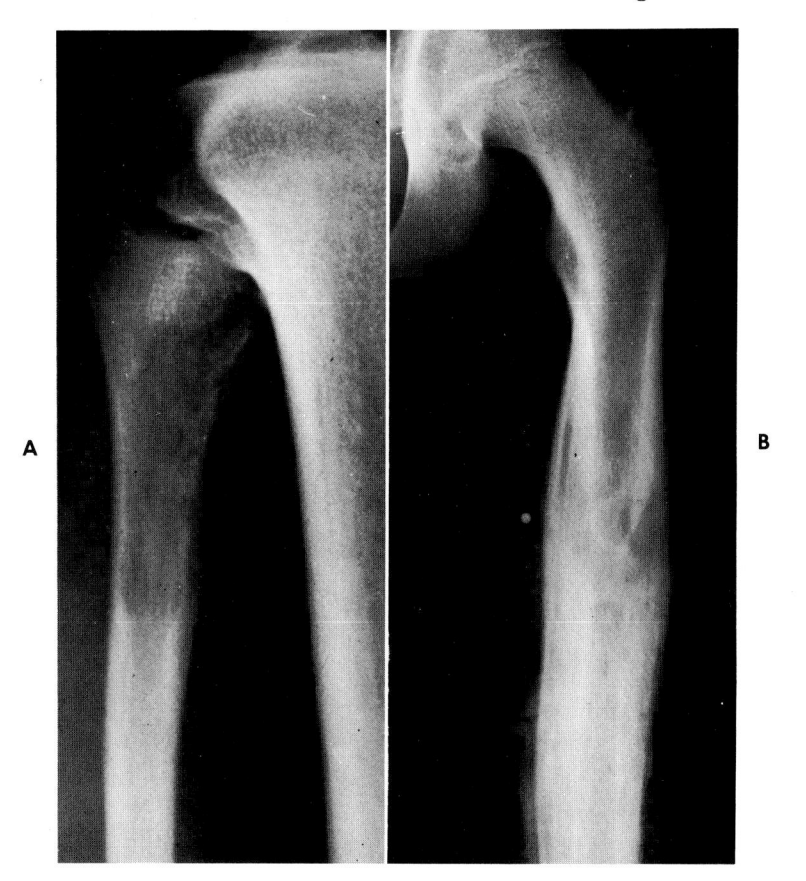

Fig. 18-1. A, Roentgenogram of a mottled and rarefied lesion in the upper fibula, which proved to be a Ewing's sarcoma. The tumor had not as yet provoked any obvious periosteal reaction. B, Another, more advanced, Ewing's sarcoma of a femur showing prominent periosteal new bone apposition as a reaction to penetration of the cortex by the neoplasm. The cortical defect represents the biopsy site. Shortly after this film was taken, pulmonary metastases were already in evidence.

from biopsy specimens may be difficult, if the area sampled shows extensive degeneration (manifested usually in shrinkage of tumor cells and other distortion of their cytologic details), necrosis, and secondary leukocytic reaction. Furthermore, the sorting out of neoplasms of more or less undifferentiated round-cell cytology entails many subtleties,[23] which require good, thin slide preparations for their resolution. In these circumstances, a biopsy impression of Ewing's sarcoma may at times represent no more than a presumption. Even when pertinent cases are followed to autopsy,[4,41] the validity of a final opinion of Ewing's tumor depends largely upon the skill and thoroughness with which the prosector has searched for other neoplasms of round-cell cytology, particularly neuroblastoma, undifferentiated carcinoma extensively metastatic to bone from a small cryptic primary focus, malignant lymphoma involving bone marrow predominantly, and occasionally even multiple myeloma.

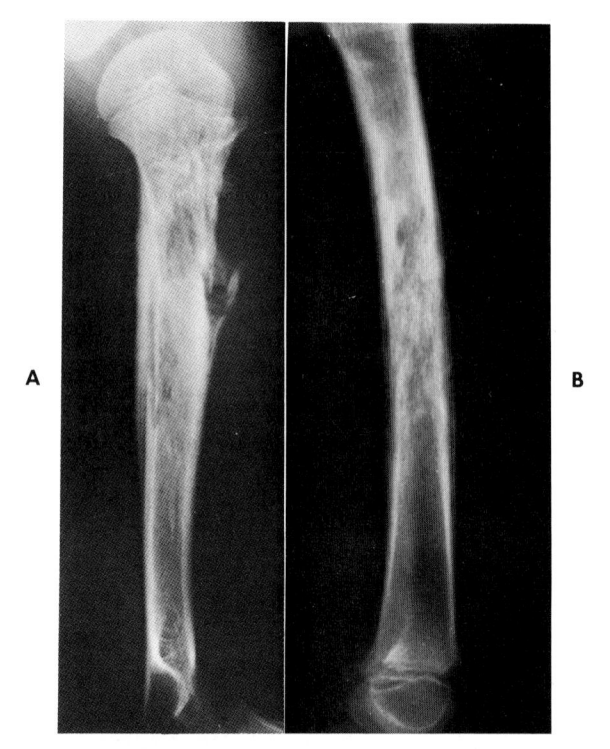

Fig. 18-2. **A,** Roentgenogram of a lesion in the upper metaphysis and shaft of the humerus in a young patient. The lesion simulated Ewing's tumor initially but proved to be a focus of osteomyelitis. **B,** Roentgenogram of a destructive lesion in the shaft of the femur of a child, which suggested Ewing's tumor to most observers, although the impression from the biopsy slides was rather that of a metastatic neoplasm, probably neuroblastoma. Cases such as this emphasize again that in the matter of diagnosis of Ewing's sarcoma an unverified roentgen impression may have little validity.

From its undifferentiated cytologic pattern as described at the outset, I am inclined to infer as a working hypothesis that the tumor cells of Ewing's sarcoma may be derived from the mesenchymal connective tissue framework of the bone marrow. This view finds some support in a recent electron microscopic study.[13] I have not been impressed by the evidence advanced by Ewing and his disciples in support of the idea that the tumor cells are derived from angioendothelium, nor have I found in my own material that perivascular orientation of the tumor cells and in the presence of pseudorosettes constitute significant features of the cytologic picture.

Be that as it may, the clinician responible for the actual management of a revelant case is not overly preoccupied with theoretic considerations in regard to histogenesis, but is more concerned with specific problems in diagnosis and therapy. For the purpose of outlining the pertinent clinical features, I will rely mainly upon observations gleaned from analysis of my own case material, although, with minor variations, these are essentially in accord with those remarked upon in other comparable surveys.

Clinical features
Age and sex incidence

Ewing's sarcoma is most commonly observed in adolescents or young adults, that is, in the age group between 10 and 25 years, although an occasional instance may be seen in a younger child or an older adult. In the last 21 cases from which I have seen material in recent years, the ages ranged from 4 to 23 years. In considering the age factor in differential diagnosis, one should bear in mind that in young children below the age of 5 particularly, neuroblastoma is a strong possibility; that in adults past 35 or 40 years, metastatic carcinoma must be suspected; and that in older adults past 50 years, multiple myeloma also becomes a major possibility.

The majority of patients are likely to be males, although this difference in sex incidence was not as strikingly reflected in our material as it is in the series of cases reported by Coley,[3] for example.

Localization

In most instances, only a single skeletal lesion was clinically recognized and demonstrated roentgenographically at the time of the patient's admission to the hospital. In an occasional case, however, roentgenographic examination of the rest of the skeleton already revealed one or more additional (clinically silent) foci of bone involvement or even early pulmonary metastases. The presenting lesions were commonly situated in trunk bones, as well as in the long limb bones, e.g., in one or another part of an innominate bone, a rib, a scapula, a clavicle, or a vertebra. Insofar as the limb bones are concerned, it is usually the shaft rather than the end of the bone that is affected. Also, while the large bones are often involved (the femur, tibia, and humerus, particularly) it is rather surprising how often the fibula is the site of the presenting tumor.

Clinical findings

In regard to the role of trauma as a possible instigating factor, it may be said that analysis of our data did not furnish any convincing evidence in favor of a causal relationship between trauma and the development of a Ewing's sarcoma.

Survey of the clinical histories of the patients in our series shows that pain was the one consistent complaint. With few exceptions, the pain was of at least some months' standing, and in several cases it had been present for at least one year before admission. In most instances, it had become increasingly severe and persistent during some weeks or months immediately before admission. Along with the local pain, there were often complaints related to spread of the tumor beyond the limits of the affected bone and varying with the location of the presenting lesion. For instance, patients in whom some part of an innominate bone was involved usually complained of disability relating to the hip joint and sometimes also of radiating pain down the lower limb. In connection with presenting lesions near the end of a long bone, there were sometimes complaints of lameness or stiffness of the corresponding joint, and, in one case in which the lesion was situated near the lower end of the femur, there were repeated serous effusions into the knee joint. In cases in which the presenting lesion was in a lumbar vertebra, there were, in addition to the local pain, complaints ascribable to implication of nerve trunks in the area, such as pain radiating down the limbs, and tingling sensations and weakness in the leg. Location of the presenting lesion in a rib was found associated with pleural effusion in one case. Other locations of the presenting lesion (for instance, in the skull) are associated with their own special clinical disabilities.

Just as local pain was the dominant clinical complaint, so the presence of a local tumor mass was the major clinical finding at the time of initial examination. A more or less prominent tumor mass was palpable at the site of the presenting bone lesion in most instances. This finding emphasizes the strong tendency of Ewing's sarcoma to break out through the cortex of the bone and spread into the surrounding soft tissues. Conspicuously large tumor masses were palpable in cases in which the tumor appeared in an innominate bone. Spreading internally toward the pelvic cavity, the tumor could sometimes be palpated as an elastic, irregular, globular mass, through the rectum if the tumor was low down, or in the lower quadrant of the abdomen if it was situated higher up. Spreading externally, a tumor springing from an innominate bone sometimes produced a large tumor mass palpable in the groin or in the gluteal region. In one of our cases in which the presenting lesion was in the shaft of a humerus there was likewise a very large extraosseous tumor mass connected with the bone. When the presenting tumor was in a superficially located bone such as a clavicle or a rib, the mass produced by extraosseous spread could likewise be seen as well as palpated.

Tenderness to pressure at the site of the lesion was recorded in practically all cases. Frequently, the subcutaneous veins overlying the presenting lesion were found to be prominent. However, it was only occasionally that increased local heat was mentioned in connection with the physical examination.

A survey of the temperature charts and the laboratory findings in our cases revealed what appeared to be significant information of clinical value. Many of our patients had been in the hospital for almost a week before specimens were secured for biopsy. During this time they had slight fever, with daily rises in temperature to about 101° F. These patients also presented a secondary anemia (with a red blood cell count of about 3,500,000) and sometimes also a leukocytosis. In addition, they usually showed a high sedimentation rate of the blood. Altogether, these findings proved to be significant in judging immediate prognosis. Specifically, the patients in whom some fever and secondary anemia were noted had a fulminating course ending in death within a few months after admission to the hospital. On the other hand, those patients who had no fever on admission and no anemia or increased sedimentation rate tended to survive for a year or more after admission.

Roentgenographic findings
Roentgenographic appearance of the presenting bone lesion

The presenting bone lesion is, as already indicated, the one causing the complaints that led the patient to enter the hospital. This was often the only lesion discernible, even when the entire skeleton was examined. One need only review the presenting lesions in a series of cases to appreciate the difficulty of making a definitive diagnosis of Ewing's sarcoma by x-ray examination alone. If the extent of bone involvement in the presenting lesion is still small and no lesions are found elsewhere, the film may be misconstrued as that of an inflammatory lesion. However, in most cases the film of the presenting lesion suggests a malignant tumor, although it may be misinterpreted as some malignant tumor other than Ewing's sarcoma.

The only fairly consistent roentgenographic finding is evidence of destruction or lysis of bone, in itself a rather nondescript feature. In some cases the presenting lesion may appear merely as a small zone of mottled rarefaction reflecting destruction of the spongiosa and, to a lesser degree, of the overlying cortex associated with only a trace of periosteal new bone reaction to the neoplastic tissue that has penetrated the cortex. This picture (which may also include some areas of condensation) is very likely to suggest an inflammatory lesion (pyogenic or tuberculous osteomyelitis) rather than a tumor, although within a month or two one is likely to observe evidence of rapid extension of the pathologic area within and beyond the bone, so that one begins to suspect the presence of a malignant neoplasm. It should be emphasized that, although the early roentgenogram shows only a relatively small area of bone destruction, this cannot be taken to indicate the actual extent of involvement of the bone, the marrow spaces of which may already be riddled by neoplastic tissue.

When the initial roentgenogram of the presenting lesion shows rather clearly that one is dealing with a malignant tumor, one usually notes a large area of bone destruction and often a large overlying soft tissue mass as well. The affected area in the bone may show some expansion, but this is not pronounced. It appears irregularly rarefied and mottled from the presence of smaller or larger foci of relatively radiolucency and shows disruption of the cortical outline over a variable distance. Reactive deposition of new bone by the periosteum, where the neoplastic tissue is penetrating the cortex, is very conspicuous.

When the shaft of a long bone is the site of Ewing's sarcoma, one does not commonly observe the concentric "onionpeel" layers of laminated periosteal new bone held to be characteristic of the roentgenologic appearance of this tumor. If the observer necessarily expects to find this allegedly pathognomonic sign, he is likely to miss the diagnosis in many cases. Moreover, even when it is present, it is not necessarily indicative of Ewing's sarcoma. It should be noted, also, that occasionally the pattern of periosteal new bone formation in an advanced lesion of Ewing's sarcoma may be that of more or less transverse radiopaque streaks, so that the picture of the destructive bone lesion and of the overlying soft tissue mass may be suggestive of osteogenic sarcoma.

Altogether, the only conclusion that can be drawn in regard to the roent-

262   *Bone tumors*

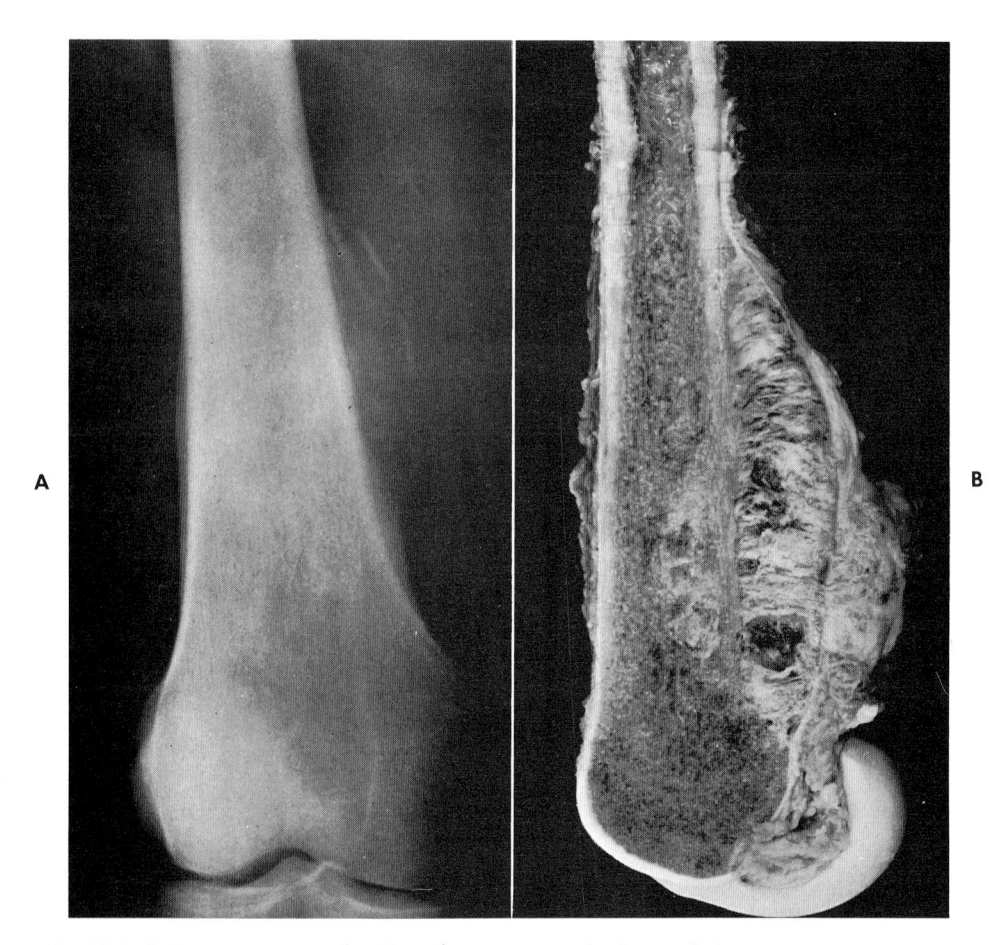

Fig. 18-3. **A,** Roentgenogram of a Ewing's sarcoma in the lower shaft of a femur of a young woman who had complained of pain and some swelling for many months. Even at this late date, the extent of involvement of the spongiosa and marrow is only vaguely indicated, although it is clear from the pattern of periosteal new bone reaction that the neoplasm has already extended well beyond the confines of the cortex. **B,** Amputation specimen of the Ewing's sarcoma shown in **A.** The tumor has permeated the cortex over a wide area and has flourished beneath the raised periosteum. Ablation was done in this case with full awareness that it offered only a slim chance for cure. The surgeon elected to amputate through the thigh rather than disarticulate in the hope of utilizing a good prosthesis. Unfortunately, examination of the fatty marrow in the shaft at the level of amputation showed the presence of a microscopic focus of tumor.

genographic appearance of the presenting lesion are that bone destruction (osteolysis) is the dominant feature of Ewing's sarcoma and that there is no typical appearance for this lesion. In general, Ewing's sarcoma is a tumor difficult to diagnose on a roentgenographic basis, often being mistaken in its early stages for an inflammatory lesion and in its later stages for other malignant tumors, including metastatic neoplasms. In many cases it may be quite difficult to make a differential diagnosis on a roentgenographic basis between Ewing's tumor and chondrosarcoma, "osteolytic" osteogenic sarcoma, malignant lymphoma, or meta-

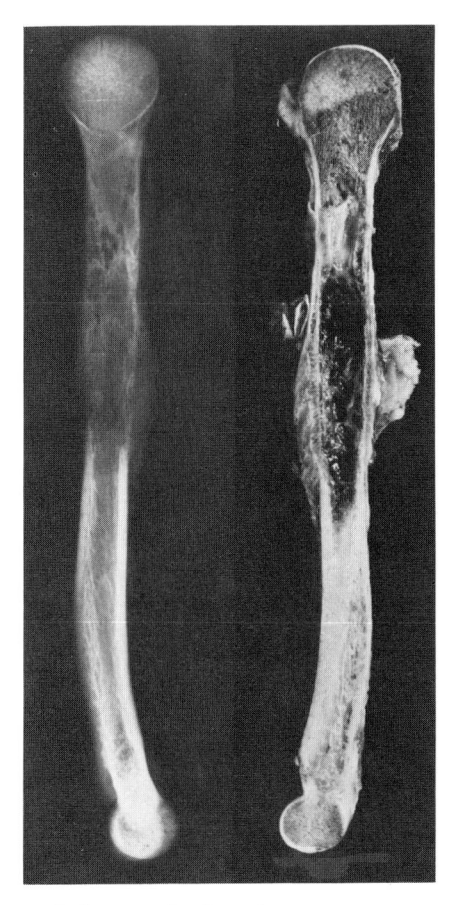

Fig. 18-4. Roentgenogram and photograph of another amputation specimen showing a Ewing's sarcoma that developed in the shaft of a humerus. The patient, a young man in his twenties, had complained of pain for about nine months. Dissection of the specimen showed that the tumor was already invading the deltoid muscle at its insertion. He remained ostensibly well for over four years after disarticulation but then developed a number of pulmonary metastases that proved fatal, despite attempts at local resection of the initial ones.

static neoplasms (including metastatic neuroblastoma). It should be noted also that a solitary lesion of eosinophilic granuloma of bone may be mistaken for Ewing's sarcoma. To make certain that a suspected tumor is Ewing's sarcoma, tissue examination is essential, but it must be emphasized that the pathologist may easily be mistaken in his opinion, especially if the tissue available is meager or extensively modified by necrosis and secondary inflammation. However, in this connection, the error is more likely to be that of mistaking other lesions (anaplastic carcinoma, metastatic neuroblastoma, malignant lymphoma) for Ewing's sarcoma, than the reverse.

Roentgenographic appearance of the "metastatic" bone lesions

Whether the additional lesions found roentgenographically on initial examination, or subsequently, represent metastases from the presenting lesion or independent multicentric foci does not concern us here. Roentgenographically, these additional lesions, like the presenting lesion, show evidence of lysis of bone. They appear first as rather faint, slightly mottled areas of rarefaction. As the resorption of the bone increases, the small, multiple, roundish foci of rarefaction become more distinct and may merge into larger, more clear-cut areas of radiolucency. In flat bones, such as those of the skull or the ilium, multiple, clear-cut, punched-out areas of rarefaction may appear in consequence of lytic destruction of the spongiosa and overlying cortex. In some instances a pathologic fracture of a long bone from destructive resorption may become manifest. It is important to bear in mind, in any event, that the actual extent of involvement of the skeleton at any one time is never adequately reflected roentgenographically. This is true even in fatal cases in which a number of destructive lesions have been demonstrated roentgenographically in bones other than the one containing the presenting lesion. At autopsy, if many additional bones are opened, they, too, will be found to have been far more extensively invaded than was suspected from roentgenographic study of the skeleton shortly before death.

Pathologic features
Gross description

Our experience supports the idea that Ewing's sarcoma arises in the marrow spaces of the interior of the affected bone, rather than in the haversian spaces of the cortex or beneath the periosteum. Also, as has been indicated, anatomic examination of an affected bone will reveal much more extensive involvement than the roentgenographic or clinical findings would suggest. Well-preserved tumor nodules appear whitish and cellular, although at bulky tumor sites there is a strong tendency to necrosis and hemorrhage. For a detailed discussion of the gross pathologic anatomy and of the spread of tumor as seen at autopsy, the reader is referred to our 1947 paper.[22] In general, apart from visceral metastases, especially to the lungs, one can expect to find at autopsy that a major part of the skeleton, in addition to the bone containing the presenting lesion, is affected. The question that cannot be answered definitely is whether the wide dissemination over the skeleton represents metastatic spread or, rather, development independently in multiple sites, although I strongly favor the latter view.

Microscopic findings

Although Ewing's sarcoma does have a characteristic cytologic pattern, secondary changes may obscure it or make it difficult to demonstrate in an individual specimen taken for biopsy, even if this has been obtained by surgical incision. Thus, a given specimen may show large fields in which the appearance of the individual tumor cells has been altered by degeneration and necrosis, areas in which the neoplastic tissue as a whole has been modified by hemorrhage and reparative reaction to it, and even areas in which reactive inflammatory changes dominate the picture. It is because such secondary changes are not relegated to the background that the reputation of Ewing's sarcoma for variability and in-

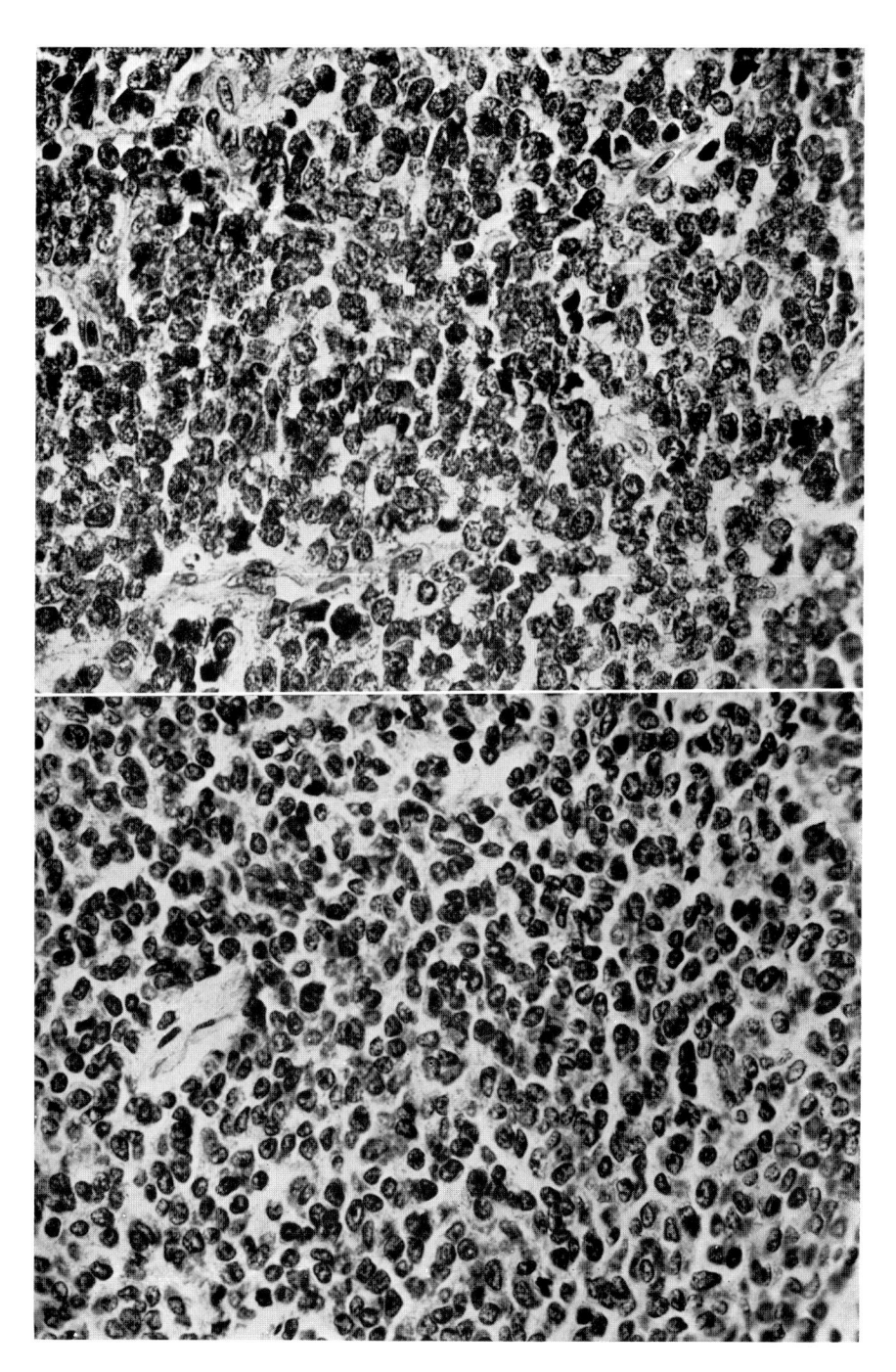

Fig. 18-5. Photomicrographs of two representative instances of Ewing's sarcoma, illustrating its basic cytologic pattern, unmodified by hemorrhage or by degeneration and necrosis. The tumor cells are closely packed and uniform in appearance (as compared with reticulum-cell sarcoma) (Fig. 20-8). They have an indistinct cytoplasmic outline and scattered chromatin within the nuclei, which often gives them a relatively dark or smoky appearance. (×475.)

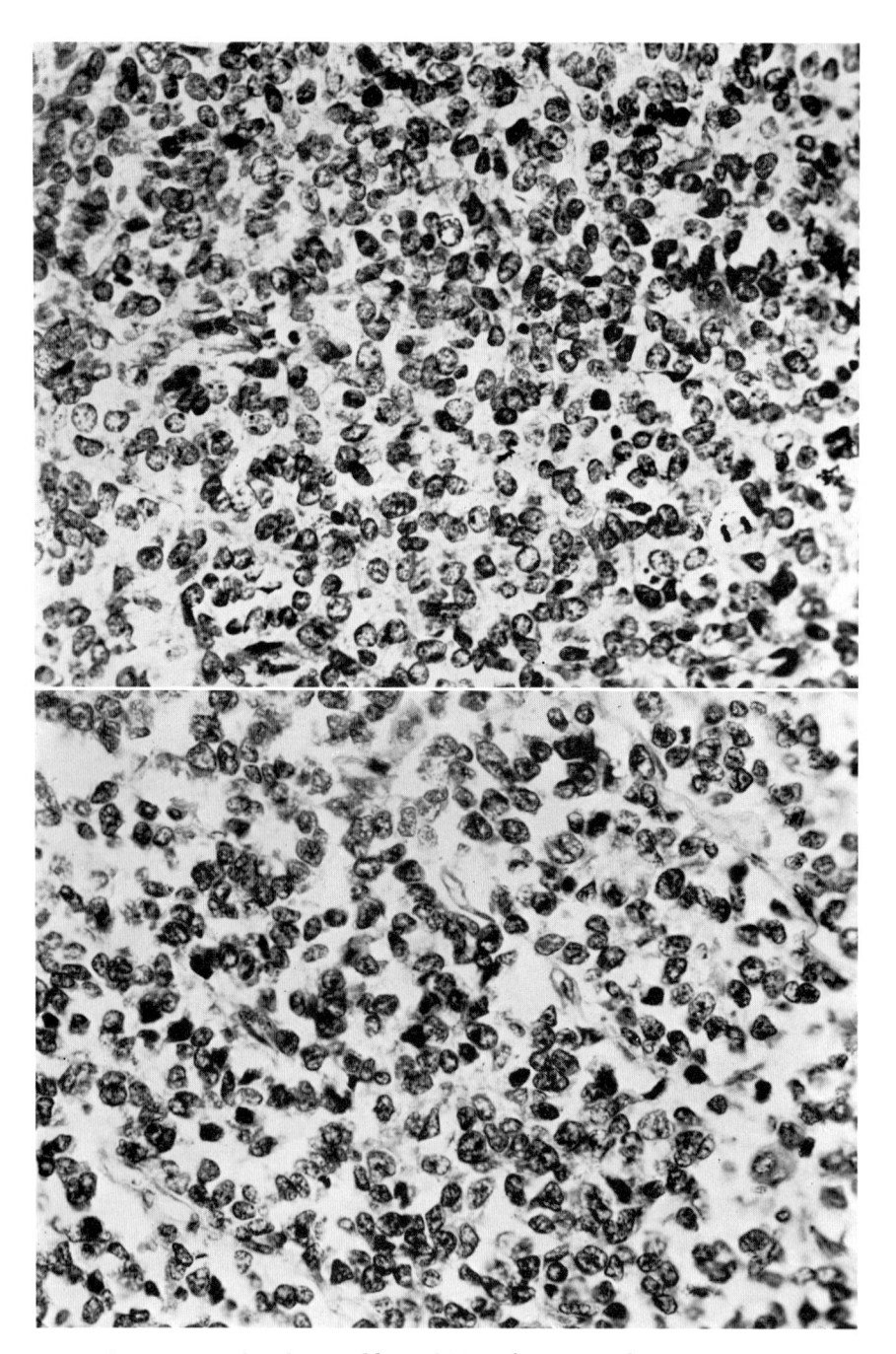

Fig. 18-6. Photomicrographs of two additional Ewing's tumors, showing variation in pattern. (×475.)

constancy of its cytologic pattern in biopsy specimens from case to case has developed and persists.

However, secondary changes in the neoplastic tissue do not present the only difficulty with which one is confronted in attempting to make a diagnosis of Ewing's tumor on the basis of a biopsy specimen. The diagnosis "Ewing's sarcoma" often has become a mere refuge when one is confronted by a puzzling malignant tumor in a bone, and is likely to be applied rather loosely and by default of a better opinion unless one's anatomic concept of Ewing's sarcoma is a definite one.

The characteristic cytology of Ewing's sarcoma is manifested in the presence of fields of tumor cells that lack clearly delimited cell boundaries, and whose nuclei are crowded together and are of fairly uniform appearance. These nuclei are round or ovoid, are about twice as great in diameter (or, in the case of the ovoid ones, perhaps three times as great in their longer axis) as the nucleus of a lymphocyte, and have finely divided or powdery chromatin and often one or more nucleoli. As a rule, the individual nuclei appear enmeshed in and are slightly separated by a loose, more or less vacuolated cytoplasmic fabric. In some fields, however, they may be found crowded together (perhaps to such an extent that many of them are even pressed into an oval shape), and in such fields there is but little cytoplasm between them. It should also be noted that in the fields presenting the general cytologic picture just described, vascularity is usually not a prominent feature (Figs. 18-5 and 18-6).

In regard to the reticulin fibrils in Ewing's sarcoma, it appears that these are not a consistent or prominent feature of the histologic picture. There is considerable variability in these fibrils, from lesion to lesion and even from part to part of the same tumor section. Some lesions, in part or throughout, present merely a few scattered argyrophil fibrils in an entire low-power field. Other lesions show more numerous fibrils, but these are irregularly distributed and are noted between smaller and larger groups of tumor cells. In no instance did we regularly observe large fields of tissue showing a lattice or meshwork of reticulin fibrils outlining not merely cell groups, but the individual tumor cells as well. Altogether, it would appear that there is no characteristic histologic pattern for Ewing's tumor insofar as these argyrophil fibrils are concerned.

A histochemical aid in the differentiation from reticulum-cell sarcoma particularly has been suggested by Schajowicz,[32] who maintains that the cells of Ewing's tumor contain glycogen, whereas those of reticulosarcoma do not. In my own experience to date, I have not found the PAS stain particularly helpful in the resolution of this problem.

Differentiation from neuroblastoma with skeletal metastases

That sympathetic neuroblastoma (sympathicoblastoma) commonly metastasizes to bones has been known for a long time. Hutchison[19] and Tileston and Wolbach[39] have pointed out that a malignant adrenal tumor is often the primary lesion in infants and children who clinically present tumorous involvement of cranial bones, proptosis, and enlargement of the preauricular and other regional lymph nodes. From the cases reported by these authors, and from those that they collected from the literature (cases now assignable to adrenal neuroblastoma), it is evident that metastases to bones other than those of the skull are often found, and that metastases to the liver, kidneys, and lymph nodes are also rather common.

Further observations have clearly indicated that, although the adrenal medulla is the most common site of origin for neuroblastomas, it is by no means the only one. Cases have been reported in which neuroblastomas arose from sympathetic nervous tissue elsewhere in the body, notably from the sympathetic chains, but sometimes even from the sympathetic tissue of organs. While infants and young children are the most common subjects, occasional instances have been reported in which sympathetic neuroblastomas developed in adults. Also, it has become clear that insofar as the skeleton is concerned, the clinically presenting, destructive bone lesion (if there is one) may be in a long bone or some bone other than the skull.

In respect to cytology, Tileston and Wolbach[39] stressed the diagnostic significance of the finding of tumor cells arranged in rosettes. It was Wright[42] who pointed out that these tumors take their origin from the pluripotential cells of the sympathetic nervous system, and that the rosettes are ball-like aggregations of tumor cells enclosing a small central meshwork of filamentous neurofibrils, some of which can be seen to constitute processes of the cells making up the periphery

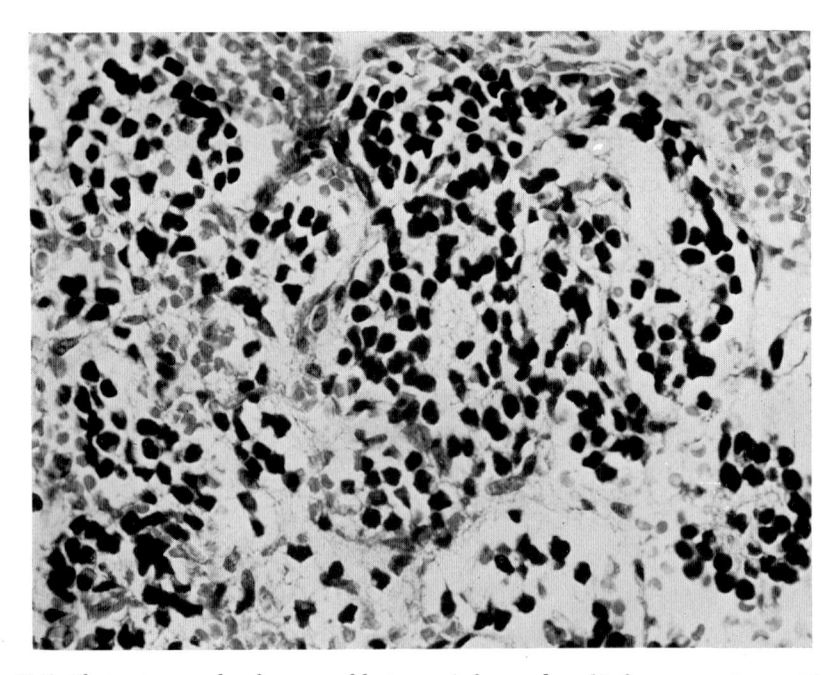

Fig. 18-7. Photomicrograph of a neuroblastoma (of an adrenal) for comparison with Figs. 18-5 and 18-6. The "ghost" outlines in the background are those of red blood cells. (×475.)

of the rosette. In addition, he pointed out that, aside from rosettes, one may be able to find masses of tumor cells interspersed with and penetrated by fibrils running parallel in bundles. However, the demonstration of neurofibrils, either in parallel bundles or as a meshwork in the center of the rosettes, may be difficult. In such instances, few fibrils may have been laid down or, as a result of degeneration or postmortem change, the fibrils may have become transformed into hyaline or granular material and be difficult to demonstrate. This is especially true of the fibrils of the rosettes. Under such circumstances, whatever rosettes are present appear as formations in which several rows of cells surround a finely granular, eosin-staining mass without a central lumen.

In any particular case, rosettes may be fairly numerous in both the primary growth and the metastases, conspicuous in the primary growth and sparse in the metastases, or difficult to find in either. As to the type cell of the tumor, there are differences from lesion to lesion, depending on the predominant level of maturation. In the most primitive type, this cell maintains the lymphocytoid character of the parent stem cell. It is usually a small round cell (strongly resembling a small lymphocyte) with a dense hyperchromatic nucleus practically filling the

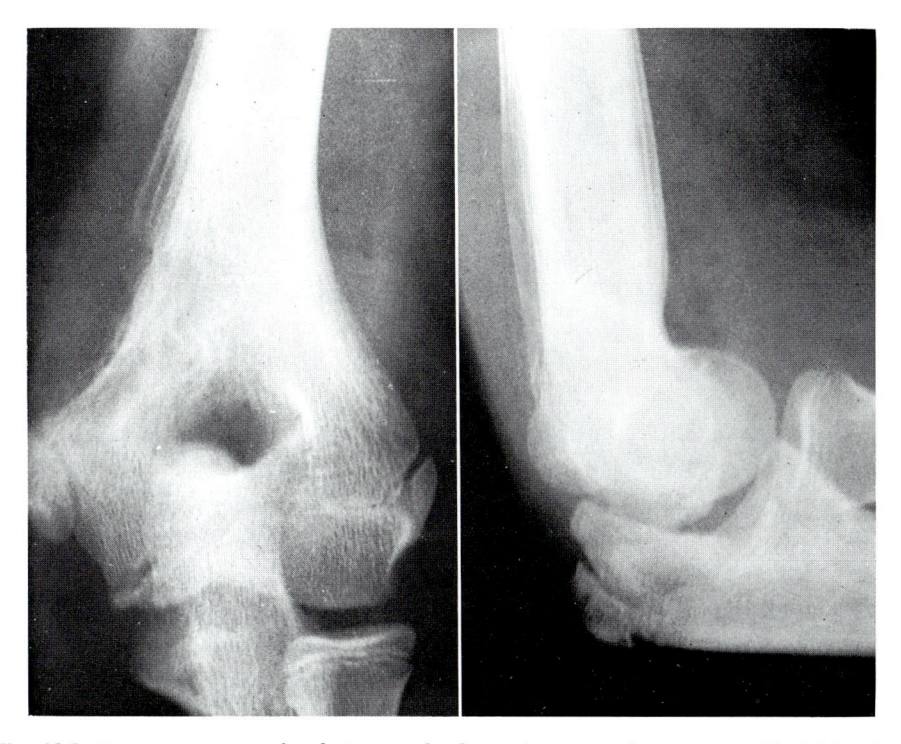

Fig. 18-8. Roentgenograms of a lesion in the lower humerus of a 10-year-old child, which clinically presented a difficult problem in differentiation between osteomyelitis and Ewing's sarcoma. At the time of biopsy, the surgeon encountered soft, whitish material that he thought was pus. However, sections of the bone fragments from the medullary cavity showed small foci of Ewing's tumor within the marrow.

entire cell so that there is little cytoplasm. Some of the cells, although maintaining this general character, may be oval, while others, especially at the periphery of the rosettes, may be piriform. In more differentiated sympathetic neuroblastomas, the cells, although mainly round, are distinctly larger than those just described, may have vesicular nuclei and a clear ring of cytoplasm about the nucleus, and often have some cytoplasmic processes. In still further matured neuroblastomas, some tumor fields may even show sympathetic ganglion cells.

With this background, we are in a better position to understand Willis' point of view concerning neuroblastoma in relation to Ewing's sarcoma. Prior to the publication of the relevant articles by Willis[41] and by Colville and Willis,[4] it seems not to have been adequately stressed that care must be taken to exclude the possibility that one may actually be dealing with a sympathetic neuroblastoma metastatic to the skeleton in cases that apparently represent Ewing's sarcoma of bone. In both cases cited there was a presenting bone tumor that had the usually accepted clinical and roentgenographic characteristics of Ewing's sarcoma. The clinical course, and in particular the susceptibility of the tumor to radiation therapy, seemed further to support this diagnosis. However, in both cases it was revealed at autopsy that the presenting bone tumor (in a femur) represented a metastasis from a neuroblastoma, primary in an adrenal in one instance and in the left lumbar sympathetic chain in the other. In each instance rosettes were found only in the primary growth and not in the biopsy specimens.

On the basis of these experiences, Willis expressed great wariness about accepting a diagnosis of Ewing's sarcoma made on clinical and roentgenographic grounds alone. He cast doubt also upon the reliability of biopsy in this connection, and analyzed, largely to reject them, the findings in the relatively few cases publisher prior to 1940, which had been interpreted as Ewing's sarcoma proved by autopsy. His paper of 1940 bears careful reading for its astute evaluation of the reported autopsied cases of Ewing's sarcoma, even if it does appear that in some instances he has perhaps been overcritical.

A number of additional relevant observations of practical importance deserve brief mention here. As is now well known, the urinary excretion of catecholamines (VMA) in patients with neuroblastoma is of diagnostic help. Secondly, occasional neuroblastomas, even those with bone metastases, may manifest spontaneous maturation to (benign) ganglioneuroma, if the patient survives long enough.[15] Finally, with reference to treatment and prognosis, the highest survival rate is observed in young children below the age of two years; in older patients, the results of treatment are likely to be comparatively poor, unless the primary tumor happens to be situated in the mediastinum and can be completely excised.[35]

Differentiation from carcinoma and other malignant tumors with skeletal involvement

The problem of the differential diagnosis of Ewing's sarcoma does not end with sympathicoblastoma, but may be raised also by metastatic carcinoma. That

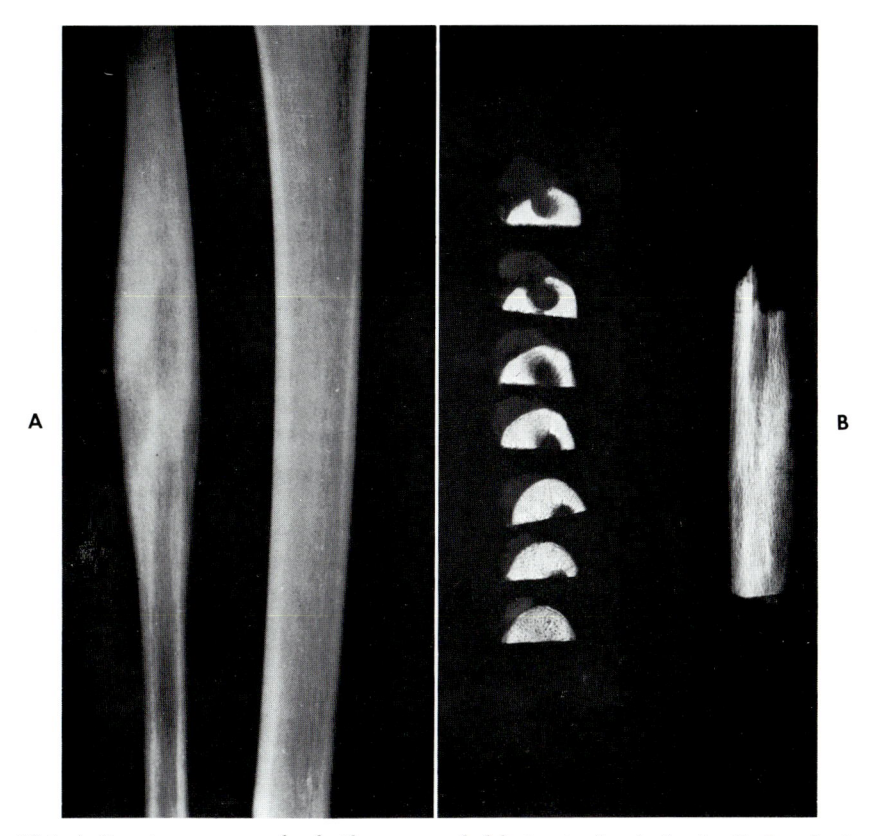

Fig. 18-9. **A,** Roentgenograms of a fusiform expanded lesion in the shaft of a fibula, which was thought clinically to be Ewing's sarcoma. The surgical procedure was excision biopsy of the involved segment. **B,** Roentgenograms of serial transverse slices of one half of the resected thickened fibula, showing that the oblique rarefied tract illustrated in **A** reflects the presence of a chronic bone abscess. The periosteal new bone has developed as a reaction to extension of this abscess to the outer surface of the cortex.

a solitary destructive bone lesion, which is proved by biopsy to represent a metastasis, may be the first clinical indication that the patient is suffering from a carcinoma hardly needs to be stated. It is also common to find that, while the primary neoplasm is silent, the histologic picture of the neoplastic tissue in the biopsy specimen affords a clue to the site of the primary growth. On the other hand, there is often insufficent cytologic differentiation to suggest the site of the primary lesion. Diagnostic difficulties arise particularly in those cases in which the primary growth is silent and in which the neoplastic tissue in the metastatic focus is so undifferentiated as to present a more or less uniform pattern of round cells. Although this problem does sometimes arise in connection with biopsy diagnosis or even in connection with the evaluation of the autopsy findings in a suspected case of Ewing's sarcoma, it does not constitute a frequent or serious difficulty in the hands of an experienced pathologist. Still, Hirsch and Ryerson[18] have pointed out that bronchial carcinomas (particularly small ones composed of undifferentiated cells) may metastasize widely to the bones before being recognizable in the lung and thus raise problems of differential diagnosis from Ewing's sarcoma. This point of view has also been stressed by Sternberg,[36] who cited a case in which a skeletal metastasis was regarded as Ewing's sarcoma, although he himself held that involvement of bone was secondary to an undifferentiated small-cell carcinoma of the breast.

Finally, it may be relevant to point out that occasionally, in the course of evaluation of a biopsy specimen, one may have to make a differential diagnosis between Ewing's sarcoma on the one hand and Hodgkin's disease or lymphosarcoma on the other. However, the latter conditions are so rarely primary in bone that one is not often confronted by this problem as a practical difficulty, and when they are not primary there, the general clinical picture in which involvement of lymph nodes occupies the foreground helps to clarify the problem.

Treatment and prognosis

The problem of giving counsel in regard to treatment of a tumor diagnosed as Ewing's sarcoma from a satisfactory biopsy specimen presents a disheartening dilemma. It has been demonstrated repeatedly that while adequate x-ray therapy may bring about remakable amelioration of complaints referable to the presenting tumor site, such patients generally die of "improvement," usually within the ensuing two or three years, and manifest at autopsy widespread skeletal involvement and also visceral extension, notably to the lungs. On the other hand, if one advocates ablation or radical surgical resection (for a tumor in an accessible site), one can likewise offer the patient or his family but meager hope for cure or even survival for as long as five years. The consensus of current opinion is that Ewing's sarcoma carries a grave prognosis even under favorable auspices, and that, irrespective of the type of treatment employed, the expectancy for survival beyond a few years is rather slim. Some of the older surveys[26] claiming a cure rate of 10% or even 20% must be taken with a grain of salt.

That there are occasional cures, however, seems clear from the available evidence, and I have personal knowledge of several. One was in a patient who was alive and well twenty years after amputation of a lower limb for a tumor in a fibula, diagnosed as Ewing's sarcoma (Fig. 18-11); I reviewed the biopsy slide and was willing to accept the tumor as a Ewing's tumor (rather than a reticulum-cell sarcoma). Another was in a 12-year-old girl with a Ewing's tumor in a radius, treated by irradiation. She was well and symptom free more than seven years later at last report. A third extraordinary instance, reported by Sirsat,[34] was that of a 4-year-old boy who had a Ewing's tumor in the distal femur that was irradiated. Six years later the limb was amputated because of recurrent tumor, which was discovered to be a chondrosarcoma (presumably a sequel of therapeutic irradiation); sections, otherwise, showed necrosis of bone, calcification, and other indications of radiation osteitis, but no trace of the original neoplasm. This would seem to be a Pyrrhic victory, but on second thought, exchange of a Ewing's tumor for a chondrosarcoma is not a bad trade. It seems to me that Ew-

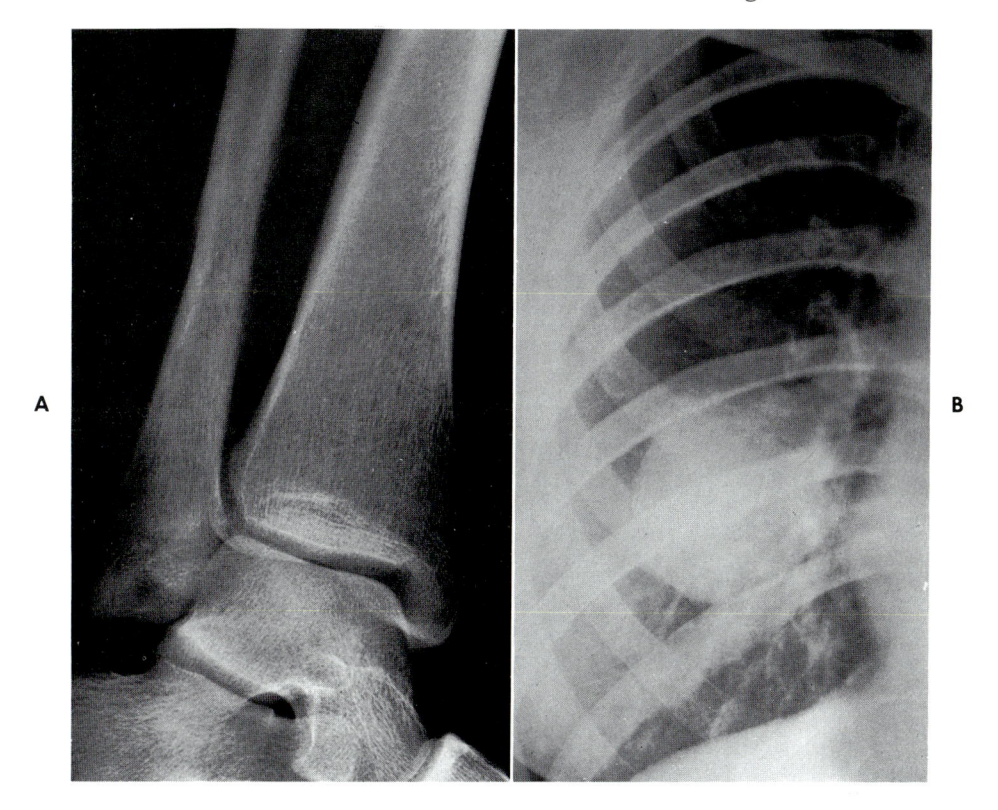

Fig. 18-10. **A,** Roentgenogram of a relatively early lesion of Ewing's sarcoma in the lower fibula of a 19-year-old girl, showing slight but definite mottled rarefaction of the spongiosa and cortex, along with rather subtle periosteal reaction (more clearly seen in the original). Amputation was resorted to without delay, in spite of which pulmonary metastasis appeared about a year later, as shown in **B.**

ing's sarcoma must be regarded essentially as a multicentric tumor, tending sooner or later to spread over the skeleton, but that there may well be exceptional instances in which the neoplastic process is more limited or even confined to a single bone. This might account for the few cures that have been observed.

That one must be circumspect about speaking of "cures" is evidenced by a well-documented case I am familiar with, that of a young patient with Ewing's tumor in a fibula treated successfully by roentgen irradiation, supplemented by sustained chemotherapy (4-5-fluorouracil). Even more remarkable was successful resection of a solitary metastatic pulmonary node some four years later. It was not until seven years had elapsed that the tumor reappeared in the fibula (now radiation fast) and before long spread throughout the skeleton and lungs, despite belated amputation. The entire clinical course extended almost nine years. The unusual case with seven-year survival reported by Heald, Soto-Hall and Hill[17] also highlights the point that pulmonary metastasis does not necessarily indicate an early fatal outcome.

In recent years I have favored irradiation as the treatment of choice, rather

274   Bone tumors

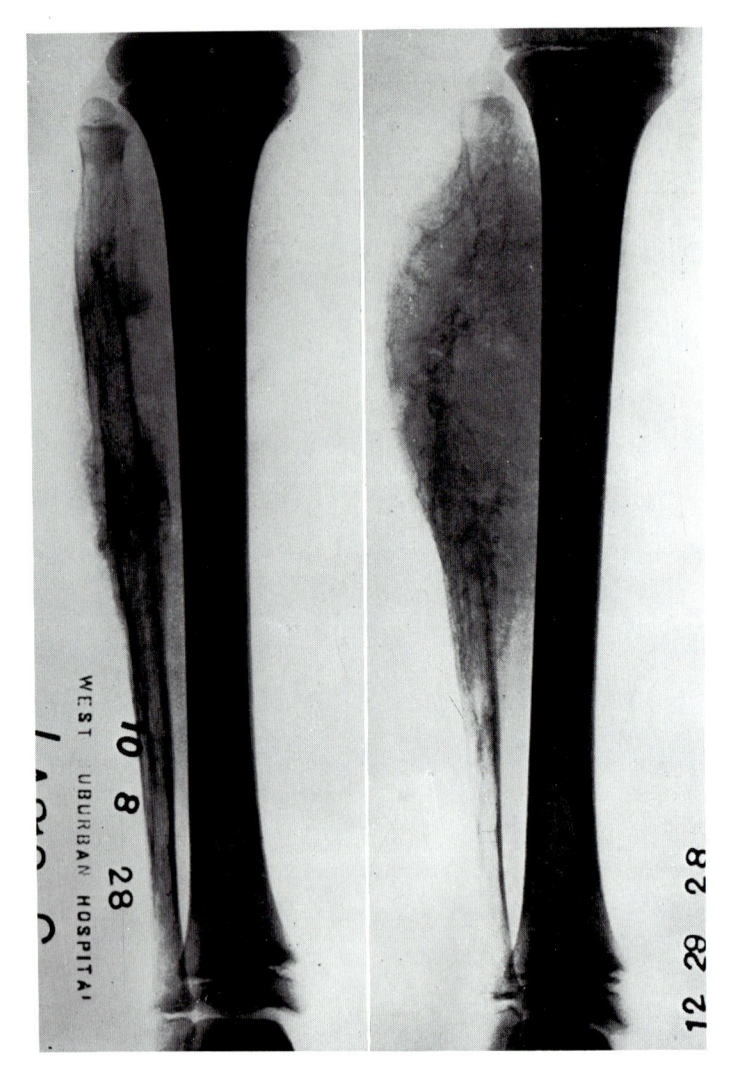

Fig. 18-11. Roentgenograms of a Ewing's sarcoma of a fibula showing rapid progression of the neoplasm over a period of less than three months. Amputation was performed, and the patient was known to be alive and well over 25 years later. I have reviewed the biopsy slide and am satisfied that the neoplasm was a Ewing's tumor and not a reticulum-cell sarcoma. This case is significant in that it represents one of the very few cures in Ewing's sarcoma of which I have personal knowledge.

than radical surgery, even for tumors in surgically accessible sites. The field of treatment should extend well beyond the limits of the roentgenographically discernible defect. Irradiation may be expected to destroy the presenting tumor (if it has not already grown to bulky size) and to ameliorate the patient's complaints. It will not prevent the appearance of tumor foci elsewhere in the skeleton or eventual pulmonary metastasis, any more than surgery will. Since, with few exceptions, the anticipated survival period before dissemination is only a few years, five at the outset, there seems to be little point in subjecting the patient (and the family) to the trauma of the loss of a limb.

The serious nature of this problem in therapy has led to the experimental clinical trial of systemic chemotherapy to supplement local irradiation[21] (actinomycin D[33], cyclophosphamide, vincristine, and 4-5-fluorouracil have been used), and even of adjuvant total-body irradiation (300 rads).[20,27] While these continuing efforts seem justified, it is too early to tell whether they will succeed in increasing the long-term survival rate.

References

1. Barden, R. P.: The similarity of clinical and roentgen findings in children with Ewing's sarcoma (endothelial myeloma) and sympathetic neuroblastoma, Am. J. Roentgenol. 50:575, 1943.
2. Bethge, J. F. J.: Die Ewingtumoren oder Omoblastome des Knochens. Die Differential-diagnose gegenüber den Knochenmetastasen der Neuroblastome des Sympathicus, Brunns' Beitr. Klin. Chir. 187:304, 1953.
3. Coley, B. L.: Tumors of bones and joints. In Bancroft, F. W., and Murray, C. R., editors: Surgical treatment of the motorskeletal system, Philadelphia, 1945, J. B. Lippincott Co., p. 349.
4. Colville, H. C., and Willis, R. A.: Neuroblastoma metastases in bones, with a criticism of Ewing's endothelioma, Am. J. Pathol. 9:421, 1933.
5. Connor, C. L.: Endothelial myeloma, Ewing; report of 54 cases, Arch. Surg. 12:789, 1926.
6. Dahlin, D. C., Coventry, W. B., and Scanlon, P. W.: Ewing's sarcoma. A critical analysis of 165 cases, J. Bone Joint Surg. 43-A:185, 1961.
7. Ewing, J.: The classification and treatment of bone sarcoma. Report of the International Conference on Cancer, London, Bristol, 1928, John Wright & Sons, Ltd., pp. 365-376 (see Endothelial myeloma, p. 371).
8. Ewing, J.: Diffuse endothelioma of bone, Proc. N. Y. Pathol. Soc. 21:17, 1921.
9. Ewing, J.: Further report on endothelial myeloma of bone, Proc. N. Y. Pathol. Soc. 24:93, 1924.
10. Ewing, J.: Neoplastic diseases. A treatise on tumors, ed. 4, Philadelphia, 1940, W. B. Saunders Co., pp. 360-370.
11. Ewing, J.: A review of the classification of bone tumors, Surg. Gynecol. Obstet. 68:971, 1939 (see Endothelioma, p. 975).
12. Foote, F. W., Jr., and Anderson, H. R.: Histogenesis of Ewing's tumor, Am. J. Pathol. 17:497, 1941.
13. Friedman, B., and Gold, H.: Ultrastructure of Ewing's sarcoma of bone, Cancer 22:307, 1968.
14. Gharpure, V. V.: Endothelial myeloma (Ewing's tumor of bone), Am. J. Pathol. 17:503, 1941.
15. Goldman, R. L., Winterling, A. N., and Winterling, C. C.: Maturation of tumors of the sympathetic nervous system. Report of long-term survival in 2 patients one with disseminated osseous metastases and review of cases from the literature, Cancer 18:1510, 1965.
16. Hamilton, J. F.: Ewing's sarcoma (endothelial myeloma), Arch. Surg. 41:29, 1940.
17. Heald, J. H., Soto-Hall, R., and Hill, H. A.: Ewing's sarcoma, Am. J. Roentgenol. 91:1167, 1964.
18. Hirsch, E. F., and Ryerson, E. W.: Metastases of the bone in primary carcinoma of the lung; a review of so-called endotheliomas of the bones, Arch. Surg. 16:1, 1928.
19. Hutchison, R.: On suprarenal sarcoma in children with metastases in the skull, Quart. J. Med. 1:33, 1907-1908.
20. Jenkin, R. D. T., Rider, W. D., and Sonley, M. J.: Ewing's sarcoma. A trial of adjuvant total-body irradiation, Radiology 96:151, 1970.
21. Johnson, R., and Humphreys, S. R.: Past failures and future possibilities in Ewing's sarcoma. Experimental and preliminary clinical results, Cancer 23:161, 1969.
22. Lichtenstein, L., and Jaffe, H. L.: Ewing's sarcoma of bone, Am. J. Pathol. 23:43, 1947.
23. Lumb, G., and Mackenzie, D. H.: Round-cell tumors of bone, Brit. J. Surg. 43:380, 1955.
24. McCormack, L. J., Dockerty, M. B., and Ghormley, R. K.: Ewing's sarcoma, Cancer 5:85, 1952.
25. Melnick, P. J.: Histogenesis of Ewing's

sarcoma of bone; with post-mortem report of a case, Am. J. Cancer **19**:353, 1933.
26. Meyerding, H. W., and Valls, J. E.: Primary malignant tumor of bone, J.A.M.A. **117**:237, 1941 (see pp. 240-241).
27. Millburn, L. F., O'Grady, L., and Hendrickson, F. R.: Radical radiation therapy and total body irradiation in the treatment of Ewing's sarcoma, Cancer **22**:919, 1968.
28. Neely, J. M., and Rogers, F. T.: Roentgenological and pathological considerations of Ewing's tumor of bone, Am. J. Roentgenol. **43**:204, 1940.
29. Oberling, C.: Les réticulosarcomes et les réticulo-endothéliosarcomes de la moelle osseuse (sarcomes d'Ewing), Bull. Assoc. franç. p. l'étude du cancer **17**:259, 1928.
30. Oberling, C., and Railenau, C.: Nouvelles recherches sur les réticulosarcomes de la moelle osseuse (sarcomes d'Ewing), Bull. Assoc. franç. p. l'étude du cancer **21**:333, 1932.
31. Parker, F., Jr., and Jackson, H., Jr.: Primary reticulum cell sarcoma of bone, Surg. Gynecol. Obstet. **68**:45, 1939.
32. Schajowicz, F.: Ewing's sarcoma and reticulum cell sarcoma of bone; with special reference to the histochemical demonstration of glycogen as an aid to differential diagnosis, J. Bone Joint Surg. **41-A**:349, 1959.
33. Senyszyn, J. J., Johnson, R. E., and Curran, R. E.: Treatment of metastatic Ewing's sarcoma with actinomycin D, Cancer Chemotherapy Reports, Part I, **54**:103, 1970.
34. Sirsat, M. V.: Some uncommon tumors in childhood, Indian J. Child Health, pp. 7-11, 1961 (see Case III).
35. Stella, J. G., Schweisguth, O., and Schlienger, M.: Neuroblastoma; a study of 144 cases treated in the Institute Gustav-Roussy over a period of 7 years, Am. J. Roentgenol. **108**:324, 1970.
36. Sternberg, C.: Zur Frage des sogenannten Ewing's Tumor, Frankfurt, Z. Pathol. **48**:525, 1935.
37. Stout, A. P.: A discussion of the pathology and histogenesis of Ewing's tumor of bone marrow, Am. J. Roentgenol. **50**:334, 1943.
38. Swenson, P. C.: The roentgenologic aspects of Ewing's tumor of bone marrow, Am. J. Roentgenol. **50**:343, 1943.
39. Tileston, W., and Wolbach, S. B.: Primary tumors of the adrenal gland in children. Report of a case of simultaneous sarcoma of the adrenal gland and of the cranium, with exophthalmos, Am. J. Med. Sci. **135**:871, 1908.
40. Wang, C. C., and Schulz, M. D.: Ewing's sarcoma; a study of fifty cases treated at the M. G. H. 1930-1952 inclusive, N. Engl. J. Med. **248**:571, 1953.
41. Willis, R. A.: Metastatic neuroblastoma in bone presenting the Ewing syndrome, with a discussion of "Ewing's sarcoma," Am. J. Pathol. **16**:317, 1940.
42. Wright, J. H.: Neurocytoma or neuroblastoma, a kind of tumor not generally recognized, J. Exp. Med. **12**:556, 1910.
43. Wyatt, G. M., and Farber, S.: Neuroblastoma sympatheticum; roentgenological appearances and radiation treatment, Am. J. Roentgenol. **46**:485, 1941.

Chapter 19

Plasma-cell myeloma (multiple myeloma)

Interest in the various aspects of this remarkable neoplasm continues unabated, and its literature flourishes like a green bay tree. Comprehensive monographs on the subject are now available, notably that of Waldenstrom.[87] In particular there has been intensified investigation of gamma globulin (immunoglobulin) synthesis and structure by electrophoretic and ultracentrifugation techniques, any detailed consideration of which is beyond the scope of this discussion. For this, the reader is referred to the papers by Osserman,[66] Osserman and Takatsui,[68] Putnam,[73] and Waldenstrom[87,89] among others.[1,24,49] With clarification of the nature of the proteins found in the sera of patients with myeloma, stemming from basic research in the gamma globulins, has come increasing complexity and the development of a descriptive language relating to chemical composition and physical constants, in which only experts can speak to one another. Whether the proteins found in myeloma are entirely normal or to some extent abnormal is still a moot point apparently. Suffice it to state here that the neoplastic plasma cells elaborate excessive globulins of one kind or another, which are dumped into the blood, then excreted in the urine (specifically the light chain fractions), and sometimes deposited in the tissues as well, as a base, presumably for amyloid or paraamyloid.

Also noteworthy is the development of several transplantable plasma-cell neoplasms in mice, the study of which, as Osserman points out, may ultimately prove to be of importance in the delineation of genetic factors and other possible pathogenic mechanisms responsible for plasma-cell neoplasia.

This chapter will deal mainly with the pathologic anatomy of plasma-cell myeloma, which is now fairly well understood,[13,48] although attention also will be directed to clinical and roentgen diagnosis and to clinical-pathologic correlation whenever this is possible. There will also be brief consideration of currently favored therapy in various circumstances, as a guide to the management of myeloma patients.

Multiple myeloma is a clinically and pathologically distinctive malignant neoplasm of the skeleton primarily, which seems clearly to originate from the he-

278   Bone tumors

matic cells in the bone marrow, and only occasionally in other extraskeletal sites. As such, it may be logically classified among the family of tumors of hematopoietic derivation, along with myeloid leukemia (chronic myelosis) and the malignant lymphomas involving bone marrow. The identification of the specific ancestral cells of multiple myeloma, however, is still a moot point, although the consensus of opinion implicates the marrow plasma cells, or perhaps more prim-

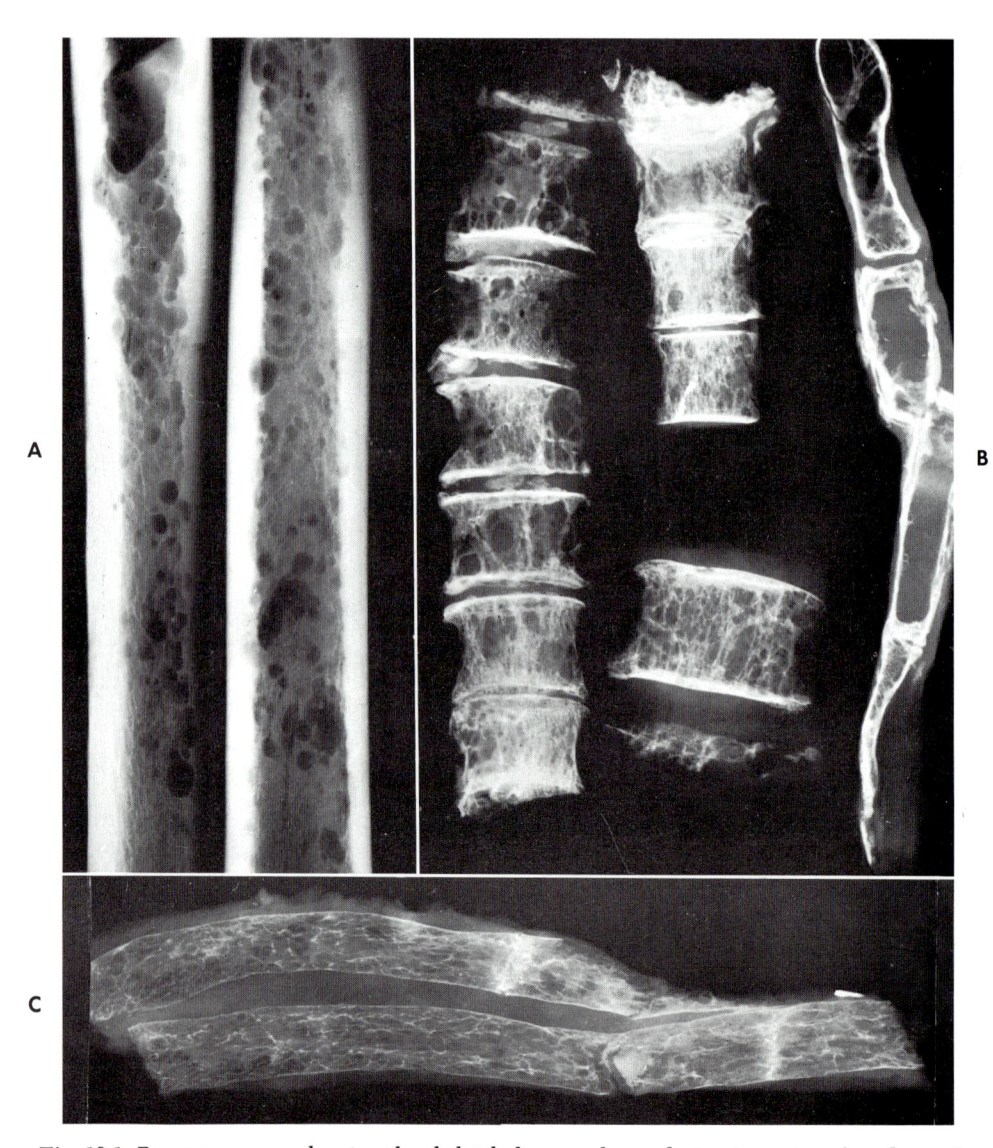

Fig. 19-1. Roentgenograms showing the skeletal changes observed at autopsy in a far-advanced case of multiple myeloma. **A,** In the shaft of the femur. **B,** In the vertebral column and in the sternum, the body of which shows a previous pathologic fracture. **C,** In the ribs, which are reduced to thin shells honeycombed by myeloma.

itive hemocytoblasts or reticulum cells. In my opinion, the old tendency to subclassify multiple myelomas, presumably on the basis of cytologic variation, into plasma cell, myeloid, erythroid, and lymphoid types, was unsound and served only to create confusion. It seems much more likely that multiple myeloma as discussed here is a neoplasm of unitary cell type, and that variations in cytologic appearance reflect stages in the maturation of the basic tumor cells, best designated noncommittally as myeloma cells.

The neoplasm is much more common than is generally suspected, and undoubtedly many cases go unrecognized, more so in private practice than in hospitals, mainly through unfamilarity with the varied clinical manifestations of the condition. Also, the widespread application of electrophoresis as a routine clinical laboratory procedure has uncovered an increasing number of cases of asymptomatic myeloma. This would indicate that the pool of myeloma patients is greater than it once was thought to be and, collaterally, that by the time a pa-

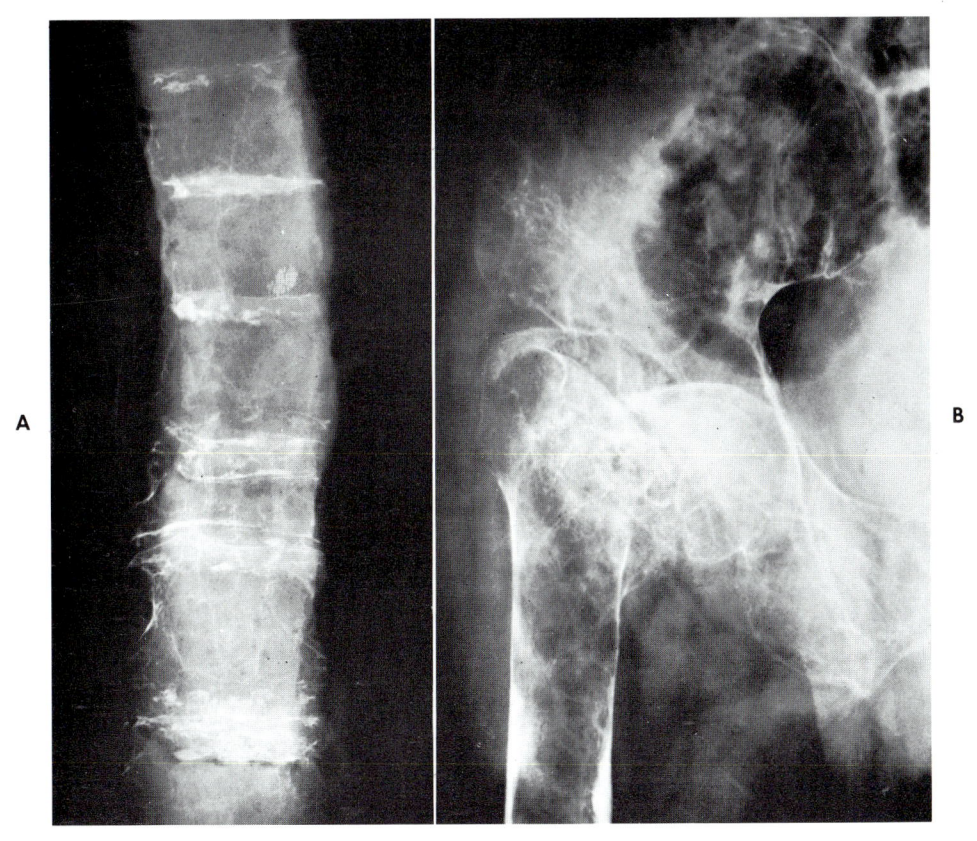

Fig. 19-2. Roentgenograms in another far-advanced case of multiple myeloma. **A**, Compression fracture of vertebra associated with extreme osteoporosis. **B**, Pathologic fracture of neck of femur, as well as striking osteoporosis and myelomatous transformation of innominate bone and upper femur.

tient is admitted to the hospital, he may present a late or end stage of a long neoplastic process.

Anatomically, practically every bone may ultimately come to be involved, more or less, in a given case. The progress of the disease may be steady and rapid, sometimes from the beginning and sometimes after a static period. One gathers also that in some cases, before the disease spreads over the skeleton, it may flourish in one bone (as a so-called solitary myeloma) for months or even years. Though at autopsy the skeleton may be found riddled with foci of myeloma, it is only infrequently that gross myelomatous foci are found in viscera and other extraskeletal parts. Nevertheless, even in the absence of gross infiltrations, microscopic examination sometimes reveals the presence of smaller or larger numbers of myeloma cells within the spleen, the liver, or the lymph nodes, and occasionally in other organs as well. Also, in some cases myeloma cells invade the bloodstream. Ordinarily, under these circumstances, relatively few myeloma cells are found in the blood smears. However, in an occasional case they may be so numerous as to create a leukemic blood picture (so-called plasma-cell leukemia).

Clinical features
Age and sex incidence

Multiple myeloma has its greatest incidence between 40 and 60 years of age, and though it is not uncommon to encounter it in the thirties, it is definitely unusual under the age of 30 years. A few unequivocal instances occurring in adolescents or children have been reported, and I can recall one such instance in a 17-year-old boy who presented the first manifestations of the disease at the age of 13 years. Some others, less convincing, in the literature may actually be instances of Schüller-Christian disease, stem-cell leukemia, Ewing's sarcoma, or neuroblastoma that has metastasized to the skeleton.

As is well known, multiple myeloma is more prevalent in males.

Clinical complaints

Evaluation of our clinical records showed that the major difficulties (occurring singly or in combination) that brought the patients to the hospital were, in order of decreasing frequency: (1) pain, especially of the back and thorax, (2) substantial loss of weight, (3) pathologic fracture of some bone, and (4) a palpable tumor appearing in relation to a superficial flat bone. Other complaints not directly resulting from skeletal alterations were referable to anemia, abnormal bleeding, neurologic manifestations, and renal involvement.

The pain occurring in the back and the thorax was often vague and generalized and accompanied by a feeling of weakness. However, in the presence of compressed or collapsed vertebral bodies, it had a more localized, persistent, and disabling character and was frequently associated with some manifestations of compression of the spinal cord or at least of issuing nerve roots. The loss of weight amounted to 30 pounds or even more in some cases. As the disease progressed, there was a tendency, even in those who showed no appreciable loss of weight on admission, toward increasing debilitation and terminal emaciation. Pathologic fracture as expressed in compression collapse of one or more vertebral bodies was not uncommon, but in some cases a femur or a humerus, for instance, presented a pathologic fracture extending through an area of exuberant myelomatous involvement. If one or more tumor masses are palpable on the skeleton, they are most likely to be found in relation to a clavicle or to one or several ribs. However, a tumor may sometimes be palpable in relation to such superficial bone sites as the calvarium or the facial bones, the sternum, a scapula, or an innominate bone.

Presenting skeletal lesions

There are some cases of multiple myeloma in which the patients complain of rather generalized bone pain without specific localization, in spite of wide-

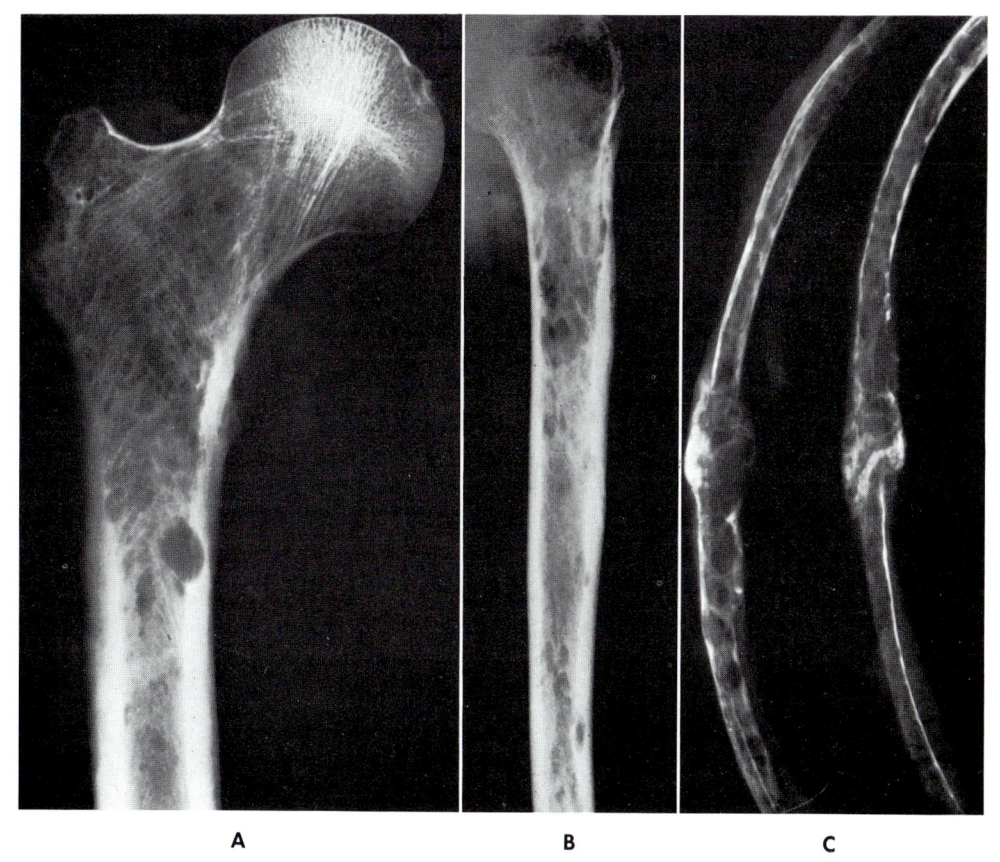

Fig. 19-3. Roentgenograms from additional cases of multiple myeloma coming to autopsy. **A,** Femur showing a circumscribed lytic defect where a tumor focus encroached upon and eroded the cortex. **B,** Humerus showing moth-eaten and also more discrete areas of rarefaction. **C,** Extensively involved ribs showing thinned cortices, honeycombed rarefaction, and pathologic fractures.

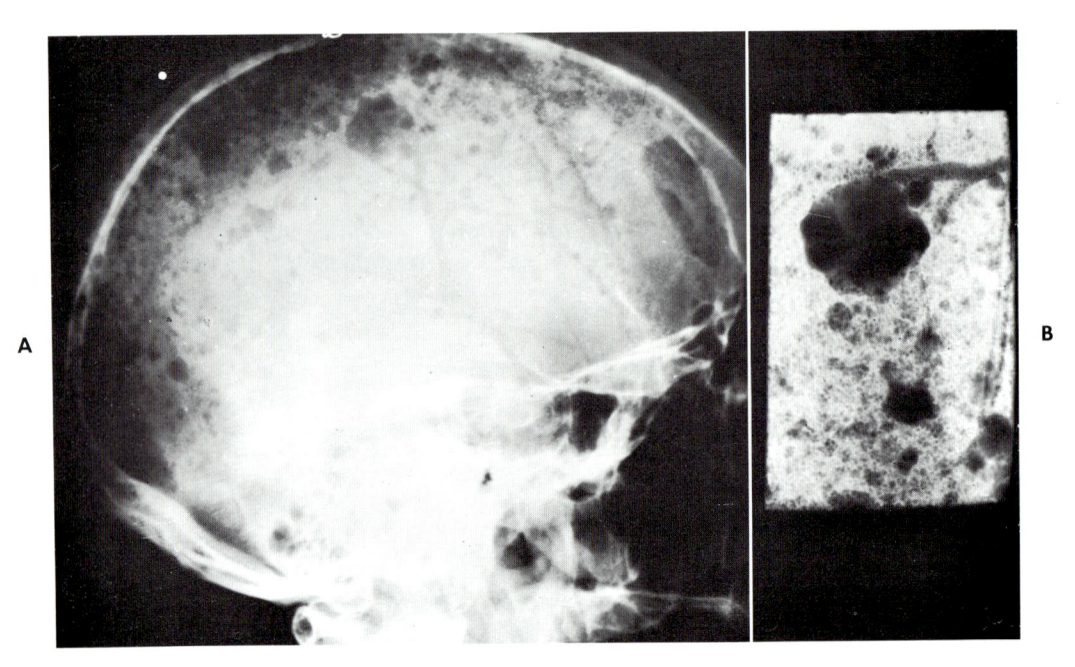

Fig. 19-4. A, Calvarium from an autopsied case of multiple myeloma showing multiple lytic defects of varying size. **B,** Roentgenogram of an excised block of the same calvarium indicating the rather sharp delimitation of the myelomatous defects. As noted, however, this is not a constant finding in multiple myeloma, even in cases showing obvious involvement of other bones.

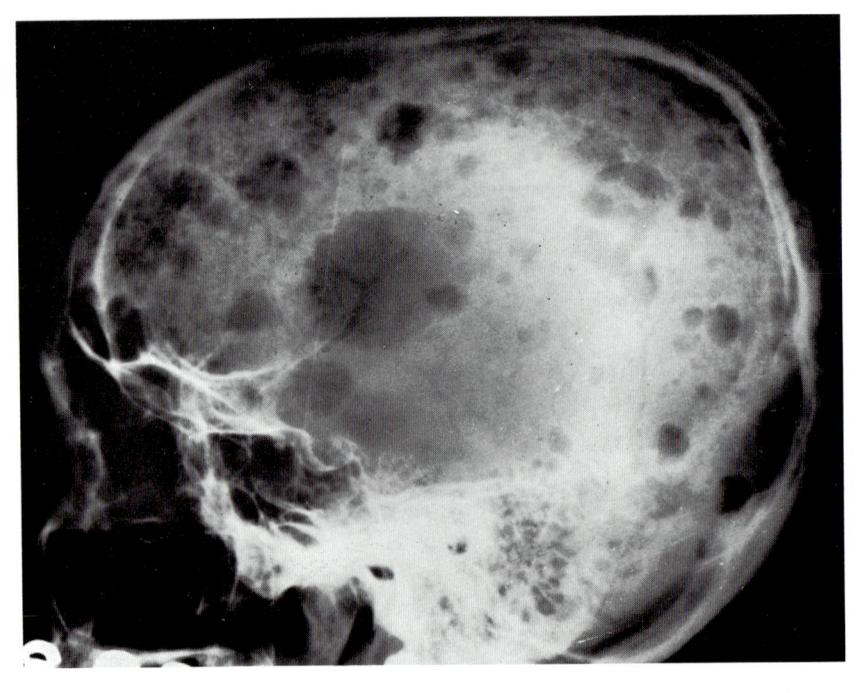

Fig. 19-5. Another instance of multiple myeloma in which there is obvious involvement of the calvarium. It must be borne in mind, however, that occasionally metastatic carcinoma may simulate this picture.

spread skeletal involvement. Usually, however, it is difficulty with some particular bone or skeletal region that first directs attention to the presence of the disease. The involved site most often responsible for difficulties in those whose initial skeletal complaints were localized was the vertebral column. Indeed, in approximately one half of these patients the difficulties were referable to the spine. The lumbar region was most often affected, next the dorsal, and least often the cervical region. Patients having complaints referable to the vertebral column often showed roentgenographic evidence of compression or collapse of one or more vertebral bodies on admission to the hospital, and a number of them presented signs of resulting compression of the cord as well. It seems worth mentioning that, with involvement of the lumbar region of the spine, disability and sciatic pain were common complaints even in the absence of compressed or collapsed vertebral bodies.

The long bones, particularly the femur, represent another clinically important site of localization, and occasionally one may encounter a strikingly large focus of myeloma in a femur or a humerus that is vulnerable to pathologic fracture. When it occurs in a superficially located bone, the presenting lesion is also likely to be clinically palpable. Thus, not infrequently, such a tumor can be felt on a rib or a clavicle. Actually, however, even a bone of a foot or a hand may sometimes be the site of the presenting lesion.

Clinical course and prognosis

In many cases the disease pursues an insidious course in the beginning, the patient complaining merely of some weakness, loss of weight, or vague pain in the back or the chest. Sometimes, a fracture of some bone (commonly a rib or a limb bone), weakened by an exuberant focus of tumor within it, is the first major difficulty. In other instances the disease may be ushered in dramatically by sudden onset of severe root pain or even paraplegia resulting from compression or collapse of one or more vertebral bodies. Taking our cases altogether, we found that the duration of symptoms prior to hospitalization ranged from as snort a time as a few weeks to as long as two years, the average duration being about nine months.

Whatever the initial complaints that bring the patients to the hospital, the progress of skeletal involvement thereafter, as judged by successive roentgenograms, is rather variable and frequently unpredictable. The patients who present a far-advanced stage of the disease when first observed usually (though not invariably) survive no more than some weeks or months. As for those with still limited involvement roentgenographically, in some, one observes tremendous progression within just a few months, while in others, one gains the impression that the neoplasm progress relatively slowly or remains static for months or even a number of years before entering its terminal phase. This variability of tempo is not explainable on a cytologic basis alone. The average period of survival following the onset of symptoms was about two years in our cases, which is in accord with the general impression, but there are striking deviations from this average.

Two patients in whom transverse myelitis developed succumbed within one and three months, respectively, although it is true that neither of them received the possible benefit of laminectomy for decompression. On the other hand, we did an autopsy in a case in which the history of the disease dated back over nine years, and another patient (presenting tumor in an ilium initially) was still alive and comparatively well after ten years. While these instances are exceptional, it is well known that the clinical course of multiple myeloma may occasionally be protracted and characterized by long remissions, which are frequently attributed to roentgen treatment but which may be spontaneous. Cases in point have been reported by Gross and Vaughan,[32] Kirsch,[45] Batts,[4] and Davison and Balser.[19] Davison and Balser cited an extraordinary case that came to autopsy sixteen years after the onset of symptoms. It is true also that patients in whom the tumor is apparently localized in some one bone in the beginning not infrequently go on for a number of years before the tumor becomes disseminated over the skeleton.

In most cases, as the disease progresses there is a tendency toward demineralization and devastation of the skeleton, associated with increasing anemia and cachexia, provided the clinical course is not cut short, as it frequently is, by such complications as intercurrent infection (especially pneumonia in bedridden patients), concomitant cancer of some other kind, cardiac failure, renal insufficiency, ascending infection of the urinary tract, or amyloidosis.

Problems of diagnosis

There are numerous clues to the diagnosis of multiple myeloma coming from many quarters—clinical, roentgenographic, hematologic, biochemical—and the recognition of the condition prior to biopsy or postmortem examination frequently requires their fullest utilization. It is true that the diagnosis of multiple myeloma will be fairly obvious if many bones, including the calvarium, are veritably riddled by osteolytic defects (the picture usually stressed in the texts) and if, in addition, Bence Jones proteinuria is discovered. Unfortunately, this skeletal picture represents the exception rather than the rule, in our experience at least, and Bence Jones proteinuria is as likely to be absent as present. One often observes merely some vaguely defined rarefactions in some of the bones or a single exuberant tumor in a single bone without obvious involvement of the skeleton generally, and sometimes (when myelomatous infiltration of the bone marrow is diffuse) skeletal changes may not be apparent at all roentgenographically in spite of complaints referable to the skeleton. In such equivocal or initially obscure cases, the lead may come from the discovery of anemia, the presence of myeloma cells in blood smears, hypercalcemia, hyperproteinemia (and certain peculiar hematologic manifestations resulting from increase of serum globulins), evidences of renal damage of a peculiar type, or even from the finding of unusual tumorlike amyloid deposits. It must be recognized, however, that these pertinent findings are not all present in every case or necessarily present in the early stages of the evolution of any given case, nor are they necessarily pathognomonic in themselves. It is only by utilizing all the logical approaches that one is likely to arrive at a combination of significant findings constituting probable or conclusive evidence of the presence of multiple myeloma.

For anatomic confirmation, puncture of the sternal marrow should be freely employed. A high degree of reliability is claimed for this procedure, though there are undoubtedly cases of multiple myeloma in which sternal marrow spreads fail to yield significant information. Biopsy of some obviously affected and readily accessible bone will resolve any possible doubt as to the diagnosis, since the histologic recognition of a myeloma entails no difficult problems in differential diagnosis as a rule.

Skeletal alterations and their roentgenologic reflection

No single description can do justice to the gross appearance of the bones in all cases of multiple myeloma coming to autopsy. At one extreme there is the occasional case in which the bones appear normal as to surface and contour and those removed do not even offer any striking lack of resistance when being cut open. On inspection of the cut surfaces of these bones, one finds that the spongy trabeculae are still numerous and that the cortices are not significantly thinned. However, the marrow is modified and replaced more or less diffusely by rather whitish tissue that, on histologic examination, is proved to be myeloma tissue. In conformity with these findings, the skeletal roentgenograms taken during life in such a case may show at most some diffuse porosity of the bones. They certainly show nothing even remotely suggestive of the roentgenographic picture one has been taught to regard as representative of multiple myeloma. This was the skeletal status in a case of atypical amyloidosis and myeloma that we studied. It reemphasizes the fact that in every case of atypical amyloidosis, despite the lack of evidence of multiple myeloma in the clinical roentgenograms, bones must be opened and their marrow examined histologically to establish or rule out the presence of myeloma.

In another occasional case, while the bones show smooth and undistended contours, they cut with abnormal ease. When cut, such bones show thinning of the cortices from the medullary side, as well as great reduction of the spongy trabeculae. This is the result of encroachment on the osseous tissue by a whitish gray tissue that has substantially replaced the marrow and that stands out in some places as discrete foci of tumor. The clinical roentgenograms of the bones in such a case hardly suggest the conventional idea of the roentgenographic picture of multiple myeloma but do reflect the tumor encroachment on the osseous tissue by showing vague mottled or vacuolated rarefactions and thinned cortices.

In many cases, however, the cortex becomes gravely weakened or even destroyed by the tumor tissue in one or several places in one or even in many bones. Thus, there is a bulge in the contour of the bone at such a site, and the tumor tissue that has spread out of the bone is found distending the periosteum but still restrained by it; or, having violated the periosteum, it may even be found invading the local musculature. Exuberant growth of the myeloma at one bone site, with destruction of the cortex and spread of the tumor beyond the bone in this area, often produces the lesion that first calls attention to the disease, though the marrow of the skeleton as a whole may already be riddled through by tumor tissue. For instance, a patient with multiple myeloma may first present himself because of a localized palpable and often painful enlargement of a rib, a clavicle, a jaw bone, an ilium, or even a long bone of an extremity—particularly a femur or a humerus. The patient showing such a lesion in a femur or a humerus may already have a pathologic fracture at the site of the presenting lesion.

However, it is remarkable how often one finds multiple myeloma presenting itself clinically because an exuberant focus of the disease has developed in a vertebral body (or several contiguous bodies). The affected body or bodies are found substantially destroyed; indeed, the tumor tends to transgress them, often producing pressure on the spinal cord or the local nerve trunks, with symptoms resulting. In such cases, roentgenographic examination of the rest of the skeleton (including the skull) often fails to reveal the clear-cut, punched-out rarefactions conventionally held to distinguish the roentgenographic picture of multiple myeloma. It is in such cases (especially if one dorsal or lumbar body alone is clearly affected) that the true nature of the disease often goes unrecognized for long periods, the lesion frequently being interpreted as a local one, i.e., as a hemangioma, a giant-cell tumor, a fracture due to Kümmell's disease, or, if grossly destructive, as a focus of metastatic cancer. The true nature of the disease may become clear if marrow is obtained by sternal puncture or if serial roentgenograms of the rest of the skeleton finally demonstrate widespread lesions in other bones suggesting multiple myeloma, or if serum electrophoresis shows one or more peaks or spikes of myeloma protein, but sometimes it is discovered only at autopsy. Eventually, in the far-advanced stage of the disease, the bones of the trunk and the limbs may become so extensively porotic and deformed from riddling by neoplastic tissue as to present the appearance of washed-out honeycombed shells roentgenographically. However, this extreme expression of skeletal devastation is observed only occasionally, even at autopsy (Fig. 19-1).

In regard to the calvarium, great emphasis is usually laid on the diagnostic value of several or even many roundish, punched-out rarefactions revealed in roentgenograms of the skull. It is true that when roentgenograms show clear-cut and widespread involvement of the rest of the skeleton in the form of numerous punched-out rarefactions, the calvarium, too, is quite likely to show these, though not infrequently it fails to display them. But it is precisely when one turns to the roentgenograms of the calvarium because those of the other bones do not show the conventional picture of multiple myeloma that the calvarium, too, fails to show it. Whether or not the calvarium shows rarefactions, histologic examination will reveal that the marrow of the diploic spaces has been substantially replaced by the tumor tissue. At sites of clear-cut rarefaction, one will find that the tumor tissue is present as a nodule that has encroached on and destroyed the diploic bone, sometimes also thinning the tables, but in our experience the tables are seldom perforated even in such sites. Actually, the riddling of the calvarium by tumor deposits, which produces numerous circular punched-out defects, is not invariably an indication of multiple myeloma, since it sometimes occurs in carcinomatosis.

It is noteworthy also, as Lowbeer[52] has emphasized, that occasionally myeloma in bone may provoke an unusual osteosclerotic reaction discernible grossly, radiographically, and microscopically. Obviously, such tumor foci may suggest osteoblastic carcinoma metastases prior to laboratory investigation and biopsy.

Hematologic observations of diagnostic importance

The significant frequency with which anemia is encountered in multiple myeloma is well known. The anemia reflects progressive neoplastic encroachment on the myeloid marrow, bleeding into tumor tissue, and frequently also the effects of general debilitation and renal damage. About 70% of our patients presented appreciable reduction of hemoglobin and erythrocyte levels when first observed, and in about one half of them the anemia was already of moderate or severe grade. The trend in most cases followed over a period of several or many months is toward slow but steady decline of the hemoglobin and erythrocyte values, often to appallingly low levels. Transfusions even when repeated, appear to have merely a temporary sparing effect. In a notable case under observation for approximately a year, the hemoglobin value fell as low as 2.6 gm. and the erythrocyte count to 1,000,000, remaining at about these levels for six months until death resulted from cachexia, renal insufficiency, and terminal bronchopneumonia. The profound anemia was reflected anatomically in intense hemosiderosis of liver, spleen, marrow, and lymph nodes. Incidentally, the blood smears showed as many as twenty to thirty normoblasts per hundred white cells counted. The anemia of this particular patient was normocytic, as anemia usually is in cases of myeloma, the color index being slightly below 1.0, but the anemia of some myelomatous patients may be macrocytic in type, simulating pernicious anemia.

The depletion and irritation of the leukopoietic marrow in cases of myeloma are not infrequently reflected by the appearance in the blood smears of a few myelocytes or even myeloblasts, and occasionally these immature leukocytes may be present in such large numbers as to produce a leukemoid picture. Thus, multiple myeloma, from a hematologic point of view, at least, sometimes simulates myeloid leukemia at first, especially if a purpuric tendency is present. Sometimes, also, the number of eosinophils may be found increased as another indication of irritation of the marrow. The total leukocyte count shows no consistency and may be normal, somewhat depressed, or slightly increased.

It is pertinent to mention also that any of the following phenomena may be observed in cases of multiple myeloma: excessive rouleau formation in blood smears, autohemagglutination of the red cells in dry and wet films, clumping with Hayem's solution, failure of clot retraction, abnormal viscosity of the blood, and rapid sedimentation rate. It has been shown also that serums from myelomatous patients often have an anticomplementary property, although by no means do all such serums give this reaction. These phenomena in general have been ascribed to the presence of hyperproteinemia, and their discovery may afford the first clue to the diagnosis of multiple myeloma.

Another important aid in the diagnosis of myeloma through hematologic methods is the finding of myeloma cells or so-called atypical plasma cells in blood smears. The frequency with which such cells are discovered and properly identified (beyond their provisional designation as "blast" cells) seems to depend largely on the thoroughness and skill of the observer, and in suspected cases of myeloma, blood smears should be scrutinized by a qualified hematologist.

In most instances in which they are found, the myeloma cells are present in relatively small or, at most, moderate numbers, but occasionally there may be such an outpouring of them into the bloodstream as to give rise to a frankly leukemic blood picture. Thus, in one of our cases (in which transverse myelitis was the cause of death) the leukocyte count during the terminal phase of the disease rose steadily from 6,000 to 40,000, and 30% to 54% of the leukocytes were identified as plasma cells. Such cases of multiple myeloma in which the tumor cells readily invade the bloodstream are well known and have been collected and discussed under the head of plasma-cell leukemia by Muller and McNaughton,[63] Piney and Riach,[72] Osgood and Hunter,[65] Patek and Castle,[70] and others. The pertinent cases coming to autopsy indicate conclusively that so-called plasma-cell leukemia has its anatomic foundation in skeletal multiple myeloma

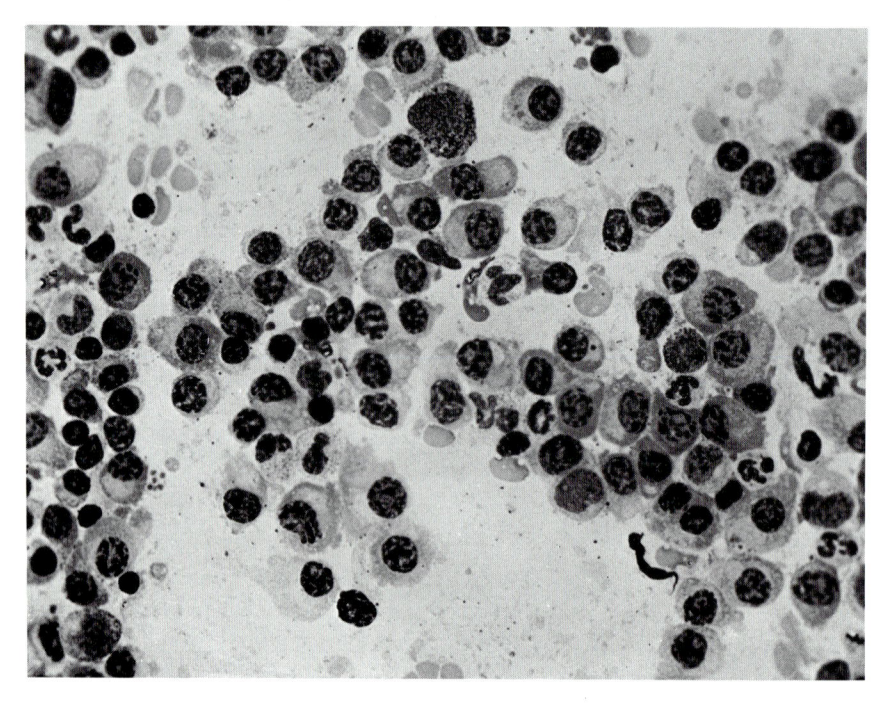

Fig. 19-6. Bone marrow spread obtained by sternal marrow puncture of a patient with multiple myeloma. (Wright's stain; ×200.)

and cannot logically be considered, as Osgood and Hunter have suggested, as a disease primarily of the blood. The development of "leukemia'" in such cases represents a phase, and often a terminal phase, in the evolution of the disease. It is worth noting that cases of multiple myeloma characterized by frank invasion of the bloodstream apparently exhibit a strong tendency toward extraskeletal spread in the form of diffuse and occasionally nodular infiltrations of the spleen, the liver, and the lymph nodes, and sometimes also of the kidney, the pancreas, the skin, or other organs.

Still another indispensable diagnostic aid is, of course, bone marrow examination. Sternal puncture has high diagnostic value in cases of multiple myeloma, although it may not necessarily yield positive information in every instance. Certainly, it is a procedure that should be employed whenever the presence of myeloma is suspected, and especially when biopsy of some obviously affected bone is not feasible. In most instances of multiple myeloma, according to Wintrobe, cellular marrow spreads will reveal myeloma cells making up 3% to 96% of the total number of cells (Fig. 19-6).

Significant biochemical changes in cases of multiple myeloma
Hypercalcemia

The occurrence of hypercalcemia with multiple myeloma was noted as early as 1927, while the observation that hypercalciuria and a negative calcium balance may be present dates back even further. Hypercalcemia occurs in about one half of the cases of multiple myeloma. The increased calcium values may range as high as 18 mg. per 100 cubic centimeters of serum. It should be noted that in such cases the kidneys tend to show deposits of calcium granules in the tubular epithelium and interstitial connective tissue. Occasionally the metastatic calcification may be quite heavy and widespread, involving, in addition, the interstitium of the lungs, the lining of the stomach, and even other tissues.

The increase of calcium in the serum reflects the lytic resorption of the bones and the tendency toward renal failure in many of the cases. It apparently develops independently of hyperproteinemia, since the highest calcium levels that we observed were in cases in which the serum protein concentration was normal. Apparently, in some instances the tendency toward hypercalcemia is perpetuated and accentuated by secondary hyperplasia of the parathyroid glands developing in response to chronic renal insufficiency.

Hypercalcemia per se is, to be sure, not diagnostic of multiple myeloma even when it is associated with rarefying skeletal lesions, since it also occurs characteristically with hyperparathyroidism and occasionally with osteoclastic carcinoma extensively metastasizing to the skeleton. However, hypercalcemia associated with either hyperproteinemia or Bence Jones proteinuria is clearly indicative of multiple myeloma. It is precisely because of the presence of hypercalcemia, nephrocalcinosis, and resorptive skeletal changes that some cases of multiple myeloma have been misinterpreted, at least temporarily, as instances of hyper-

290 *Bone tumors*

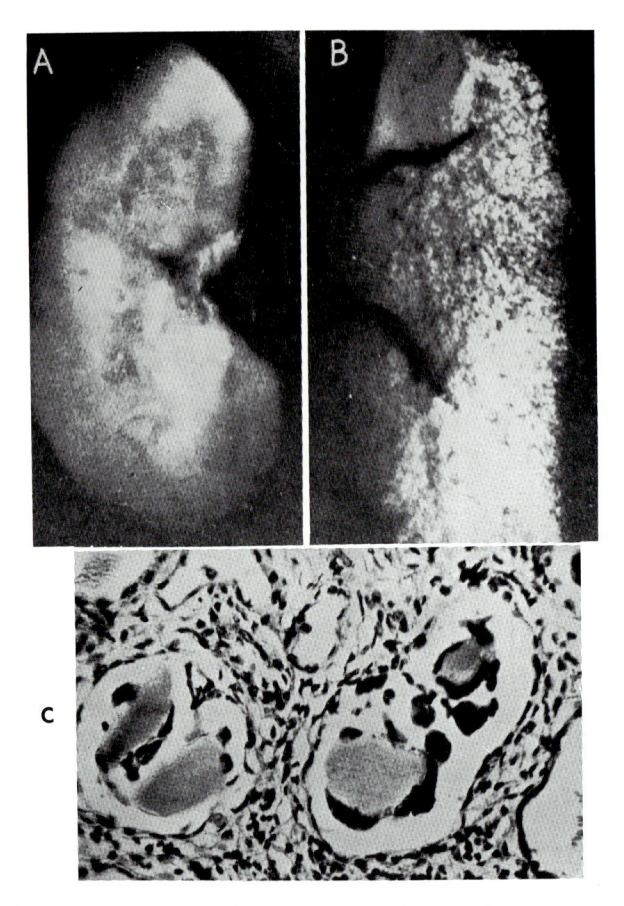

Fig. 19-7. **A** and **B**, Roentgenograms from an autopsied case of multiple myeloma featured by extremely rapid demineralization and hypercalcemia, illustrating metastatic calcification in kidney, **A**, which showed deposits of calcareous material within some of its calices and in lungs, **B**, which showed grossly evident, yellow, gritty deposits of calcium, particularly in the lower lobes. **C**, Photomicrograph from another case of multiple myeloma showing obstruction of renal tubules by protein-containing casts about which there is foreign body giant-cell reaction. (×200.) (After Lichtenstein, L., and Jaffe, H. L.: Arch. Pathol. 44:207, 1947.)

parathyroidism, and the patients even subjected to surgical exploration in a search for a parathyroid adenoma.

The serum phosphatase activity tends to be normal, no matter how extensive the skeletal involvement may be. It is true that if the serum phosphatase activity is measured shortly after the occurrence of a pathologic fracture, it may be found slightly increased, but the increase does not attain the level that is usually reached in advanced stages of hyperparathyroidism.

Hyperproteinemia

One of the peculiar and characteristic features of some cases of myeloma is the presence of hyperproteinemia, specifically hyperglobulinemia. Indeed, the occurrence of abnormal protein in the blood of patients with multiple myeloma was noted as early as 1899 by Ellinger.[24] Hyperglobulinemia is observed in about one half or more of the cases of multiple myeloma. The formaldehyde-gel and Takata reactions provide convenient crude tests for hyperglobulinemic serums, but when positive they should be supplemented by quantitative methods. The serum albumin does not contribute to the hyperproteinemia, being normal, as a rule, when the globulin value is normal and actually diminished when the globulin value is increased. The reason that the serum albumin values are consistently low in the cases of myeloma characterized by hyperglobulinemia seems to be that, in these cases particularly, damage of the renal tubules tends to develop, and thus the loss of albumin may conceivably be part of the complex of renal insufficiency.

Hyperglobulinemia per se is, of course, not necessarily indicative of multiple myeloma, since it is known to occur with other conditions also—particularly with chronic infections, notably lymphogranuloma venereum, sarcoidosis and kala-azar, and occasionally with cirrhosis of the liver, chronic nephritis, etc. However, hyperglobulinemia should always suggest the possibility of myeloma and, if found in association with hypercalcemia or Bence Jones proteinuria, speaks definitely for myeloma.

The protein composition of myeloma serums has been the subject of active investigation in recent years. The early studies of Magnus-Levy[55] and others have been greatly extended by the application of modern electrophoretic methods, which have unraveled some of the complexities of the subject. Detailed analysis of these findings may be found in recent reviews[25,68,87] and is beyond the scope of this discussion.

The multiplicity of Bence Jones proteins and the difficulty of separating them from other normal and abnormal serum proteins make further progress in their identification and assay difficult. Nor does the complexity of the problem end there. The observations of Wintrobe and Buell,[92] von Bonsdorf, Groth, and Packalen,[84] and Shapiro, Ross, and Moore[78] indicate that the serums of myelomatous patients may on occasion contain still another peculiar abnormal protein substance of high molecular weight and great viscosity, differing from Bence Jones protein and showing a tendency to spontaneous precipitation and crystallization. Also noteworthy is the finding in occasional cases of peculiar lipoproteins, of cryoglobulin (a cold-precipitable serum protein), of pyroglobulins, so-called, and of unusual proteins that seemingly interfere with fibrin formation. There will undoubtedly be other bizarre proteins reported in the future.

Bence Jones proteinuria

In current immunochemical parlance, Bence Jones protein consists of light (or low molecular weight) chains of polypeptides of gamma globulin derivation. As is well known, the occurrence in the urine of protein giving the Bence Jones reaction, dating back a century, is the earliest recorded observation in connection with the neoplasm now commonly designated multiple myeloma. It is also generally recognized that the presence of this reaction strongly favors the diagnosis of multiple myeloma (with certain reservations), but that, on the other hand, it may be absent in established cases of myeloma. It is said to be present in at least 65% of all cases of multiple myeloma, although some perseverance may be necessary for its detection, since (1) it may be undetectable in casual specimens but present in a 24-hour specimen, (2) it may be present at certain times but not at others (that is, its excretion may be intermittent rather than continuous), and (3) it may be absent early in the course of the disease and become evident later on. On the other hand, there are undoubtedly instances of myeloma in which no detectable Bence Jones protein is ever excreted. In one of our cases twenty-five examinations for Bence Jones proteinuria were made over a period of a year, all of them yielding negative results, including that made on urine taken from the bladder at autopsy.

In regard to the specificity of Bence Jones proteinuria, it is universally stated that Bence Jones protein may occasionally be found in the urine in certain conditions other than multiple myeloma, especially in leukemia and in carcinoma metastatic to the skeleton. However, citations of actual experience to that effect are scarce in the literature. We have never encountered it in other conditions ourselves, although we have not made any systematic study of the Bence Jones reaction in skeletal diseases other than myeloma. There are a few pertinent observations, however—namely, those of Boggs and Guthrie,[10] Geschickter and Copeland,[30] and Bayrd and Heck[6]—purporting to show that rarely in chronic leukemia and metastatic carcinoma of bone, and still more rarely in certain other diseases of bone (e.g., senile osteomalacia, gunshot wound, polycythemia), the urine may contain protein giving the Bence Jones reaction. With these exceptions, the finding of Bence Jones proteinuria is, for all practical purposes, indicative of multiple myeloma.

Increased uric acid in the blood

This represents still another significant, though not specific, change occurring with multiple myeloma. It has been commented on by Stewart and Weber[80] and has been observed by Tarr and Ferris,[82] and also by us[48] in several instances. In the opinion of Stewart and Weber, the uric acid increment results from the catabolism of nucleoproteins derived from the myeloma cells—an explanation that seems quite plausible. Multiple myeloma is, of course, not the only tumor responsible for hyperuricemia; it is well known, for example, that hyperuricemia may also occur with the leukemias.

Extraskeletal myelomatous infiltrations

As noted, the extraskeletal occurrence of grossly discernible myelomatous foci is decidedly uncommon, although there can be no doubt that in occasional cases of multiple myeloma coming to autopsy (particularly in those in which the bloodstream had been invaded by myeloma cells) one may find single or even multiple tumor foci within the internal organs. Microscopic infiltrations, particularly of the spleen, the liver, or the lymph nodes, are somewhat less unusual, but in our experience even these are lacking in most cases of multiple myeloma. Not infrequently, what may appear to be independent extraskeletal tumor foci occurring, for example, in the dura, the pituitary gland, the oropharynx, the nasopharynx, the larnyx, the thyroid gland, the pleura and the retroperitoneal, mediastinal, and subcutaneous tissues may actually represent direct outgrowth of tumor of contiguous bones. Also, in evaluating the reported cases of supposed multiple myeloma characterized by extensive and widespread tumor deposits in the internal organs, it is important to bear in mind that some of them may actually have been instances of metastasizing occult carcinoma, malignant lymphoma, or stem-cell leukemia.

Nevertheless, cases of myeloma demonstrating the presence of extraskeletal tumor foci are prominently featured in the literature precisely because of their unusual nature, and infiltration of practically any organ that might be named has been noted at one time or another. Thus, Mallory cited a case of multiple myeloma in which a single metastatic nodule was found in a lung (and also in a bronchial lymph node), and similar instances of pulmonary metastasis have been noted also by Hallermann,[34] Carlisle,[12] Piney and Riach,[72] and Batts.[4] Metastases have been observed in the heart by Piney and Riach and by Carlisle, who commented on the finding of two discrete bean-sized nodules of myeloma within the wall of the right auricle. Nodular infiltrations of an enlarged spleen have been observed by Osgood and Hunter,[65] and Churg and Gordon[15] described a remarkable case in which the spleen (weighing 650 grams) presented innumerable tumor nodules studding and substantially replacing the pulp. In the latter case, infiltration of some of the intraabdominal lymph nodes and of the portal areas and sinusoids of the liver was also noted. Piney and Riach described the finding of a tumor node, the size of a plum, within the pancreas, and Patek and Castle,[70] with regard to a patient exhibiting "plasma-cell leukemia," commented on the observation of a soft, reddish brown tumor node, 1.5 cm. in diameter, in the tail of the pancreas. In this case, incidentally, infiltration of the liver, the spleen, the kidneys, and the abdominal lymph nodes was also noted microscopically. A metastasis in the form of a cherry-sized tumor node has been observed in an adrenal gland by Piney and Riach, and adrenal metastases have been noted by others. Involvement of the kidney has been noted by Carlisle,[12] Morse,[62] Donhauser and de Rouville,[21] and Newns and Edwards.[64] Newns and Edwards described the finding of an essentially circumscribed rounded tumor, 4 cm. in diameter, replacing part of the lower pole of a kidney and bulging into its pelvis.

Involvement of the tonsils was noted in an extraordinary case reported by Jackson, Parker, and Bethea,[39] in which a "plasmacytoma" in that region had been removed fully eight years before generalized involvement of bone could be detected, although the neoplasm had extended to the cervical lymph nodes in the interim. Striking involvement of the intestinal tract has been described by Carlisle, who found numerous tumor deposits in the submucosa of the duodenum and small bowel, the mucosa being tautly stretched over these protuberances. Ovarian metastases have been noted by Herrick and Hektoen,[37] and bilateral tumorous involvement of the male gonads has been observed by Ulrich.[83] Cutaneous involvement in the form of multiple raised nodular infiltrations (scattered over the scalp, the region of the clavicle, and the arm) has been described by Duvoir and associates,[22] and Kin[44] reported a comparable case in which the nodular infiltrations (over the face and the back) were large, umbilicated, and ulcerated, presenting the general picture of so-called mycosis fungoides. Piney and Riach described a most unusual case of multiple myeloma with "leukemia" in which the patient presented a diffuse nodular eruption over the trunk and limbs, looking not unlike neurofibromatosis clinically. The patient also presented a peculiar helmet-like thickening extending down from the infiltrated scalp of the region of the forehead, in front of the ears, and to the nape of the neck. Incidentally, in this case, as in some of the others characterized by a leukemic blood picture, histologic examination showed infiltration of multiple sites, including the cervical lymph nodes, the kidneys, the liver, and the heart.

Whether myeloma-cell infiltrations of the liver, the spleen, or lymph nodes represent hematogenous metastases of tumor occurring in the bones or, rather, tumor foci independently formed as a result of activation and neoplasia of potential blood-forming cells within the organs in question does not concern us here directly. Sometimes infiltration of the spleen and the liver may already be manifested grossly by whitish streaks or nodules, or, in the case of lymph nodes, by diffuse enlargement and cellularity, but more often it is detected only on microscopic examination. Our experience with reference to its frequency does not parallel that of Lowenhaupt,[53] who claimed to have found "plasma cells" of myelomatous nature in every one of the spleens from twelve patients who came to autopsy, in all of the lymph nodes examined, and in three of the livers as well. Similarly, Gordon and Churg[31] felt that they had established the presence of extraskeletal tumor foci in twenty-two of thirty cases studied. It should be pointed out, however, that the indubitable identification of isolated small nests of cells presumed to be myeloma cells and their clear-cut differentiation from cells of histiocytic or inflammatory nature commonly encountered in the spleen and the lymph nodes, particularly, may be exceedingly difficult. Furthermore, as Mallory rightly emphasized, small collections of immature blood cells representing foci of compensatory extramedullary hemopoiesis are observed rather frequently in cases of multiple myeloma, and these may also be mistaken for nests of myeloma cells.

Significant renal changes in cases of multiple myeloma

In the patient with multiple myeloma there are certain cytologic renal changes of almost pathognomonic distinctiveness. These changes may be manifested clinically in more or less heavy albuminuria, though not necessarily Bence Jones proteinuria, and in diminished power of the kidney to concentrate and to clear nitrogenous constituents. Only exceptionally do they result in the development of edema or hypertension. It has been emphasized on that account (Foord[27] and others) that the finding of "atypical nephritis" should always suggest the possibility of multiple myeloma. When the renal damage is limited in extent, it results clinically in no more than persistent albuminuria. On the other hand, when it is more severe, it often leads ultimately to progressive renal insufficiency. Occasionally it leads to the relatively early appearance of azotemia, which dominates the clinical picture before the presence of multiple myeloma is even suspected.

Already in 1921, Löhlein[51] noted the deposition of crystalloid hyalin-like casts in the renal tubules of a subject with multiple myeloma coming to autopsy. Many of the casts plugging the tubules were surrounded by polymorphonuclear leukocytes, and often also by giant cells, which Löhlein thought were derived from proliferated tubular epithelium. There was some dilatation of the tubules and also some interstitial scarring, but the glomeruli and the blood vessels were not remarkable. The specificity of these essential changes was confirmed by

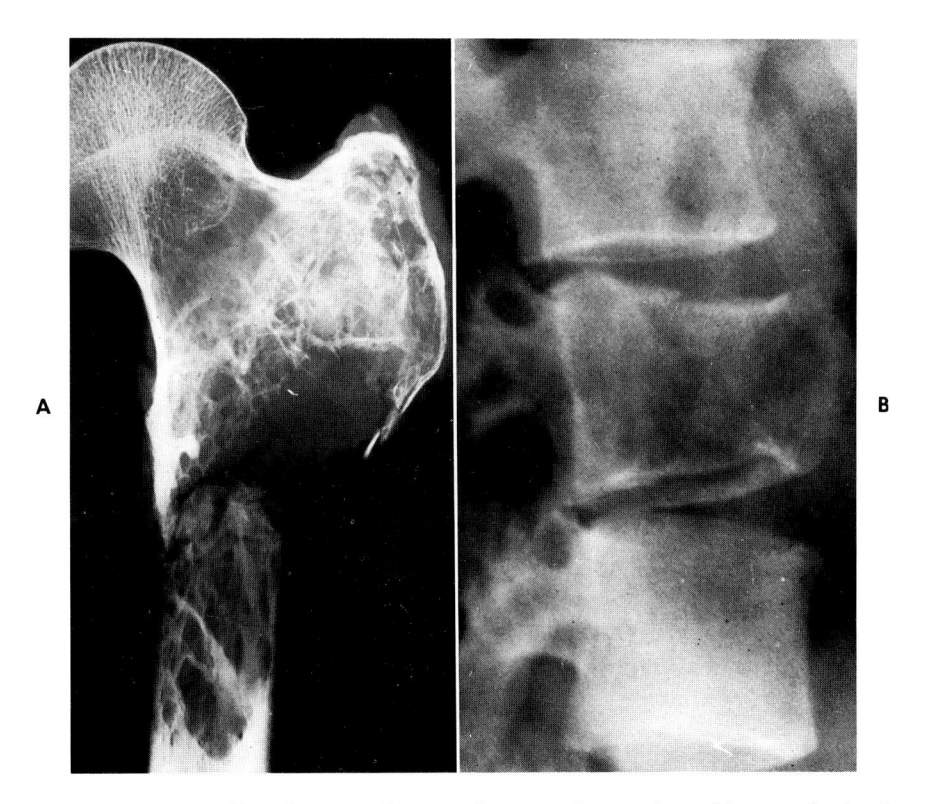

Fig. 19-8. A, An ostensibly solitary myeloma in the upper femur of an old man. The break in continuity reflects a pathologic fracture that followed open biopsy. (Aspiration biopsy often serves to establish a diagnosis in dealing with readily accessible lesions.) Although roentgen survey had revealed no other obvious lesions, microscopic foci of myeloma were found in several other bones sampled at autopsy. This was true also of two other comparable instances (not illustrated) in which the clinical films had shown only a single large myeloma focus, in a sacrum and in an iliac bone, respectively. B, Another, initially solitary, myeloma focus within a third lumbar vertebral body. The lesion was irradiated on the premise that it might represent a giant-cell tumor, and it was not until two and one-half years later that a shower of myelomatous foci appeared throughout the skeleton.

Perla and Hutner,[71] Ehrich,[23] Bell,[8] Fishberg,[26] Forbus and associates,[28] Morison,[60] Blackman and associates,[9] Newns and Edwards,[64] and others. Indeed, Mallory and his colleagues spoke of the "myeloma kidney" and maintained that it is often possible to make a diagnosis of multiple myeloma from observing the kidney sections alone.

On reviewing the sections of kidneys obtained in our own autopsy material, we,[48] too, were impressed by the constant finding of rather dense eosinophilic hyalin-like plugs of proteinaceous material in the renal tubules, particularly in the lower portions of the nephrons. In about half of the kidneys examined, one could find foreign body giant cells or clumps of polymorphonuclear leukocytes, or both, about the casts, although at times one had to search for them (Fig. 19-7, C). In some instances the proteinaceous plugs were rather scattered, but in others they were numerous. It is pertinent in this connection to recall the exceptional case reported by Holman, in which the tubular obstruction was extensive enough to result in complete urinary suppression. It is noteworthy that the characteristic tubular plugs were found by us in cases in which the Bence Jones reaction had been negative as well as in those in which it had been positive. It seems altogether probable that abnormal proteins other than Bence Jones protein are also precipitated out in the tubules. We observed no significant glomerular changes in our material.

Some of the kidneys also exhibited a number of other changes worthy of mention. In some, slight to moderate arteriosclerotic contraction was noted (which must be evaluated in the light of the fact that these subjects were older adults). In several, pyelonephritis was present, having followed on compression of the spinal cord and ascending infection of the urinary tract. In a few, what appeared to be amyloid in granular or droplet form was present within the tubular epithelium and lumens, though not in the glomeruli. In one (in a case of far-advanced myeloma featured by rapidly progressing, extreme demineralization of the skeleton and hypercalcemia, the calcium amounting to almost 18 mg.) evidence of deposition of calcium was observed grossly as well as microscopically. In this kidney (there was also heavy metastatic calcification of the lungs) one could recognize yellowish streaks within some of the pyramids, and fine yellowish calcific gravel was present in many of the calices and within the urinary bladder as well (Fig. 19-7, A and B).

Amyloidosis in relation to multiple myeloma

Another arresting feature of the pathologic anatomy of multiple myeloma is the presence of amyloid in some cases. Atkinson[2] found amyloidosis complicating myeloma in 40 of 643 cases of myeloma collected from the literature. On this basis the incidence is about 6%. In our own material it was about 10%. The immunologic aspects of amyloidosis, about which there has been a good deal of speculation, are still the subject of active investigation.[59]

As far as the skeleton is concerned, if amyloid is found, it usually appears in the form of scattered deposits detectable only microscopically in the neoplastic

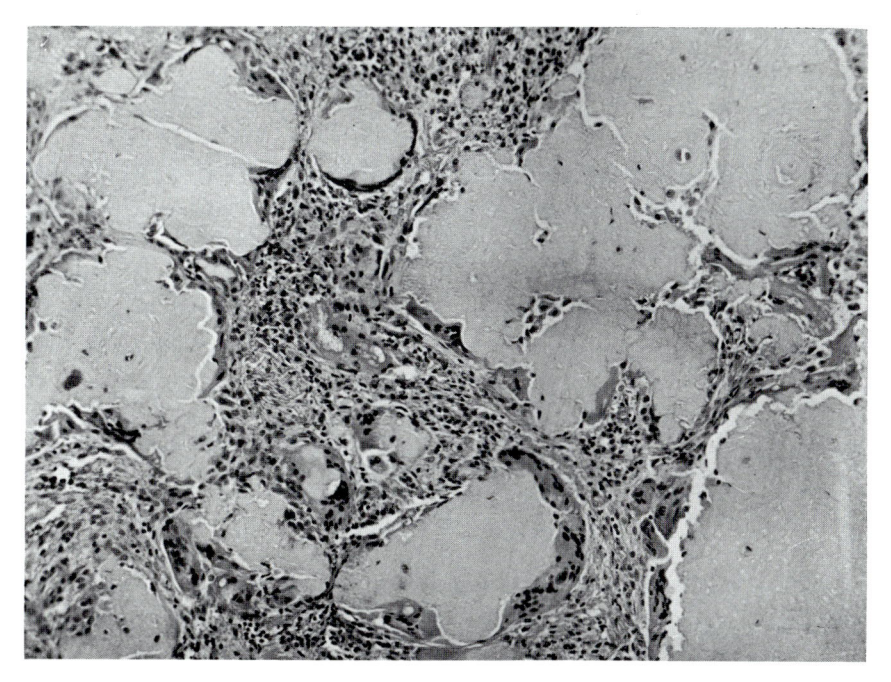

Fig. 19-9. Photomicrograph showing amyloid deposits within a focus of multiple myeloma. The tumor cells in the background cannot be distinguished at this low magnification. (×125.)

tissue of the affected bones. In an occasional case, however, one finds not only the microscopic deposits but large agglomerations of amyloid intermingled with and substantially replacing myelomatous foci. In Freund's case[29] the amyloid took the form of multiple calcifying amyloid tumors, one of which, breaking out of the seventh dorsal vertebral body, had produced extradural compression of the cord. The presence of multiple myeloma as a basis for the amyloid tumors in this case was recognized only on microscopic examination, there having been no grossly discernible tumor nodes within the bones but rather a diffuse infiltration of the marrow. In this case the amyloid was entirely limited to the skeleton. On the other hand, we have observed a case of so-called atypical amyloidosis in which autopsy failed to reveal evidence of amyloid in the myelomatous tissue itself, though practically all the extraskeletal tissues and organs, including the voluntary muscles and the skin, were heavily infiltrated with amyloid.

In general, one of the striking features of amyloidosis appearing in association with multiple myeloma is the frequency with which amyloid is deposited in unusual sites, either more or less diffusely or in the form of tumorlike masses that may attain large bulk. In contrast to the commonplace amyloidosis of parenchymatous organs (particularly the liver, the spleen, the adrenal glands, and the kidneys), one may find amyloid deposited in great quantity in bones, in muscles, in joint capsules and in the skeletal connective tissues generally, in the skin and subcutaneous tissue, in the buccal and anal mucous membranes, in the tongue, in the heart, in the lungs, in the intestines, in the genitourinary tract, and in other tissues. Indeed, so often is multiple myeloma the basis for so-called atypical or idiopathic amyloidosis that the possibility of myeloma should be investigated in every case, even though the bones present no apparent evidence of tumor either roentgenographically or on gross inspection at autopsy.

These cases of unusual amyloidosis are all of great interest, but we may single out certain ones for special comment. In one of our cases involvement of the skin and subcutis led to remarkable scleroderma-like thickening and the occurrence of amyloid-containing verrucae, which were found on the eyelids, about the anus, on the oral mucous membrane, and along the margins of the enlarged, rubbery, ulcerated tongue. Also noteworthy are the cases in which the mucosa or the muscular coat of the small intestine is extensively infiltrated by amyloid, since this deposition may lead at times to clinically puzzling intestinal obstruction. Of particular interest, also, are the cases standing out because of the presence of multiple, smaller or larger, localized amyloid masses attached to the periosteum of the bones, especially near their articulations, and situated also in the skeletal muscles of the trunk and the extremities and about and within joint capsules. In relation to the latter, the amyloid may extend to the synovium and sublining tissue and, at times, even erupt into the joints. Among the regions that may be selected are the hands, the antecubital fossae, the shoulders, and the articulations of the clavicle. The presence of such joint swellings, associated with pain and limitation of motion, sometimes leads to a clinical diagnosis of rheumatoid arthritis, which may be entertained for years before the nature of the condition is recognized. The amyloid masses seen in these cases are described as having a firm, grayish yellow or pinkish, lardaceous or glassy appearance somewhat suggestive of the flesh of fish. Microscopically they present as amorphous, poorly cellular, generally eosinophilic aggregates, about which one may observe foreign body giant cells (Fig. 19-9). It is noteworthy also that this amyloid material, either in part or throughout, may fail to give the usual metachromatic staining reactions with one or another, or perhaps all, of the dyes commonly employed for the detection of amyloid.

Relationship of apparently solitary myeloma and multiple myeloma

As has been stated, there are occasional cases of myeloma in which the first skeletal manifestation is that of an exuberant tumor focus within some one bone (commonly a femur or a humerus, but sometimes a vertebral body, an innominate bone, a bone of the calvarium, or some other bone) and in which clear-cut roentgenographic evidence of implication of other bones does not appear for a number of years (Fig. 19-10, B and C). We have observed a number of such cases, only a few of which will be cited here to highlight the problem in interpretation. In one of them, attention was at first centered on an apparently solitary neoplastic focus in the third lumbar vertebral body. Indeed, this lesion was irradiated as a possible hemangioma or giant-cell tumor. It was not until two and one-

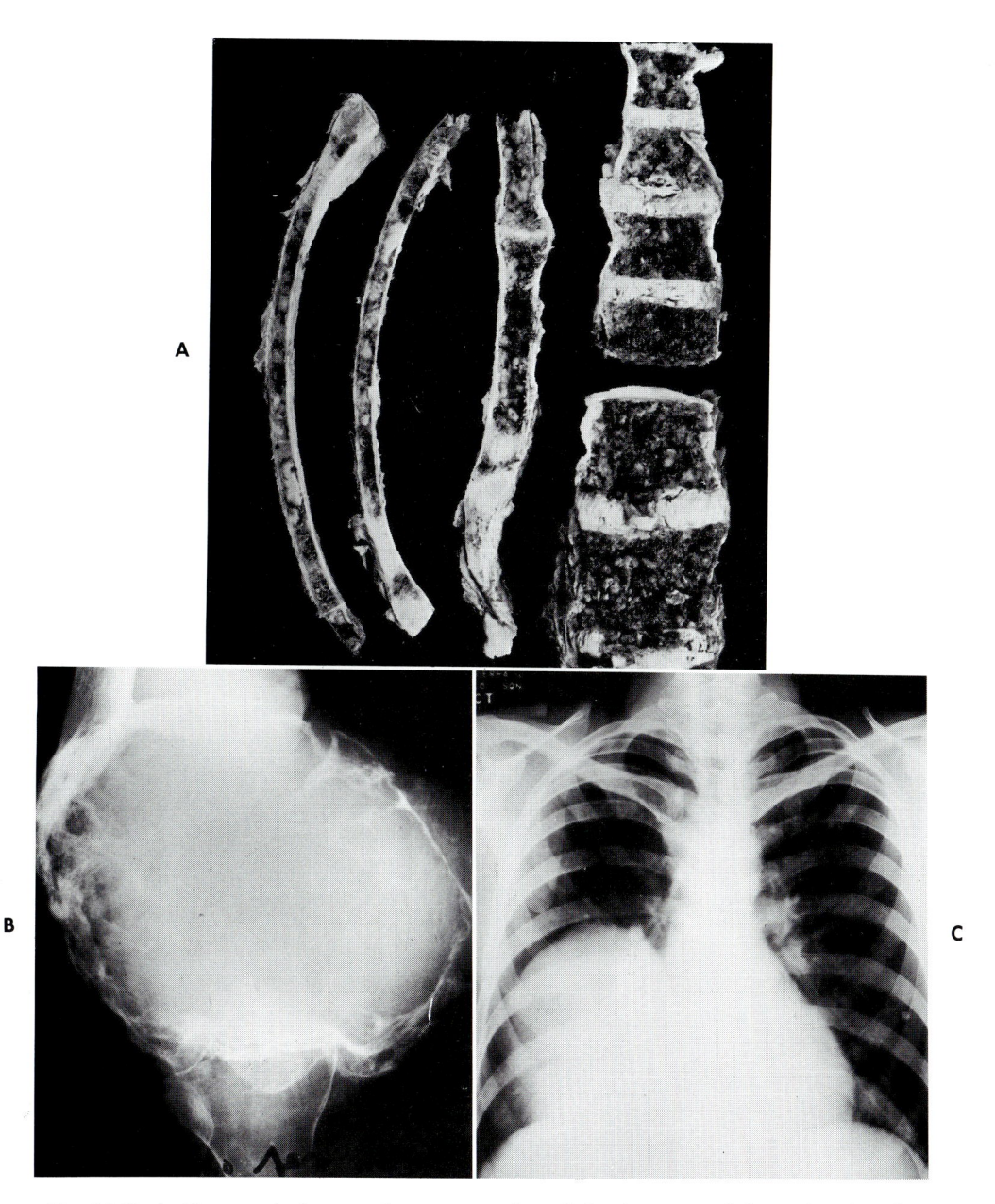

Fig. 19-10. A, Photograph showing the presence of small focal tumor nodules within the ribs, sternum, and vertebral column of an autopsied case of multiple myeloma. It should be borne in mind, however, that there are instances of multiple myeloma in which the infiltration of the bone marrow is diffuse and in which there may be no grossly discernible tumor foci. B and C, Roentgenograms of a remarkably large, ostensibly solitary myeloma that metastasized to the right lung. (Courtesy Drs. Sotelo-Ortiz and Guerra, Hermosillo, Mexico.)

half years after the onset of symptoms that a veritable shower of foci of myeloma appeared throughout the skeleton. In another case the presenting focus (identified by biopsy as a myeloma) was a large tumor apparently localized within the upper end of the right femur. This tumor had transformed the upper part of the shaft, the intertrochanteric region, and the neck into a ballooned-out, rarefied, and coarsely honeycombed lesion simulating a peculiar cyst or giant-cell tumor. Roentgenograms of the pelvis and the upper ends of the femurs (the only roentgenograms taken at the time) showed, otherwise, merely equivocal involvement of the right ilium and suggestive rarefaction shadows within the greater trochanter region of the left femur. This patient received radiation therapy at another hospital, with clinical improvement resulting. The case was subsequently included among those reported by Coley,[16] who likewise interpreted it as one of solitary myeloma. From him we learned that the patient died after a terminal wasting illness suggesting dissemination of tumor, but not until she had survived almost ten years after the onset of complaints referable to the tumor of the femur.

Many comparable cases of supposedly solitary myeloma have been reported, including some with entirely inadequate follow-up records, and have attracted attention because they tended to controvert the usual poor prognosis for myeloma in general. In regard to these initially localized myelomas, it is hardly possible to determine from the available evidence whether the tumor in any given instance was entirely confined to the skeletal focus first attracting attention or whether it was already present elsewhere in the skeleton but clinically and roentgenographically silent. It has been claimed by the advocates of the former view that the negative result of roentgenographic examination of the remainder of the skeleton affords proof of the solitary nature of the myeloma in question. However, it is well known that the marrow throughout the skeleton may be extensively permeated by myeloma without this being evident roentgenographically. Also cited as proof of actual one-bone localization is the absence of anemia and of Bence Jones proteinuria, but these are hardly trustworthy indications. The long period of latency is also cited as evidence, but, as we have seen, there is no certainty, when dealing with such a tumor, that foci of myeloma may not appear throughout the skeleton at any time. Indeed, as such cases are followed, the number of survivors falls off steadily from year to year, so that at the end of a ten-year period of observation few ostensibly solitary myelomas are left.

The foregoing comment is not intended to convey the impression that genuine solitary myeloma or plasmacytoma of bone does not exist. Apparently it does, although the condition is very unusual in relation to the incidence of multiple myeloma. On the basis of meticulously autopsied cases, such as those reported by Harding and Kimball,[35] Rutishauser,[77] and Raven and Willis,[74] one certainly has to concede this. Even more convincing is the survey by Wright[94] of a small group of patients who survived from sixteen to thirty-five years after radical surgery for solitary plasmacytoma.

Cytologic character of multiple myeloma

The tumor tissue in multiple myeloma (when its appearance is not modified by hemorrhage, degeneration and necrosis, fracture of the bone, or extension of the tumor into the soft parts) tends characteristically to be composed of large aggregates or veritable sheets of more or less compacted cells without any discernible intercellular material and without conspicuous supporting stroma. However, where the bone marrow is being invaded by tumor, one observes marrow cells intermingled with tumor cells that, as they proliferate, tend to crowd out and eventually replace the marrow constituents. In selecting material for sectioning, one should choose some blocks of solid tumor tissue (relatively free of secondary changes) that do not require decalcification, since treatment with acid tends to shrink the cells and to darken and obscure nuclear detail. In the matter of staining histologic preparations, eosin-methylene blue seem particularly well suited to bringing out cytologic detail.

It has been recognized and must be emphasized that the cytologic picture is not the same in all specimens of multiple myeloma. Roughly, however, the tumors can be fitted into two general cytologic groups. On the one hand there are those in which the tumor cells are quite uniform, predominantly small, and have a superficial resemblance to plasma cells. The tumor cell is roundish and has a stippled nucleus substantially filling the cell. The darkish chromatin particles spotting the nucleus are dispersed centrally as well as peripherally, and one actually observes nothing resembling a cartwheel in the sense of spokes radiating from a hub. The cytoplasm tends to be uniformly eosinophilic, though in occasional tumors one may observe lighter-staining perinuclear demilunes. Interspersed among these cells there may be some cells that, though of the same general character, are larger in respect to both cytoplasm and nucleus. There may also be occasional cells with double nuclei, but there is no tendency to cellular irregularity otherwise. It is to the myeloma showing this cytologic character that the name "plasma-cell myeloma" or "plasmacytoma" is commonly applied (although these names have come to be rather indiscriminately applied to most myelomas, even to those in which the tumor cells have only the remotest resemblance to plasma cells).

In the other group of myelomas the cytologic picture tends to be dominated by cells larger than those resembling plasma cells, but it may be a rather variegated picture. The dominant cells in the tumor generally exceed the myeloblast in size and, on the whole, show farily abundant cytoplasm and have a large, round, oval, or even reniform, pale stippled nucleus. The latter is not necessarily eccentric and indeed is often centrally placed. In some tumors the nuclei of certain of the cells may contain a well-defined pinkish or reddish round body resembling a nucleolus. The cytoplasm is generally eosinophilic but sometimes takes a more basophilic or polychromatic tinctorial hue, and in some tumors it also presents paler demilunes around the central face of the nucleus. Occasionally the cytoplasm is vacuolated or contains refractile rod-shaped bodies, considered by some to be of protein nature. In any particular tumor site examined, one may also

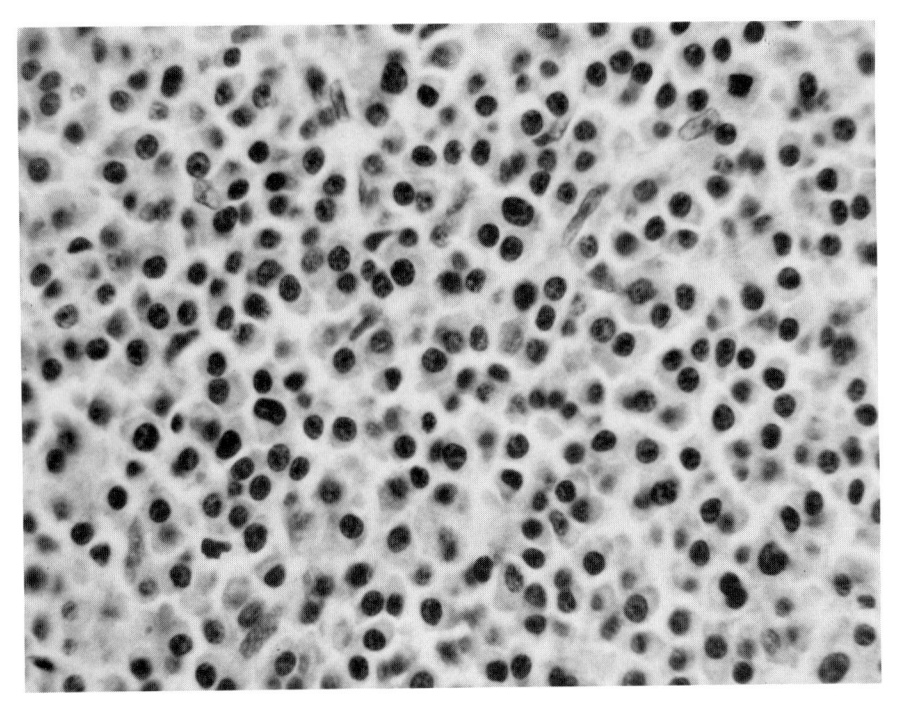

Fig. 19-11. Photomicrograph of tissue obtained by needle aspiration biopsy of a large tumor focus in a sacrum. (This lesion was the only one observed at the time in the clinical x-ray films, although subsequent autopsy revealed additional foci of myeloma in other bones.) (×500.)

find some of the smaller cells resembling plasma cells or, on the other hand, find cells that are much larger than the dominant ones and frequently show nuclear atypism. Specifically, such atypical cells may present large and hyperchromatic nuclei of bizarre shape or two or more nuclei (Fig. 19-12).

It is pertinent at this point to consider whether or not the large and small tumor cells, respectively, represent essentially different types of cells as far as their derivation is concerned. This question may not be of as great practical moment as it would be if, for instance, it had been established that the myelomas of relatively mature histologic appearance respond more favorably to treatment or necessarily pursue a more prolonged course than do the others; it is, however, germane to a better understanding of the nature of the neoplastic process. We are inclined to doubt whether there is any essential difference, save one of maturity, between the large and small tumor cells, since the predominantly large-cell myelomas contain smaller cells in some places, to which it is possible to trace transitions, and the predominantly small-cell myelomas contain occasional large cells. We would emphasize instead the unity of multiple myelomas and explain cytologic variations within them as expressions of their relative maturity or immaturity. This is the concept that has been advocated by Wallgren[90] in particular. One may draw a parallel with malignant lymphomas, among which one observes some composed of relatively small, mature lymphocytic cells, others com-

Plasma-cell myeloma (multiple myeloma) 303

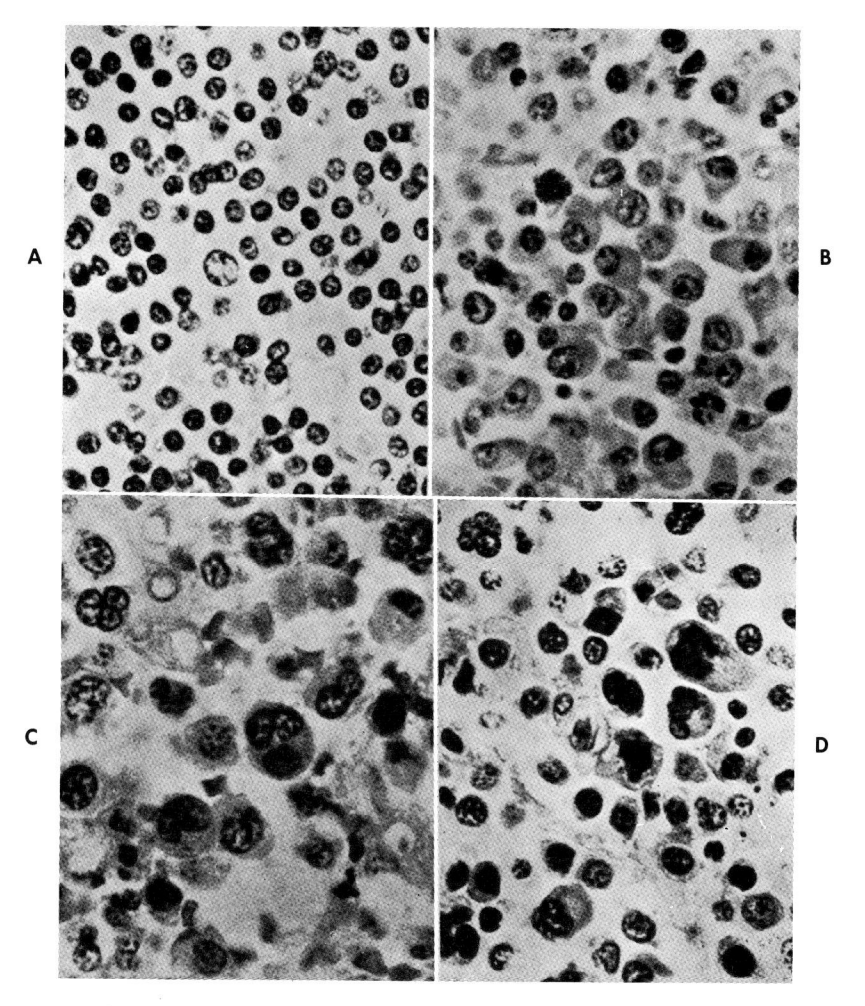

Fig. 19-12. Photomicrographs further illustrating the cytologic appearance of multiple myeloma. **A**, Myeloma composed of predominantly small, uniform tumor cells that have a superficial resemblance to plasma cells. Such tumors are frequently designated as plasma-cell myeloma or plasmacytoma. **B**, Another myeloma whose cytologic pattern is dominated by cells considerably larger than those resembling plasma cells, some of which show mitotic figures. **C** and **D**, Fields from another myeloma whose cytologic picture is also dominated by comparatively large cells although there is a sprinkling of smaller cells with nuclei not unlike those of so-called plasma cells. A number of the tumor cells have two or more nuclei, some of which are markedly hyperchromatic.

posed of somewhat larger, less mature lymphoblastic cells, and still others composed of quite large, immature reticulum cells of more variable appearance, all of them derived from a common lymphoid stem cell.

The identification of the common ancestral cell of multiple myeloma, however, is still a moot point. Some have held that the tumor cells of multiple myeloma are abnormal hematic cells whose origin may be traced to the primitive reticulum cell of the bone marrow, and this theory has much to recommend it.

I have observed material from a number of ostensibly solitary tumors in which one could clearly trace transitions from reticulum cells to myeloma cells, and I designate these provisionally as *reticulomyelomas* to direct attention to them. Others have been impressed in certain cases by the alleged resemblance of the tumor cells to myeloblasts or myelocytes, to lymphoblasts or lymphocytes, to erythroblasts, to mature or immature marrow plasma cells, to megakaryoblasts, or to hemocytoblasts.

Be that as it may, it should be emphasized that multiple myeloma presents a characteristic clinicoanatomic picture, centered around the skeletal manifestations of the disease and their sequelae, and that, with rare exceptions, this picture is readily distinguishable from that presented by any of the other neoplasms of hemopoietic derivation. So distinctive is multiple myeloma as a single and basically uniform disease complex that one is at a loss to understand why in some quarters it has been subclassified, presumably on the basis of cell type, into plasma-cell, myeloid, erythroid, and lymphoid myeloma. Indeed, there can be little doubt that multiple myeloma as discussed in this chapter is a disease of unitary cell type, the variations in cytologic appearance reflecting stages in the maturation of the basic tumor cell. Specifically, regarding the histogenesis of multiple myeloma, we are inclined to hold with Wallgren,[90] Wood and Lucké,[93] Wintrobe,[91] and others that this neoplasm consists of distinctive tumor cells that are probably of myeloid formative or hematic origin (though not clearly resembling any normal marrow cells or their immediate precursors) and are best designated noncommittally as myeloma cells.

Cognizance must also be taken of the idea stemming from both von Rustizky[85] and Lubarsch[54] that multiple myeloma represents a systematized disease of the hemopoietic apparatus and, as such, is not a true neoplasm but rather a hyperplasia related to the "leukemias." There can be no serious objection to holding that multiple myeloma is akin to chronic myelosis and malignant lymphoma in the sense that it, too, belongs to the general family of neoplasms of hematic origin, although, as has already been indicated, it presents definite clinicoanatomic characteristics that sharply delimit it from these diseases. However, it is difficult to understand, even on theoretic grounds, how multiple myeloma can be regarded as anything but a malignant neoplasm in the face of widespread formation of tumors within the skeleton, the tendency toward perforation of the cortices of affected bones and extension into the adjacent soft parts, the capacity of its cells to invade the bloodstream and to metastasize to the viscera generally in addition to involving the hemopoietic organs, and the consistent trend toward a fatal termination.

Treatment

Problems in therapy are concerned mainly with palliation, particularly the relief of distressing bone pain, general supportive measures, and the handling of such complications as fractures and compression of the spinal cord. In regard to general supportive measures, the use of repeated transfusions to combat anemia when this is present and the avoidance of prolonged bed care should be emphasized. The consensus of radiotherapists seems to be that roentgen therapy, if judiciously employed, frequently, though not invariably, has value in palliation but that it has relatively little influence otherwise on the course of the disease, except possibly when one is dealing with what appears to be a solitary myeloma.

Over the years a succession of chemotherapeutic agents has been used for multiple myeloma, including stilbamidine, pentamidine, urethane, and others that have fallen by the wayside because of undesirable side effects or because their long-range results did not engender any great enthusiasm. This seems to apply also to the use of radioactive phosphorus and of steroids. The agent currently favored is melphalan (phenylalanine mustard, Alkeran) administered either intermittently[38] or on a sustained maintenance basis,[87] although the development of leukopenia and thrombocytopenia may be a limiting factor. It is said to bring about clinical improvement and to prolong life.[38] Cyclophosphamide (Cytoxan), another orally administered analogue of nitrogen mustard, has also been given extensive clinical trial.[18] Some investigators feel that the addition of prednisone to the alkylating agent enhances its beneficial effect, and the adjuvant use of fluoride also has its advocates.[49]

Aside from treatment of fractures, especially those of long bones, surgical intervention has a place in the relief of transverse myelitis resulting from extradural compression, which is accomplished by laminectomy. In regard to the latter, Jacox and Kahn,[40] and Batts[4] have shown that this procedure, if followed by roentgen therapy, may permit complete recovery of function and even survival thereafter for a number of years. They emphasized that laminectomy should always be done before roentgen therapy is given, in order to prevent further damage to the cord by swelling subsequent to irradiation. Also, the question of ablation of a limb for myeloma sometimes arises, but only in connection with the comparatively rare, ostensibly solitary myeloma of a long bone. In cases of this type, as noted, one can never be certain that tumor is not present in other bones in spite of their negative roentgenographic appearance. It is pertinent, however, to recall the remarkable cases of long-term survival after radical surgery cited by Wright,[94] and in particular the case reported by Stewart and Taylor,[81] in which the patient was alive and well at follow-up thirty-five years later. In this instance, forequarter amputation was done for a huge myeloma that had largely destroyed the upper third of the shaft of a humerus and was freely invading the muscles of the upper arm.

Summary

Multiple myeloma represents a clinically and pathologically distinctive malignant disease of the skeleton primarily, which apparently takes its departure from the hematic cells in the bone marrow and occasionally in other extraskeletal sites. Anatomically, practically every bone may ultimately come to be involved more or less in a given case. The skeletal progress of the disease may be steady and rapid, sometimes from the beginning and sometimes after a static period. In some cases, also, before the disease becomes spread over the skeleton, it may flourish in one bone (as a so-called solitary myeloma) for months or even years. Though at autopsy the skeleton may be found riddled through with foci of myeloma, it is only infrequently that gross foci are found in the viscera and other extraskeletal parts. Nevertheless, even in the absence of gross infiltrations, microscopic examination sometimes reveals smaller or larger numbers of myeloma cells within the spleen, the liver, or lymph nodes, and occasionally in other organs as well. Also, in some cases, myeloma cells may invade the bloodstream. Ordinarily, under these circumstances, relatively few myeloma cells are found in the blood smears, but in an occasional case they may be so numerous as to create a leukemic blood picture (so-called plasma-cell leukemia).

Although there are these points of resemblance to other neoplasms of hematic origin, it should be emphasized that multiple myeloma presents a characteristic clinicoanatomic picture centered around the skeletal manifestations of the disease and their sequelae, and that with rare exceptions this picture is readily distinguishable from that presented by any of the other neoplasms of hemopoietic derivation. Differentiation from macroglobulinemia (Waldenstrom) may require untracentrifugation as well as serum electrophoresis. In this connection we have stressed the diagnostic significance of hypercalcemia, hyperglobulinemia (and its associated hematologic manifestations) and Bence Jones proteinuria, the not infrequent presence of atypical amyloidosis in association with myeloma, and the well-known cytologic renal changes of almost pathognomonic distinctiveness. The latter results commonly in more or less heavy albuminuria and often in renal insufficiency of a peculiar type. In regard to amyloidosis it was indicated that multiple myeloma is so often the basis for atypical amyloid deposits that the possibility of myeloma should be investigated in every case of idiopathic amyloidosis, even though the bones present no evidence of tumor either roentgenographically or on gross inspection at autopsy.

The tumor tissue in multiple myeloma tends characteristically to be composed of large aggregates of more or less compacted cells without any discernible intercellular material and without conspicuous supporting stroma. It has been recognized and must be emphasized that the cytologic picture is not the same in all specimens of multiple myeloma. Roughly, however, the tumors can be fitted into two general cytologic groups. On the one hand there are those in which the tumor cells are quite uniform and predominantly small and have a superficial resemblance to plasma cells. It is to the myeloma showing this cytologic appearance that the name "plasma-cell myeloma" or "plasmacytoma" is commonly applied. In the other group of myelomas the cytologic picture tends to be dominated by cells larger than those resembling plasma cells, but may be a rather variegated one. The dominant cell shows fairly abundant cytoplasm and has a large, round, oval, or even reniform, pale stippled nucleus. In any particular tumor site examined, one may also find some of the smaller cells resembling plasma cells, or, on the other hand, one may find cells that are much larger than the dominant ones and frequently show nuclear atypism. Specifically, such atypical cells may present large and hyperchromatic nuclei, giant nuclei of bizarre shape, or two or more nuclei.

We are inclined to doubt whether there is any essential difference, save one of maturity, between the large and the small tumor cells. So distinctive is multiple myeloma as a single and basically uniform disease complex that one is at a loss to understand why in the past it was subclassified, presumably on the basis of cell type, into plasma-cell, myeloid, erythroid, and lymphoid myeloma. Indeed, there seems to be little doubt that multiple myeloma as discussed here is a disease of unitary cell type, the cytologic variations reflecting stages in the maturation of the basic tumor cell. Specifically, regarding the histogenesis of multiple myeloma, we are inclined to hold with Wallgren and others that this neoplasm consists of distinctive tumor cells that are probably of myeloid-formative or hematic origin (though not clearly resembling any normal marrow cells or their immediate precursors) and are best designated noncommittally as myeloma cells.

On the clinical side, in our cases of multiple myeloma, we found that the great majority of the patients were between 40 and 60 years of age, though some were in their thirties, and one was only 13 years old when the first manifestations of the disease appeared. Our data indicate that multiple myeloma may be more prevalent in males than in females, but do not support the often repeated statement that the condition is at least twice as frequent in males. In regard to the roentgenographic findings, we found that the picture conventionally held to distinguish multiple myeloma—that of many bones, including the calvarium, riddled by clear-cut punched-out osteolytic defects—represents the exception rather than the rule and applies only to certain cases in which the disease is far advanced. Indeed, very often one observes merely some vaguely defined rarefactions in a number of the bones or a single exuberant tumor focus in some one bone (commonly a femur or a humerus, but sometimes a vertebral body, a rib, or a clavicle, an innominate bone, a bone of the calvarium, or some other bone) without obvious involvement of the skeleton generally. Sometimes (when myelomatous infiltration of the marrow is diffuse) skeletal changes may not be apparent at all roentgenographically, or the replacement of the marrow by tumor may be reflected merely by some osteoporosis. As for the calvarium, this not infrequently fails to show numerous punched-out rarefactions, even when roentgenograms show clear-cut and widespread involvement of the rest of the skeleton. In such equivocal or initially obscure cases, one must utilize fully all the available diagnostic clues to arrive at a combination of significant findings constituting probable or conclusive evidence of the presence of multiple myeloma. Marrow obtained by sternal puncture is often of great value in establishing the diagnosis, as is electrophoretic study of the serum proteins.

Multiple myeloma has too variable a clinical course to permit any dogmatic statement in regard to prognosis. It is true that the average length of survival after the onset of symptoms is not likely to be more than about two years. However, there are occasional patients with multiple myeloma, particularly those in whom the disease was apparently localized at the outset, whose course may be protracted over a number of years, sometimes as long as ten years or more.

Problems in therapy are concerned mainly with palliation, particularly the relief of distressing bone pain, and general supportive measures, together with the handling of such complications as fractures of bones and compression of the spinal cord. Chemotherapy for disseminated myeloma, employing alkylating agents combined with steroids and possibly other adjuvants, is held to be of distinct value.

References

1. Dixon, F. J., Jr., and Kunkel, H. G., editors: Advances in immunology, New York, 1967, Academic Press, Inc., vol 7 (see chaps. 1 and 2).
2. Atkinson, F. R. B.: Multiple myelomata, Med. Press 195:312, 327, 1937.
3. Bailey, C. O.: Am. J. Roentgenol. 36:980, 1936.
4. Batts, M., Jr.: Multiple myeloma, Arch. Surg. 39:807, 1939.
5. Bayne-Jones, S., and Wilson, D. W.: Immunological reactions of Bence-Jones proteins, Bull. Johns Hopkins Hosp. 33:37, 1922.
6. Bayrd, E. D., and Heck, F. J.: Multiple myeloma, J.A.M.A. 133:147, 1947.
7. Bezier, L. H., Hall, B. E., and Giffin, H. Z.: Am. J. Med. Sci. 203:829, 1942.
8. Bell, E. T.: Renal lesions associated with multiple myeloma, Am. J. Pathol. 9:393, 1933.
9. Blackman, S. S., Jr., Barker, W. H., Buell, M. V., and Davis, B. D.: On pathogenesis of renal failure associated with multiple myeloma, J. Clin. Invest. 23:163, 1944.
10. Boggs, T. R., and Guthrie, C. G.: Bull. Johns Hopkins Hosp. 23:353, 1912.
11. Bulger, A. A., Dixon, H. H., Barr, D. P., and Schregardus, O.: J. Clin. Invest. 19:1143, 1930.
12. Carlisle, V.: Myelomatosis with visceral metastasis in native of Southern Rhodesia, S. Afr. Med. J. 12:298, 1938.
13. Carson, C. P., Ackerman, L. V., and Maltby, J. D.: Plasma cell myeloma. A clinical, pathologic, and roentgenologic review of 90 cases, Am. J. Clin. Pathol. 25:849, 1955.
14. Christopherson, W. M., and Miller, A. J.: A re-evaluation of solitary plasma-cell myeloma of bone, Cancer 3:240, 1950.
15. Churg, J., and Gordon, A. J.: Multiple myeloma with unusual visceral involvement, Arch. Pathol. 34:546, 1942.
16. Coley, W. B.: Multiple myeloma, Ann. Surg. 93:77, 1931.
17. Craddock, C. G., Jr., Adams, W. S., and Figueroa, W. G.: Interference with fibrin formation in multiple myeloma by an unusual protein found in blood and urine, J. Lab. Clin. Med. 42:847, 1953.
18. Craver, L. F., and Miller, D. G.: Multiple myeloma, Ca 16:142, 1966.
19. Davison, C., and Balser, B. H.: Myeloma and its neural complications, Arch. Surg. 35:913, 935, 1937.
20. Devine, J.: Analysis of Bence-Jones protein, Biochem. J. 35:433, 1941.
21. Donhauser, J. L., and de Rouville, W. H.: Multiple myeloma, with special reference to soft tissue metastasis, Arch. Surg. 43:946, 1941.
22. Duvoir, M., Pollet, L., Layani, F., Dechaune, M., and Gaultier, M.: Myélomes multiples avec tumeurs cutanées, Bull. Mém. Soc. Méd. Paris 54:687, 1938.
23. Ehrich, W.: Die Nierenerkrankung bei Bence-Jonesscher Proteinurie, Z. Klin. Med. 121:396, 1932.
24. Ellinger, A.: Dtsch. Arch. Klin. Med. 62:254, 1899.
25. Fahey, J. L.: Antibodies and immunoglobulins. Normal development and changes in diseases, J.A.M.A. 194:255, 1965.
26. Fishberg, A. M.: Hypertension and nephritis, ed. 4, Philadelphia, 1939, Lea & Febiger, p. 369.
27. Foord, A. G.: Hyperproteinemia, autohemagglutination, renal insufficiency and abnormal bleeding in multiple myeloma, Ann. Intern. Med. 8:1071, 1935.
    Foord, A. G., and Randall, L.: Hyperproteinemia, autohemagglutination and renal insufficiency in multiple myeloma, Am. J. Clin. Pathol. 5:532, 1935.
28. Forbus, W. D., Perlzweig, W. A., Parfentjev, I. A., and Burwell, J. C., Jr.: Bence-Jones protein excretion and its effect

upon kidney, Bull. Johns Hopkins Hosp. **57**:47, 1935.
29. Freund, E.: Über diffuses Myelom mit Amyloidtumoren, Frankfurt. Z. Pathol. **40**: 400, 1930.
30. Geschickter, C. F., and Copeland, M. M.: Multiple myeloma, Arch. Surg. **16**:807, 1928.
31. Gordon, A. J., and Churg, J.: Visceral involvement in multiple myeloma, N. Y. State J. Med. **49**:282, 1949.
32. Gross, R. E., and Vaughan, W. W.: Plasma cell myeloma, Am. J. Roentgenol. **39**:344, 1938.
33. Gutman, A. B., Moore, D. H., Gutman, E. B., McClellan, V., and Kabat, E. A.: Fractionation of serum proteins in hyperproteinemia, with special reference to multiple myeloma, J. Clin. Invest. **20**:765, 1941.
Moore, D. H., Kabat, E. A., and Gutman, A. B.: Bence-Jones proteinemia in multiple myeloma, J. Clin. Invest. **22**:67, 1943.
34. Hallermann, W.: Zur Kenntnis des primären multiplen Myeloms, Dtsch. Arch. Klin. Med. **165**:57, 1929.
35. Harding, W. G., Jr., and Kimball, T. S.: Solitary myeloma (plasmacytoma) of femur, Am. J. Cancer **16**:1184, 1932.
36. Hektoen, L.: Specific precipitin for Bence-Jones protein, J.A.M.A. **76**:929, 1921.
37. Herrick, J. B., and Hektoen, L.: Med. News **65**:239, 1894.
38. Hoogstraten, B., Costa, J., Cuttner, J., Forcier, J., Leone, L. A., Harley, J. B., and Glidewell, O. J.: Intermittent melphalan therapy in multiple myeloma, J.A.M.A. **209**:251, 1969.
39. Jackson, H., Jr., Parker, F., Jr., and Bethea, J. M.: Am. J. Med. Sci. **181**:169, 1931.
40. Jacox, H. W., and Kahn, E. A.: Multiple myeloma with spinal cord involvement, Am. J. Roentgenol. **30**:201, 1933.
41. Jaffe, H. L.: Hyperparathyroidism, Bull. N. Y. Acad. Med. **16**:291, 1940.
42. Johnson, L. C., and Meador, G. E.: The nature of benign "solitary myeloma" of bone, Bull. Hosp. Joint Dis. **12**:298, 1951.
43. Kekwick, R. A.: Serum proteins in multiple myelomatosis, Biochem. J. **34**:1248, 1940.
44. Kin, S. S.: Beitrag zur Kenntnis der Kahlerschen Krankheit mit Mycosis fungoides, besenders über die Genese der Geschwulstzellen, Arch. Jap. Chir. **16**:79, 1939.
45. Kirsch, I. E.: Plasma-cell myeloma of bone of over 12 years' duration, Med. Bull. Vet. Admin. **18**:96, 1941.
46. Lawrence, J. H., and Wasserman, L. R.: Multiple myeloma: study of 24 patients treated with radioactive isotopes (P^{32} and Sr^{89}), Ann. Intern. Med. **33**:41, 1950.
47. Lewis, L. A., and Page, I. H.: Serum proteins and lipoproteins in multiple myelomatosis, Am. J. Med. **17**:670, 1954.
48. Lichtenstein, L., and Jaffe, H. L.: Multiple myeloma. A survey based on thirty-five cases, eighteen of which came to autopsy, Arch. Pathol. **44**:207, 1947.
49. Little, J. R., and Loeb, V., Jr.: Immunoglobulin abnormalities and current status of treatment of multiple myeloma, J.A.M.A. **208**:1688, 1969.
50. Loge, J. P., and Rundles, R. W.: Urethane (ethyl carbamate) therapy in multiple myeloma, Blood **4**:201, 1949.
51. Löhlein, M.: Beitr. Pathol. **69**:295, 1921.
52. Lowbeer, L.: Occurrence of osteosclerosis in multiple myeloma, Lab. Med., Bull. Pathol. **10**:396, 1969.
53. Lowenhaupt, E.: Proliferative lesions in multiple myeloma, with special reference to those of spleen, Am. J. Pathol. **21**:171, 1945.
54. Lubarsch, O.: Virchows Arch. **184**:213, 1906.
55. Magnus-Levy, A.: Multiple myeloma, Z. Klin. Med. **126**:62, 1933.
56. Mallory, T. B.: N. Engl. J. Med. **215**:1133, 1936.
57. Mallory, T. B.: N. Engl. J. Med. **221**:983, 1939.
58. Mallory, T. B.: Medical progress; pathology, N. Engl. J. Med. **224**:559, 1941.
59. Mandema, A., Ruinen, L., Scholten, J. H., and Cohen, A. S., editors: Amyloidosis, Excerpta Medica Monograph, The Netherlands, 1969.
60. Morison, J. E.: Obstruction of renal tubules in myelomatosis and in crush injuries, J. Path. Bact. **53**:403, 1941.
61. Morissette, L., and Watkins, C. H.: Multiple myeloma, Proc. Staff Meet., Mayo Clin. **17**:433, 1942.
62. Morse, P. F.: J. Cancer Res. **5**:345, 1920.
63. Muller, G. L., and McNaughton, E.: Multiple myeloma (plasmacytomata) with blood picture of plasma cell leukemia, Folia Haematol. **46**:17, 1931.
64. Newns, G. R., and Edwards, J. L.: Case of plasma-cell myelomatosis with large renal metastasis and widespread renal tubular obstruction, J. Path. Bact. **56**:259, 1944.
65. Osgood, E. E., and Hunter, W. C.: Plasma cell leukemia, Folia Haematol. **52**:369, 1934.
66. Osserman, E. F.: Plasma-cell myeloma. II.

Clinical aspects, N. Engl. J. Med. 261:952, 1006, 1959.
67. Osserman, E. F., and Lawlor, D. P.: Abnormal serum and urine proteins in 35 cases of multiple myeloma, as studied by filter paper electrophoresis, Am. J. Med. 18:402, 1955.
68. Osserman, E. F., and Takatsui, K.: Plasma cell myeloma: gamma globulin synthesis and structure. A review of biochemical and clinical data, with the description of a newly-recognized and related syndrome, "H-Gamma-2Chain (Franklin's) disease," Medicine 42:385, 1963.
69. Pasternack, J. G., and Waugh, R. L.: Solitary myeloma of bone, Ann. Surg. 110:427, 1939.
70. Patek, A. J., and Castle, W. B.: Plasma cell leukemia, Am. J. Med. Sci. 191:788, 1936.
71. Perla, D., and Hutner, L.: Nephrosis in multiple myeloma, Am. J. Pathol. 6:285, 1930.
72. Piney, A., and Riach, J. S.: Multiple myeloma, Folia Haematol. 46:37, 1931.
73. Putnam, F. W.: Plasma cell myeloma and macroglobulinemia. I. Physiochemical, immunochemical, and isotopic turnover studies of the abnormal serum and urinary proteins, N. Engl. J. Med. 261:902, 1959.
74. Raven, R. W., and Willis, R. A.: Solitary plasmocytoma of spine, J. Bone Joint Surg. 31-B:369, 1949.
75. Reinhard, E. H., Moore, C. V., Bierbaum, O. S., and Moore, S.: Radioactive phosphorus as therapeutic agent, J. Lab. Clin. Med. 31:107, 1946.
76. Rosenthal, N., and Vogel, P.: Value of sternal puncture in diagnosis of multiple myeloma, J. Mt. Sinai Hosp. 4:1001, 1938.
77. Rutishauser, E.: Zur Frage der solitären Myelome, Centralbl. allg. Path. u. path. Anat. 58:355, 1933.
78. Shapiro, S., Ross, V., and Moore, D. H.: Viscous protein obtained in large amount from serum of patient with multiple myeloma, J. Clin. Invest. 22:137, 1943.
79. Snapper, I.: Stilbamidine and pentamidine in multiple myeloma, J.A.M.A. 133:157, 1947.
80. Stewart, A., and Weber, F. P.: Quart. J. Med. 7:211, 1938.
81. Stewart, M. J., and Taylor, A. L.: Observations on solitary plasmacytoma, J. Path. Bact. 35:541, 1932.
82. Tarr, L., and Ferris, H. W.: Multiple myeloma associated with nodular deposits of amyloid in muscles and joints and with Bence Jones proteinuria, Arch. Intern. Med. 64:820, 1939.
83. Ulrich, H.: Multiple myeloma, Arch. Intern. Med. 64:994, 1939.
84. Von Bonsdorf, B., Groth, H., and Packalen, T.: On presence of high-molecular crystallizable protein in blood serum in myeloma, Folia Haematol. 59:184, 1938.
85. Von Rustizky, J.: Deutsch. Z. Chir. 3:162, 1873.
86. Waldenstrom, J.: Acta Chir. Scand. 87:365, 1942.
87. Waldenstrom, J.: Diagnosis and treatment of multiple myeloma, New York, 1970, Grune & Stratton, Inc.
88. Waldenstrom, J.: The incidence and cytology of different myeloma types, Lancet 1:1147, 1961.
89. Waldenstrom, J.: Studies on conditions associated with disturbed gamma globulin formation (gammopathies), Harvey Lectures, Series 56:211, 1961.
90. Wallgren, A.: Untersuchungen über die Myelomkrankheit, Uppsala, 1920, Almquist & Wiksells; Baltimore, William Wood & Co.
91. Wintrobe, M. M.: Clinical hematology, Philadelphia, 1961, Lea & Febiger, p. 1069.
92. Wintrobe, M. M., and Buell, M. V.: Hyperproteinemia associated with multiple myeloma, Bull. Johns Hopkins Hosp. 52:156, 1933.
93. Wood, A. C., and Lucké, B.: Multiple myeloma of plasma-cell type, Ann. Surg. 78:14, 1923.
94. Wright, C. J. E.: Long survival in solitary plasmacytoma of bone, J. Bone Joint Surg. 43-B:767, 1961.

Chapter 20

Skeletal manifestations of other tumors of hematopoietic origin

In this rather concise consideration of a complex subject, the emphasis, as noted, is placed entirely upon skeletal manifestations in keeping with the scope of this text. For a comprehensive discussion of the leukemias, both acute and chronic, and of the various expressions of malignant lymphoma in their broader aspects, the reader is referred to the standard hematology texts of Wintrobe and others and to selected reviews dealing with these subjects.

Chronic myeloid leukemia

It is well known that in chronic myeloid leukemia (chronic myelogenous leukemia, chronic myelocytic leukemia, chronic myelosis) the bone marrow throughout the skeleton is regularly and more or less extensively replaced, as one might expect, by proliferating cells of the myeloid series. However, there may be no symptoms directly referable to this skeletal involvement, except for the finding in many cases of localized tenderness (elicited by pressure) over the sternum, a clinical sign emphasized by Craver[7] as being of some diagnostic value. Roentgenographically also, one fails as a rule to detect any discernible evidence of diffuse marrow infiltration. This is true even of roentgenograms of autopsy specimens, of the vertebral column for instance, which afford optimum clarity of detail (Fig. 20-1). On gross inspection of such specimens, a uniform grayish coloration of the marrow is generally the only significant alteration noted. It should be noted however, as Snapper[31] has emphasized, that in rare instances of the disease one may observe the formation of smaller or larger, discrete localized tumor nodes within one or more affected bones, e.g., the ribs, the vertebrae, a femur, or an innominate bone, as the case may be.[8,31,35] Also, occasionally patients with chronic granulocytic leukemia (about 3%) may develop destructive bone lesions as an early manifestation of blastic transformation to a phase resembling acute leukemia.[4]

It may be relevant here to comment briefly upon the occasional finding of diffuse osteosclerosis and myelofibrosis in association with splenomegaly and a blood picture simulating that of myeloid leukemia. It was formerly held that the

312 Bone tumors

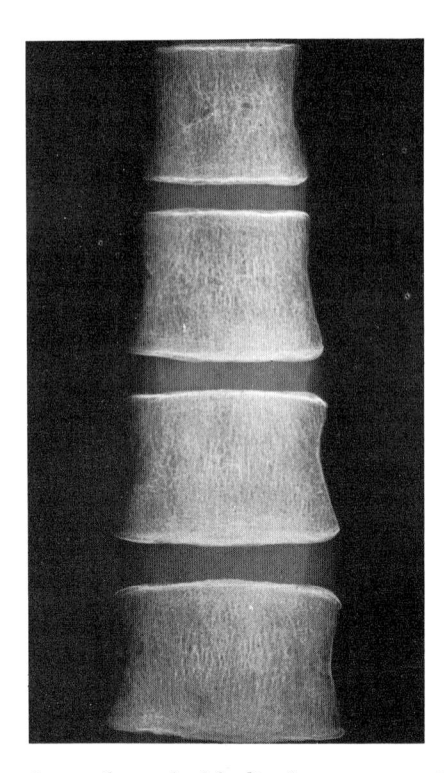

Fig. 20-1. Roentgenogram of several vertebral bodies from an autopsied case of chronic myeloid leukemia. The roentgenogram shows no discernible alteration, even though the marrow everywhere is diffusely infiltrated.

skeletal changes indicated might represent a burned-out end stage of a true leukemia. However, in subsequent papers[3,16,17,28] dealing with such cases, this view was challenged, and the prevailing interpretation is rather that of a primary or idiopathic osteosclerosis and marrow fibrosis leading to myeloid exhaustion, extensive compensatory extramedullary hemopoiesis in the lymph nodes, liver, and spleen (so-called agnogenic myeloid metaplasia), and the concomitant appearance of immature leukocytes and erythrocytes in the peripheral blood.

Acute leukemias

In the acute leukemias (which may be of lymphoblastic, myeloblastic, monocytic, or more undifferentiated "stem-cell" type), the clinical and especially roentgenographic manifestations of skeletal involvement take on diagnostic importance and are commonly observed, particularly in infants and children. This is rather what one might expect in dealing with a group of relatively aggressive and rapidly progressive or even fulminant, hematic neoplasms. In such cases, osseous involvement is frequently manifested clinically in bone pain and tenderness, limitation of motion, and ostensible arthritic symptoms attributable to juxta-articular leukemic infiltration. Before the presence of leukemia is recognized, these skeletal manifestations, considered in association with anemia and fever,

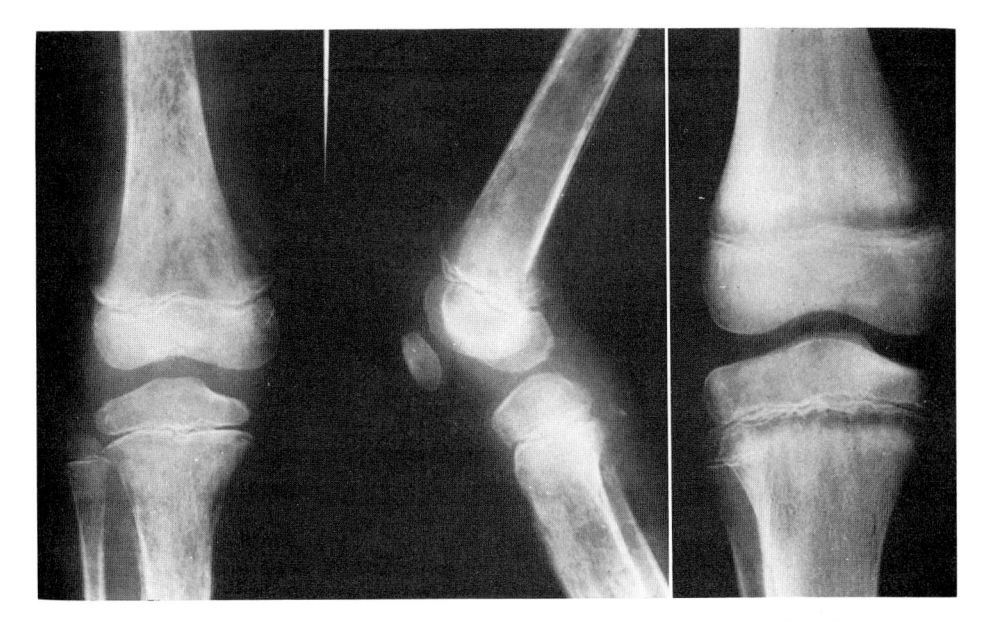

Fig. 20-2. Roentgenograms reflecting skeletal changes of acute leukemia in a child.
Fig. 20-3. Early skeletal changes in leukemia in a child. Note irregular rarefaction zones adjacent to epiphyseal cartilage plates (suggestive of the diagnosis, though not pathognomonic).

may plausibly suggest osteomyelitis, brucellosis, sepsis, rheumatic fever, or Still's disease, as the case may be. On roentgen skeletal survey, if attention is not focused altogether upon a single region, distinctive changes may be observed in a significantly large number of cases in the long bones, the pelvis, the vertebral column, the calvarium, and even the hand bones. These roentgenographic findings have been discussed at length by Silverman[30] and Kalayjian, Herbut, and Erf,[18] among others. Specifically one may observe multiple, ill-defined or more clearly punched-out areas of rarefaction in affected bones, for example in the shafts of long bones, where the spongiosa or corticalis has been focally destroyed. In some instances, these osteolytic lesions may be found in association with concomitant, focal, or more diffuse reactive osteosclerosis. In relation to these osseous defects also, there is often discernible periosteal new bone apposition ("onion-peel" effect), developing as a reaction to penetration of the cortex by leukemic cells. Among the other significant changes that have been described in acute leukemia are the presence of juxtaepiphyseal transverse radiolucent bands, pathologic fractures and dislocations, compression of one or more vertebral bodies, and partial destruction of epiphyses, especially collapse of a capital femoral epiphysis (Figs. 20-2 and 20-3).

Specific mention should also be made of the striking skeletal changes observed in chloroma (an unusual aggressive form of acute or subacute leukemia occurring particularly though not exclusively in children), in which the tumor deposits present an evanescent greenish coloration said to be due to protoporphyrin. In chloroma, one may encounter not only conspicuous periosteal new bone formation, but also sizable subperiosteal and parosteal tumor masses developing in relation to the vertebral column, ribs, calvarium, and other bones. In the skull particularly, there may be extension into the base of the cranial vault, the paranasal sinuses, and especially the orbits, giving rise to proptosis and conspicuous tumorous protrusions, comparable to those sometimes observed in children with disseminated neuroblastoma.[19,20] I have observed material from a pertinent case in an adult in whom the clinical picture was at first dominated by signs of optic nerve impairment (shown eventually to have resulted from aggressive infiltration at the base of the brain by chloroma). It was not until some months had elapsed that hematologic examination including sternal marrow puncture revealed the presence of myeloblastic leukemia (Fig. 20-4).

As has already been indicated, plasma-cell leukemia, so-called, seems clearly to represent a leukemic phase, often a terminal one, of multiple myeloma. As such, the pathologic changes associated with it have been discussed under the head of multiple myeloma (Chapter 19).

Mention should also be made of mastocytosis characterized by mast-cell hyperplasia in the skin (urticaria pigmentosa, clinically) and also systemically in the spleen, liver, lymph nodes, bone marrow, and other reticulum-bearing organs. In some instances, mast-cell foci in the bone marrow may produce roentgenographically discernible alterations. For a survey of the literature to date on this unusual and interesting condition, the reader is referred to a paper by Bendel and Race.[2] Several instances of bone involvement have also been reported by Barer and his associates.[1]

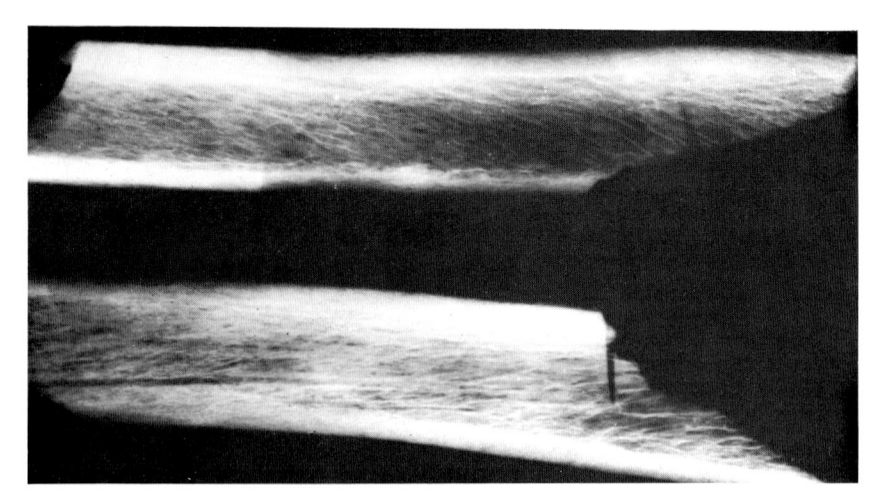

Fig. 20-4. Roentgenogram of a segment of the shaft of a femur from an autopsied case of chloroma (myeloblastic leukemia). This aggressive neoplasm had extended through the cortex and periosteum into the adjacent soft parts. This is not apparent in the x-ray film, which does, however, show appreciable rarefaction of the femur and moth-eaten erosion of its cortex in places.

"Lymphosarcoma"

This section deals briefly with the skeletal changes observed in lymphocytic, lymphoblastic, and reticulum-cell lymphoma, whether or not these are associated with a blood picture of lymphatic leukemia. The latter, in keeping with the concept of Gall and Mallory,[13] is interpreted not as a pathologic entity, but rather as an incidental phase, often a late or terminal one, in the evolution of malignant lymphoma (or lymphosarcoma in the older terminology).

On the whole, extensive infiltration or replacement of the bone marrow by proliferating tumor cells is not nearly as constant in lymphosarcoma as it is in chronic myeloid leukemia. Moreover, it is only in occasional instances that osseous involvement is sufficiently outspoken to be recognized roentgenographically, and published estimates of their incidence range from about 7% to 25%. While one may sometimes observe a compressed vertebral body (Fig. 20-5) or a lytic defect in one bone or another, e.g., the calvarium or a limb bone, involvement of the bone marrow when present does not lead as a rule to grossly discernible, discrete tumor nodes and therefore becomes clearly evident in most instances only on microscopic examination. The tumor deposits microscopically may occasionally take the form of focal nodular aggregates, but more often they

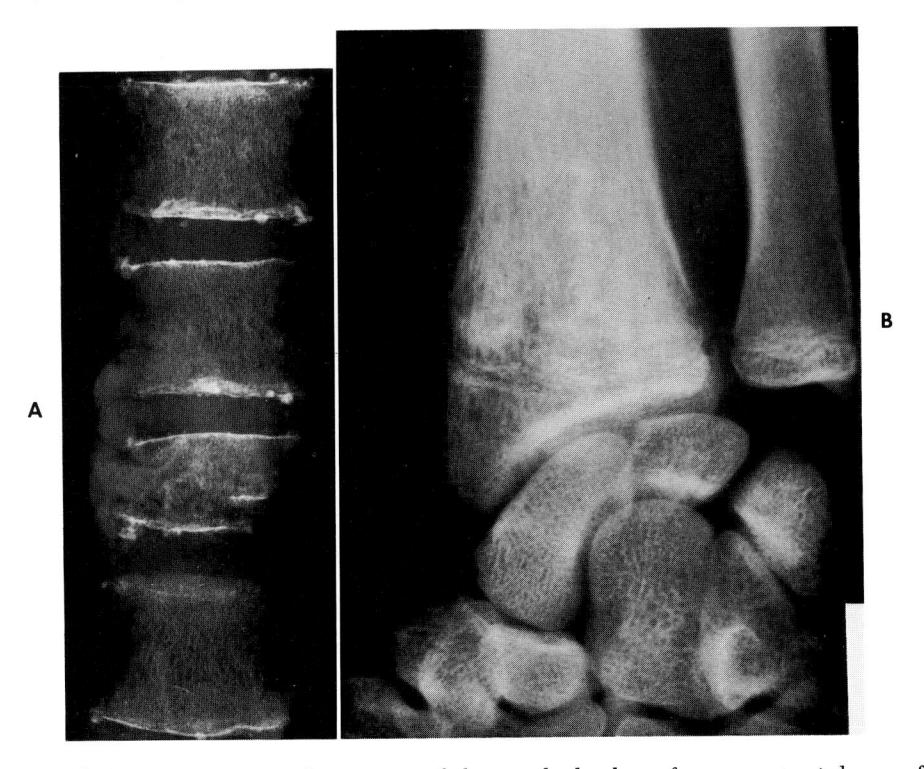

Fig. 20-5. A, Roentgenogram of a segment of the vertebral column from an autopsied case of chronic lymphatic leukemia. The roentgenogram shows a compressed vertebral body. B, Roentgenogram of a focus of malignant lymphoma in the distal radius of a boy of 16. Skeletal survey failed to show any other bone lesions, and there was no apparent involvement of liver, spleen, or lymph nodes.

316   Bone tumors

are less circumscribed and rather diffusely infiltrating. The extent of marrow replacement by tumor is likewise variable and may be rather limited or, on occasion, so pronounced as to have resulted clinically in myelophthisic anemia. The cytology of the tumor foci in the bone marrow in any particular case reflects that of the neoplastic processes generally, and as noted, depending upon their stage of maturation, the cells may be predominantly lymphocytic, lymphoblastic, of reticulum-cell type, or occasionally more polymorphous in character. It may be mentioned in passing that the occurrence of bone marrow involvement in lymphosarcoma need occasion no surprise, since even in normal bone marrow one not infrequently finds isolated collections of lymphocytes, if one searches for them.

The presence of localized skeletal lesions of sufficient size and destructiveness to be detectable roentgenographically is more likely to be encountered in dealing with the reticulum-cell sarcomas than with the more differentiated lymphosarcomas. In surveying their extensive material pertaining to malignant lymphoma,

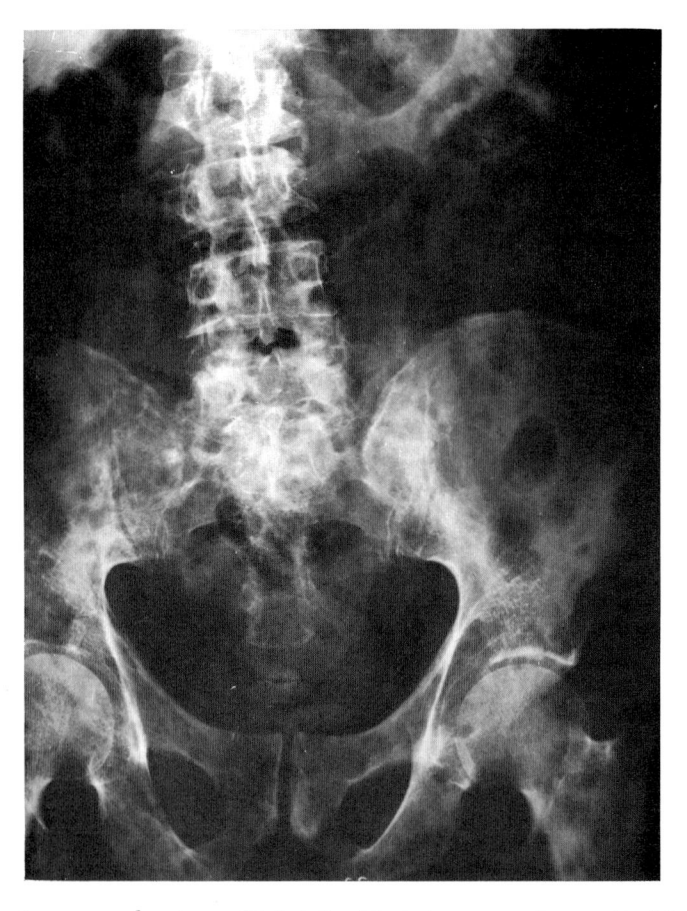

Fig. 20-6. Roentgenogram showing multiple lytic defects in a case of generalized lymphosarcomatosis, simulating those of multiple myeloma. Extensive skeletal involvement such as this is exceptional, however.

Gall and Mallory[13] found that clinically discernible skeletal lesions, representing in many instances an apparently solitary manifestation of the disease, had been noted in one fourth of the patients with "clasmatocytoma" (a subdivision of reticulum-cell sarcoma). Such skeletal foci were observed less frequently in lymphoblastic lymphoma and were distinctly unusual in lymphocytic lymphoma. It is pertinent to note also that clinically significant skeletal involvement may be encountered in some instances of follicular lymphoblastoma. Thus Meyer,[24] in surveying six cases in point, found roentgenographically discernible osseous involvement in two, in one of which there was an obvious destructive focus in the lower shaft of a femur. In the same connection, it is relevant to cite the remarkable case of "polymorphous-cell sarcoma" reported by Kenney,[21] which apparently represents an instance of reticulum-cell sarcomatosis developing as an end stage of giant-follicular lymphoblastoma and involving the lymph nodes and the gastrointestinal tract as well as the bones. Virtually the entire skeleton showed osteoporosis and vaguely mottled, moth-eaten rarefactions and, in fact, the patient's presenting complaints related to the occurrence of multiple pathologic fractures (Fig. 20-6).

Primary reticulum-cell sarcoma of bone

The occasional finding of apparently localized skeletal involvement as the sole, or at least initial, manifestation of what appears to be reticulum-cell sarcoma (clasmatocytoma, monocytoma) deserves further consideration because of the possibility of clinical cure in such cases by appropriate therapy. As established by Parker and Jackson[26] and subsequently confirmed by others, there can be no doubt that such instances do occur from time to time, and that cures can be obtained by radical surgery in selected cases in which the tumor is situated in an accessible site (usually a limb bone) and has not as yet come to involve the regional lymph nodes or spread to distant parts. There is further evidence to indicate that roentgen therapy in moderate dosage may effectively destroy such tumors. There is also sound evidence to indicate that even in pertinent cases in which fatal dissemination does occur eventually, clinical remission for a number of years may be obtained by resorting to surgical ablation and/or irradiation. The publication in recent years of sizable groups of documented cases from a number of large centers has fully substantiated the soundness of the concept of primary reticulum-cell sarcoma of bone and has afforded much information of value in regard to diagnosis and treatment.

In 1939, Parker and Jackson,[26] on the basis of a study of seventeen pertinent cases, many of them culled from the Bone Sarcoma Registry, directed attention to the tumor under consideration, which they held to be distinctive and, in particular, different from Ewing's sarcoma. They further expressed the view that this neoplasm was derived from the reticulum cells of the marrow of the affected bone and that its cell type was identical with that of reticulum-cell sarcoma of lymph nodes and other hematopoietic tissues. In regard to cytologic detail, it was emphasized that many of the tumor cells present ovoid, reniform, or horseshoe-shaped nuclei, suggesting ameboid activity. In this connection, it is significant also that the tumor cells at times display a striking tendency to phagocytose leukocytes. These are features, one might add, that hardly characterize the cytology of Ewing's sarcoma. It is also pertinent to point out in regard to nomenclature that the designations of primary reticulum-cell sarcoma of bone,[26] clasmatocytic lymphoma,[13] and monocytoma[38] seem clearly to have reference to essentially the same neoplasm.

Clinically, the tumor under discussion presents as a painful, often extensive but localized, destructive lesion prone to pathologic fracture. When it arises in a long bone, as is often the case, the end of the bone and much of the shaft tend to be involved. The roentgenographic picture may be suggestive of the diagnosis to an observer who has had personal experience with the lesion, as emphasized by Sherman and Snyder,[29] but, on the whole, it lacks any sharp or specific distinctiveness that would enable one to distinguish it clearly from that of other, more

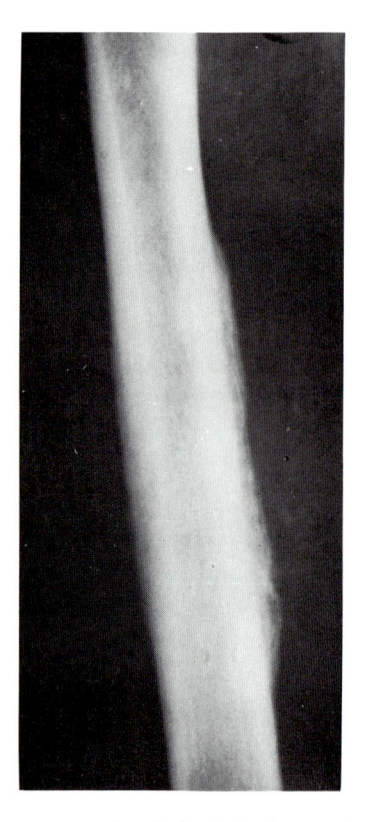

Fig. 20-7. Roentgenogram of a tumor in the shaft of the femur of an adult woman. This tumor proved on biopsy to be a reticulum-cell sarcoma. The picture here is not one of destructive mottling, but rather that of localized cortical thickening, with periosteal new bone reaction. The extent of marrow involvement is not too clear. Roentgen irradiation afforded complete relief of symptoms; the patient was well two years later, and her progress is still being followed.

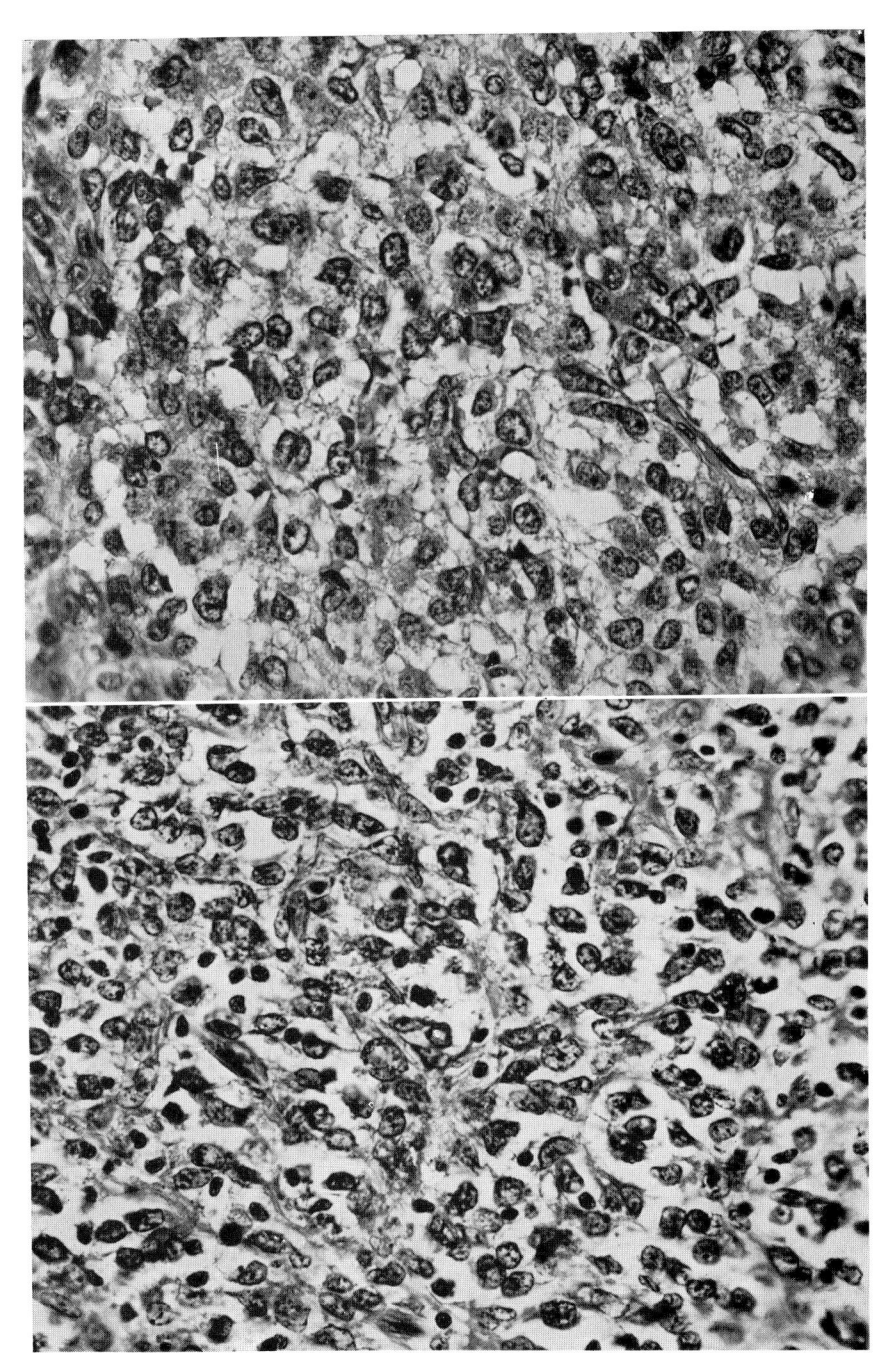

Fig. 20-8. Photomicrographs of two representative instances of primary reticulum-cell sarcoma of bone marrow. The picture is not unlike that of reticulum-cell sarcoma elsewhere. On the other hand, it differs in a number of essential respects from that of Ewing's sarcoma. (Compare with Fig. 18-5 taken at the same magnification, ×475.)

differentiated lymphomas, Ewing's tumor, or osteolytic osteogenic sarcoma. Roentgenograms of a lesion that has not been irradiated previously are likely to show vaguely mottled rarefaction and possibly some widening of the affected bone area. There may be insidious penetration of the cortex by tumor and extension into the contiguous soft parts or into a neighboring joint (e.g., a knee or a shoulder joint), without provoking any conspicuous periosteal new bone apposition. In order to establish a definitive diagnosis of the presenting tumor, one must resort to biopsy. Before instituting treatment, however, a roentgen skeletal survey should be made, and any enlarged superficial lymph nodes that may be present should also be examined.

Since the second edition of this book was published, I have had occasion to observe material from some twenty additional instances of primary reticulum-cell sarcoma of bone. Although the pertinent data have little statistical validity, they happen to be in line with trends observed in substantially larger published series. Most of the patients were comparatively young, in the second, third, and fourth decades, although some were older adults in their sixties. Most of the presenting lesions were in long limb bones, although occasional ones were encountered elsewhere. In several instances of long bone involvement, pathologic fracture had ensued prior to treatment. X-ray irradiation was recommended in all instances in which treatment had not already been instituted.

In regard to therapy, Parker and Jackson[26] advocated prompt radical surgery (amputation of the affected limb in most instances), as a curative measure, followed by prophylactic irradiation of the regional lymph nodes. They further expressed the view that roentgen therapy in itself, in lieu of surgery, is inadequate. Of the seventeen patients whose cases were discussed by them, seven who had received appropriate treatment were alive and apparently free of tumor ten years or more later. In those patients who survived for a shorter period, there were indications of subsequent involvement of regional lymph nodes and eventual widespread dissemination of the tumor. That this sanguine experience is not unique is evidenced, for example, by the reports of Hatcher,[14] reflecting the experience of the University of Chicago Clinic, and of Coley,[5] citing that of the Memorial Hospital. In both series of cases cited, survival well beyond five years was observed in as many as half of the patients treated. The recent experience of Wang and Fleischli[37] at the Massachusetts General Hospital is comparable.

The validity of the opinion expressed by Parker and Jackson that roentgen therapy for reticulum-cell sarcoma of bone is necessarily inadequate may now be questioned with some justification. Aside from empiric clinical observations indicating the apparent effectiveness of irradiation per se, both Hatcher and Coley have cited pertinent instances in which examination of an affected bone that had been irradiated prior to excision failed to show any viable residual tumor. In this connection also, I have had occasion to examine a tibia that had been the site of a reticulum-cell sarcoma, as established by biopsy. The patient had previously received a total tumor dose of approximately 2,000 r, following which amputation was nevertheless performed with a view to cure (skeletal survey did

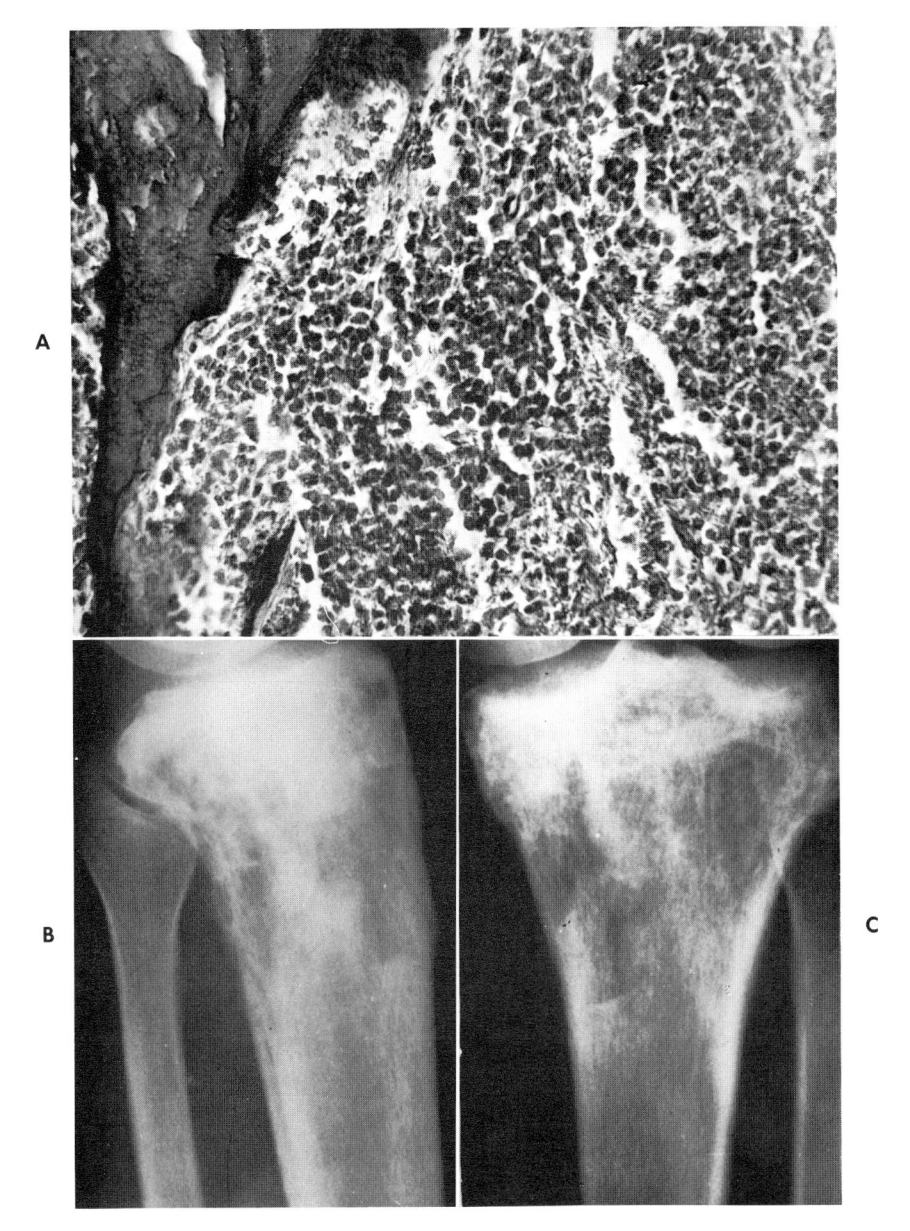

Fig. 20-9. **A**, Photomicrograph of a representative field of an irradiated necrotic reticulum-cell sarcoma in the upper end of a tibia, the roentgen pictures of which are illustrated in **B** and **C**. After biopsy examination, the tumor received 2000 r. In all of the numerous sections examined, one observed merely the ghost outlines of necrotic tumor cells. (×225.) **B** and **C**, Lateral and anteroposterior views of the irradiated reticulum-cell sarcoma shown in **A**. This patient was apparently well and free of tumor at the follow-up four years later.

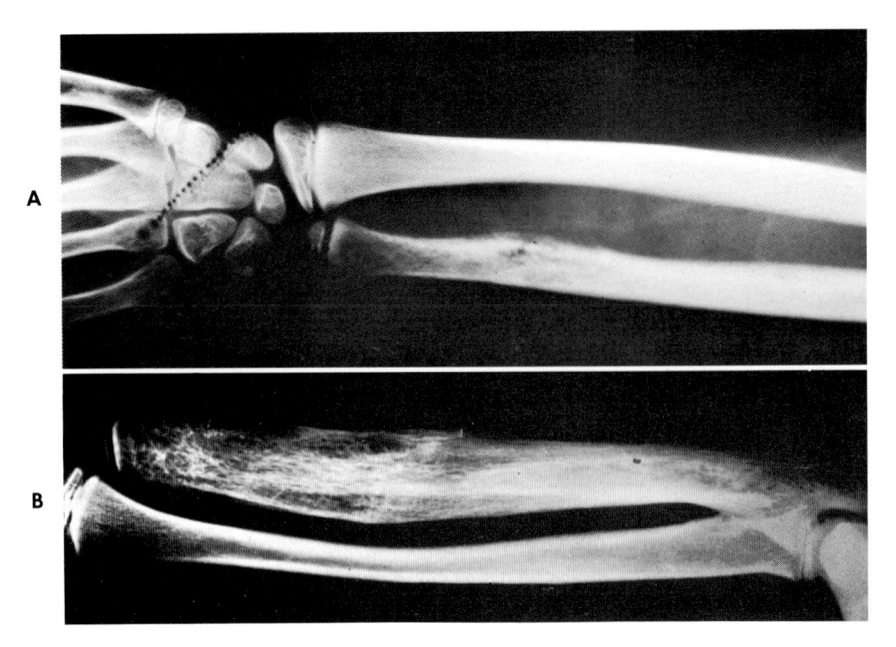

Fig. 20-10. A, Roentgenogram of a focus of reticulum-cell sarcoma in the lower ulna of a child aged 8, showing pathologic fracture. B, Roentgenogram of another irradiated focus of reticulum-cell sarcoma in the distal half of an ulna. (The diagnosis was based upon a preirradiation biopsy.) The patient subsequently manifested another tumor focus in a tibia.

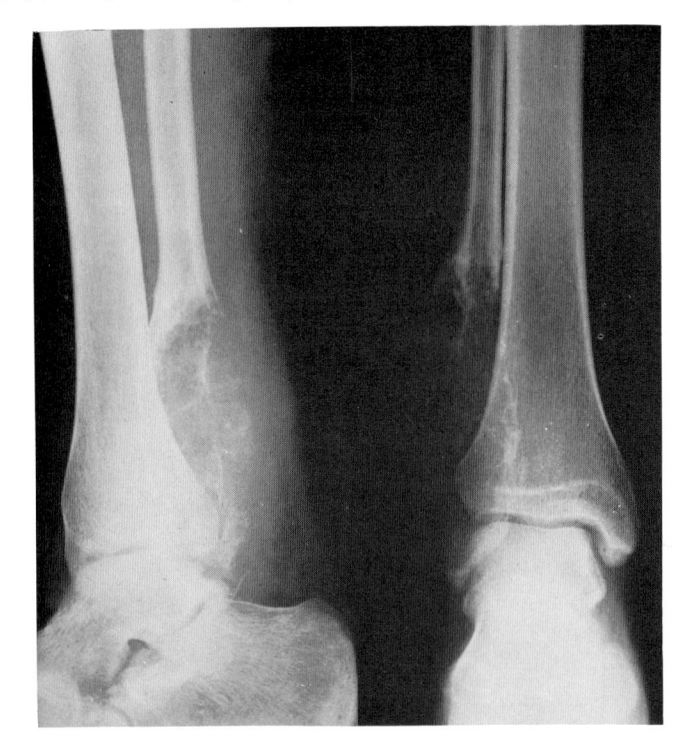

Fig. 20-11. Roentgenogram of a primary reticulum-cell sarcoma of the lower fibula in a young patient. In this instance, there was local recurrence after roentgen irradiation, and, eventually, below-knee amputation had to be done. (In our experience of recent years, failure of irradiation is the exception, rather than the rule.)

not reveal any additional lesions), since some doubt had been raised as to the efficacy of the roentgen therapy. It is therefore significant to note that, although the medullary cavity of the affected proximal end of the tibia was extensively permeated by necrotic tumor, nowhere in any of the numerous sections examined did this tumor tissue appear viable (Fig. 20-9). Coley, Higinbotham, and Groesbeck[6] have also stressed the relatively high degree of radiocurability in those patients in whom clinically discernible distant metastases have not occurred prior to therapy. Specifically, they estimated the five-year survival rate for this group at 73.7% and the ten-year rate as high as 55%. In any individual patient, however, one must be cautious in the matter of prognosis, even though the therapeutic response is gratifying, since the appearance of tumor foci elsewhere may be delayed as much as five to ten years or more. Incidentally, Coley, Higinbotham and Groesbeck advocated a total tumor depth dose as high as 3,000 to 4,000 r (even though a substantially smaller dose in the neighborhood of 2,000 r can be effective) in the belief that this tends to minimize the possibility of local recurrence. Wang and Fleischli[37] and Newall and Friedman[25] advocated a dose as high as 4,500 to 5,000 r (supervoltage) covering the entire bone area, adjacent soft tissues, and regional lymph nodes. That this is not without some hazard is evidenced by a case I saw recently in which an 18-year-old girl, who had had a reticulum-cell sarcoma of the upper tibia apparently cured by roentgen irradiation, developed a fibrosarcoma there sixteen years later.

It is relevant to remark at this point, by way of summary, that altogether, the natural course of the tumors under discussion is certainly not that of Ewing's sarcoma. In particular, the localized character of many of these tumors, their tendency to involve regional lymph nodes eventually, and their gratifying response to appropriate therapy resulting in a high percentage of five-year to ten-year cures are quite unlike the behavior of Ewing's tumors, in which cures are seldom obtained even following prompt surgical ablation and in which roentgen therapy achieves only local amelioration without significantly inhibiting early dissemination throughout the skeleton or pulmonary metastasis. The differentiation, therefore, between primary reticulum-cell sarcoma of bone and Ewing's sarcoma is of more than academic import and rests upon a more substantial basis than subtle cytologic differences. With reference to biopsy diagnosis, it should be possible in most instances to make a clear distinction, although this may be difficult at times, particularly if the specimen does not include well-preserved tumor or if the histologic preparations are not of good technical quality.

Hodgkin's disease

Hodgkin's disease exclusively limited to a single bone marrow focus or even to the marrow as a whole, without concomitant involvement of hematopoietic tissues elsewhere, must be very rare, if it exists at all, and I have never observed such an instance. In the same connection, it may be noted that Gall and Mallory,[13] in their extensive survey of malignant lymphoma (of all types) covering 193 cases of Hodgkin's disease and thirty-six of Hodgkin's sarcoma, did not re-

324 Bone tumors

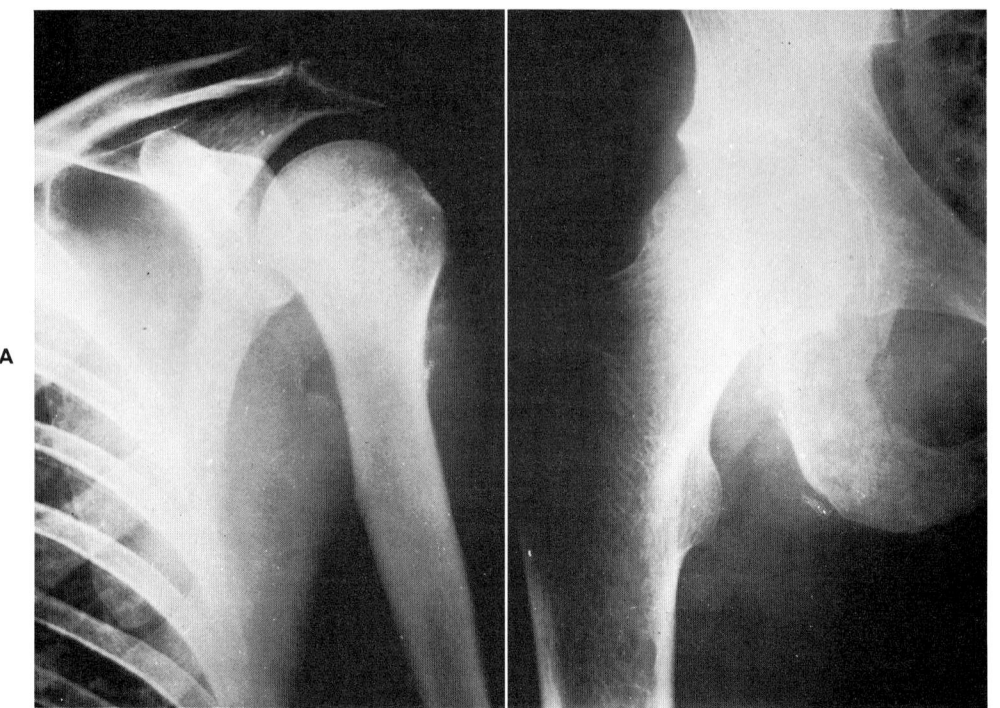

Fig. 20-12. **A,** Roentgenogram showing a lesion in the upper end of a humerus that proved on biopsy to represent a focus of Hodgkin's disease. Evidence of periosteal new bone reaction is the only clue afforded by the x-ray film, which indicates the malignant nature of the lesion. This patient also presented marked widening of the mediastinum. **B,** Another, rather nondescript, lesion in an ischium, which likewise proved to be a focus of Hodgkin's disease. From the mottled rarefaction and erosion of the cortex, one might suspect a malignant lesion, although not necessarily Hodgkin's disease. This patient also presented a collapsed vertebral body.

cord a single instance in which initial localization in some one bone was observed. However, bone marrow involvement as part of the picture of more or less disseminated Hodgkin's disease is rather common, although here again, as in other expressions of malignant lymphoma, there are many cases in which this cannot be detected on roentgenographic skeletal survey. Thus, as indicated by Falconer and Leonard,[11] published estimates of the incidence of skeletal lesions in Hodgkin's disease as determined by roentgen examination fall in the range from 7% to 26% (averaging about 15%), whereas comparable estimates as determined by autopsy[32] range between 40% and 78%. This wide deviation may reflect random sampling, but more likely it is the fact that some examiners are more thorough than others in their search for skeletal foci. The higher figure is more in keeping with my experience; I find that as random cases of generalized Hodgkin's disease come to autopsy one case is likely to show no discernible foci at all within the bone marrow (at least of the vertebral column, sternum, and ribs);

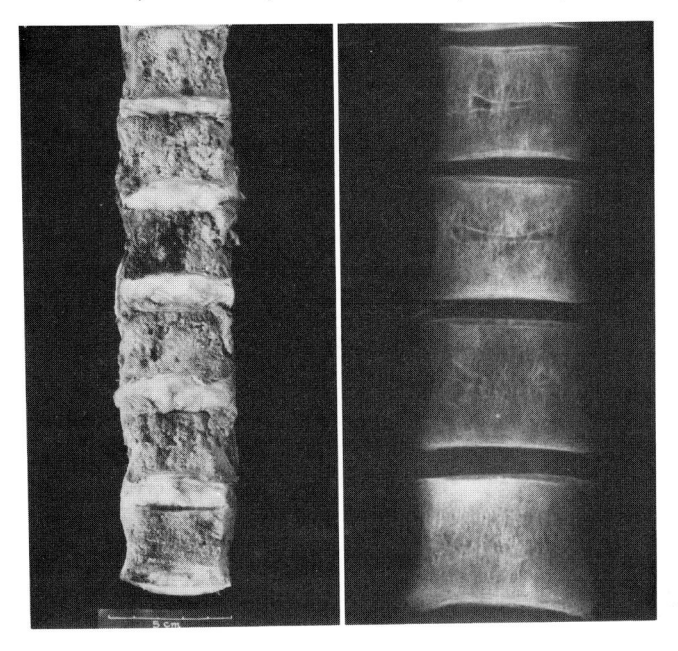

Skeletal manifestations of other tumors of hematopoietic origin   325

Fig. 20-13. A case of Hodgkin's disease in which, although every vertebral body is riddled with tumor, there is no roentgenographic indication of extensive skeletal involvement. (See also Fig. 20-14.)

a second, a limited number of grossly evident, yellowish foci within a number of bones; and a third, riddling of the skeleton by many such foci.

As noted, roentgen examination of the involved bones fails to reflect this involvement in most instances, despite the sharp detail afforded by roentgenograms of actual specimens (Figs. 20-13 and 20-14). It is only when the lesions happen to destroy or erode cortical bone or, having penetrated the cortex, provoke periosteal new bone apposition, or, in the case of the spine, bring about compression or collapse of a vertebral body, that there is any tangible evidence of their presence. When such lesions are detected (and they may be encountered in innominate bones, the vertebral column, and in flat bones, as well as long bones), their roentgenographic appearance is rather nondescript, and while one may think in terms of some neoplasm, one is not likely to suspect the correct diagnosis prior to biopsy unless the patient also happens to present mediastinal widening, enlarged superficial lymph nodes, or a palpable abdominal or retroperitoneal mass (Fig. 20-12).

The recognition of Hodgkin's disease in a bone biopsy specimen often presents a difficult problem, because the picture tends frequently to be masked or distorted by necrosis and secondary inflammatory reaction. This may be true not only of needle aspiration biopsies, but also of tissue obtained by open operation. To cite a case in point, I recall a biopsy specimen from a collapsed vertebral body (discovered after an injury) in which the underlying lesion was so obscured by extensive necrosis that it was virtually impossible to venture any defin-

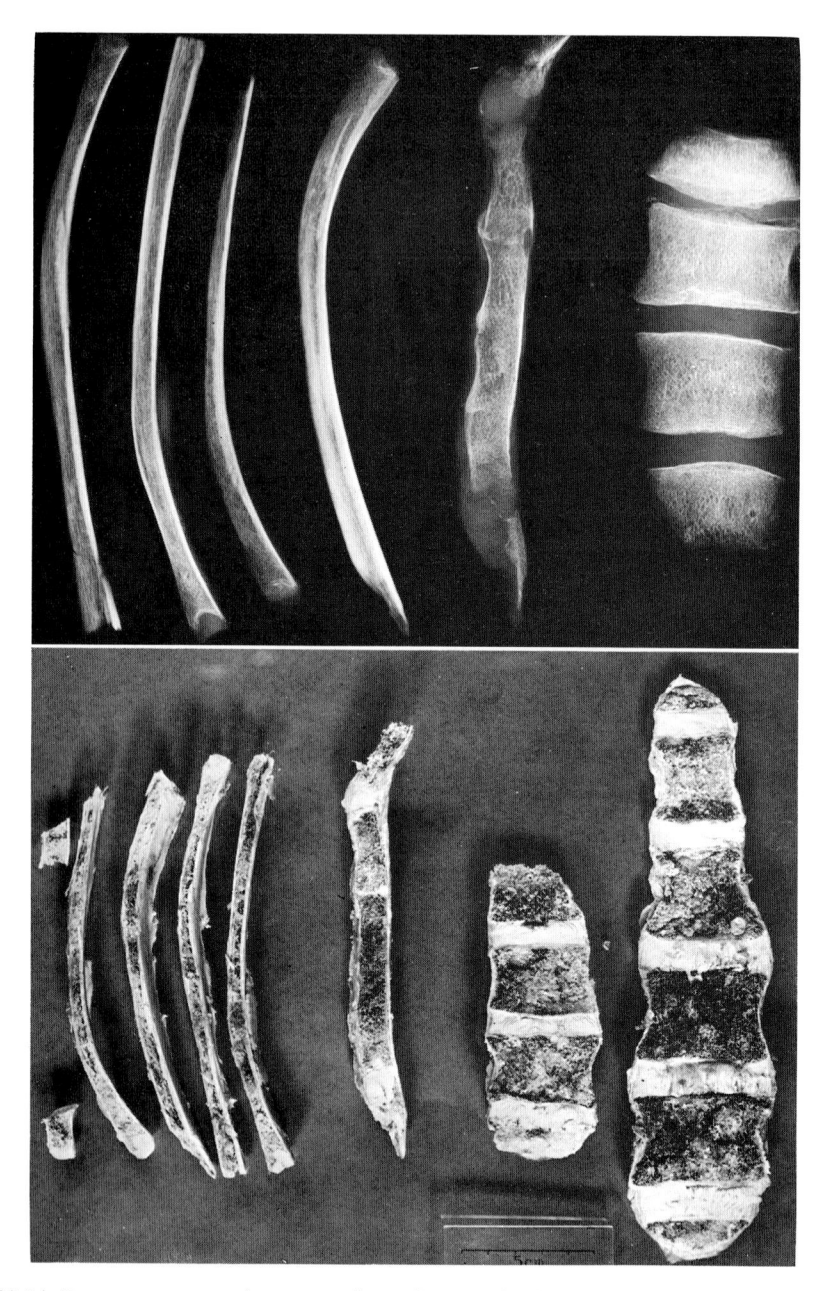

Fig. 20-14. Roentgenogram and corresponding photograph of portions of the vertebral column, sternum, and several ribs from an autopsied case of Hodgkin's disease showing extensive skeletal and visceral involvement. Although these bones were riddled with tumor foci, there is no tangible evidence of their presence in the roentgenogram of the specimen.

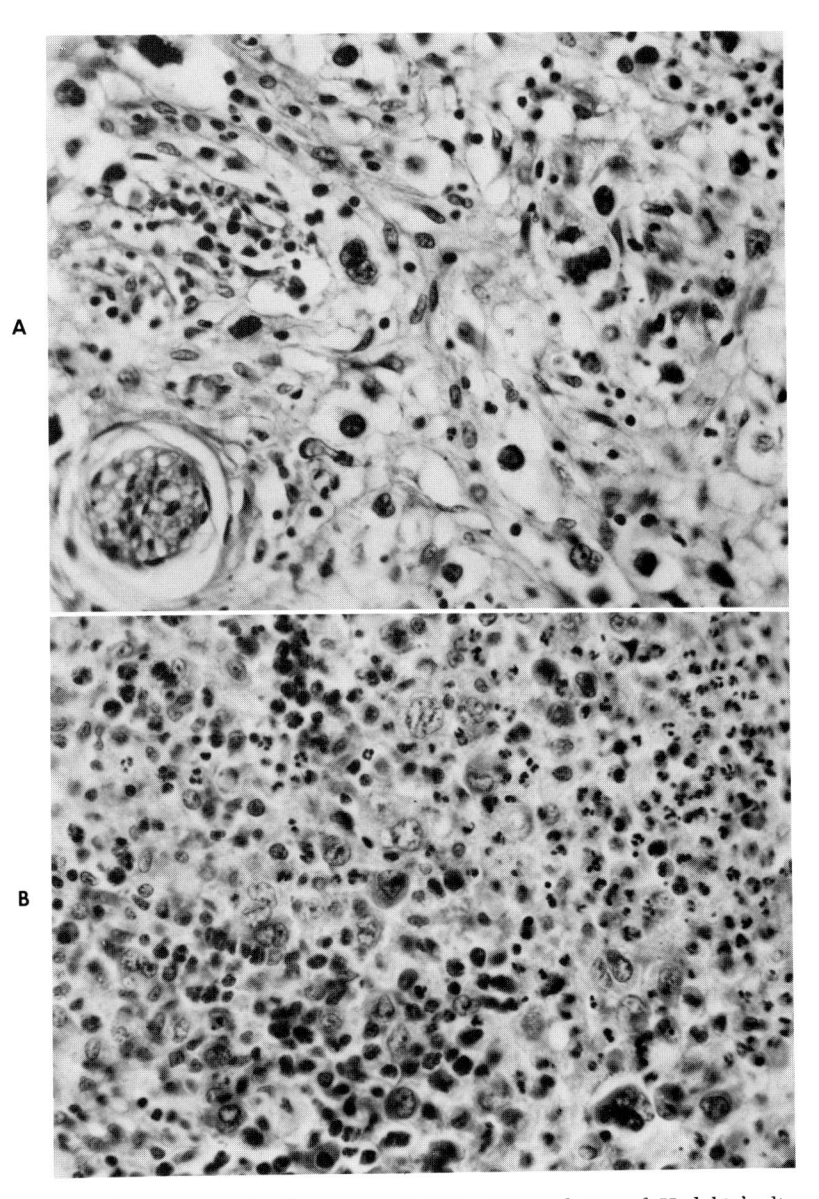

Fig. 20-15. **A,** Photomicrograph of a preserved field within a lesion of Hodgkin's disease in a vertebral body (autopsied case). The classical picture of Hodgkin's disease as seen in lymph nodes is usually not observed in bone marrow sites, and the diagnosis may sometimes be rather difficult. (It is interesting to note the fortuitous finding of a small nerve bundle in the field in the lower left-hand corner.) (×325.) **B,** Photomicrograph of an unusual lesion of Hodgkin's disease in a sternum, which simulated a focus of eosinophilic granuloma (the polymorphonuclear leukocytes in the field were eosinophils), although the large cells, some of which are multinuclear, did suggest a malignant neoplasm. It was not until the patient developed a packet of enlarged lymph nodes that the diagnosis of Hodgkin's disease became obvious. (×220.)

itive diagnosis. It was not until some time afterward, when the patient developed a packet of enlarged axillary nodes, that examination of the latter established the diagnosis of Hodgkin's disease, and at autopsy some months later, widespread visceral as well as skeletal involvement was demonstrated. At other times, it is true, one may discern multinucleated cells apparently of reticular origin, associated with an inflammatory reaction and appreciable fibrosis, but again it may not be a simple task on the basis of such evidence alone to distinguish clearly between Hodgkin's disease and other expressions of malignant lymphoma (Fig. 20-15, A).

References

1. Barer, M., Peterson, L. F. A., Dahlin, D. C., Winkelmann, R. K., and Stewart, J. R.: Mastocytosis with osseous lesions resembling metastatic malignant lesions in bone, J. Bone Joint Surg. 50-A:142, 1968.
2. Bendel, W. L., Jr., and Race, G. J.: Urticaria pigmentosa with bone involvement, J. Bone Joint Surg. 45-A:1043, 1963.
3. Carpenter, G., and Flory, C. M.: Chronic non-leukemic myelosis: report of a case with megakaryocytic myeloid splenomegaly, leukoerythroblastic anemia, generalized osteosclerosis and myelofibrosis, Arch. Intern. Med. 67:489, 1941.
4. Chabner, B. A., Haskell, C. M., and Canellos, G. P.: Destructive bone lesions in chronic granulocytic leukemia, Medicine 48:401, 1969.
5. Coley, B. L.: Neoplasms of bone and related conditions. Their etiology, pathogenesis, diagnosis, and treatment, New York, 1949, Paul B. Hoeber, Inc. (see p. 335 and Fig. 201).
6. Coley, B. L., Higinbotham, N. L., and Groesbeck, H. P.: Primary reticulum-cell sarcoma of bone, Radiology 55:641, 1950.
7. Craver, L. F.: Tenderness of sternum in leukemia, Am. J. Med. Sci. 174:799, 1927.
8. Craver, L. F., and Copeland, M. M.: Changes of the bones in the leukemias, Arch. Surg. 30:639, 1935.
9. Edwards, J. E.: Primary reticulum cell sarcoma of the spine. Report of a case with autopsy, Am. J. Pathol. 16:835, 1940.
10. Ewing, J.: A review of the classification of bone tumors, Surg. Gynecol. Obstet. 68:971, 1939 (see pp. 975-976).
11. Falconer, E. H., and Leonard, M. E.: Skeletal lesions in Hodgkin's disease, Ann. Intern. Med. 29:1115, 1948.
12. Forkner, C. E.: Leukemia and allied disorders, New York, 1938, The Macmillan Co.
13. Gall, A. E., and Mallory, T. B.: Malignant lymphoma, Am. J. Pathol. 18:381, 1941.
14. Hatcher, C. H.: Treatment of bone sarcoma, Rocky Mountain Med. J. 45:999, 1948 (see section on Reticulum-cell sarcoma).
15. Ivins, J. C., and Dahlin, D. C.: Reticulum-cell sarcoma of bone, J. Bone Joint Surg. 35-A:835, 1953.
16. Jackson, H., Jr., Parker, F., Jr., and Lennon, H. M.: Agnogenic myeloid metaplasia of the spleen, N. Engl. J. Med. 222:985, 1940.
17. Jordan, H. E., and Scott, J. K.: A case of osteosclerosis with extensive extramedullary hemopoiesis and a leukemic blood picture, Arch. Pathol. 32:895, 1941.
18. Kalayjian, B. S., Herbut, P. A., and Erf, L. A.: The bone changes of leukemia in children, Radiology 47:223, 1946.
19. Kandel, E. V.: Chloroma, Arch. Intern. Med. 59:691, 1937.
20. Kemp, T. A., and Williams, E. R.: Chloroma, Brit. J. Radiol. 14:157, 1941.
21. Kenney, W. E.: Polymorphous-cell sarcoma, the malignant phase of giant-follicle lymphoma, with generalized skeletal involvement and multiple pathological fractures, J. Bone Joint Surg. 27:668, 1945.
22. Lichtenstein, L., and Jaffe, H. L.: Ewing's sarcoma of bone, Am. J. Pathol. 23:43, 1947.
23. McCormack, L. J., Ivins, J. C., Dahlin, D. C., and Johnson, E. W., Jr.: Primary reticulum-cell sarcoma of bone, Cancer 5:1182, 1952.
24. Meyer, O. O.: Follicular lymphoblastoma. A report of 6 cases, Blood 3:921, 1948.
25. Newall, J., and Friedman, M.: Reticulum-cell sarcoma. Part II: Radiation dosage for each type, Radiology 94:643, 1970.
26. Parker, F., Jr., and Jackson, H., Jr.: Primary reticulum-cell sarcoma of bone, Surg. Gynecol. Obstet. 68:45, 1939.
27. (a) Richter, M. N. In Downey, H., editor:

Handbook of hematology, vol. IV, Section on leukemia, pp. 2287-3035.
(b) Mettier, S. R., and Lucas, W. T.: Leukemia in infants and children, ibid. pp. 3039-3048.
(c) Watson, C. J.: Lymphosarcoma and leucosarcoma, ibid. pp. 3051-3106.
28. Rosenthal, N., and Erf, L. A.: Clinical observations on osteopetrosis and myelofibrosis, Arch. Intern. Med. 71:793, 1943.
29. Sherman, R. S., and Snyder, R. E.: The roentgenological appearance of primary reticulum-cell sarcoma of bone, Am. J. Roentgenol. 58:291, 1947.
30. Silverman, F. N.: The skeletal lesions in leukemia, Am. J. Roentgenol. 59:819, 1948.
31. Snapper, I.: Medical clinics on bone diseases, ed. 2, New York, 1949, Interscience Publishers, Inc., pp. 266-267.
32. Steiner, P. E.: Hodgkin's disease, Arch. Pathol. 36:627, 1943.
33. Strange, V. M., and deLorimier, A. A.: Reticulum-cell sarcoma primary in the skull, Am. J. Roentgenol. 71:40, 1954.
34. Sturgis, C.: Hematology, Springfield, Ill., 1948, Charles C Thomas, Publisher.
35. Townsend, S. R.: A single myeloid bone tumor associated with a blood picture of chronic myelocytic leukemia, Can. Med. Assoc. J. 40:352, 1939.
36. Valls, J., Muscolo, D., and Schajowicz, F.: Reticulum-cell sarcoma of bone, J. Bone Joint Surg. 34-B:588, 1952.
37. Wang, C. C., and Fleischli, D. J.: Primary reticulum cell sarcoma of bone, with emphasis on radiation therapy, Cancer 22:994, 1968.
38. Wintrobe, M. M.: Clinical hematology, ed. 6, Philadelphia, 1967, Lea & Febiger.

Chapter 21

Lipoma and liposarcoma of bone

The occasional occurrence of a lipoma of bone in the sense of a circumscribed benign tumor of adult fat cells within fatty bone marrow should be noted. A number of lipomas within vertebral bodies have been reported by Makrycostas,[16] but Schmorl[21] was inclined to discount these as conspicuous circumscribed foci of fatty marrow rather than genuine neoplasms. Be that as it may, they are not discernible roentgenographically and are of no practical importance. Several other case reports in the older literature have been cited by Dawson.[7] Haas also made casual mention of "a few authentic cases" of lipoma of bone marrow, but cited no specific references that can be verified. In 1951, Dickson and associates[8] published a well-documented instance of an intramedullary lipoma situated in the lower end of a tibia and cited two additional cases in the older literature. Within recent years several additional pertinent cases have been recorded by Caruolo and Dahlin,[3] by Child,[5] and by Skinner and Fraser.[23] I have also seen material from a case in point reported by Mueller and Robbins,[18] in which the lipoma was situated within the distal tibia, and from another in the upper humerus (Fig. 21-1). These comparatively rare medullary lipomas are of no great practical moment apparently, except insofar as they may be mistaken clinically for more serious neoplasms.

Mention also should be made in passing of the condition of lipomatosis involving soft tissues and bones, usually of a lower extremity, as reported by Kaufmann and Stout.[15] It apparently represents an unusual congenital developmental anomaly, analogous to hemangiomatosis.

The development in bone of primary malignant neoplasms of fat-cell derivation has also been established, particularly by the well-documented, recently published cases of Dawson,[7] Mastragostino,[17] and Catto and Stevens.[4] Considering that liposarcoma in soft tissues is one of the more common mesenchymal tumors, the comparative rarity of its counterpart within bone is rather surprising, although it is entirely possible that some of the poorly differentiated pleomorphic liposarcomas are not recognized as such. It may be recalled that in the 1930's, a series of some eight malignant neoplasms in bone held to represent liposarcomas were reported by Ewing,[11] Stewart,[24] and others at the Memorial Hospital, but

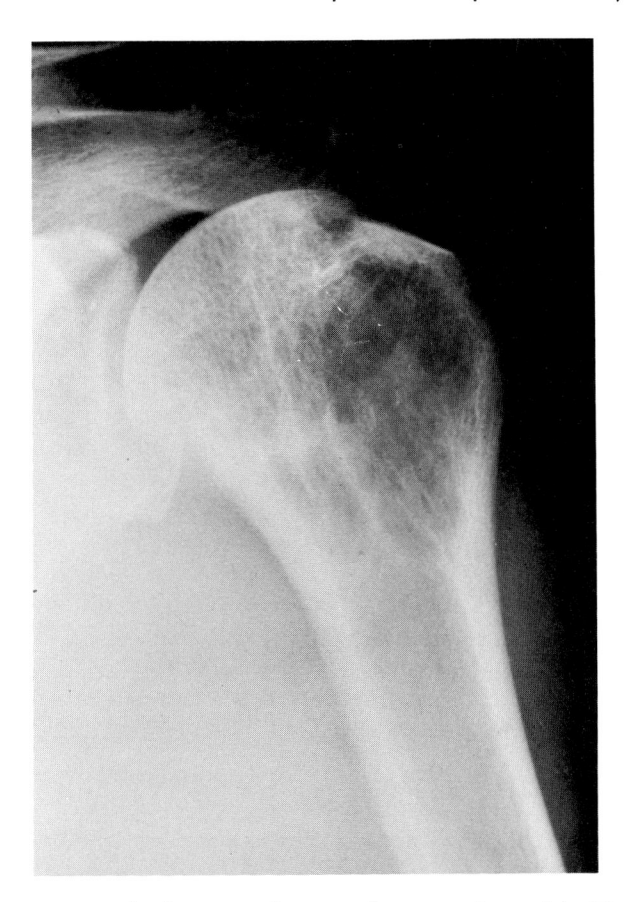

Fig. 21-1. Roentgenogram of a lipoma in the upper humerus of an adult. The rarefied defect is so nondescript, and the tumor so unusual, that one would hardly surmise its nature prior to biopsy.

the precise nature of these particular tumors became a subject of controversy and is still apparently questionable.

Briefly, however, in the case reported by Dawson, the evidence presented in support of the interpretation of primary liposarcoma should convince even the most skeptical observer. Incidentally, this was the only neoplasm of its kind seen in the University Laboratory at Edinburgh over a period of twenty-six years. It developed in the lower shaft of a femur of a 28-year-old woman, invaded the contiguous soft parts, and proved fatal from pulmonary metastasis, despite prompt disarticulation. The case reported by Catto and Stevens from Glasgow as liposarcoma of bone is equally convincing. This tumor developed in the upper tibia of a 16-year-old girl, who also succumbed from pulmonary metastases only five months after amputation. The first of the two cases reported by Mastragostino[17] as instances of primary liposarcoma of bone may well be another in point and suggests that the prognosis may not necessarily be ominous. This tumor developed in the upper shaft of a fibula of a 30-year-old man and was resected; there

332 Bone tumors

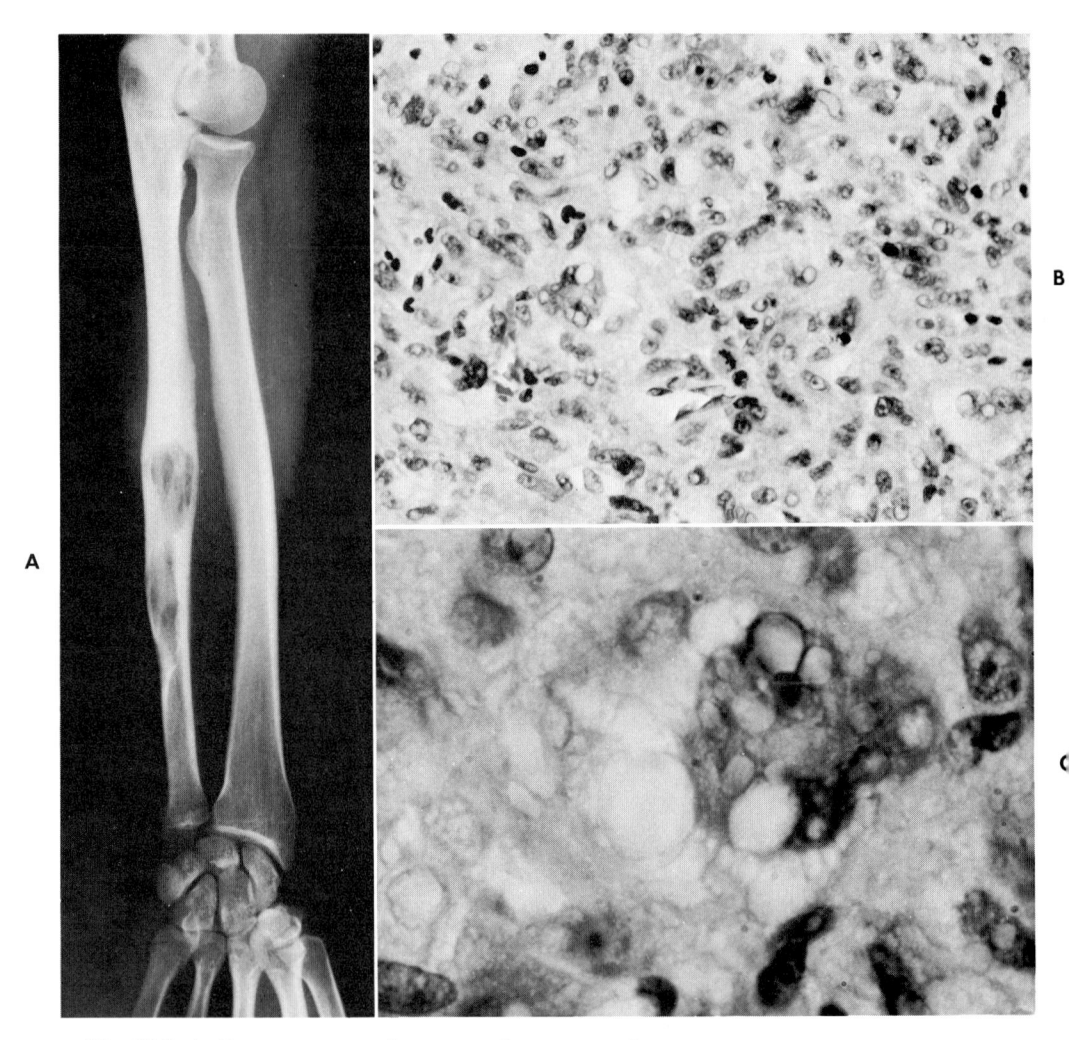

Fig. 21-2. **A**, Roentgenogram of an unusual primary malignant tumor in the lower shaft of an ulna, which was interpreted pathologically as a liposarcoma (**B** and **C**). Evidence of muscle invasion was found on frozen section at the time of surgery, so that an above-elbow amputation was done. **B**, Low-power photomicrographs of the tumor illustrated in **A**. Note the vacuolization of many of the cells. Elsewhere the tumor was more spindly. **C**, Higher magnification showing one of the larger vacuolated lipoblasts, which stained vividly with oil-red-O and other lipid stains. (From Goldman, R. L.: Am. J. Clin. Pathol. 42:503, 1964.)

was no recurrence during the ensuing four-year period of follow-up. The second tumor reported by Mastragostino involved the lower end of the femur in a 56-year-old woman and was designated as angiolipoblastoma because of prominent vasoformative areas; it could conceivably have represented a malignant mesenchymoma. Some other possible cases have been tabulated by Catto and Stevens and, for the sake of brevity, will not be specifically cited here.

Still another apparently clear-cut instance of primary liposarcoma of bone was reported from our own laboratory by Goldman.[14] Thus tumor developed in-

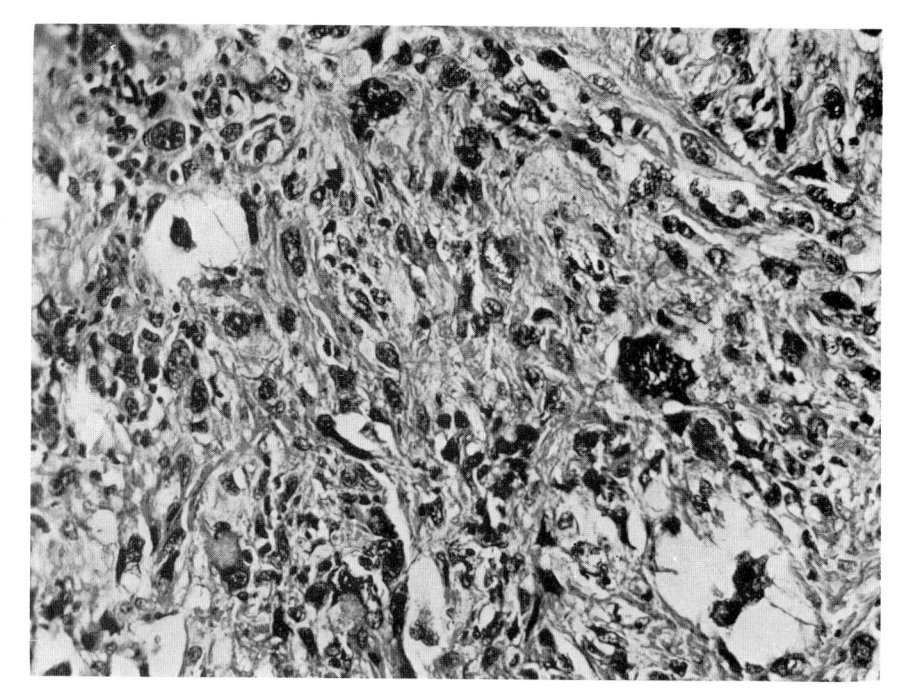

Fig. 21-3. Photomicrograph of a field of a primary sarcoma in the intertrochanteric region of the femur of a young man in his twenties. The cytology of this tumor and especially the presence of large, bizarre, vacuolated tumor giant cells strongly suggested the possibility of liposarcoma. (×220.)

sidiously in the shaft of an ulna of a 33-year-old man (Fig. 21-2, A) and was found on frozen section at the time of surgery to have penetrated the cortex and invaded contiguous muscle tissue, so that supracondylar amputation was deemed the procedure of choice. Too little time has elapsed to have a valid opinion as to the eventual outcome. On microscopic examination, this neoplasm contained many fields of immature, small and large, often bizarre lipoblasts showing conspicuous globules of fat readily stained by oil-red-O (Fig. 21-2, B and C).

Liposarcoma may also be a prominent component of a malignant mesenchymoma arising within bone. Some years ago, I had occasion to observe a fat-containing mesenchymoma of bone arising within the upper tibia, which, in spite of prompt amputation, metastasized freely to the lungs and mediastinum shortly thereafter. In this case, both the primary tumor and its metastases contained abundant unmistakable embryonal fat associated with prominent aggregates of lymphoid cells, osteogenic sarcoma being the other major component. The large fields of fat tissue were clearly recognizable as such, even in the gross, being pale yellow and distinctly greasy. It appears to me that, if neoplastic tissue of malignant fat-cell origin can develop as a major integral part of a primary mesenchymoma of bone, there is no good reason a priori why it should not occasionally take the form of a pure liposarcoma. The only surprising thing is that it does not happen more often.

References

1. Barnard, L.: Primary liposarcoma of bone, Arch. Surg. **29**:560, 1934.
2. Barnard, W. G.: Abstract, Cancer Rev. **6**: 434, 1931.
3. Caruolo, J. E., and Dahlin, D. C.: Lipoma involving bone and simulating malignant bone tumor. Report of case, Proc. Staff Meet. Mayo Clin. **28**:361, 1953.
4. Catto, M., and Stevens, J.: Liposarcoma of bone, J. Path. Bact. **86**:248, 1963.
5. Child, P. L.: Lipoma of the os calcis, Am. J. Clin. Pathol. **25**:1050, 1955.
6. Coley, B.: Neoplasms of bone and related conditions. Their etiology, pathogenesis, diagnosis and treatment, New York, 1949, Paul B. Hoeber, Inc., pp. 341-344.
7. Dawson, E. K.: Liposarcoma of bone, J. Path. Bact. **70**:513, 1955.
8. Dickson, A. B., Ayres, W. W., Mason, M. W., and Miller, W. R.: Lipoma of bone of intraosseous origin, J. Bone Joint Surg. **33-A**:257, 1951.
9. Duffy, J., and Stewart, F. W.: Primary liposarcoma of bone; report of a case, Am. J. Pathol. **14**:621, 1938.
10. Ewing, J.: The classification and treatment of bone sarcoma. Report of the International Conference on Cancer, London, 1928, Baltimore, 1928, William Wood & Co., pp. 365-376.
11. Ewing, J.: A review of the classification of bone tumors, Surg. Gynecol. Obstet. **68**: 971, 1939.
12. Fender, F. A.: Liposarcoma; report of a case with intracranial metastases, Am. J. Pathol. **9**:909, 1933.
13. Geschickter, C. F., and Copeland, M. M.: Tumors of bone, ed. 3, Philadelphia, 1949, J. B. Lippincott Co., p. 623.
14. Goldman, R. L.: Primary liposarcoma of bone, Am. J. Clin. Pathol. **42**:503, 1964.
15. Kaufmann, S. L., and Stout, A. P.: Lipoblastic tumors of children, Cancer **12**:912, 1959.
16. Makrycostas, K.: Ueber das Wirbelangiom, -lipom und -osteom, Virchows Arch. **265**: 259, 1927.
17. Mastragostino, S.: Tumori Lipoblastici Primitivi dello Scheletro, Chir. d. vig. di movimento **44**:18, 1957.
18. Mueller, M. C., and Robbins, J. L.: Intramedullary lipoma of bone; report of a case, J. Bone Joint Surg. **42-A**:517, 1960.
19. Rehbock, D. J., and Hauser, H.: Liposarcoma of bone; Report of two cases and review of literature, Am. J. Cancer **27**:37, 1936.
20. Retz, J. D., Jr.: Primary liposarcoma of bone; report of a case and review of the literature, J. Bone Joint Surg. **43-A**:123, 1961.
21. Schmorl, G.: Die gesunde und kranke Wirbelsaüle im Röntgenbild, Leipzig, 1932, Georg Thieme, p. 77.
22. Schwartz, A., Shuster, M., and Becker, S. M.: Liposarcoma of bone. Report of a case and review of the literature, J. Bone Joint Surg. **52-A**:171, 1970.
23. Skinner, B. G., and Fraser, R. C.: Medullary lipoma of bone, J. Can. Assoc. Radiol. **8**:19, 1957.
24. Stewart, F. W.: Primary liposarcoma of bone, Am. J. Pathol. **7**:87, 1931.
25. Stout, A. P.: Tumor seminar, J. Missouri M. A., pp. 259-291, April, 1949 (see p. 280).

Chapter 22

Chordoma

Chordoma is one of the rarer primary neoplasms of the skeleton and of the vertebral column particularly. It apparently results from neoplastic proliferation of notochordal remnants persisting within the nucleus pulposus of intervertebral discs, and probably also of aberrant chordal vestiges within the vertebral bodies themselves.[7] As is well known, this tumor develops most often at the ends of the axial skeleton, that is, in the sacrum and/or coccyx, or in the vicinity of the sphenooccipital synchondrosis or the clivus of Blumenbach (where occasionally also a nonmalignant excrescence of notochordal tissue, the so-called "ecchordosis physaliphora," may be encountered). In fact, the sacrococcygeal and the basicranial sites account for fully 90% of all the reported instances of chordoma. It should be noted, however, that occasional instances have been encountered also in the lumbar and even the dorsal and cervical regions of the vertebral column (although one must be certain in such cases that one is not dealing actually with chondrosarcoma). Survey of the literature of recent years shows reports continuing to appear of relatively unusual chordomas at the lumbar, dorsal, and cervical levels of the vertebral column, as well as of the more common ones in the sacrococcygeal region and the cephalad end of the axial skeleton. Among these, the paper by Congdon[2] furnishes a good deal of pathologic detail of value, supported by clinical correlation. A number of electron microscopic studies of the ultrastructure of chordoma are now on record, but these have not been particularly informative.

Whatever its situation may be, chordoma is a locally invasive tumor that tends to destroy and replace the bone at its site of development. By the time it comes to clinical notice, it usually has extended also into the contiguous soft parts, giving rise eventually to bulky intrapelvic, intraabdominal, or intracranial growths, as the case may be.

In the majority of instances the tumor grows relatively slowly, often over a period of years, and manifests no disposition to metastasize, even late in the course of its evolution and after one or more unsuccessful attempts at local excision. It should be noted, however, that there are occasional instances of chordoma, particularly in the sacrococcygeal region, that pursue a more aggressive course and give rise to widespread visceral metastases.[4,15,16] However, even those tumors that remain localized to the end and fail to metastasize, sooner or later prove fatal from encroachment on vital structures.

As noted, chordoma is so infrequently encountered that the experience of any single observer is likely to be limited to a few cases. Considerable interest has been evinced, however, in these extraordinary neoplasms, and surveys of more than 100 cases culled from the literature have been made by Mabrey[9] and by Gentil and Coley,[6] among others. These are useful for historical background and clinical orientation particularly. From such compilations one gathers that, while the neoplasm may sometimes appear in infancy or childhood, it is encountered most often in later adult life. The symptoms produced by any particular chordoma depend naturally upon its localization and the direction of its spread. In the basicranial region, of course, these relate to manifestations of increased intracranial pressure associated with an expanding lesion in the posterior fossa. With involvement of the vertebral column more caudally, one encounters manifestations of pressure on the spinal cord and its nerve roots (severe pain, paraplegia, incontinence, etc.). The sacrococcygeal tumors, in particular, that have attained appreciable size and invaded the pelvic structures may in addition infiltrate and compress the rectum and the urinary bladder, giving rise oftentimes to intestinal obstruction, hemorrhage, urinary difficulty, and other serious complications.

Roentgenographically, chordoma, in the sacrococcygeal region at least, appears as an expanded, rarefied destructive lesion, which is said also to present some evidence of calcification. While this roentgen picture may suggest chordoma to one who is alert to the possibility, it is hardly conclusive in itself, and definitive diagnosis must await pathologic examination of an adequate sample of tumor tissue. In this connection, Gentil and Coley,[6] in their report of seven cases of chordoma, have stressed the diagnostic value of needle aspiration biopsy to obviate surgical exposure of the neoplasm.

The pathologic data contained in the relevant articles in the literature relate mainly to microscopic details, but one gathers that the tumor tissue in most pertinent specimens is essentially solid in the gross, although the bulkier tumors may exhibit areas of cystic softening, as well as foci of hemorrhage and necrosis. If the neoplasm is not too far advanced nor modified by previous surgical intervention, one may find, further, that it is invested by a fibrous capsule and presents a lobulated or bossed surface. What is more significant is that on section it is likely to present a distinctly mucinous or gelatinous character, although this feature appears more pronounced in some specimens than in others.

The key to an understanding of the peculiar cytology of chordomas is afforded by information relating to the development of notochordal tissue in the early fetus. Embryologically, the notochord, which represents the primitive axial skeleton common to all vertebrates and the forerunner of the cartilage anlage of the vertebral column, appears to be intimately associated in its development with both ectodermal and mesodermal tissues. This consideration, according to Robbins,[13] is significantly reflected in the cytology of chordomas in general. Thus, in

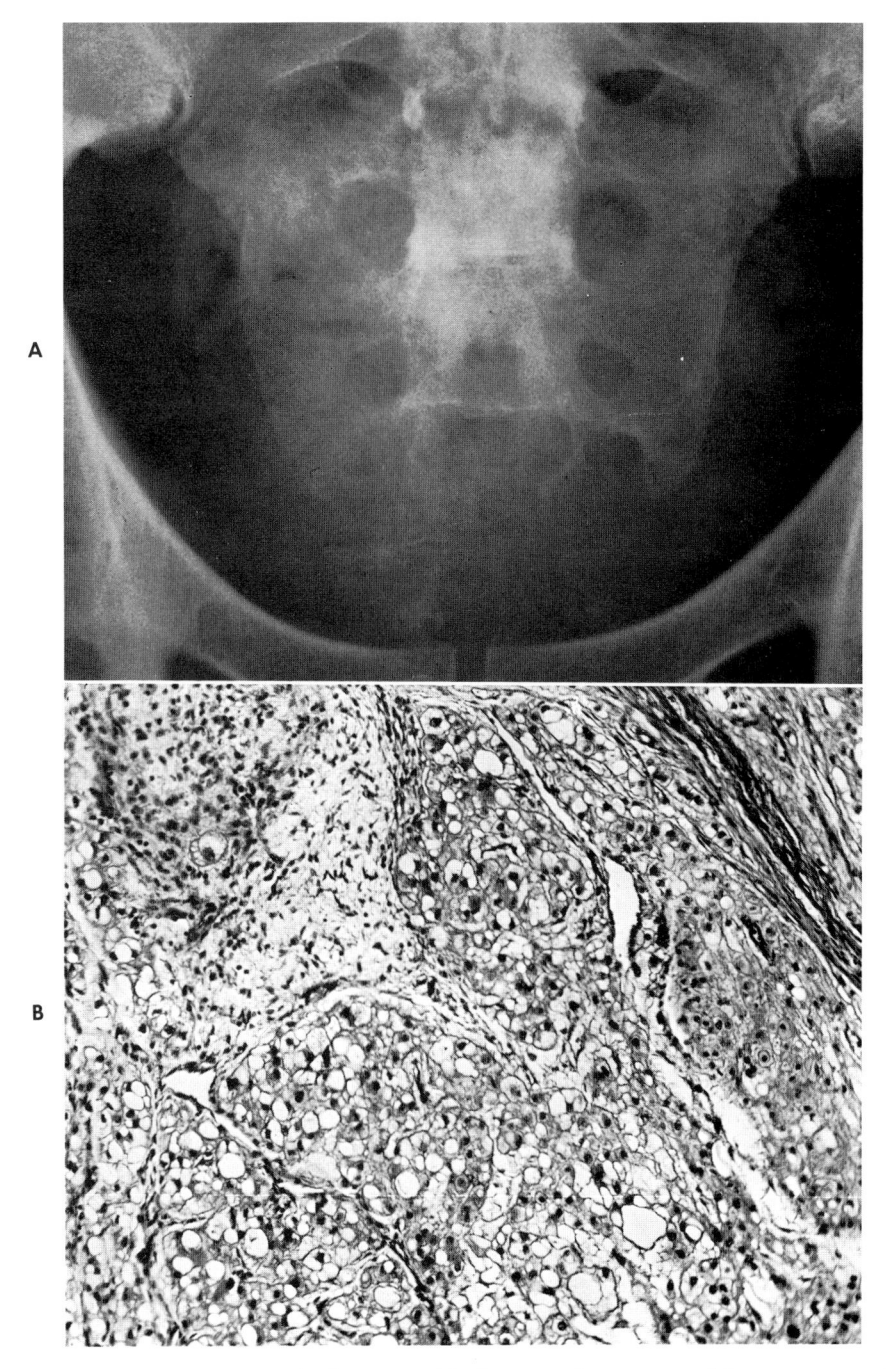

Fig. 22-1. **A,** Roentgenogram of a lytic tumorlike lesion in the coccyx and lower sacrum, which proved to be a chordoma. The appearance of the lesion is rather nondescript, although its location might lead one to suspect the presence of a chordoma. The patient, a 38-year-old man, had complained of obstipation and presented a palpable mass over the coccyx, which could also be felt through the compressed rectum. **B,** Photomicrograph of a representative field of the chordoma illustrated in **A,** showing the presence of peculiar vacuolated mucin-containing (physaliferous) tumor cells. (×110.)

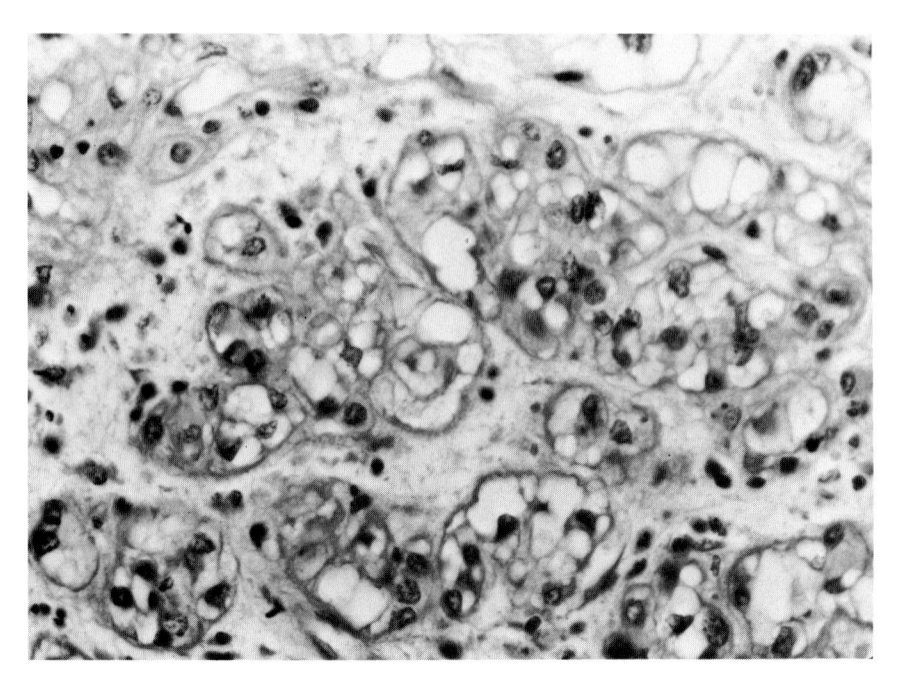

Fig. 22-2. Photomicrograph of another sacrococcygeal chordoma, at higher magnification, showing the strikingly vacuolated character of many of the tumor cells, which are arranged in nests and cords. (×400.)

any given instance, the tumor may be composed of epithelial-like structures or, on the other hand, may closely resemble spindle-cell sarcoma, and frequently both types of cell growth may be observed in the same neoplasm. To be sure, the degree of differentiation, the rapidity of growth, and the extent of anaplasia are also factors influencing the cytology of any particular chordoma. Thus, at one extreme, one may observe well-differentiated chordomas containing regular cavities lined by cuboidal epithelium, closely resembling the primitive notochordal tube, and at the other, distinctly anaplastic chordomas whose recognition as such may occasion considerable difficulty. In most instances, one is likely to observe cords, lobules, or sheets of unusual syncytial cells resembling epithelial cells, separated by matrix containing an abundance of mucin. Great emphasis in the matter of specific diagnosis has been placed upon this mucinous intercellular matrix within which the tumor cell aggregates are dispersed, and, even more so, upon the presence of peculiar large, distended, and vacuolated tumor cells commonly designated as physaliphorous cells.

It remains to point out two obvious pitfalls in the matter of differential diagnosis. First, in regard to chordomas presenting relatively sparse tumor cells scattered within a distinctly mucinous stroma, a diagnosis of colloid carcinoma (of the rectum) may sometimes be entertained by the unwary who have not taken cognizance of the existence of a large destructive lesion in the sacrum and coccyx. Second, in regard to chordomas whose matrix may acquire a chondroid appear-

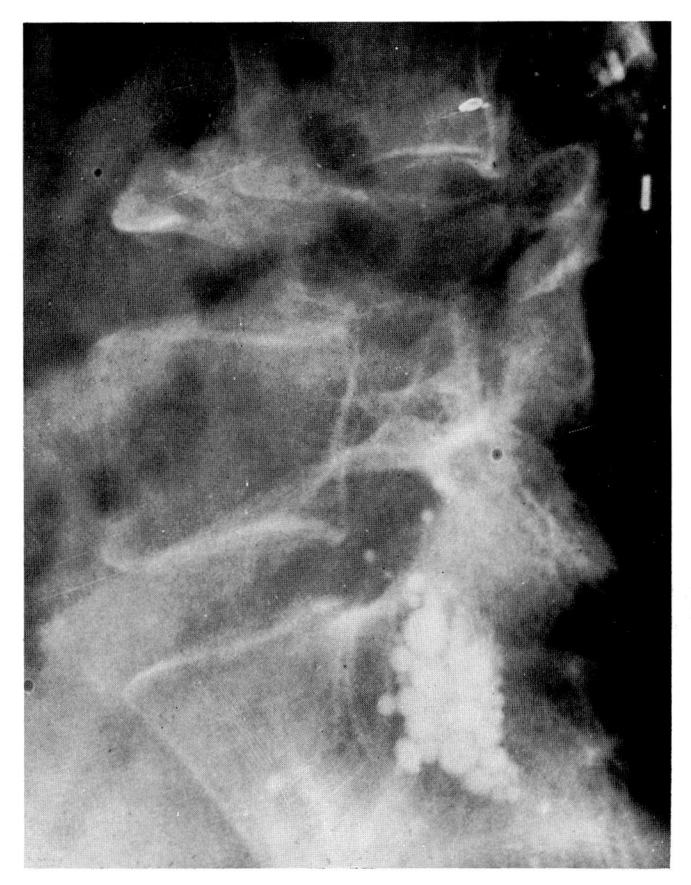

Fig. 22-3. Far-advanced chordoma of L-4, which has destroyed almost the entire body, leaving only the inferior ventral corner. (Pantopaque studies were done because of spinal-cord compression.)

ance in places, reminiscent of intervertebral disc tissue, and its cells, a rounded contour, the pathologist's impression may be that of chondrosarcoma. Adequate sampling of the available tumor tissue, however, should clearly resolve this difficulty.

In regard to therapy, the consensus of opinion is to the effect that irradiation is not likely to bring about any appreciable regression of the tumor, except perhaps in children,[10] and it should be reserved for palliation in far-advanced cases. On the other hand, complete surgical extirpation is usually not feasible because of the location of the neoplasm. In the case of sacrococcygeal chordomas, the sacrum is already more or less extensively involved by the time the presence of the tumor is recognized. One is therefore confronted by a situation involving a choice between two unsatisfactory alternatives. Nevertheless, most observers are agreed that surgical removal of as much of the tumor as possible should be attempted, since even partial resection, repeated when necessary, may result in relief of pain and of disability from pressure and may likewise appreciably prolong life

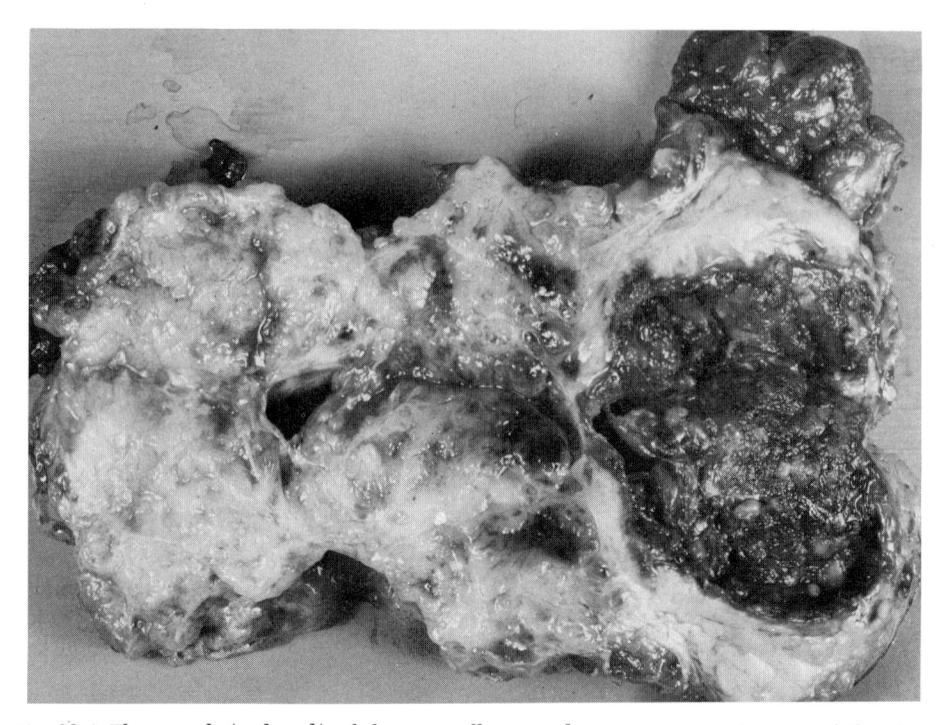

Fig. 22-4. Photograph (reduced) of the surgically excised tumor mass in the case of the chordoma of the coccyx illustrated in Fig. 22-1. The specimen represents the extraosseous extension of the neoplasm, and postoperative roentgenograms showed that relatively little of the involved sacrococcygeal bone was removed. The tumor tissue presented a gelatinous appearance modified by surgically induced hemorrhage in places. (Courtesy Dr. K. F. Ernst, Letterman General Hospital, San Francisco, Calif.)

expectancy. As noted, however, the ultimate prognosis is doleful, since sooner or later the tumor proves fatal from the effects of encroachment upon vital structures, although this eventuality may sometimes be delayed several or many years. Much clinical information of value may be obtained from a recent article by Kamrin, Potanos, and Pool,[8] in which they survey as many as thirty cases.

For chordomas developing in the coccyx (or even involving the distal sacral segments, as well), early recognition and consideration of radical block excision with a view to clearance are of paramount importance. That the situation is not altogether hopeless is evidenced by the outcome in a patient who was operated on at our hospital. The tumor was still well delimited, although it had already substantially destroyed the coccyx and was encroaching upon the sacrum. In this instance meticulous block excision extending through the distal sacral segment apparently effected a cure; at all events, the patient was well, over five years later presented no indication whatsoever of local recurrence, and had surprisingly little residual disability (Fig. 22-5). It was not until nine years after surgery that the tumor recurred locally. Another encouraging case in point is that reported by Birrell,[1] in which, following excision of a small coccygeal chordoma, there was no recurrence after nine years' observation.

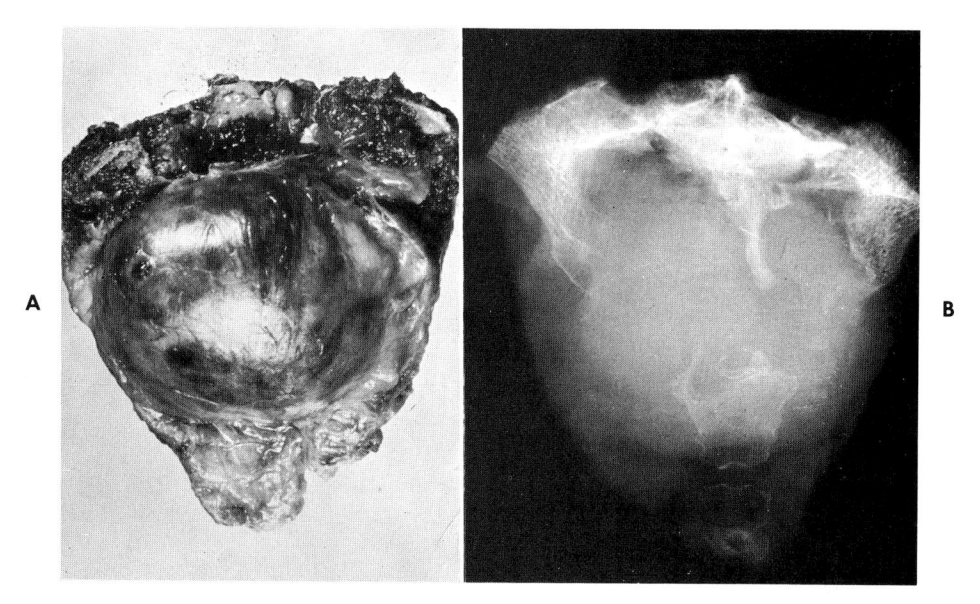

Fig. 22-5. **A**, Photograph of a successfully resected chordoma (viewed on its ventral aspect) that had destroyed much of the coccyx and extended into the distal sacral segment. (See text for details of this case.) **B**, Roentgenogram of the surgical specimen illustrated in **A**.

In the management of chordomas that are no longer amenable to successful treatment by surgery, cognizance should be taken of the claim of Friedman[5] that the result of high-voltage irradiation is substantially better than can be obtained by conventional technics. Therapists using supervoltage radiation may push the dose as high as 5,000 to 6,000 r to achieve symptomatic relief and some appreciable reduction in the size of the tumor mass.[8,11,15] That this entails some hazard is evidenced by the case reported by Fox, Batsakis, and Owano[4] in which, following irradiation of a chordoma at the level of D-12, a sarcoma developed three and one-half years later.

References

1. Birrell, J. H. W.: Chordomata; review of 19 cases of chordomata including 5 vertebral cases, Aust. N. Z. J. Surg. **22:**258, 1953.
2. Congdon, C. C.: Benign and malignant chordomas. A clinico-anatomical study of twenty-two cases, Am. J. Pathol. **28:**793, 1952.
3. Dahlin, D. C., and MacCarty, C. S.: Chordoma. A study of 59 cases, Cancer **5:**1170, 1952.
4. Fox, J. E., Batsakis, J. G., and Owano, L. R.: Unusual manifestations of chordoma, J. Bone Joint Surg. **50-A:**1618, 1968.
5. Friedman, M.: Technique of treatment of chordoma of a lumbar vertebra with 2 million volt x-rays using a rotation technique, Bull. Hosp. Joint Dis. **14:**180, 1953 (see also Radiology **64:**1, 1955).
6. Gentil, F., and Coley, B. L.: Sacrococcygeal chordoma, Ann. Surg. **127:**432, 1948.
7. Horwitz, T.: Chordal ectopia and its possible relationship to chordoma, Arch. Pathol. **31:**354, 1941.
8. Kamrin, R. P., Potanos, J. N., and Pool, J. L.: An evaluation of the diagnosis and treatment of chordoma, J. Neurol. Neurosurg. Psychiatry **27:**157, 1964.
9. Mabrey, R. E.: Chordoma: A study of 150 cases, Am. J. Cancer **25:**501, 1935.
10. Montgomery, A. H., and Wolman, I. J.: Sacrococcygeal chordomas in children, Am. J. Dis. Child. **46:**1263, 1933.

11. Pearlman, A. W., and Friedman, M.: Radical radiation therapy of chordoma, Radiology **108**:333, 1970.
12. Peña, C. E., Horvat, B. L., and Fischer, E. R.: The ultrastructure of chordoma, Am. J. Clin. Pathol. **53**:544, 1970.
13. Robbins, S. L.: Lumbar vertebral chordoma, Arch. Pathol. **40**:128, 1945.
14. Shepherd, J. A.: Sacrococcygeal chordoma, Brit. J. Surg. **42**:576, 1955.
15. Wang, C. C., and James, A. E., Jr.: Chordoma: brief review of the literature and report of a case with widespread metastases, Cancer **22**:162, 1968.
16. Willis, R. A.: Sacral chordoma with widespread metastases, J. Path. Bact. **33**:1035, 1930.

Chapter 23

Dermal inclusion tumors in bone (so-called adamantinoma of limb bones)

This chapter deals with the tumor category that, for almost sixty years, has been designated "adamantinoma" following the lead of Fischer.[10] These are among the more unusual tumors in bone, and only about 100 cases, more or less, have been recorded to date.[15] For many years it was thought that they developed only in the tibia. While the tibia is certainly the major site of predilection, recent experience has shown that occasionally the tumors in point may appear also in the forearm bones (ulna and radius), the fibula, the femur (Fig. 23-1), and possibly other bones (I have seen a probable instance in a pubic bone). It has become clear also that the alleged resemblance to adamantinoma (ameloblastoma) of jaw bones was a superficial one (Figs. 23-2 to 23-4); hence the qualification of so-called adamantinoma.

In these circumstances, it was inevitable that the pathogenesis of this peculiar tumor category would become the subject of controversy. One hypothesis advanced by Changus, Speed, and Stewart[5] maintains that so-called adamantinomas of long bones have a vascular genesis and actually represent malignant angioblastomas. It is undoutedly true that some hemangioendotheliomas are called "adamantinoma" simply because they are found in the tibia, and one must be circumspect about this possibility, using silver stains where indicated. On reviewing my material on hemangioendothelioma of bone, I found a number of tumors in various sites that might have been regarded as so-called adamantinoma by a casual observer, had they developed in the tibia. Another interesting suggestion put forth by Hicks[13] and by Lederer and Sinclair[14] is that so-called "adamantinoma" of the tibia is really synovial sarcoma in disguise. Here again, my response is that if you think you are dealing with a spindle-cell sarcoma, be it synovial or any other, call it that and not something else.

When one strips away the instances that do not really belong in the tumor category under discussion, one is left with a hard core of distinctive neoplasms that may be appropriately designated *dermal inclusion tumors.* Many of them

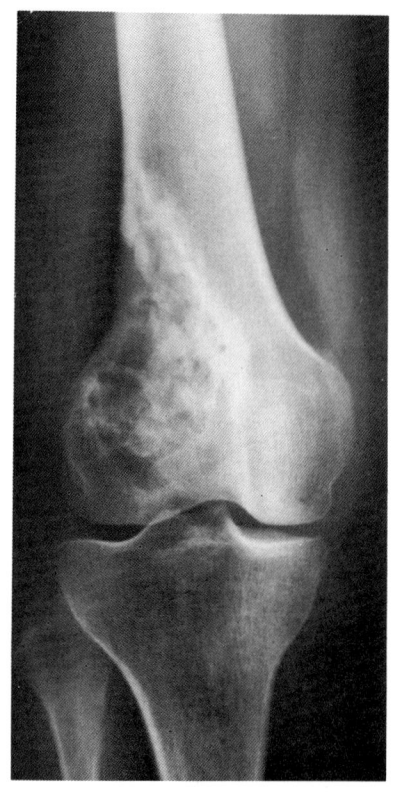

Fig. 23-1. Roentgenogram of an unusual tumor in the distal femur of a young adult, that proved to be a dermal inclusion tumor on microscopic examination (so-called adamantinoma).

resemble basal cell carcinoma (Fig. 23-4); some of them contain squamous cell nests; and occasional ones are reminiscent of adnexal skin tumors of sweat gland origin (Fig. 23-3). It seems logical to postulate that they have their origin in misplaced embryonal rests (the old Cohnheim theory). In this connection, recent electron microscopic studies[1,18] of tibial "adamantinomas" have supported the concept of an epithelial (rather than mesodermal) origin. Whether the tumors start on the outside or the inside of the affected bone and whether trauma plays a significant role[8,19] in some instances in instigating neoplastic growth during adolescence or early adult life are interesting subjects for speculation, though not of critical importance. In any event, I feel it is high time to break with tradition in the matter of nomenclature (calling a spade a spade) and to relegate the designation of "adamantinoma" (in limb bones) to the historical shelf of tumor pathology.

Clinically, one gathers that the tumors develop insidiously and slowly, often over a period of years, and manifest a tendency to gradual but progressive local invasion. From some of the recorded cases it is also known that the tumor is capable at times of extension to regional lymph nodes and even of metastasis

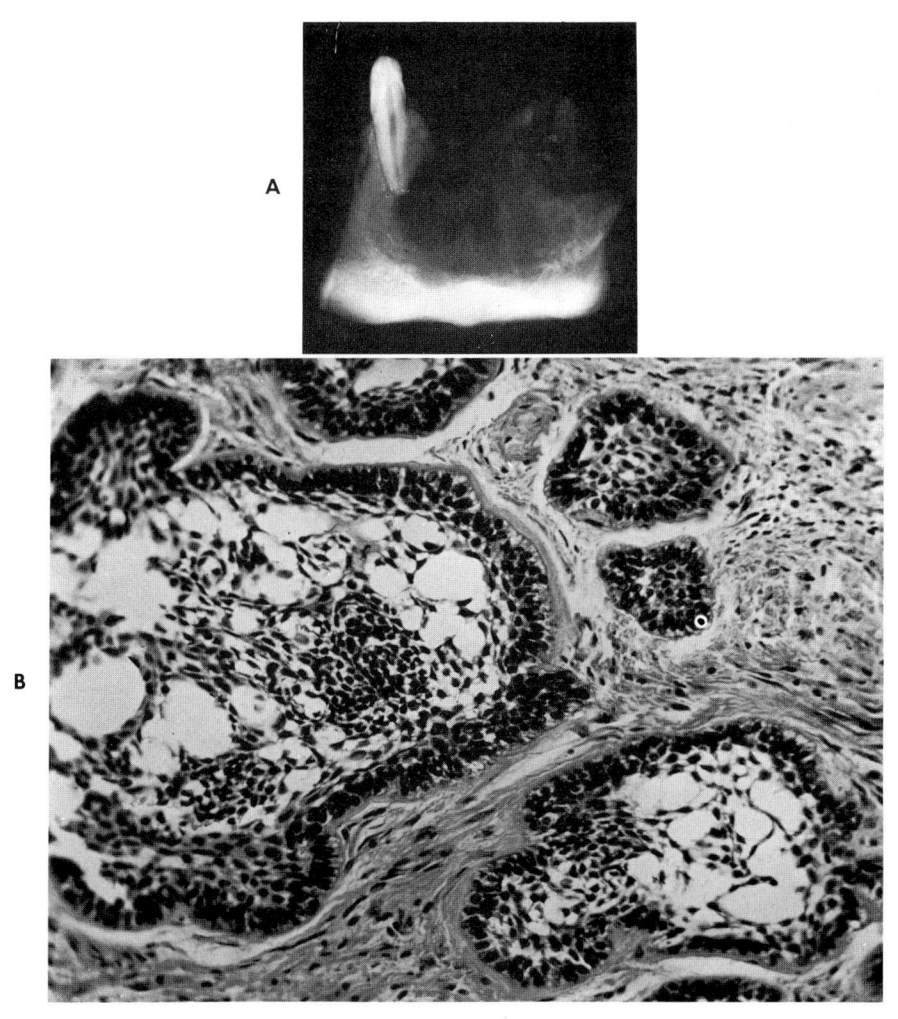

Fig. 23-2. **A**, Roentgenogram of a resected adamantinoma of a mandible. **B**, Photomicrograph of another adamantinoma of a mandible that was locally invasive and recurred twice after unsuccessful attempts at surgical extirpation. The tumor proved fatal after three years of treatment as a result of exsanguination, presumably due to erosion of a large blood vessel. No metastases were found at autopsy. This picture is presented for contrast with Figs. 23-3, *B*, and 23-4. (×200.)

to the lungs, and one must be alert to these possibilities. In a considerable number of the cases reported, though by no means all, the past history contains some reference to previous injury to the affected site, often an old healed fracture. The usual difficulties calling attention eventually to the presence of the lesion are pain and some swelling, induration of the affected limb, and occasionally pathologic fracture.

Roentgenographically, the tumor appears as a smaller or larger, finely trabeculated, expanded, rarefied lesion with a well-defined peripheral outline. The overlying cortex is likely to be attenuated and somewhat expanded, but is usually not broken through, unless there has been previous surgical intervention. Also, as a rule, one observes little, if any, spontaneous periosteal new bone reaction. If the tumor has been allowed to progress for a number of years, it may attain large size and come to involve a substantial or major part of the shaft of the affected bone. Thus, in the specimen described by Halpert and Dohn,[11] the tumor (in a tibia) measured fully 15 cm. in length; and in one reported by Anderson and Saunders,[2] it came eventually to involve as much as two thirds of the shaft (of an ulna). In such large specimens, one finds the shaft of the affected bone appreciably widened and otherwise deformed. Also, by the time amputation is resorted to, the tumor may already have extended through the cortex into the contiguous soft parts, sometimes spontaneously, but more often as a result of fracture or previous surgery. Altogether, the slow evolution of the lesion, its peculiar localization in the tibia (with few exceptions), and its roentgen picture, which is not calculated to suggest any other neoplasm in particular, should point to the possibility of a dermal inclusion tumor (so-called adamantinoma). Nevertheless, most cases are not recognized prior to biopsy, and some not even after biopsy is performed, because of unfamiliarity with the tumor or because the possibility is not considered, owing to its rarity.

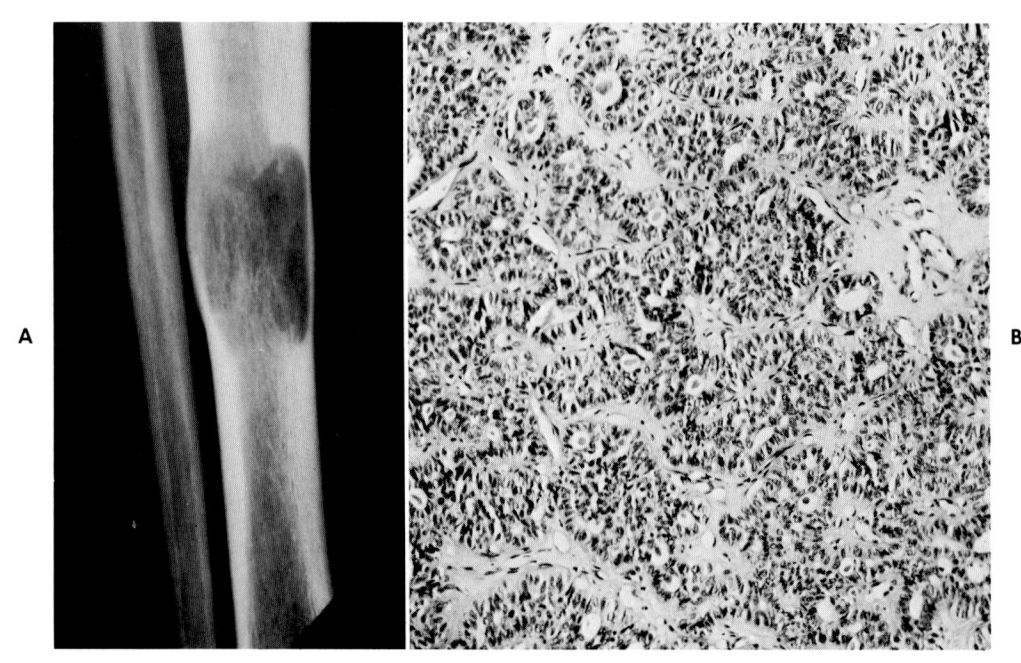

Fig. 23-3. A, Roentgenograms of a dermal inclusion tumor (so-called adamantinoma) within the shaft of a tibia of a 49-year-old woman, who had complained of pain for about one and one-half years. B, Photomicrograph of a representative field of the tumor illustrated in A. Note the numerous small alveolar or glandlike structures, many of which contain secretion. The picture is reminiscent of an adnexal skin tumor of sweat gland origin. (×150.)

On examination of biopsy material or of an amputation specimen, one observes that the tumor tissue, if its appearance has not been altered by previous treatment, is gray or gray-white and is rather firm in consistency. Its histologic appearance may vary from specimen to specimen and even in different fields of the same specimen. In places, one may observe a suggestive glandular pattern, which may be mistaken for metastatic adenocarcinoma by the unwary (Fig. 23-3). In other fields, as noted, one may be impressed by the resemblance to a basal-cell tumor growing in strands or nests, which may exhibit pseudoglandular or cystic change (Fig. 23-4). In still other fields of one specimen or another, the tumor may appear epidermoid and exhibit suggestive pearl formation, so that it may be mistaken for squamous-cell epithelioma invading bone, if one has not inquired into the pertinent clinical findings.

In regard to treatment, it should be emphasized that the tumor tissue is highly radioresistant, and that surgical excision or ablation affords the only means of cure. If a dermal inclusion tumor of a limb bone is approached for the first time and is still relatively small and localized, one may be justified in advocating block excision of the tumor focus in an attempt to salvage the limb. On the other hand, if this procedure should prove unsuccessful, or if, when the

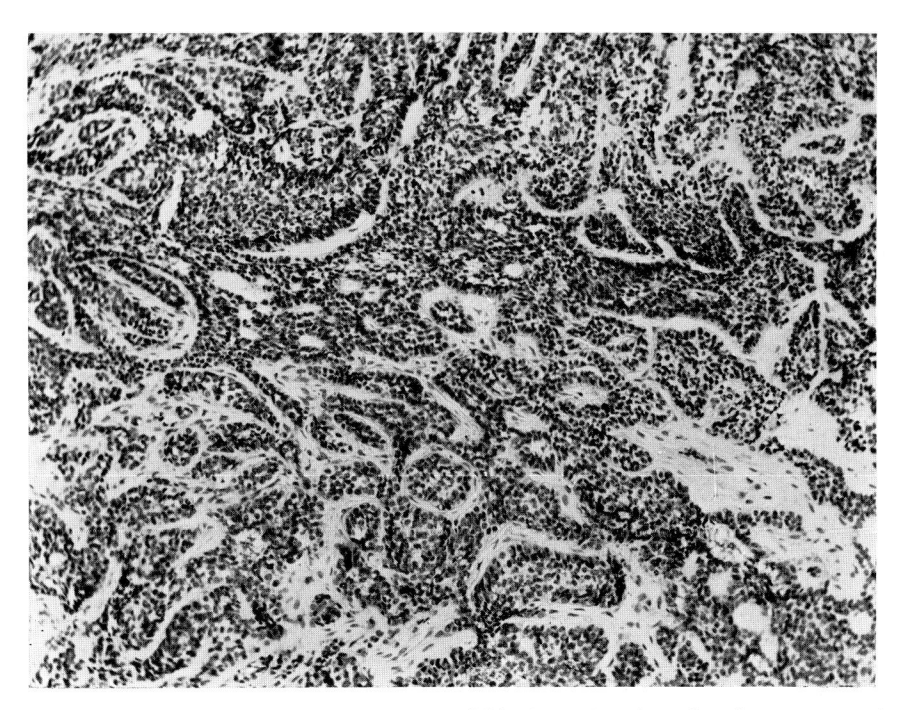

Fig. 23-4. Photomicrograph of a representative field of another dermal inclusion tumor (so-called adamantinoma) of a tibia (one of the two cases reported by Wolfort and Sloane, which eventually came to amputation after unsuccessful attempts at local resection and reconstruction). (×100.)

tumor is explored, it is found to have already invaded too widely to make resection feasible, amputation should be resorted to without undue delay. Repeated experience with such cases has clearly demonstrated the futility of compromising with the necessity for radical surgery. This point has been stressed by Anderson and Saunders,[2] Dockerty and Meyerding,[8] and Halpert and Dohn,[11] among others. Also, in the two cases reported by Wolfort and Sloane,[22] which I had occasion to review, repeated attempts at local excision of the tumor and reconstruction proved unsuccessful and led eventually to amputation for recurrent tumor, after the patients had been subjected to several years of needless disability. The feeling of complacency once held in regard to these tumors and the leisurely approach it engendered are no longer justified. As noted, clinical follow-up data are slowly accumulating to indicate that they not only tend regularly to recur (locally), but may also extend to regional lymph nodes and even metastasize to the lungs. The importance of prompt ablation of the affected extremity, once the diagnosis is clearly established, is thus heavily underscored.

References

1. Albores Saavedra, J., Díaz Gutiérrez, D., and Altamirano Dimas, M.: Adamantinoma de la tibia. Observaciones ultrastucturales, Rev. Med. hosp. Gral. Mex. 31:241, 1968.
2. Anderson, C. E., and Saunders, J. B. de C. M.: Primary adamantinoma of the ulna, Surg. Gynecol. Obstet. 75:351, 1942.
3. Baker, P. L., Dockerty, M. B., and Coventry, M. B.: Adamantinoma (so-called) of the long bones. Review of the literature and a report of three new cases, J. Bone Joint Surg. 36-A:704, 1954.
4. Campanacci, M., Giunti, A., and Leonessa, C.: Adamantinoma delle ossa lunghi, Chir, d. org. di movimento 58:385, 1969.
5. Changus, G. W., Speed, J. S., and Stewart, F. W.: Malignant angioblastoma of bone. A reappraisal of adamantinoma of long bone, Cancer 10:540, 1957.
6. Cohen, D. M., Dahlin, D. C., and Pugh, D. G.: Fibrous dysplasia associated with adamantinoma of the long bones, Cancer 15:515, 1962.
7. Coley, B. L.: Neoplasms of bone and related conditions. Their etiology, pathogenesis, diagnosis and treatment, New York, 1949, Paul B. Hoeber, Inc. (see Fig. 113).
8. Dockerty, M. B., and Meyerding, H. W.: Adamantinoma of the tibia. Report of two new cases, J.A.M.A. 119:932, 1942.
9. Elliott, G. B.: Malignant angioblastoma of long bone. So-called "tibial adamantinoma," J. Bone Joint Surg. 44-B:25, 1962.
10. Fischer, B.: Frankfurt, Ztschr. f. allg. Path. 12:422, 1913.
11. Halpert, B., and Dohn, H. P.: Adamantinoma in the tibia, Arch. Pathol. 43:313, 1947.
12. Hebbel, R.: Adamantinoma of the tibia, Surgery 7:860, 1940 (compilation of reported cases).
13. Hicks, J. D.: Synovial sarcoma of tibia, J. Path. Bact. 67:151, 1954.
14. Lederer, H., and Sinclair, A. J.: Malignant synovioma simulating "adamantinoma of tibia," J. Path. Bact. 67:163, 1954.
15. Moon, N. F.: Adamantinoma of the appendicular skeleton. A statistical review of reported cases and inclusion of 10 new cases, Clin. Orthop. 43:189, 1965.
16. Morgan, A. D., and Mackenzie, D. H.: A metastasizing adamantinoma of the tibia, J. Bone Joint Surg. 38-B:892, 1956.
17. Naji, A. F., Murphy, J. A., Stasney, R. J., Neville, W. E., and Chrenka, P.: So-called adamantinoma of long bones. Report of a case with massive pulmonary metastases, J. Bone Joint Surg. 46-A:151, 1964.
18. Rosai, J.: Adamantinoma of the tibia. Electron microscopic evidence of its epithelial origin, Am. J. Clin. Pathol. 51:786, 1969.
19. Ryrie, B. J.: Adamantinoma of the tibia, Brit. Med. J. 2:1000, 1932.
20. Thoma, K. H.: Oral surgery, ed. 5, St. Louis, 1964, The C. V. Mosby Co.
21. Willis, R. A.: Pathology of tumours, St. Louis, 1953, The C. V. Mosby Co.
22. Wolfort, B., and Sloane, D.: Adamantinoma of tibia; report of 2 cases, J. Bone Joint Surg. 20:1011, 1938.

Chapter 24

Other rare malignant tumors in bone

For the sake of completeness and to provide a frame of reference for reports in the future, this brief section will take cognizance of several additional malignant tumors of bone, although recorded experience with them is still limited apparently to a few random observations.

Leiomyosarcoma of bone

The major reference here is to a well-documented and convincing report by Evans and Sanerkin[1] in 1965 of a large, destructive, lytic tumor in the upper tibia of a man of 73, that was interpreted pathologically as a primary leiomyosarcoma of bone. They were able to demonstrate myofibrils in this spindle-cell tumor, as well as a tendency to arrangement in muscle-like bundles in the better-differentiated areas. Thorough necropsy examination failed to turn up a primary tumor elsewhere, and the possibility of secondary invasion of bone by a deep-seated soft-tissue leiomyosarcoma was likewise ruled out. To be sure, this advanced neoplasm had penetrated the cortex and invaded the parosteal tissues circumferentially, but it undoubtedly arose within the bone.

In attempting to explain the histogenesis of a tumor such as this, as the authors indicated, one must, of necessity, assume that it arose from proliferating smooth muscle cells in the media of a blood vessel, either *de novo* or conceivably through malignant change in a preexisting angioleiomyoma.

Evans and Sanerkin[1] also quote Stout as saying that he had seen a leiomyosarcoma in the fibula of an elderly woman, but gave no details. Continuing, Stout and Lattes,[6] in their A.F.I.P. Fascicle on "Tumors of the Soft Tissues," stated, apropos of leiomyosarcoma, that "in infants they may arise in the prostate and urinary bladder and *rarely in bone.*" This observation is not documented either.

In going through my consultation files, I found two relevant neoplasms. One was a (resected) tumor in a proximal fibula that I had interpreted as a low-grade, primary leiomyosarcoma of bone; this was an old case, and further details, unfortunately, are no longer available. The other was an unusual tumor in a proximal phalanx of a toe, sections of which showed a vasoformative tumor, with actively proliferating smooth muscle cells within and around the vascular channels, so that it was held to represent an early angioleiomyosarcoma.

Rhabdomyosarcoma

Rhabdomyosarcoma, when deep-seated, may sometimes erode the underlying bone, and, of course, it may spread to bone, among other sites, by metastasis. However, I have never seen it as a primary neoplasm arising within bone, nor have I found any reference to it, as such. On the other hand, it may, on rare occasions, appear as an integral component of a malignant mesenchymoma of bone (see below).

Alveolar soft-part sarcoma (malignant granular-cell tumor, malignant granular-cell myoblastoma, malignant nonchromaffin paraganglioma)

On rare occasions, one may encounter a tumor resembling alveolar soft-part sarcoma, so-called, that appears to be primary in bone. I have seen sections of one such neoplasm (in the distal femur of a young woman, in whom intensive clinical search failed to detect a primary site elsewhere). Professor M. Campanacci, of Bologna, has called my attention to several other comparable instances (as yet unpublished). One must be circumspect, however, about assuming that such tumors are necessarily primary in nature, without conclusive evidence, inasmuch as alveolar soft-part sarcomas may extend to bone from a contiguous, deep-seated extraosseous site, or may eventually spread to bone by metastasis from a cryptic primary focus elsewhere.

Malignant mesenchymoma of bone

Another unusual category of malignant tumors in bone comprises those with two or more different mesenchymal components, and malignant mesenchymoma is an acceptable, convenient designation for them.

In the chapter on liposarcoma (page 333) I gave a concise account of a mesenchymoma of bone arising in the upper tibia that was composed of malignant embryonal fat tissue and osteogenic sarcoma in both its primary and metastatic sites. This particular combination of liposarcoma and osteosarcoma was found also in the cases recently reported by Schajowicz, Cuevillas, and Silberman[4] and by Ross and Hadfield.[3] All these tumors developed in one or another lower limb bone of teen-agers. Still another reported by Sterns, Haust, and Wollin[5] appeared in a mandible, again in a boy of 15.

That the pattern can be more varied than this, however, is indicated by the composition of three other mesenchymomas of bone in my files. One in the ischium of a man of 64 showed, in addition to a major component resembling low-grade fibrosarcoma, occasional foci of bone formation and also giant-cell fields, which appeared clearly tumorous rather than reactive. Another mesenchymoma, in the pubic bone of a young man of 23, contained, in addition to fields of osteogenic sarcoma, large multinuclear "strap" cells apparently indicative of rhabdomyosarcoma, and also occasional giant vacuolated cells resembling lipoblasts.

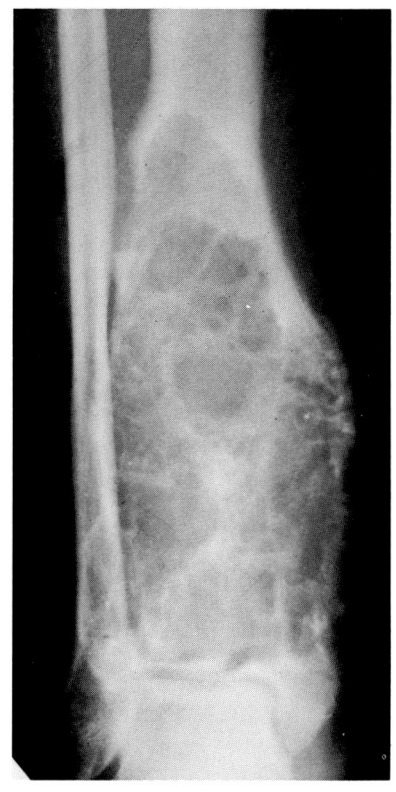

Fig. 24-1. Roentgenogram of a malignant mesenchymoma in the distal tibia of an adult, which on tissue examination showed several different connective tissue components.

Still another, in the distal tibia of an adult (Fig. 24-1), likewise showed several malignant connective tissue components other than fibrosarcoma.

It would appear from our limited experience to date that these malignant mesenchymomas of bone can be aggressive and prone to metastasize, although one can hardly lay down any reliable guidelines at this time. It is noteworthy that, in dealing with malignant mesenchymomas of soft tissues, the fatality rate in adults has been estimated[6] to be as high as 60%, and in children, 40%.

References
1. Evans, D. M. D., and Sanerkin, N. G.: Primary leiomyosarcoma of bone, J. Pathol. 90:348, 1965.
2. Lichtenstein, L.: Bone tumors, ed. 3, St. Louis, 1965, The C. V. Mosby Co. (see p. 314).
3. Ross, C. F., and Hadfield, G.: Primary osteo-liposarcoma of bone (malignant mesenchymoma), J. Bone Joint Surg. 50-B: 639, 1968.
4. Schajowicz, F., Cuevillas, A. R., and Silberman, F. S.: Primary malignant mesenchymoma of bone, Cancer 19:1423, 1966.
5. Sterns, E. E., Haust, M. D., and Wollin, D. G.: Malignant mesenchymoma of the mandible, Can. J. Surg. 12:444, 1969.
6. Stout, A. P., and Lattes, R.: Tumors of the soft tissues. Fascicle 1, Atlas of tumor pathology, Armed Forces Institute of Pathology, 1967 (see p. 127).
7. Dutt, A. K., Balasegaram, M., and Bin Din, O.: Alveolar soft-part sarcoma with invasion of bone. A case report, J. Bone Joint Surg. 51:765, 1969.

Chapter 25

Carcinoma metastatic to the skeleton

Metastatic carcinoma is by far the most common malignant bone tumor, and, as such, must weigh heavily in any consideration of differential diagnosis. The pertinent literature that has developed through the years is too voluminous to review here—literally thousands of papers have been written on the subject—nor would it be particularly profitable to do so, except to comment on some significant recent advances in therapy, notably hormonal therapy for prostatic and breast cancer and other endocrine-sensitive tumors. I will be content to record certain impressions, gleaned empirically for the most part, relating to the recognition and treatment of metastatic foci in the skeleton, particularly from such primary sites as the breast, prostate, lung, kidney, and thyroid, among others.

It appears to be valid and useful to distinguish between carcinoma involving contiguous bones by direct extension and that spreading by hematogenous dissemination. As rather well-known instances of the former, one may cite erosion of the facial bones or calvarium by burrowing squamous or basisquamous carcinoma of the skin; invasion of the maxilla or mandible by squamous-cell carcinoma of the mouth, tongue, and occasionally the lip; erosion of the maxillary, ethmoid, and nasal bones as well as of the base of the skull by tumors of the nasopharynx; invasion and partial destruction of ribs and chest wall by direct extension of carcinoma originating in the lung or breast; invasion and collapse of cervical vertebrae by Pancoast tumor; extension of advanced bladder carcinoma into the pubic bones; and also extension of advanced rectal carcinoma to the pelvic bones or sacrum and coccyx.

The incidence of metastasis to the skeleton by carcinoma in general, from whatever primary site, is probably greatly underestimated. Only a limited number of such foci manifest themselves clinically through the development of severe pain, a palpable tumor mass, pathologic fracture (usually of a rib or a long bone), or neurologic manifestations of compression of the spinal cord or its nerve roots as a result of vertebral column involvement. Many more give rise to only a vague awareness of their presence or are entirely occult. If one resorts to roentgen skeletal survey, many additional carcinoma foci may come to light, but one must recognize that roentgen examination alone has inherent limitations also and does not necessarily begin to indicate the full extent of skeletal involvement. Another

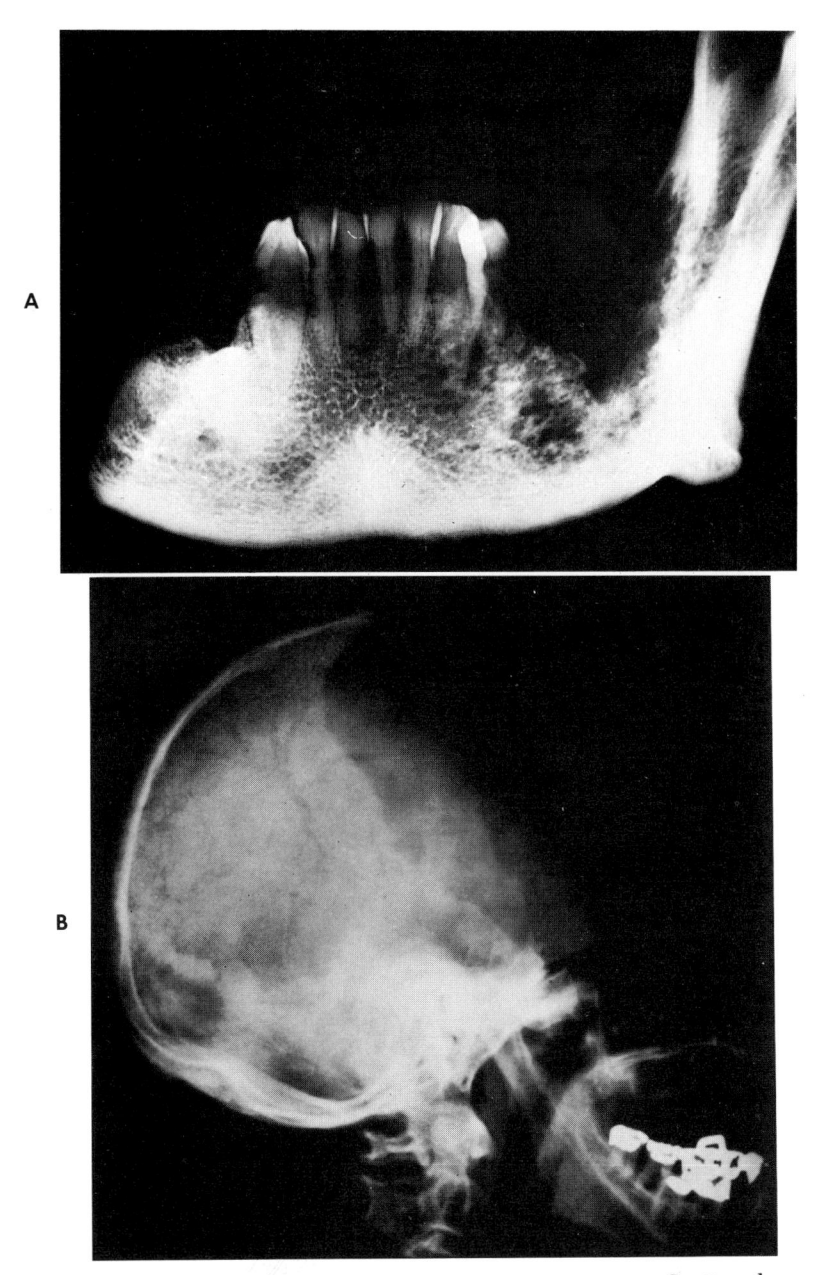

Continued.

Fig. 25-1. **A,** Roentgenogram of a resected mandible showing moth-eaten rarefaction and destruction reflecting invasion by squamous-cell carcinoma originating in the floor of the mouth. **B,** Roentgenogram showing striking osteolysis of the anterior half of the calvarium by meningioma *en placque.* I call this "the case of the disappearing calvarium." The tumor originated apparently in the nasal vault and slowly spread through the bone over a period of several years. **C,** Roentgenogram of the upper humerus of an adult showing a destructive tumor focus, which proved to be malignant melanoma on biopsy. The primary site could not be identified clinically. **D,** Roentgenogram of another focus of malignant melanoma (pigmented) in the body of T-8. The diagnosis was established by needle biopsy, and no other bone lesions were found on skeletal roentgen survey. Twenty years previously, the patient had had enucleation of an eye for melanoma of the choroid.

354 Bone tumors

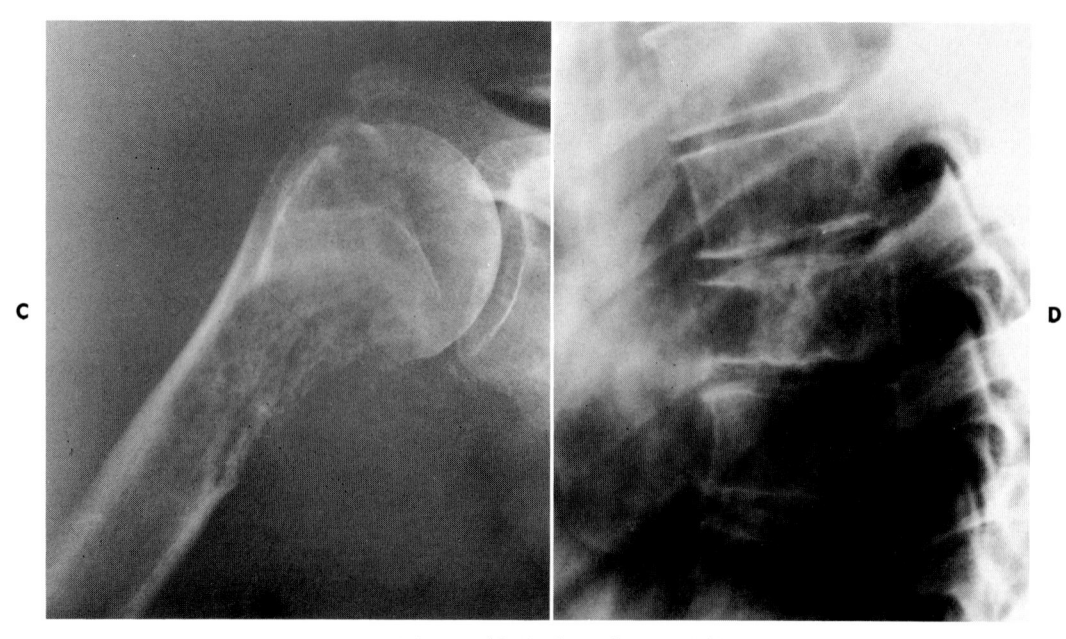

Fig. 25-1, cont'd. For legend see p. 353.

clinical aid to the recognition of early skeletal metastases recently advocated by Sklaroff and Charkes[20] is photoscanning with strontium 85. Other radioisotopes with relatively short half-lives, such as ^{87m}Sr, gallium 67, and fluorine 18, have also been introduced, and this promising approach to the detection of occult metastases is currently under active investigation.[15]

Also noteworthy here is the finding of elevated hydroxyproline excretion in the urine of adult patients with skeletal tumors. In general, the excretion of this amino acid in peptide form appears to be a measure of bone collagen turnover, but there are so many variable factors influencing this that the observation has not yet had widespread clinical application.

To what extent the spread of carcinoma to the skeleton is revealed by autopsy depends obviously upon the thoroughness with which the bones are examined, grossly and microscopically. It is unfortunately true, for one reason or another, that the skeleton is regarded by many pathologists as a sacred cow and its examination is usually limited to taking a slice of the ventral aspect of a few lumbar vertebral bodies, occasionally supplemented by inspection of the sternum or of one or two ribs. It is significant, therefore, to point out that in a survey of the metastases in carcinoma based upon an analysis of 1,000 autopsied cases, Abrams, Spiro, and Goldstein[1] found the incidence of widespread metastases, including those in the skeleton, to be substantially higher than the literature would lead one to believe. Their findings reflect the meticulous care and thoroughness in the performance of autopsies, which are traditional at the Montefiore Hospital (New York City). Specifically, in their large series of cancer pa-

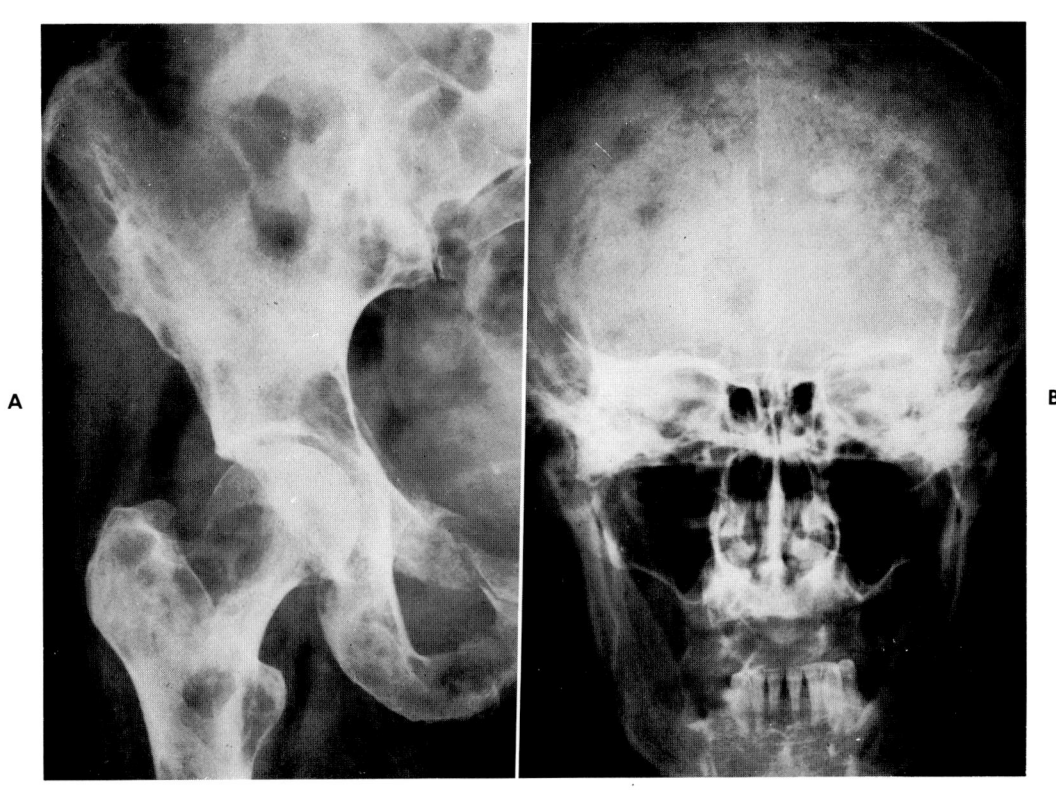

Fig. 25-2. **A**, Roentgenogram showing widespread lytic defects and a number of pathologic fractures resulting from skeletal metastasis of a breast carcinoma. **B**, Calvarium from another case of breast carcinoma showing multiple lytic defects representing metastases.

tients, 27% of the entire group showed skeletal metastases. Their analysis also revealed that over two thirds of the breast carcinomas, approximately one third of the lung tumors, and one fourth of the renal tumors had spread to one or more bones. It showed further that carcinoma in still other sites not ordinarily thought of as spreading to the skeleton had nevertheless done so in an appreciable number of instances (e.g., pancreas 13%, rectum 13%, stomach 11%, colon 9%, ovary 9%). In the same connection, it is also pertinent to point out, as is well known, that thyroid carcinoma often metastasizes to one, several, or many bones, and that more than half of all prostatic carcinomas likewise spread to the skeleton, particularly to the pelvis and lumbar vertebral column. What is perhaps not generally appreciated is that neoplasms of the testis (be they seminomas, embryonal carcinomas, or teratocarcinomas) also metastasize not infrequently to the skeleton, particularly to the spine. Malignant melanoma may likewise do so, especially in its late phase of widespread dissemination, and it is interesting to note in this connection that some of the bone metastases may be heavily pigmented while others may be virtually nonpigmented, as observed, for instance, in adjacent bodies of a vertebral column specimen. On occasion, a destructive

356 Bone tumors

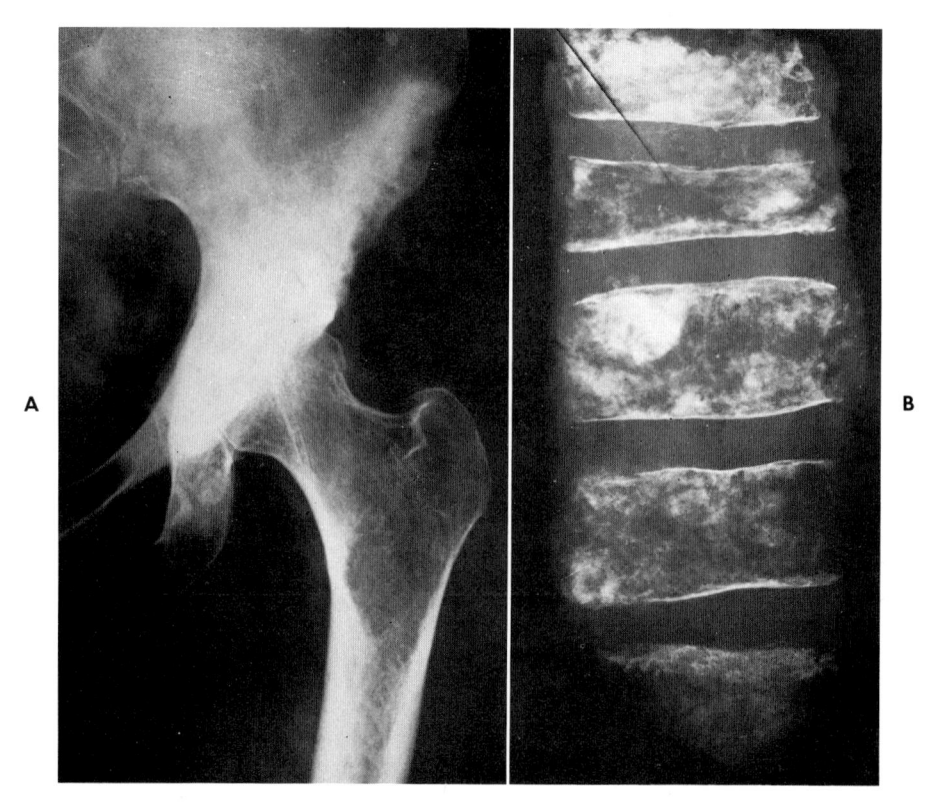

Fig. 25-3. **A,** Roentgenogram from still another instance of carcinoma of the breast with widespread skeletal metastases showing a lytic focus in the upper femur and a sclerosing one in the adjacent innominate bone. **B,** A segment of the spine from the same subject showing compression of the vertebral bodies and the presence of both osteolytic and osteoplastic metastases.

skeletal tumor may be the initial manifestation of disseminated melanoma (Fig. 25-1, C and D). Even malignant carcinoid tumors may sometimes spread to the skeleton, as may alveolar soft-part sarcoma, and, without detailing further specific instances, suffice it to state that on occasion virtually every malignant neoplasm may do so, some more often than others.

It is pertinent also to comment briefly upon the matter of localization in one part of the skeleton or another. The predilection of carcinoma metastases for the innominate bones, the vertebral column, and the ribs is well known. It is not generally appreciated, perhaps, that the calvarium also is not infrequently involved (e.g., by thyroid carcinoma) and that sometimes it may be so riddled by osteolytic defects as to simulate the picture usually held to be typical of multiple myeloma (Fig. 25-12). Also, if one is willing to search for it, involvement of long limb bones and of the bones of the shoulder girdle is not infrequently observed. As for the remainder of the skeleton, it is generally held that it is distinctly unusual to find skeletal metastases below the elbows and knees, and yet such are the vagaries of carcinoma metastasis that Dr. G. J. Hummer, of Los Angeles, has

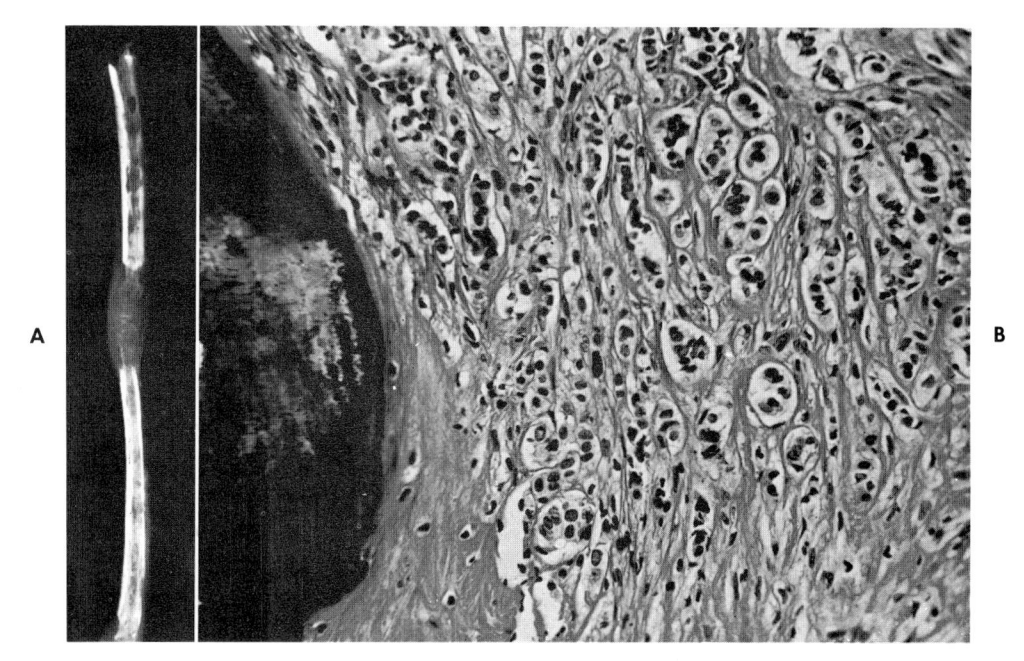

Fig. 25-4. **A**, Roentgenogram of a rib from the case illustrated in Fig. 25-3, showing multiple lytic defects including one that has destroyed a short segment of the rib. **B**, Photomicrograph of a biopsy specimen of a lytic rib lesion in a comparable case, showing replacement of the spongy bone and marrow by undifferentiated scirrhous carcinoma. (×200.)

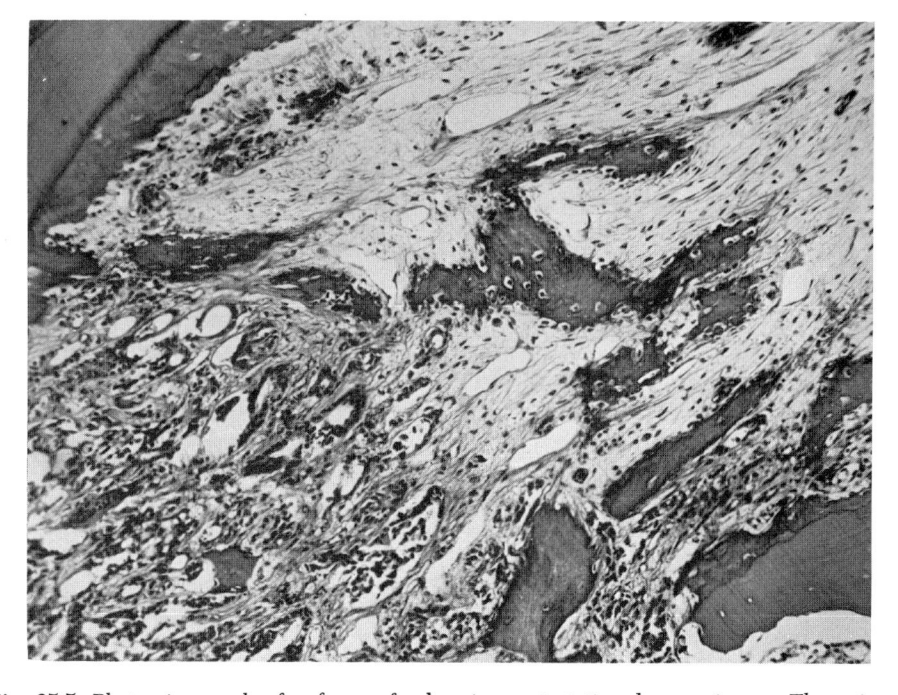

Fig. 25-5. Photomicrograph of a focus of sclerosing metastatic adenocarcinoma. The primary tumor was in the cecum. (×125.)

358   Bone tumors

had occasion to observe an instance of carcinoma of the colon that metastasized to the bones of both hands and feet. With reference to the hand and wrist particularly, some thirty-four such cases had been collected[7] as of 1963.

The roentgen picture produced by carcinoma foci in the skeleton is much too varied to permit formulation of any integrated comprehensive description. By the same token, it is difficult to surmise except in a few special instances (e.g., prostatic carcinoma and sometimes renal or thyroid carcinoma[17,18]) what the primary site of any given carcinoma may be from the roentgen appearance of its skeletal metastases. In fact, it may be difficult in any specific instance to distinguish clearly a single focus of metastatic carcinoma from a primary malignant tumor of bone, e.g., a solitary myeloma or, on occasion, even osteogenic sarcoma. All that one can say with any assurance in such cases is that one is dealing with a malignant neoplasm, and that biopsy is indicated for definitive diagnosis. For such lesions suspected of being foci of metastatic carcinoma, aspiration biopsy has been advocated rather than open biopsy, and Coley[3] has

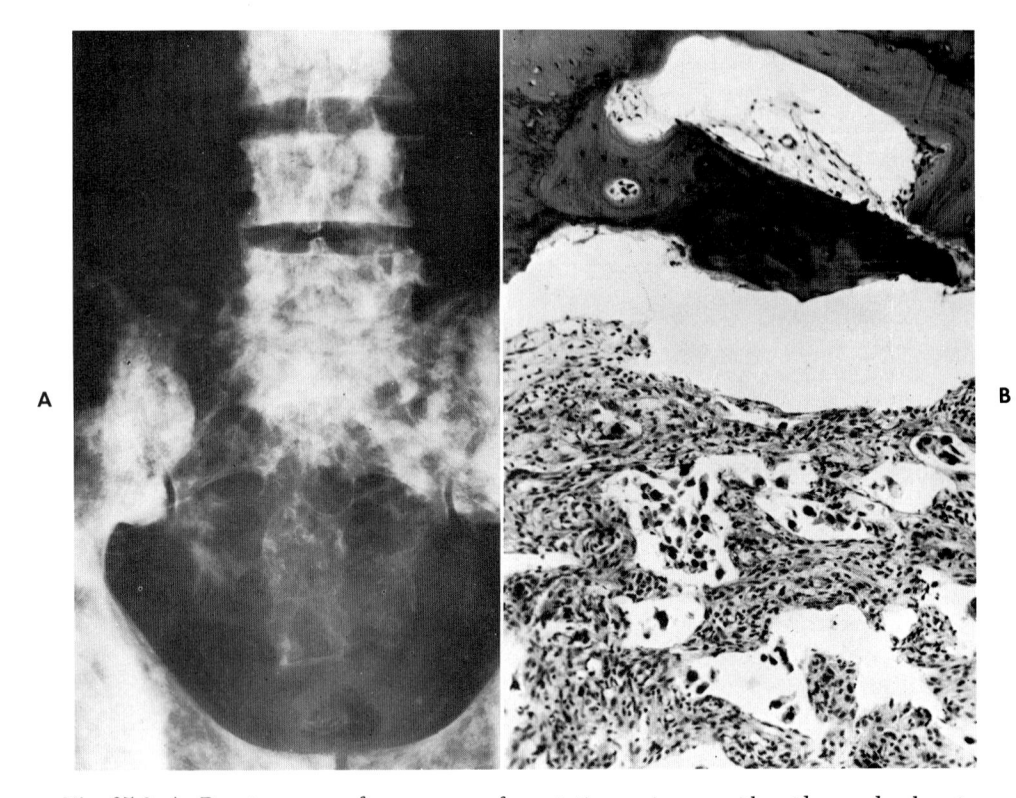

Fig. 25-6. **A,** Roentgenogram from a case of prostatic carcinoma with widespread sclerosing metastases in the spine and pelvis. This patient had received the benefit of estrogen therapy, but succumbed after several years from the effects of visceral metastasis. **B,** Photomicrograph of a needle aspiration biopsy of an involved lumbar vertebral body in another instance of prostatic carcinoma. (×100.)

claimed a high degree of accuracy for this procedure (90 of 107 cases, or 84%). Further, as is well known, multiple punched-out defects of metastatic carcinoma must be distinguished particularly from those of multiple myeloma, and this differentiation is not invariably simple, at least from the roentgenograms alone. Also, as has been pointed out elsewhere, an unrecognized small primary carcinoma (e.g., in a small-order branch bronchus or in the gastric mucosa) may sometimes give rise to widespread skeletal metastases, and the latter may then be misinterpreted as lesions of Ewing's sarcoma.

It is customary in describing carcinoma metastases in the skeleton to distinguish between those that are essentially destructive (osteolytic) and those that provoke significant reactive osteosclerosis (osteoplastic). Actually, the great majority of carcinoma metastases in bone are lytic in their effect, and only in dealing with prostatic carcinoma does one consistently observe osteosclerotic reaction, although breast and urinary bladder cancers, and, occasionally, tumors arising in other primary sites, may have this effect. Moreover, this distinction

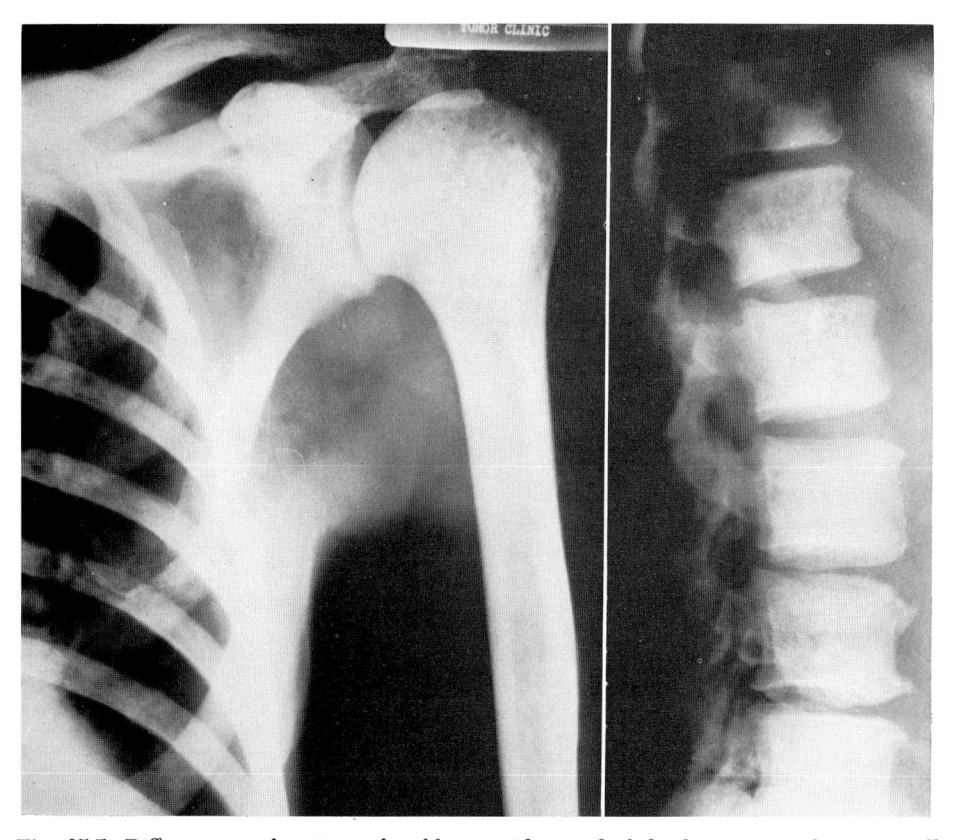

Fig. 25-7. Diffuse osteosclerosis attributable to widespread skeletal metastasis from a small gastric carcinoma, the presence of which was not recognized until autopsy was performed. The provisional clinical impression was marble bone disease or possibly endemic fluorosis.

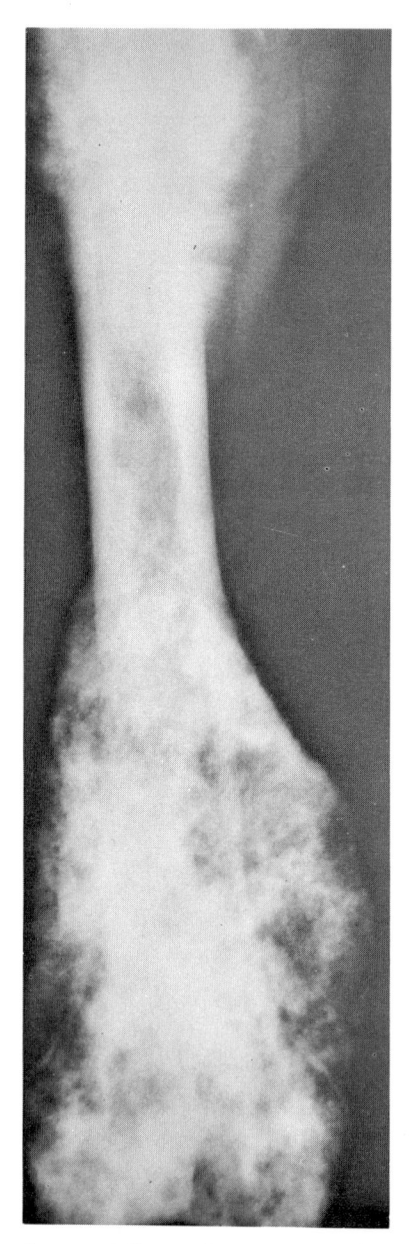

Fig. 25-8. Roentgenogram of a prostatic carcinoma metastatic to a femur, provoking such marked new bone reaction as to simulate osteogenic sarcoma.

Carcinoma metastatic to the skeleton 361

is a relative one, in the sense that a breast cancer, for instance, may give rise to osteolytic metastases in some bones and osteoplastic metastases in other bones in the same case (Fig. 25-3).

Some consideration should be given to certain blood chemical findings as they relate to diagnosis and particularly to significant alterations in the values of serum calcium, phosphorus, and phosphatase activity. The serum calcium level may remain within normal limits even in the face of obvious skeletal metastases, although, not infrequently, it is slightly elevated and occasionally, especially when the vertebral column is undergoing rapid demineralization, it may be very significantly increased to 16 mg. or more. In such cases, as in comparable instances of multiple myeloma, one may observe conspicuous calcium deposition in the renal pelvis and tubules, the lungs, and sometimes the gastrointestinal tract as well. Cognizance must also be taken of certain lung cancers, particularly, that induce significant hypercalcemia by elaborating a parathormone-like sub-

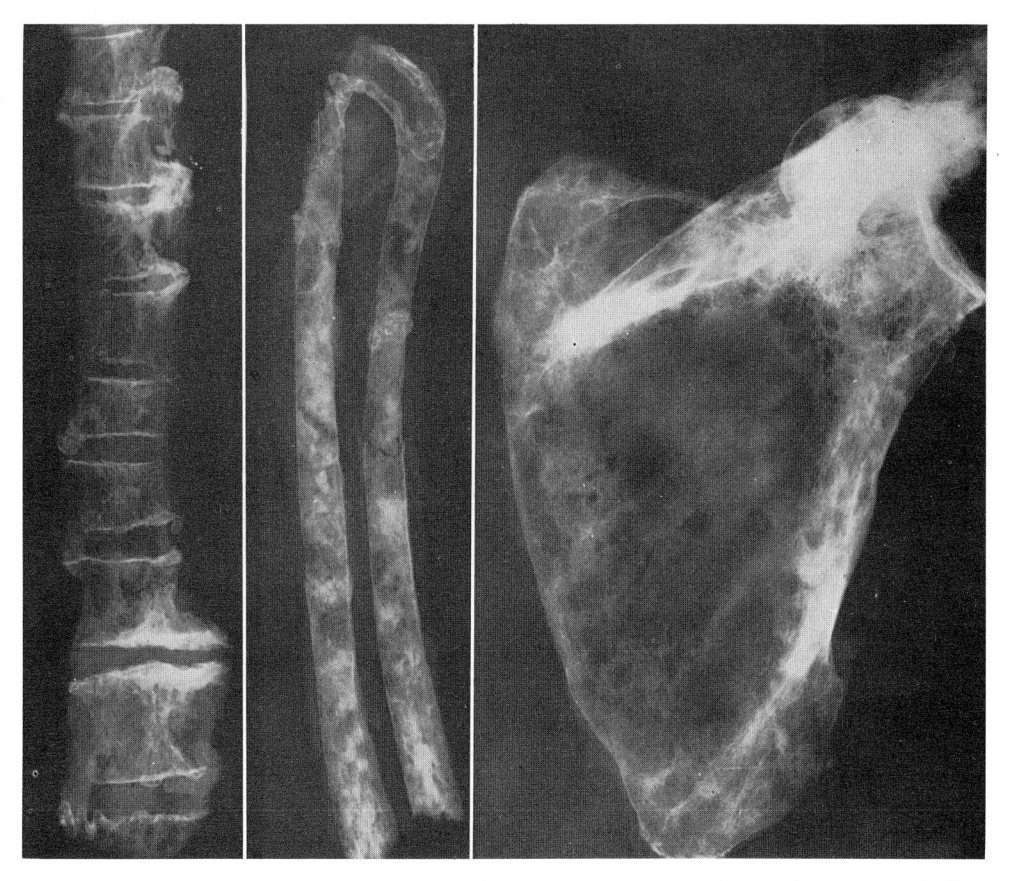

Fig. 25-9. Roentgenograms from an autopsied case of prostatic carcinoma showing punched-out lytic defects (in the scapula), as well as the usual osteoplastic metastases (in the vertebral column and ribs).

stance. Collaterally, one must note the value of steroids in such cases in bringing the serum calcium level down and thereby preventing serious renal damage and other untoward side effects (Fig. 25-17). In breast cancer, the osteolytic effect and concomitant hypercalcemia have been ascribed by Gordan[8] to the production of osteolytic phytosterols with a vitamin D–like action on bone. Incidentally, these sterols may on occasion be responsible apparently for resorptive ("cystic") lesions in the bones, which do *not* contain metastatic carcinoma.[10] The serum phosphorus level is not likely to be significantly increased unless there has been concomitant renal damage and associated phosphate retention. As for the serum alkaline phosphatase activity, slight or appreciable increases are not infrequently observed, particularly if pathologic fractures have occurred and if the skeletal metastases have provoked bone formation. One must be wary, however, of ascribing such increased values to skeletal metastases alone, unless one can rule out the possibility of liver metastases. In the presence of well-established osteoplastic metastases, particularly from prostatic cancer, appreciable though not necessarily dramatic elevations of serum alkaline phosphatase activity are to be expected, and in such cases, values of 10 to 20 or more Bodansky units are not

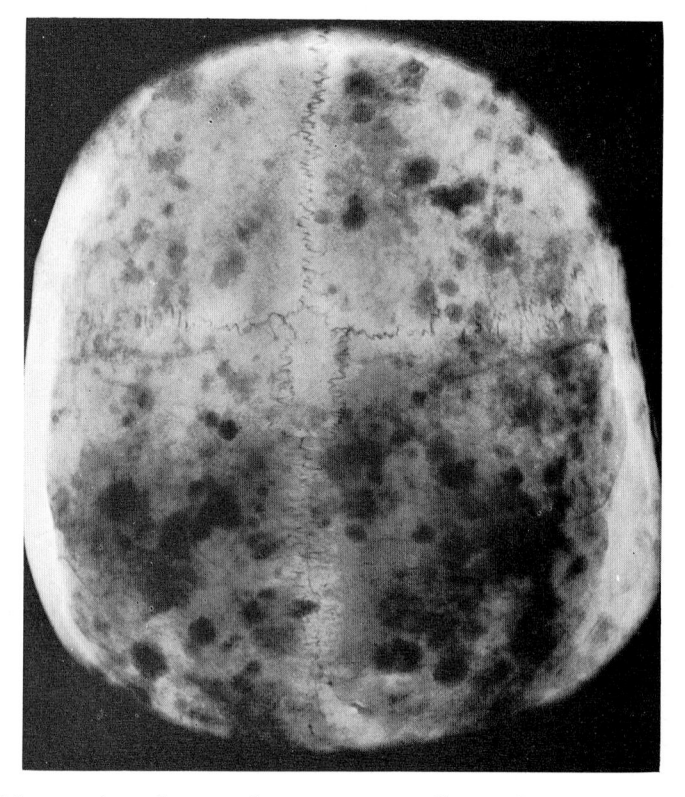

Fig. 25-10. Calvarium from the case of prostatic cancer illustrated in Fig. 25-9 showing widespread, well-defined lytic defects indistinguishable from those commonly encountered in multiple myeloma.

unusual. Also in cases of prostatic carcinoma invading the surrounding soft tissues and metastasizing to the spine and pelvis, significant elevation of the serum acid phosphatase level is commonly observed, although this does not occur in every instance, while the extent of the elevation, when present, varies from case to case. With clinical remission following estrogen therapy or castration, one may anticipate a prompt and sharp fall in the serum acid phosphatase value, although the alkaline phosphatase level may rise for a time as a reflection of tumor necrosis and accelerated calcification and ossification of osseous metastases.[12]

In regard to therapy also, attention should be directed to the well-known observation that castration, roentgen sterilization, and steroid therapy may, in some instances at least, bring about temporary regression of skeletal metastases from breast carcinoma, although the metastases elsewhere are not likely to be significantly influenced. In premenopausal women whose disease is beyond surgical or roentgen therapy, castration is held to be the most effective treatment.

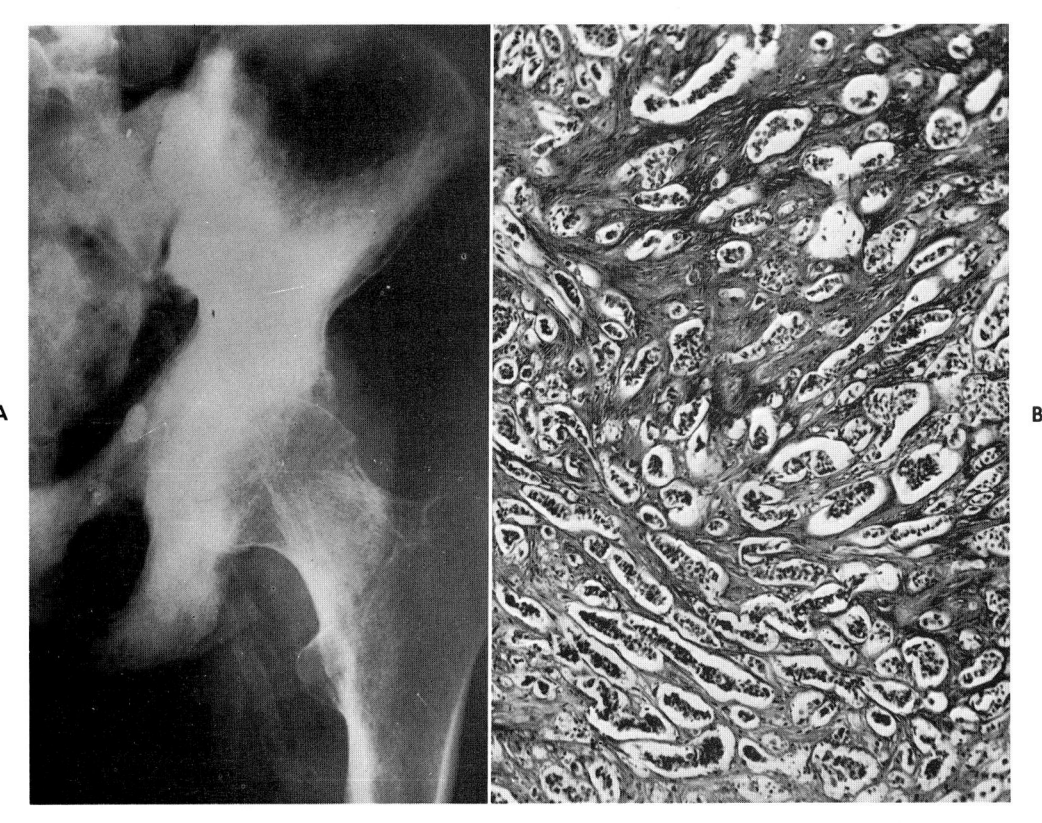

Fig. 25-11. A, Another instance of carcinoma of the prostate with osteoplastic metastases in the spine and innominate bones. B, Photomicrograph of a field from a sclerosing skeletal metastasis showing scirrhous reaction and early osseous metaplasia of the connective tissue stroma. ($\times$100.)

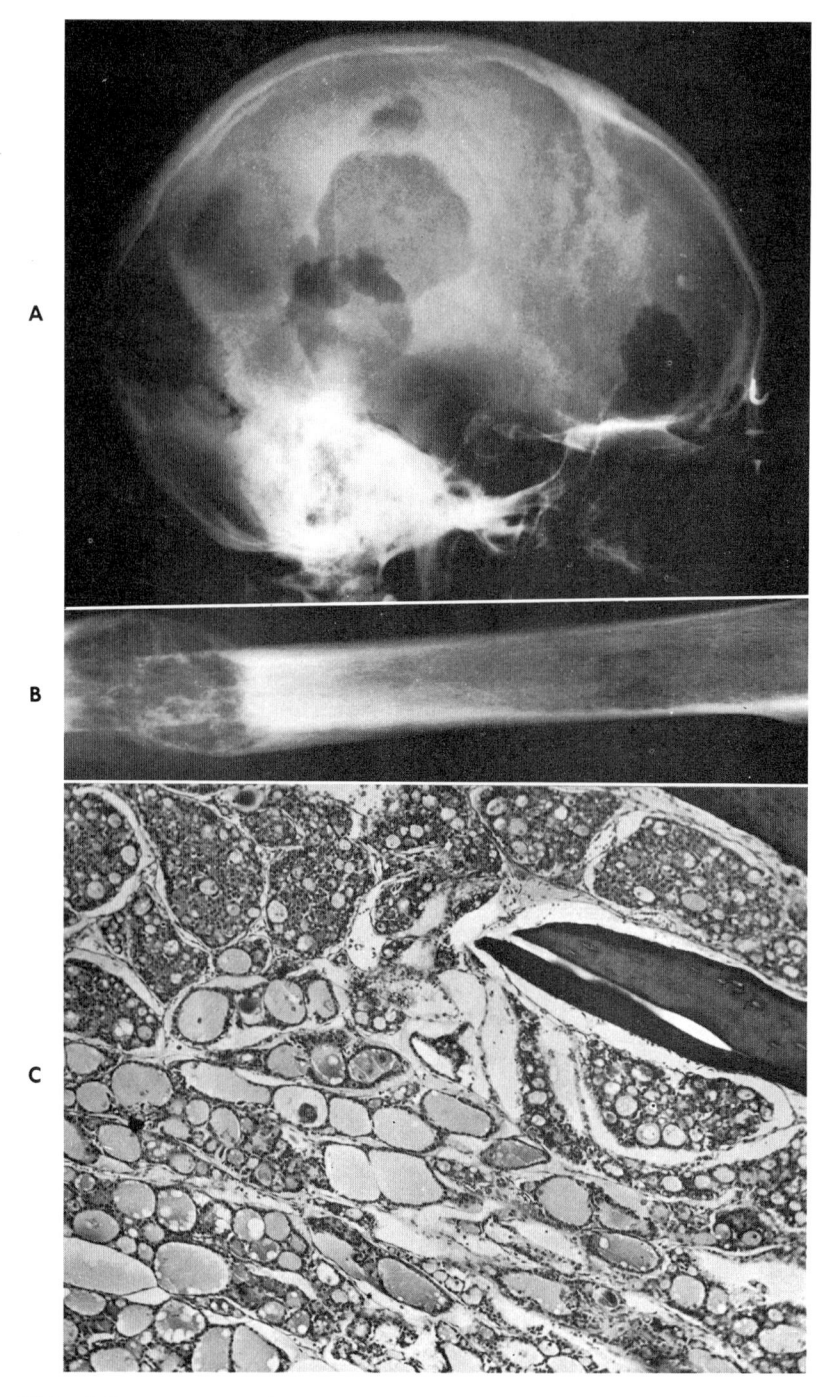

Fig. 25-12. **A,** Roentgenogram from a case of thyroid carcinoma showing striking, large circumscribed lytic metastases in the calvarium. **B,** Comparable lesions in the shaft of a femur. (Additional metastatic foci were present in other bones also.) **C,** Photomicrograph of one of the skeletal metastases showing the formation of well-differentiated, colloid-containing thyroid acini. It is in instances such as this that one is rather likely to observe the uptake of radioactive iodine. (×75.)

Also noteworthy is a very promising pilot study by Gordan, Halden, and Walter[9] of the antitumor efficacy of 7β, 17α—dimethyltestosterone (Calusterone) in women with far-advanced, hormone-refractory breast cancer. Following administration of this sex steroid, bone metastases were observed radiographically to "heal" and undergo recalcification. For a detailed account of the beneficial effects of intensive therapy with estrogens and androgens, as well as its limitations and complications, the reader is referred to a review by Crowley and Duwe.[5] With reference to prostatic carcinoma, the potentially serious side effects of estrogen therapy are such that this should be reserved for patients who have symptomatic disease. Specific mention should also be made of the demonstrated value of radioactive iodine in the prolonged palliation of selected cases of thyroid cancer with skeletal metastases, particularly those that are of the nature of functioning, colloid-producing adenocarcinoma and, as such, exhibit the capacity to pick up and retain the radioactive substance.[6,16] Also, there is clinical evidence to sug-

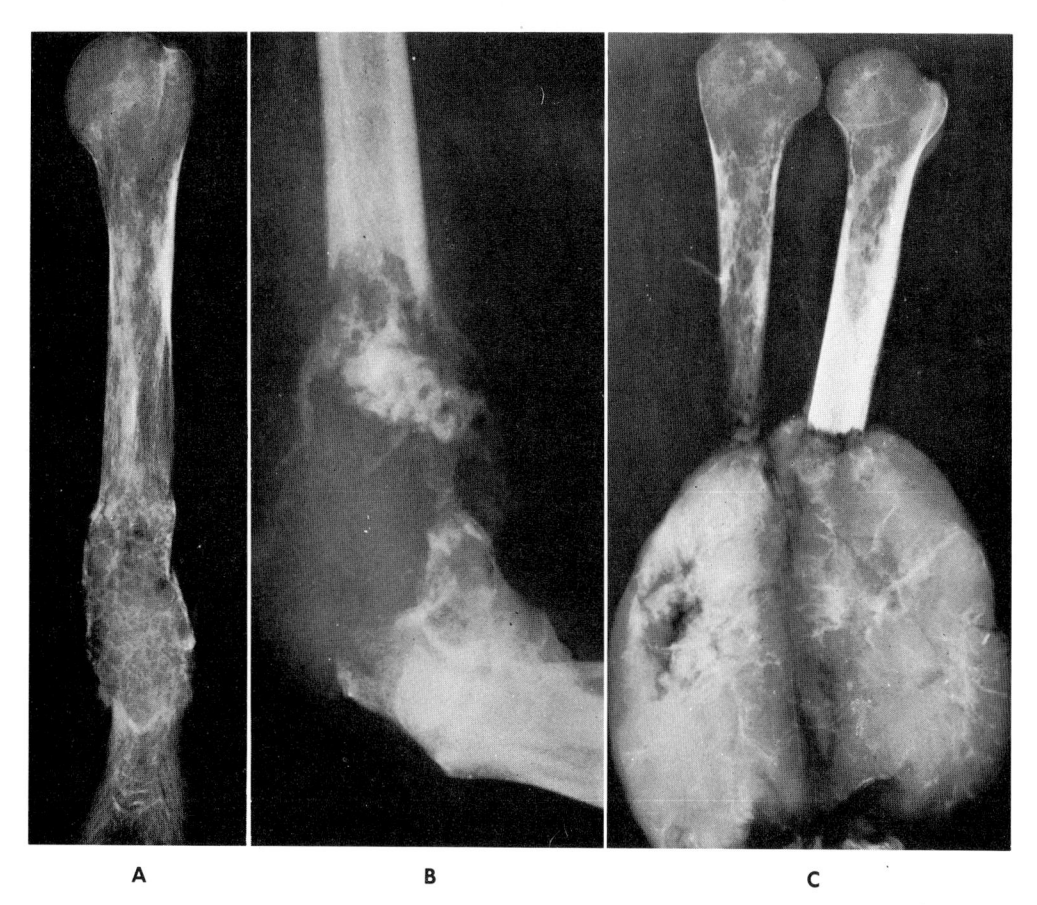

Fig. 25-13. A-C, Three instances of renal carcinoma (hypernephroma) metastatic to the humerus. A and C represent amputation specimens.

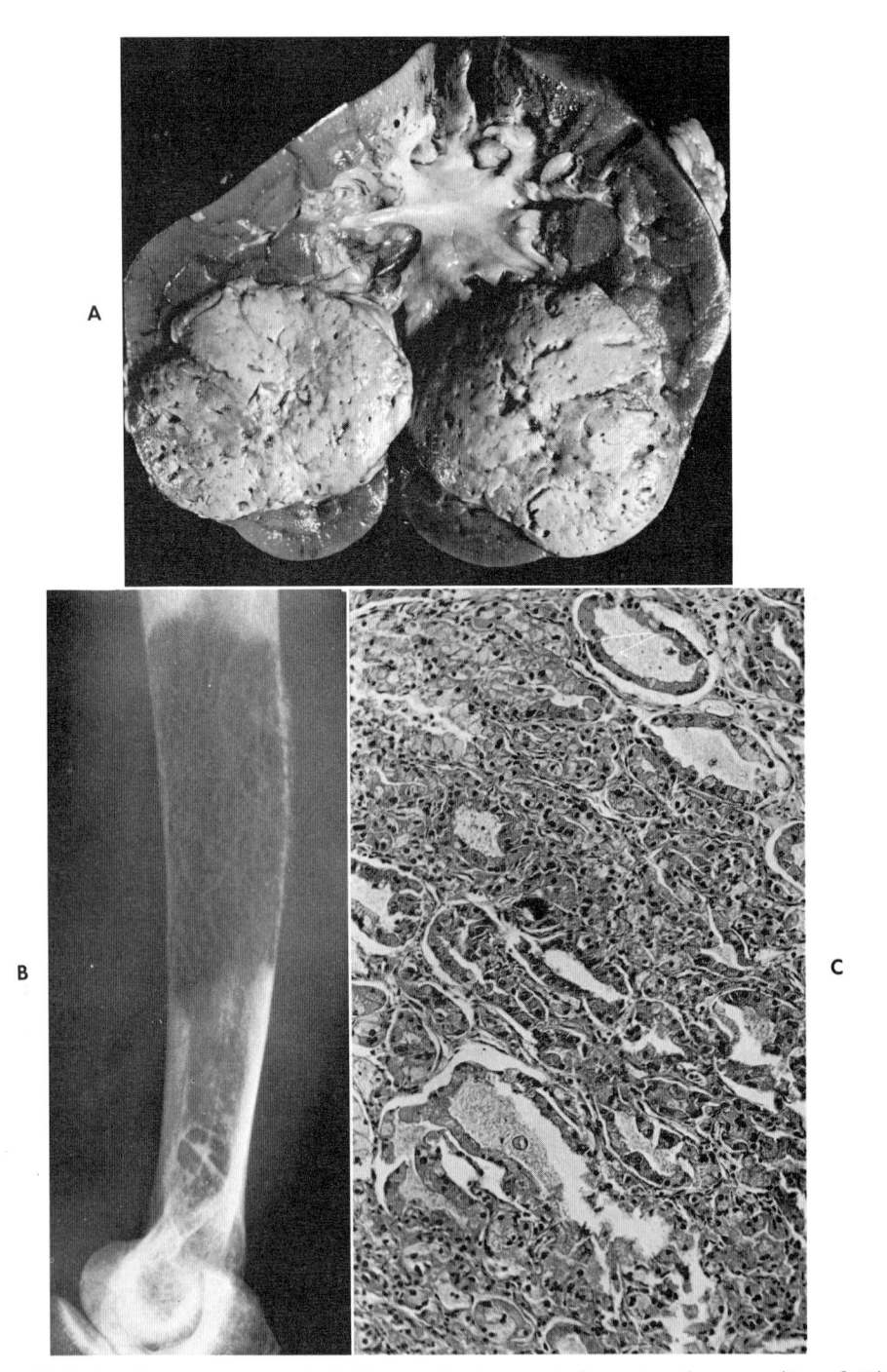

Fig. 25-14. Another instance in which biopsy of a metastatic focus in a humerus (**B** and **C**) led to the discovery of a hypernephroma of a kidney. Nephrectomy was followed by ablation of the involved upper limb in an attempt to obtain a cure (roentgen skeletal survey revealed no other discernible metastatic lesions). It is interesting to note that this patient had a remission for as long as eight years before he manifested another tumor focus in a femur.

gest that suppressive doses of thyroid extract may cause regression of many papillary and some follicular carcinomas of the thyroid.

The question of surgical eradication of an ostensibly solitary skeletal metastasis as a curative measure seldom arises, except in occasional instances of renal carcinoma (hypernephroma). This particular neoplasm may exhibit a curious tendency to spread to a single bone, particularly the humerus, at least insofar as one can ascertain from roentgen skeletal survey, and moreover it faithfully reproduces the cytology of the primary clear-cell carcinoma in its skeletal metastasis, so that it may become feasible to undertake nephrectomy followed by surgical ablation of the metastatic skeletal focus. I have observed several instances in which this was done in an attempt to obtain a cure; in one of them a remission for as long as eight years was obtained; but then other skeletal metastases appeared (Fig. 25-14). Another remarkable case in point is that cited by Bruce[2] of a hypernephroma with metastasis to a scapula treated by nephrectomy and forequarter amputation, with a ten-year survival thereafter.

As for the rest, x-ray irradiation may be resorted to for palliation of skeletal metastases. One must bear in mind, however, that the dosage should not be pushed to the point of inducing radiation necrosis or enhancing the likelihood of pathologic fracture and that the results, while distinctly worthwhile in many instances, are on the whole unpredictable.

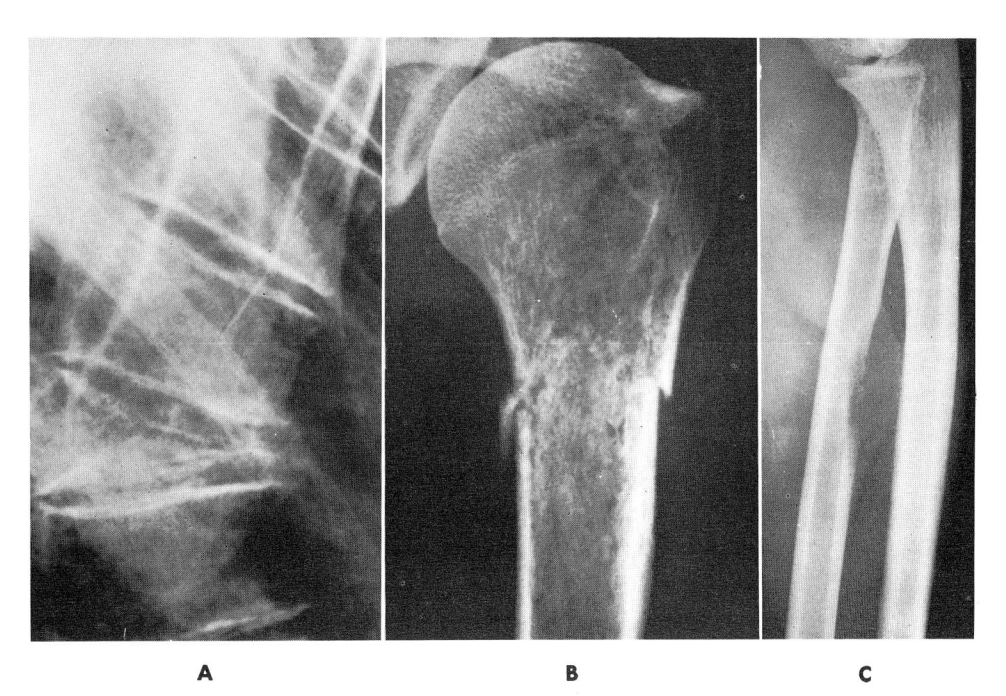

Fig. 25-15. Three instances showing more unusual skeletal metastases of carcinomas originating in the respiratory tract. **A**, In the larynx (collapsed and wedged vertebra). **B**, In the trachea (pathologic fracture of a humerus). **C**, In the lung (destructive tumor focus in the shaft of a radius as the initial clinical manifestation).

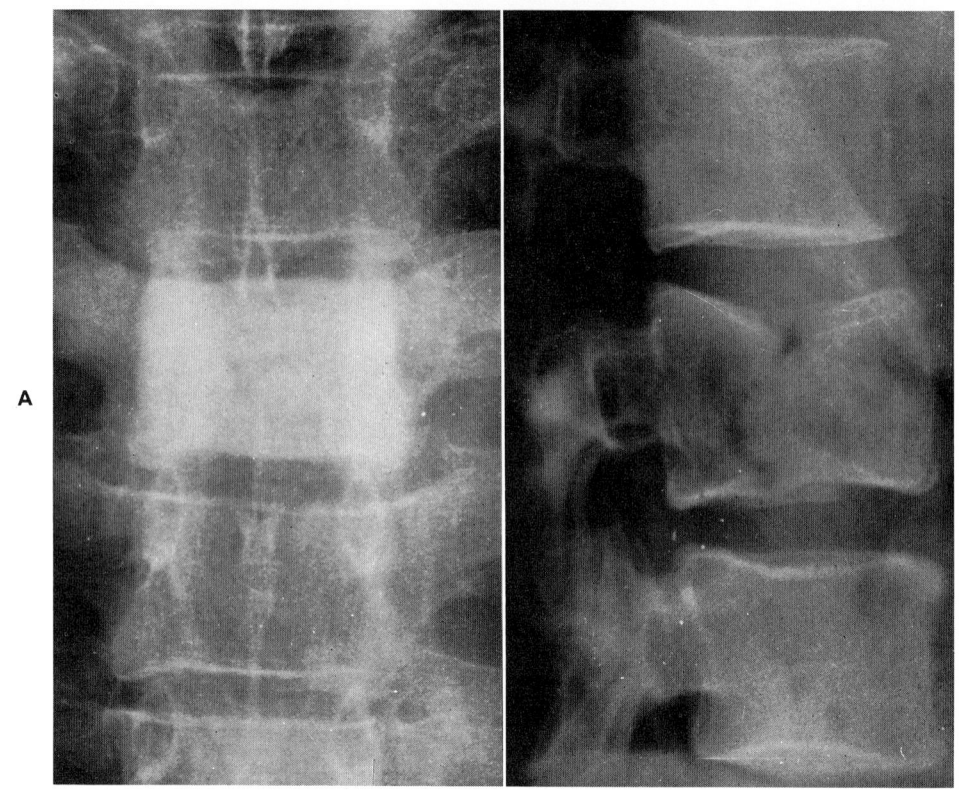

Fig. 25-16. Two additional instances showing unusual metastases in the spine. **A,** A single sclerosed body reflecting metastasis from a carcinoma of the urinary bladder. **B,** Pathologic fracture through a vertebra in a case of cancer of the pancreas. Roentgenograms taken three weeks earlier revealed no discernible lesion at the site indicated.

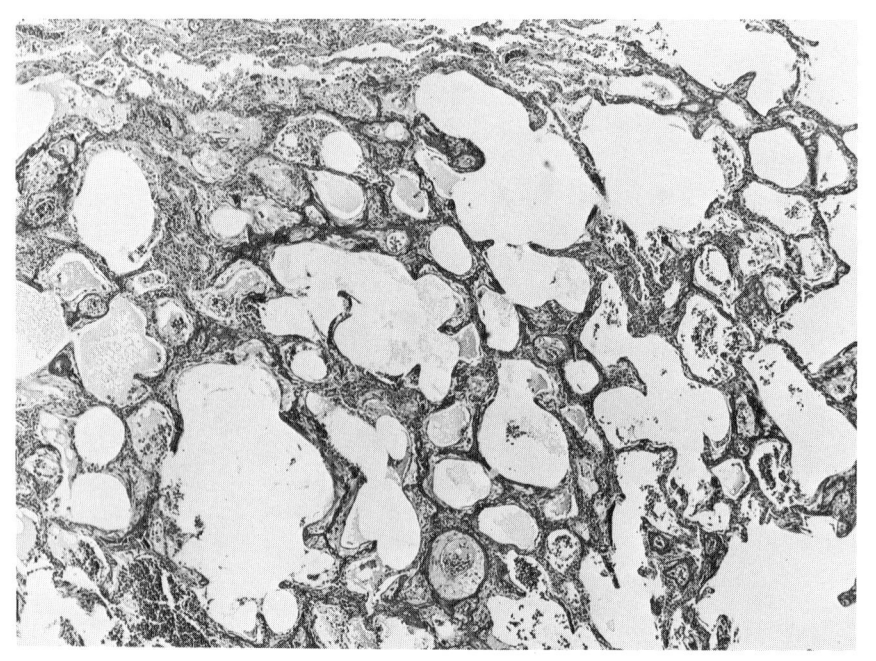

Fig. 25-17. Photomicrograph from a case of carcinoma of the lung with hypercalcemia, showing extensive calcium deposition and ossification within alveolar septae. (×48.)

References

1. Abrams, H. L., Spiro, R., and Goldstein, N.: Metastases in carcinoma. Analysis of 1,000 autopsied cases, Cancer 3:74, 1950.
2. Bruce, J.: J. Bone Joint Surg. 43-B:395, 1961.
3. Coley, B. L.: Neoplasms of bone and related conditions; their etiology, pathogenesis, diagnosis and treatment, New York, 1949, Paul B. Hoeber, Inc., p. 38.
4. Craver, L. F.: Recent advances in treatment of inoperable cancer, Bull. N. Y. Acad. Med. 28:385, 1962.
5. Crowley, L. G., and Duwe, S. A.: Current status of the management of patients with endocrine-sensitive tumors, Part II-Carcinoma of the prostate, endometrium, thyroid, kidney and miscellaneous tumors, Calif. Med. 110:139, 1969.
6. Fitzgerald, P. J., Foote, F. W., and Hill, R. F.: Concentration of I^{131} in thyroid cancer shown by radioautography, Cancer 3:86, 1950.
7. Gold, G. L., and Reefe, W. E.: Carcinoma and metastases to the bones of the hand, J.A.M.A. 184:236, 1963.
8. Gordan, G. S., Fitzpatrick, M. E., and Lubick, W. P.: Identification of osteolytic sterols in human breast cancer, Tr. Assoc. Am. Physicians 80:183, 1967.
9. Gordan, G. S., Halden, A., and Walter, R. M.: Antitumor efficacy of 7β, 17α—dimethyltestosterone (Calusterone) in advanced female breast cancer, Calif. Med. 113:1, 1970.
10. Gordan, G. S., Lichtenstein, L., and Roof, B. S.: Metabolic bone diseases associated with malignancies, Eighth European Conference on Calcified Tissues, Jerusalem, March 28, 1971.
11. Huggins, C., and Dao, T. L. Y.: Mechanism of regression of mammary cancers after adrenalectomy. Abstract paper presented at National Academy of Sciences, Washington, D. C., April, 1953 (in Science, May 1, 1953, p. 468).
12. Jaffe, H. L., and Bodansky, A.: Diagnostic significance of serum alkaline and acid phosphatase values in relation to bone disease, Bull. N. Y. Acad. Med. 19:831, 1943.
13. Kennedy, B. J., and Nathanson, I. T.: Effects of intensive sex steroid hormone therapy in advanced breast cancer, J.A.M.A. 152:1135, 1953.
14. MacDonald, I., Davis, F. E., and Jacobson, G.: Steroid hormone therapy in mammary cancer, Am. J. Roentgenol. 68:954, 1952.
15. Rubin, P.: Comment: The detection of occult metastatic cancer by radioactive bone scans, J.A.M.A. 210:1079, 1969.
16. Seidlin, S. M., Marinelli, L. D., and Oshry, E.: Radioactive iodine therapy; effect on functioning metastases of adrenocarcinoma of the thyroid, J.A.M.A. 132:838, 1946.
17. Sherman, R. S., and Ivker, M.: The roentgen appearance of thyroid metastases in bone, Am. J. Roentgenol. 63:196, 1950.
18. Sherman, R. S., and Pearson, T. A.: Roentgenographic appearance of renal cancer metastasis in bone, Cancer 1:276, 1948.
19. Sisson, M. A., and Garland, L. H.: The treatment of metastatic breast cancer in bone, Calif. Med. 75:265, 1951.
20. Sklaroff, D. M., and Charkes, N. D.: Diagnosis of bone metastasis by photoscanning with strontium 85, J.A.M.A. 188:121, 1964.

Chapter 26

Tumors of periosteal origin

Inasmuch as the periosteal covering of bones may be regarded logically as an integral part of the skeleton, this chapter has been added for the sake of completeness and to enhance the usefulness of the book. It includes the material presented in my paper[21] in *Cancer* in 1955, with some additions and changes intended to bring the discussion up to date. Prior to this survey, there appears to have been no comprehensive discussion on record of tumors developing within periosteal connective tissue, although there were some reports of unusual cases or of small groups of cases demonstrating the characteristic features of some particular periosteal tumor or other. These comparatively uncommon neoplasms constitute a group unto themselves, and their pathologic traits and clinical behavior must be determined empirically, rather than inferred by analogy. The behavior of a periosteal fibrosarcoma, for example, cannot be predicted from that of a central fibrosarcoma of bone. It is only in recent years that the field has been explored to any significant degree, and there is still much to be ascertained, as will be indicated presently.

The main purpose of this chapter is to survey and integrate the limited information now available and to highlight certain practical problems in diagnosis and treatment that require further clarification. Specific reference will be made to periosteal neurofibroma, lipoma, and chondroma as the major, though infrequent, benign tumors in point, and to fibrosarcoma, chondrosarcoma, and osteogenic sarcoma as the malignant ones. It is altogether probable that on rare occasions neoplasms of other types may arise from the periosteum, but too little is known about their incidence for them to serve as a basis for discussion.

Mention should also be made in passing of pseudotumors on the surface of affected bones induced by penetrating thorns,[26] for example, reflecting unsuspected fracture callus, or developing through innocuous localized periosteal ossification without apparent cause (Fig. A-4). Large penetrating tropical ulcers over the tibia, as seen in Africa, also provoke extensive periosteal new bone reaction as well as a variety of peculiar secondary changes within the bone itself.[20] Such lesions are not infrequently explored for biopsy because of a roentgenographic suspicion of sarcoma, especially osteogenic sarcoma, but are otherwise not relevant here.

Benign tumors
Periosteal "desmoid"

On occasion one may observe a comparatively small, circumscribed, benign fibrous growth on the surface of a large limb bone, ostensibly arising in its periosteal covering. Four pertinent instances were reported by Kimmelstiel and Rapp[19] in 1951 under the title of *Cortical Defect Due to Periosteal Desmoids*. All of these, remarkably enough, were encountered on the lower femur in the supracondylar region. It seems noteworthy also that their patients were all young males between the ages of 8 and 20 years. What has been called periosteal desmoid may well be the same lesion as subperiosteal fibrous cortical defect and, as such, is not of any clinical consequence. In any event, it should be clearly distinguished from the larger, poorly defined, and more cellular fibrosarcomas of the periosteum, which will be considered farther on. Another relevant report is that of Marek[25] dealing with two instances in point, both in boys, situated in the lower metaphysis of the femur and the tibia, respectively, for which surgery was performed.

Several years ago I had occasion to observe a comparable instance (in a 15-year-old boy) situated on the lower shaft of a femur posteriorly in the supracondylar area, a little above the attachment of the capsule of the knee joint (Fig.

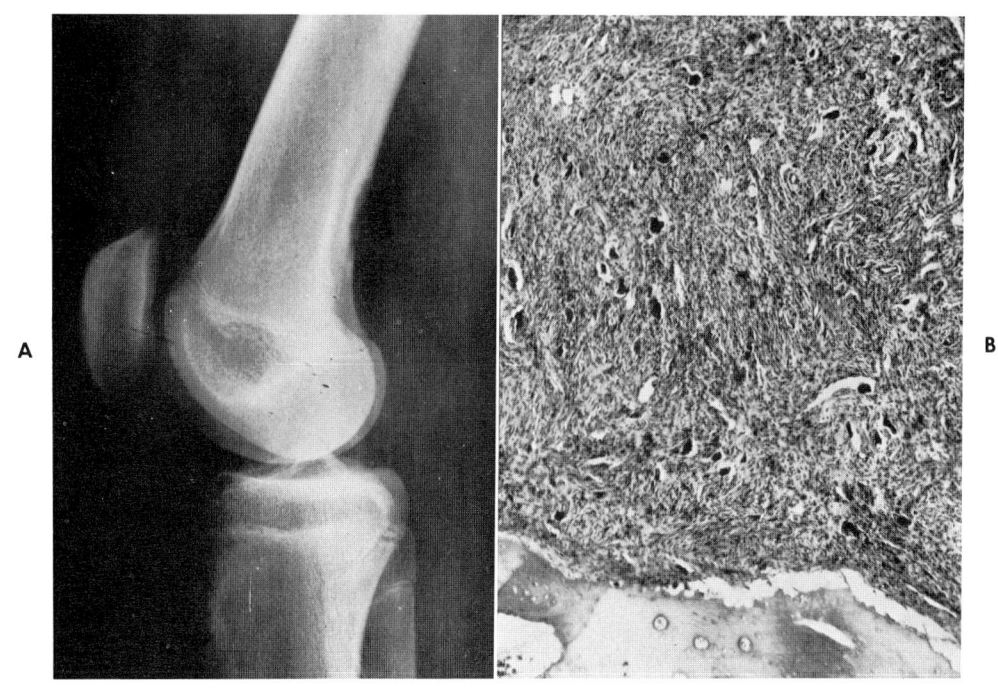

Fig. 26-1. **A**, Roentgenogram of a periosteal "desmoid" on the posterior aspect of the lower femur that has eroded a sclerotized shallow trough in the cortical bone. **B**, Photomicrograph of a representative field of the lesion illustrated in **A**. (×58.) (From Lichtenstein, L.: Tumors of periosteal origin, Cancer **8**:1060, 1955.)

26-1, A). The lesion was discovered on roentgen-ray examination after an injury and had evidently been present for some time, for it had eroded a sclerotized, somewhat scalloped, shallow trough in the underlying cortical bone in much the same way that a periosteal chondroma does (Fig. 26-3, A). Despite this feature that clearly pointed to the benign character of the lesion, the initial radiologic impression was that of a periosteal sarcoma. Fortunately, conservative surgical excision was done, and examination of the available sections (Fig. 26-1, B) showed a mature fibrocytic growth manifesting no indication of significant recent activity. Incidentally, its random content of giant cells (mainly within or in proximity to blood channels) gave this particular tumor a superficial resemblance to nonosteogenic fibroma of bone (which, of course, is a subcortical intramedullary lesion). I have also observed a very similar instance in an 8-year-old boy, in which the lesion was likewise detected roentgenographically following an injury.

Periosteal neurofibroma and neurofibromatosis

It has been well established that neurofibromas may develop within the periosteum as one of the numerous skeletal manifestations of von Recklinghausen's disease, though perhaps not as often as is generally assumed. In this situation they tend to erode the underlying cortex, appearing roentgenographically as localized blisterlike lesions between the eroded cortex and the elevated periosteum (so-called subperiosteal bone cyst). As previously indicated, Brooks and Lehman[3] have described a histologically proved, globular-shaped neurofibroma of this type on the upper end of a tibia, which was delimited peripherally by a delicate shell of periosteal new bone. Comparable instances in a number of sites have been recorded by Holt and Wright,[15] McCarroll,[24] and Hensley,[14] among others. I might add that I had occasion recently to observe a small tumor in point on a phalanx of a finger, where it had produced a blisterlike defect (Fig. 14-2). I have also seen material from a localized malignant tumor on the tibia of a 67-year-old woman that resembled a neurofibrosarcoma. Incidentally, the case reported by Lièvre[23] under the somewhat confusing title of *Ossifying Parosteal Neurinoma* seems not to be relevant here, but to represent rather an instance of parosteal bone and cartilage formation on the lower femur, ascribed with questionable justification to multipotent activity of a schwannian neoplasm.

It appears further from the observations of Weber[34] that, on occasion, periosteal neurofibromatosis may come to involve a major part of the shaft of a limb bone and result in rather striking, diffuse periosteal thickening as well as appreciable thickening and irregularity of the adjacent cortical bone. It should also be noted that if malignant change ensues in von Recklinghausen's neurofibromatosis, as it commonly does, such schwannian tumors may extensively erode and invade contiguous bones, e.g., multiple bodies of the vertebral column.

Periosteal chondroma

In 1952, J. E. Hall and I[22] drew attention to a distinctive benign cartilage tumor that was designated periosteal chondroma. This paper stressed its salient clinical, roentgenographic, and pathologic features as observed in six instances, four of which were encountered on hand or foot bones, and two in apposition to the shafts of large limb bones. Within recent years, I have encountered many additional specimens that have served to substantiate our original impressions. As previously noted,[22] periosteal chondroma is a slowly growing neoplasm of comparatively small size that develops within the periosteal connective tissue and characteristically erodes and induces appreciable sclerosis of the contiguous cortical bone. As such, its roentgenographic appearance has a certain distinctiveness that enables one to recognize the lesion if he is familiar with it and clearly to distinguish it from osteochondroma as well as from solitary enchondroma. Two pertinent instances, each of which developed on the calcaneus, were reported by Feinberg and Wilber.[11] It is interesting to note that there was a history of intermittent painful swelling for as long as eight years in one case and ten years in the other, and that in both the correct diagnosis was suspected from

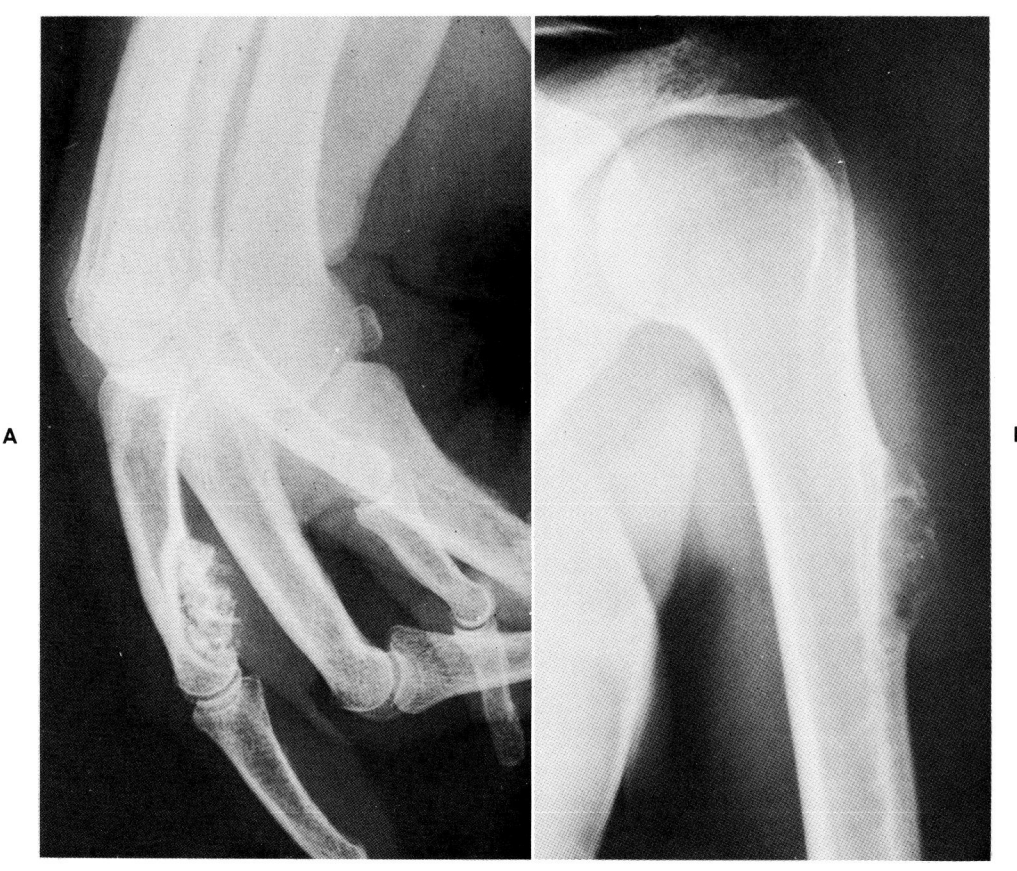

Fig. 26-2. A, Roentgenogram of a periosteal chondroma on a finger phalanx, which has eroded a deep trough in the underlying cortex. This tumor is of long standing and shows extensive secondary ossification. B, Periosteal chondroma on the upper shaft of the humerus of a young woman of 20, who had been aware of a protrusion at the site for about 10 months.

374 Bone tumors

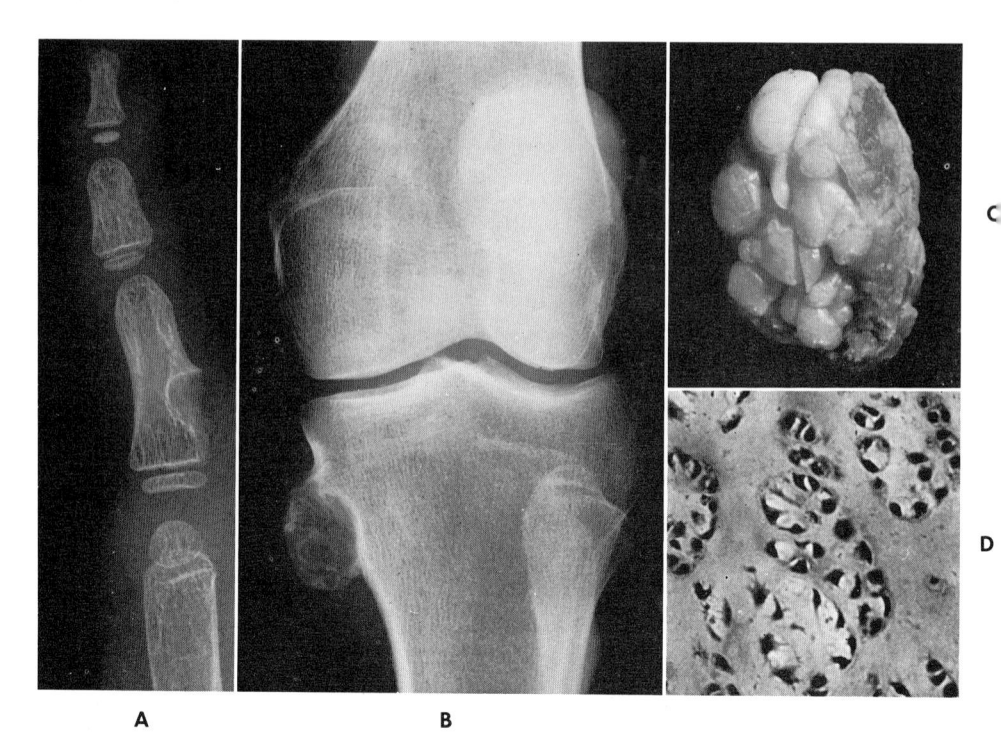

Fig. 26-3. **A**, Roentgenogram of a periosteal chondroma of the proximal phalanx of a finger of a 5-year-old child. At surgery, a firm, rubbery, whitish tumor node was found lodged in the gouged-out cortical defect. **B**, Roentgenogram of another periosteal chondroma protruding from the medial aspect of the upper tibia of a 37-year-old woman, who had been aware of the growth for ten years, according to the history. In this instance, the tumor shows spotty calcification and is outlined peripherally by a delicate shell of periosteal new bone. **C**, Photograph (enlarged) of a periosteal chondroma that was shelled out of a hollow in the cortex of a first metatarsal bone. The tumor was adherent to the periosteum and presented a glistening-white bosselated surface. **D**, A representative field of a periosteal chondroma showing its cytologic details. Although the cartilage-cell nests are more compact than they would be ordinarily in a solitary enchondroma and some of the nuclei are relatively plump, these findings should not be interpreted as indications of malignant change. (×175.) (From Lichtenstein, L.: Tumors of periosteal origin, Cancer **8**:1060, 1955.)

roentgen examination prior to surgical extirpation. A number of additional instances in point were also recorded by Jaffe[17] under the head of "juxtacortical chondroma."

The tumor may develop in children as well as in adults. The symptoms usually referable to it are pain, gradual swelling, and local tenderness. The duration of symptoms in the cases observed ranged from a few months to as long as ten years. Clinically, one finds a firm, generally small, slightly tender tumor, which, if located near a joint, may produce some limitation of motion. At surgery one observes a rubbery, firm, lobulated cartilage tumor, adherent to the periosteum. This is found to be partially nestled within the gouged-out underlying sclerotized cortex, which is extremely resistant to curettage.

Whatever its localization the tumor is composed characteristically of lobules of hyaline cartilage. Although its cartilage-cell nests are likely to be more compact than those of an enchondroma, and its cell nuclei somewhat plumper, these cytologic features are not to be construed as indications of aggressiveness or malignancy (Fig. 26-3, *C* and *D*). It is noteworthy that I have seen an unusual periosteal chondroma on a finger phalanx of an adult that was less differentiated and essentially chondroblastic in its cytology. This tumor did not behave any differently, however, than the common ones composed of facets of hyaline cartilage.

The treatment recommended in most instances is conservative surgical extirpation and curettement of the eroded, sclerotized cortical base. Block excision is feasible if the tumor has involved a long limb bone and is substantially larger than it is on the phalanx of a finger, for example. The results of treatment by either method have been uniformly satisfactory. The patients covered by our original report have been followed for many years now, and there has been no indication of any tendency to local recurrence following surgical excision.

On the other hand, Dr. J. L. Carr, of San Francisco, has called my attention to a periosteal chondroma in a 49-year-old man that recurred three years after surgical extirpation. The recurrent tumor was somewhat more cellular than the original one but was still apparently circumscribed. At the follow-up two and one-half years later, the patient was in good health and presented no evidence of tumor either at the local site or elsewhere. Whether or not the initial tumor was completely removed cannot now be ascertained. In any event, this experience, while it gives one pause, would seem to be the exception that proves the rule. The two cases of recurrent periosteal chondroma (on finger phalanges) reported recently by Nosanchuk and Kaufer[27] also highlight the necessity for meticulously complete excision (including the capsular connective tissue) and curettement of the underlying cortical bone. Similarly, in one of several instances reported by Scaglietti and Stringa,[30] there was also local recurrence necessitating wider excision; this patient was well nine years later, as were the others.

Periosteal or parosteal lipoma

The specific reference here is to the very occasional finding of a slowly enlarging, circumscribed, benign growth of lobulated simple fat, developing deep in the soft parts of an extremity in intimate contact with the periosteum of a limb bone. Whether the lipoma under these circumstances actually arises in the periosteum or merely comes in apposition to it may be difficult to determine with assurance in any particular case. It seems noteworthy, however, that in two pertinent instances in children, reported by Bartlett, the lipomas were so adherent to the thickened periosteum of the affected bone (a tibia and a humerus, respectively) as to require sharp dissection for their separation. Such tumors may eventually attain appreciable size. Their presence is reflected roentgenographically by a well-outlined, ovoid, translucent, soft-tissue mass abutting on the contiguous bone, usually a long limb bone. When fully developed, they produce discernible swelling without being especially painful, although they may sometimes cause pressure on nerves in their vicinity. Richmond,[29] for example, has described a lipoma attached to the periosteum of the neck of a radius that displaced and impaired the function of the posterior interosseous nerve. A comparable instance, though without paralysis, was recorded by Fairbank,[10] to whom we are also indebted for a survey of the older literature dating back to 1868.[2,28,31] Among the references mentioned, that of Bland-Sutton[2] in which fourteen relevant cases are cited seems particularly noteworthy. For a survey of the recent literature and detailed consideration of differential roentgen diagnosis, one may have recourse to the report of Fleming, Alpert, and Garcia.[12] Altogether, these deep-seated periosteal lipomas seem to be distinctly unusual. I have observed only a few in my own experience and am not aware of any recorded instance in which malignant change ensued.

Malignant tumors

In the interest of clarity, a sharp distinction must be made at the outset between the malignant tumors that apparently originate in the periosteum and the parosteal soft-part tumors (e.g., fibrosarcoma, liposarcoma, malignant schwannian tumors, and myosarcoma) that in the course of their growth come to erode the adjacent bone and its periosteal covering secondarily. These parosteal

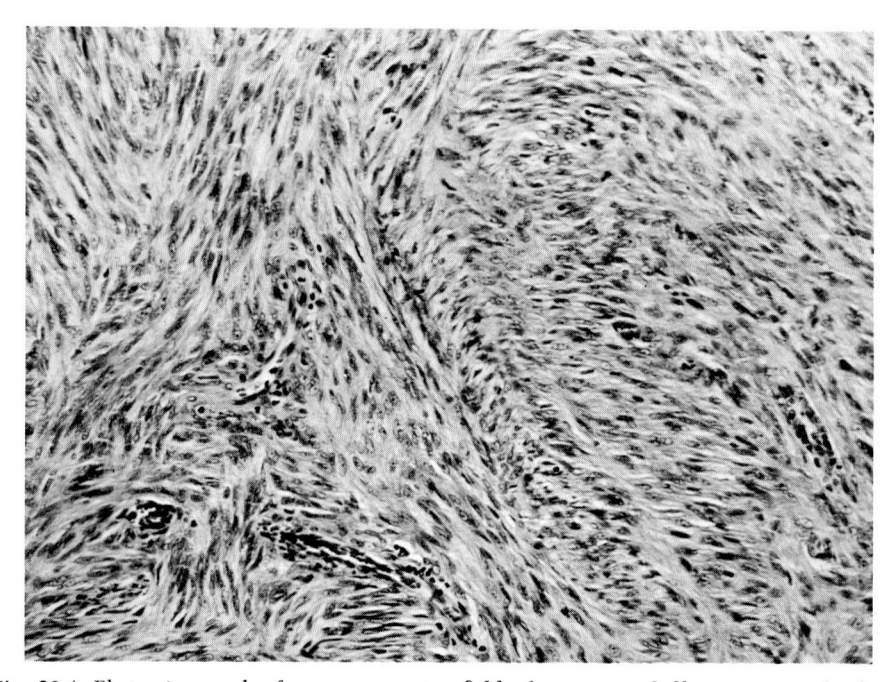

Fig. 26-4. Photomicrograph of a representative field of a periosteal fibrosarcoma. The lesion was a circumscribed tumor of limited size, apparently arising from the periosteal covering of a large limb bone. Tumors such as this can often be cured by adequate block excision, without sacrificing the affected extremity.

tumors, while interesting in their own right, are not the subject of the present discussion. This will be concerned rather with the recognition and appropriate treatment of the comparatively unusual instances of periosteal fibrosarcoma, chondrosarcoma, and osteogenic sarcoma (rapidly growing from onset and apparently different from *slowly developing* parosteal osteogenic sarcoma).

Periosteal fibrosarcoma

Malignant fibroblastic tumors are occasionally encountered that seem clearly to arise from the periosteal connective tissue and produce a slowly enlarging mass intimately attached to the external surface of the affected bone. When they have attained appreciable size prior to surgical intervention, these periosteal fibrosarcomas may sometimes erode the underlying cortical bone, although they do not, as a rule, invade the medullary cavity. Stout[33] has reported thirteen pertinent instances, of which eight developed on bones other than large limb bones, notably the scapula, the mandible, and the sacrum and coccyx. He is inclined to regard them as relatively favorable neoplasms (as compared with fibrosarcomas in other sites), inasmuch as metastasis was observed in only one of his thirteen cases. The relatively few periosteal fibrosarcomas that I have observed have been tumors of rather low-grade malignancy, exhibiting a tendency to relatively slow growth and a disposition to merely local recurrence after incomplete surgical extirpation. Initial radical surgery for such tumors would seem unnecessarily drastic unless they are so situated or so far advanced that the surgeon cannot obtain adequate clearance by more conservative measures (Fig. 26-4).

Periosteal chondrosarcoma

Malignant periosteal tumors composed entirely of cartilage are comparatively rare, although some periosteal osteogenic sarcomas may present conspicuous fields of tumor cartilage (Fig. 26-6). I have observed only a few tumors that developed on the cortical surface, ostensibly from its periosteal covering, and that could be plausibly interpreted as chondrosarcoma. One of these was a rather small, localized growth on the upper shaft of the humerus (of a young adult), that was partially walled off by a shell of periosteal new bone. Its roentgenographic appearance was, in fact, reminiscent of periosteal chondroma, although the relative cellularity of the tumor in places and its tendency to invade the contiguous cortical bone favored an impression of low-grade malignancy, so that wide block excision was recommended. This was done, and at the last follow-up about one year later the patient was well clinically and showed no sign of local recurrence. Another tumor in point is the one illustrated in Fig. 26-5, *A*. It was intimately attached to the cortex of the upper humerus, where it had produced a sclerotized trough. The radiopaque streaks within it reflect secondary ossification of actively growing tumor cartilage. The initial surgical approach was conservative and, unfortunately, long-term follow-up is not available. Still another case in point is the periosteal chondrosarcoma protruding from an iliac bone; this tumor is illustrated in Fig. 26-5, *B*.

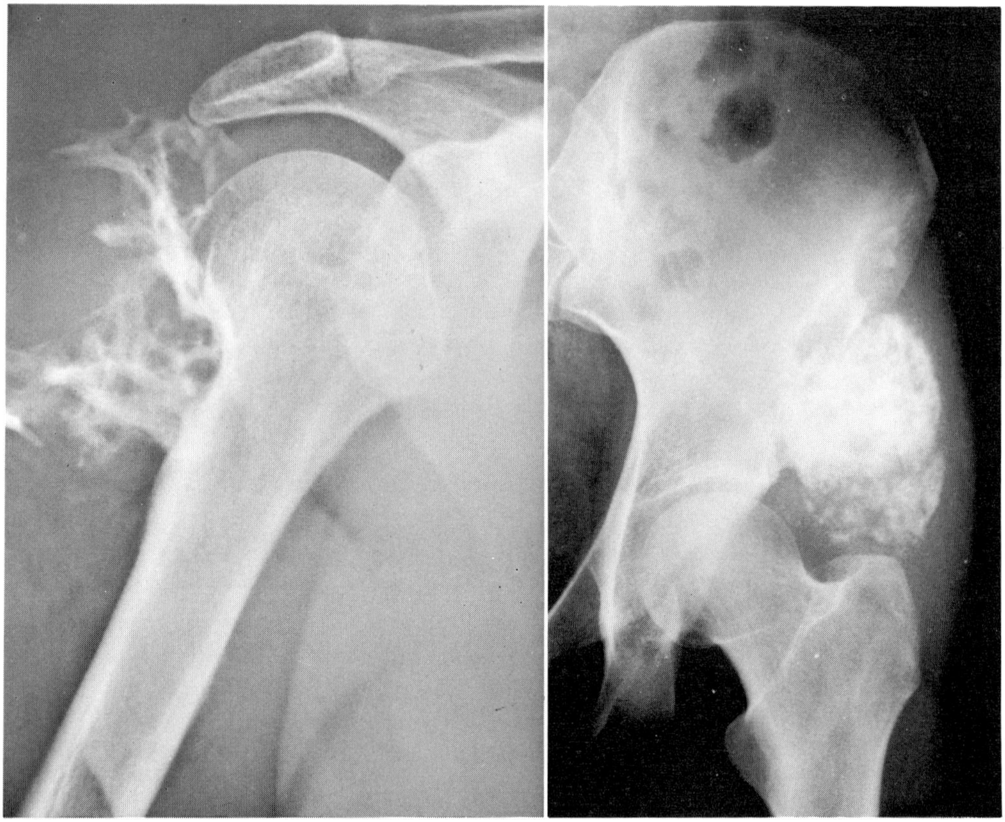

378 Bone tumors

Fig. 26-5. **A,** Roentgenogram of an unusual periosteal chondrosarcoma. **B,** Roentgenogram of a circumscribed, slowly growing periosteal chondrosarcoma protruding from the iliac bone in a woman of 32. The radiopaque areas within the tumor reflect secondary ossification of cartilage. Local excision was done, along with removal of a strip of uninvolved cortical bone around its site of attachment. The patient was well and free of tumor at the last follow-up, some 2½ years later.

The pertinent literature on periosteal (juxtacortical) chondrosarcoma continues to be meager. Jaffe in his book illustrated one on the upper humerus. It eroded the cortex but did not penetrate the medullary cavity and Cooper[6] reported one on the shaft of an ulna, which was successfully resected, although a tumor implant developed in the subcutaneous tissue of the surgical wound.

To emphasize the problem of differentiation between chondrosarcoma and osteogenic sarcoma, it may be helpful to cite the following instance of another unusual neoplasm, which developed on the lower shaft of a femur of an 18-year-old boy (Fig. 26-6, *A*). On initial biopsy it was interpreted as a periosteal chondrosarcoma, but in subsequent specimens it showed other features clearly stamping it as a cartilage-containing osteogenic sarcoma (Fig. 26-6, *C* and *D*). When first explored, this tumor presented as a somewhat nodular, rubbery, gray mass, 4 by 1.5 cm., sitting on the intact cortex of the femur, from which it came away

Tumors of periosteal origin 379

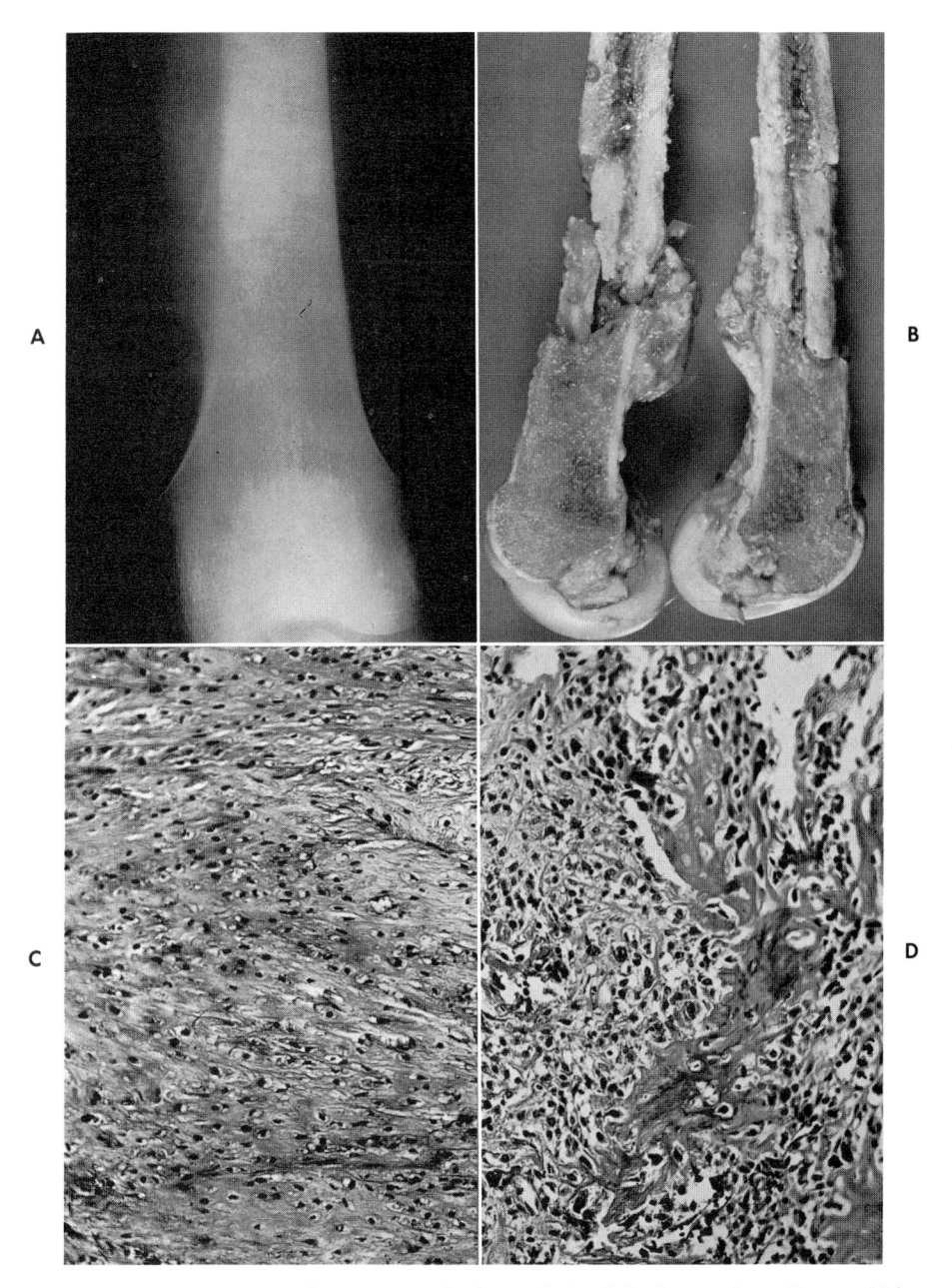

Fig. 26-6. A, Roentgenogram of a tumor on the lower shaft of the femur of an 18-year-old boy, which proved to be a periosteal osteogenic sarcoma. B, Photograph of the recurrent periosteal tumor in the case illustrated in A, as seen in the amputation specimen. The medullary cavity of the femur was found to be free of tumor. C, The appearance of the tumor as seen in the original biopsy specimen. From this, the impression gained was that of a chondrosarcoma. (×175.) D, A selected field in the amputation specimen indicating that the neoplasm was actually an osteogenic sarcoma. (×200.) (From Lichtenstein, L.: Tumors of periosteal origin, Cancer 8:1060, 1955.)

with ease. The available sections of this, as noted, showed a dominant picture of rather cellular tumor cartilage undergoing focal calcification and osseous transformation. Examination of the recurrent neoplasm, however, revealed, in addition to abundant cartilage, fields of malignant spindle connective tissue, forming osteoid in places. Following an unsuccessful attempt at wide block excision, infection developed and amputation was resorted to. Study of the residual tumor in the amputation specimen also conveyed the impression of osteogenic sarcoma. Although some penetration of the outer cortex was noted, the marrow cavity of the femur was free of tumor, thus confirming the periosteal origin of the neoplasm.

Another instance illustrating the same problem in differentiation was that of a rapidly growing, malignant periosteal neoplasm surrounding the distal tibia, which seemed clearly to be chondrosarcoma on biopsy. Local resection was attempted unsuccessfully and sections again showed abundant cartilage, but also occasional microscopic foci of osteoid and bone formation within malignant stroma. The amputation specimen confirmed the fact that the tumor was basically an osteogenic sarcoma, although at least 90% of it was composed of malignant cartilage.

Periosteal osteogenic sarcoma (parosteal or juxtacortical osteogenic sarcoma)

Considerable interest has been evinced recently in this category of unusual neoplasms. They develop apparently through progressive active proliferation of bone-forming periosteal connective tissue and appear on the surface of large limb bones rather than in their interior. The distal femur particularly is a site of predilection, through occasionally the tibia, the humerus, the fibula, or some other long bone may be affected. They are further distinguished from the conventional intramedullary osteogenic sarcomas by their more favorable course and substantially higher survival rate. In the matter of appraisal, however, it must be recognized that not all periosteal osteogenic sarcomas are comparable. They appear to fall into two separate and distinct groups, comprising the rapidly growing ones that are clearly malignant from the start and those that seem to develop through subtle, slow, and gradual malignant change in certain lesions of juxtacortical osseous (and sometimes also cartilaginous) metaplasia. The former may be regarded as the periosteal counterpart of central or intramedullary osteogenic sarcoma, and it appears to be characteristic of them that they contain abundant cartilage. The latter may well be analogous to the comparatively rare sarcomas that develop through malignant change in lesions of myositis ossificans, as Jaffe and Selin[18] have intimated (Chapter 16).

The initially malignant periosteal osteogenic sarcomas are encountered so infrequently that relatively little is known as yet about their clinical behavior and appropriate treatment. There are no informative precedents, for example, to indicate whether one can resort with impunity to the expedient of block resection in an attempt to spare the affected limb, or whether, on the other hand, ablation is mandatory. I have had occasion to observe only a few instances in point. One of them is the periosteal tumor previously mentioned, whose periphery was composed predominantly of cartilage so that its basic osteogenic character was not clearly recognizable at the outset (Fig. 26-6). Another was a painful, progressively enlarging neoplasm that developed on the upper shaft of the tiba of a 5-year-old child over a period of observation of no more than two to three months. In the roentgenogram one could discern a localized area of cortical thickening, the outer convex surface of which appeared fuzzy, ill defined, and relatively radiolucent. The available biopsy sections showed condensed cortical bone interspersed with patches of newly formed osteoid and tracts of ominous-looking cellular fibroblastic connective tissue. The opinions expressed by the group of pathologists who studied the slides originally, namely, periosteal osteogenic sarcoma, ossifying periosteal fibrosarcoma, and periosteal osteoma, serve to highlight

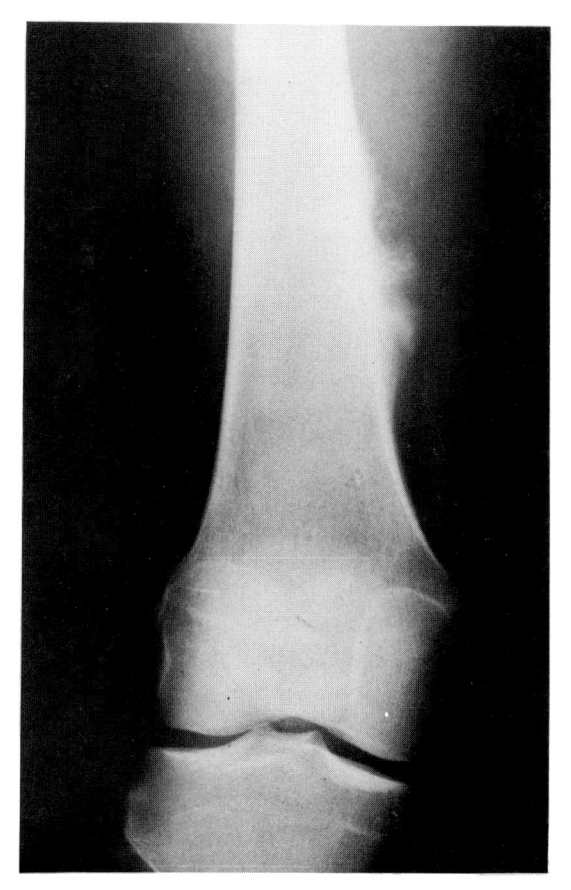

Fig. 26-7. Roentgenogram of another periosteal osteogenic sarcoma developing on the cortex of the distal femur in a 15-year-old girl who had complained of pain and swelling for about five months. This tumor also contained abundant cartilage, but was basically osteogenic in character.

the problems in interpretation. Because of uncertainty as to the potential seriousness of this lesion, the recommendation of block excision was ventured, with the proviso that amputation without further temporizing should be considered in the event of aggressive local recurrence. Still another tumor in point is the one illustrated in Fig. 26-7, which developed on the lower femoral shaft of a 15-year-old girl who had been aware of a swelling for about five months. This malignant neoplasm also contained abundant cartilage, but was basically osteogenic in character.

The insidiously developing malignant tumors have already been discussed in the chapter on osteogenic sarcoma under the head of ossifying parosteal sarcoma (juxtacortical osteogenic sarcoma, parosteal osteogenic sarcoma, parosteal "osteoma"). For the sake of brevity, the views expressed will not be reiterated here.

References

1. Bartlett, E. I.: Periosteal lipoma; report of two cases, Arch. Surg. 21:1015, 1930.
2. Bland-Sutton, J.: Tumours, innocent and malignant; their clinical characters and appropriate treatment, ed. 4, London, 1906, Cassell & Co., Ltd., p. 21.
3. Brooks, B., and Lehman, E. P.: The bone changes in Recklinghausen's neurofibromatosis, Surg. Gynecol. Obstet. 38:587, 1924.
4. Carr, J. L.: Personal communication.
5. Coley, W. B.: Myositis ossificans traumatica. A report of three cases illustrating the difficulties of diagnosis from sarcoma, Ann. Surg. 57:305, 1913.
6. Cooper, R. R.: Juxtacortical chondrosarcoma: a case report, J. Bone Joint Surg. 47-A:524, 1965.
7. Dahlin, D. C.: Personal communication, Sept. 8, 1956.
8. Dwinnell, L. A., Dahlin, D. C., and Ghormley, R. K.: Parosteal (juxtacortical) osteogenic sarcoma, J. Bone Joint Surg. 36-A:732, 1954.
9. Ewing, J.: A review of the classification of bone tumors, Surg. Gynecol. Obstet. 68:971, 1939.
10. Fairbank, H. A. T.: A parosteal lipoma, J. Bone Joint Surg. 35-B:589, 1953.
11. Feinberg, S. B., and Wilber, M. C.: Periosteal chondroma (a report of two cases), Radiology 66:383, 1956.
12. Fleming, R. J., Alpert, M., and Garcia, A.: Parosteal lipoma, Am. J. Roentgenol. 87:1075, 1962.
13. Geschickter, C. F., and Copeland, M. M.: Parosteal osteoma of bone: a new entity, Ann. Surg. 133:790; disc., 807, 1951.
14. Hensley, C. D., Jr.: The rapid development of a "subperiosteal bone cyst" in multiple neurofibromatosis; a case report, J. Bone Joint Surg. 35-A:197, 1953.
15. Holt, J. F., and Wright, E. M.: The radiologic features of neurofibromatosis, Radiology 51:647, 1948.
16. Jaffe, H. L.: Fibrous dysplasia of bone; a disease entity and specifically not an expression of neurofibromatosis, J. Mt. Sinai Hosp. 12:364, 1945.
17. Jaffe, H. L.: Juxtacortical chondroma, Bull. Hosp. Joint Dis. 17:20, 1956.
18. Jaffe, H. L., and Selin, G.: Tumors of bones and joints. In Ashford, M., editor: The musculoskeletal system: a symposium presented at the Twenty-Third Graduate Fortnight of the New York Academy of Medicine, October Ninth to Twentieth, 1950, New York, 1952, The Macmillan Co., pp. 338-339.
19. Kimmelstiel, P., and Rapp, I.: Cortical defect due to periosteal desmoids, Bull. Hosp. Joint Dis. 12(2):286, 1951.
20. Kolawole, T. M., and Bohrer, S. P.: Ulcer osteoma—bone response to tropical ulcer, Am. J. Roentgenol. 109:611, 1970.
21. Lichtenstein, L.: Tumors of periosteal origin, Cancer 8:1060, 1955.
22. Lichtenstein, L., and Hall, J. E.: Periosteal chondroma; a distinctive benign cartilage tumor, J. Bone Joint Surg. 34-A:691, 1952.
23. Lièvre, J. A., Verne, J. M., and Lièvre, J. A., Mme.: Un type de tumeur osseuse: le neurinome parostal ossificant, Presse Med. 61:441, 1953.
24. McCarroll, H. R.: Clinical manifestations of congenital neurofibromatosis, J. Bone Joint Surg. 32-A:601, 626, 1950.
25. Marek, F.: Fibrous cortical defect (periosteal desmoid), Bull. Hosp. Joint Dis. 16:77, 1955.

26. Maylahn, D. J.: Thorn-induced "tumors" of bone, J. Bone Joint Surg. 34-A:386, 1952.
27. Nosanchuk, J. S., and Kaufer, H.: Recurrent periosteal chondroma—report of two cases and a review of the literature, J. Bone Joint Surg. 51-A:375, 1969.
28. Power, D. A.: A parosteal lipoma, or congenital fatty tumour, connected with the periosteum of the femur, Tr. Path. Soc. London 39:270, 1888.
29. Richmond, D. A.: Lipoma causing a posterior interosseous nerve lesion, J. Bone Joint Surg. 35-B:83, 1953.
30. Scaglietti, O., and Stringa, G.: Periosteal myxoma of infancy and periosteal chondroma of adolescence, with local malignancy, Clin. Orthop. 9:147, 1957.
31. Smith, T.: Fatty tumour growing from the neck of the radius, Tr. Path. Soc. London 19:344, 1868.
32. Stevens, G. M., Pugh, D. G., and Dahlin, D. C.: Roentgenographic recognition and differentiation of parosteal osteogenic sarcoma, Am. J. Roentgenol. 78:1, 1957.
33. Stout, A. P.: Fibrosarcoma; the malignant tumor of fibroblasts, Cancer 1:30, 1948.
34. Weber, F. P.: Periosteal neurofibromatosis, with a short consideration of the whole subject of neurofibromatosis, Quart. J. Med. 23:151, 1930.

Appendix A

Some nonneoplastic lesions of bone that may be mistaken for tumors

The emphasis upon early diagnosis of malignant tumors as a means of reducing mortality has also been carried over into the field of bone tumors. Unfortunately, this principle has limited application here inasmuch as certain malignant tumors are already far advanced when first recognized clinically, while others tend ultimately by their very nature to involve many bones, in spite of prompt vigorous therapy directed against the presenting lesion. It is true that chondrosarcoma developing through subtle malignant change in a benign enchondroma or an osteocartilaginous exostosis is not always recognized as early as it might be and that such delay may sometimes mean the difference between cure and ultimate fatality. This urgency may apply also to instances of central fibrosarcoma and of primary reticulum-cell sarcoma of bone, which can often be cured if they are appropriately treated before metastasis has developed. On the other hand, an osteogenic sarcoma frequently spreads to the lungs so early that a tumor of which the patient has been aware only a few weeks carries as serious a prognosis as one known to have been present for a number of months. Also, the chances for cure when dealing with Ewing's sarcoma or with myeloma and other tumors of hematopoietic origin (exclusive of primary reticulum-cell sarcoma) are not very bright in any event, since these neoplasms tend strongly to dissemination throughout the skeleton, even when this is not clinically or roentgenographically discernible.

It is my impression that in the matter of recognizing and treating skeletal tumors in general more mischief is done currently through overdiagnosis than through failure to recognize malignant neoplasms promptly. Much of this can be obviated by seeking expert opinion, whereby it is often possible to forestall or avert unnecessary radical surgery for lesions that are less serious than they were at first considered to be by the clinician, radiologist, or pathologist, as the case may be. As examples of benign tumors that are sometimes overdiagnosed and hence treated more radically than is necessary, one may cite instances of benign chondroblastoma and chondromyxoid fibroma mistaken for chondrosarcoma; of bulky, though not actively growing, osteocartilaginous exostoses mistaken for

Some nonneoplastic lesions of bone that may be mistaken for tumors

chondrosarcoma, as well as osteogenic sarcoma; of benign osteoblastoma mistaken for osteogenic sarcoma; and of nonosteogenic fibroma mistaken for giant-cell tumor, or even for low-grade fibrosarcoma.

It is important to recognize also that certain nonneoplastic lesions of bone may sometimes be mistaken for tumors. It is common knowledge, for example, that on occasion, infections, especially acute or subacute osteomyelitis of a long bone that has provoked rapid periosteal new bone apposition, may simulate Ewing's tumor clinically and roentgenographically (Fig. 18-2, A). In fact, even after exploration the surgeon may not be quite certain whether he is dealing with one condition or the other, inasmuch as it may be difficult under such circumstances to distinguish clearly pus from softened, necrotic tumor tissue. Similarly, a solitary lesion of eosinophilic granuloma of bone (in a rib or a long bone, for example) may also simulate Ewing's tumor clinically since it tends rather rapidly

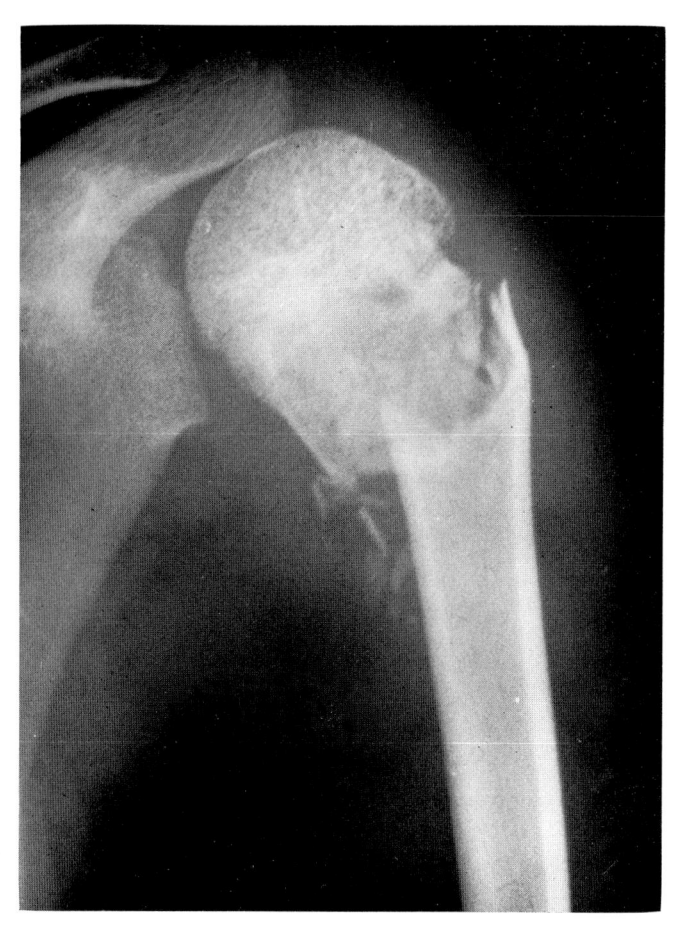

Fig. A-1. Roentgenogram of a bone cyst in its common location, the upper metaphysis of the humerus, showing a pathologic fracture. Lesions such as this are still mistaken on occasion for giant-cell tumor, though without much justification.

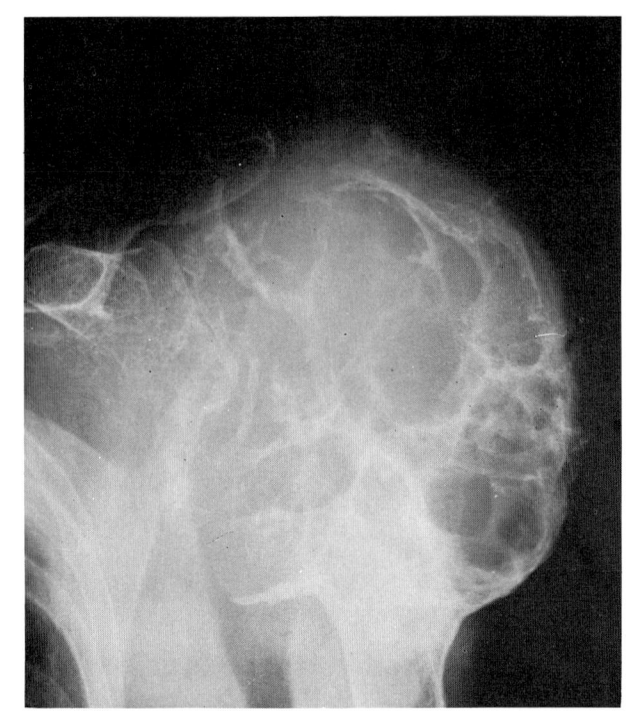

Fig. A-2. Remarkable, expanded tumorlike lesion of Gaucher's disease in an old woman, who had been aware of a mass in her left shoulder region for more than thirty years.

to break through the cortex of the affected bone and extend into the adjacent muscle tissue (Fig. A-10, A). By the same token, cases of eosinophilic granuloma of bone presenting multiple defects in the calvarium, pelvis, and long bones may at first simulate instances of metastatic tumor, especially neuroblastoma. Here again, clarification of the diagnosis must often await pathologic examination of a biopsy specimen.

By way of citing other instances in point, one may mention that occasionally the common bone cyst[9] is mistaken for giant-cell tumor with untoward consequences. I recall a pertinent case in which a bone cyst in the upper metaphysis of the humerus of a child was heavily irradiated on the premise that it represented a giant-cell tumor (despite its location and the youthfulness of the patient). In this instance a fibrosarcoma developed several years later at the site of irradiation, necessitating disarticulation of the extremity (Fig. 17-7). It is also relevant here to point out that the peculiar lesion that we designated as aneursymal bone cyst has been mistaken in the past for giant-cell tumor (atypical subperiosteal giant-cell tumor, so-called) and occasionally for osteogenic sarcoma.

Further, it is not too unusual for localized rarefied defects resulting from hyperparathyroidism to be confused with genuine gaint-cell tumors, so that attention is diverted from a search for the offending parathyroid adenoma, thereby

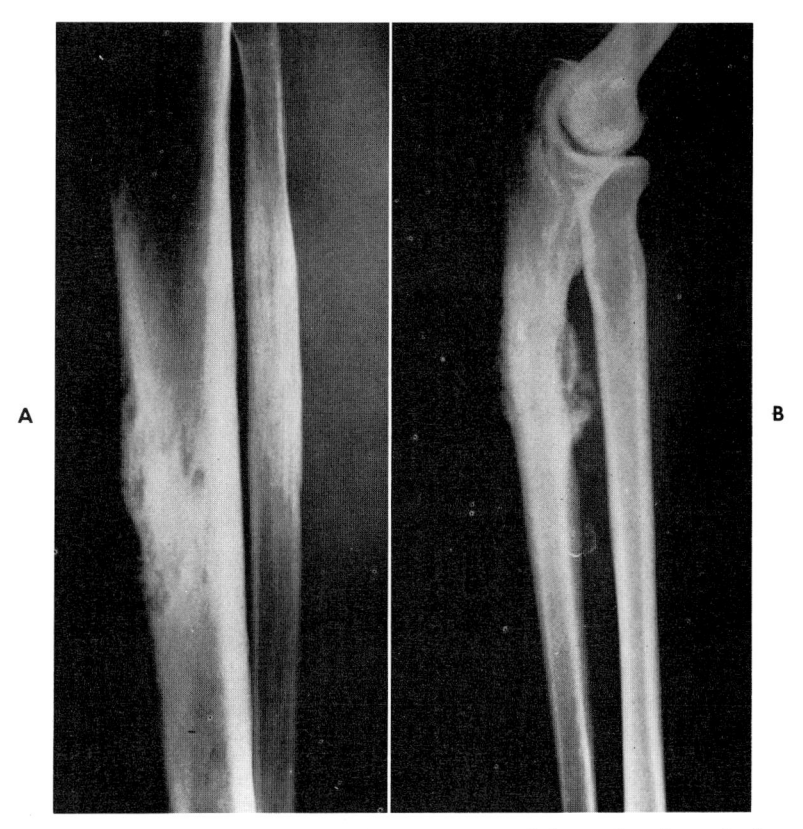

Fig. A-3. A, Roentgenogram of a lesion of gummatous syphilis in the tibia, which might be mistaken by some for a bone sarcoma. There is also apparent cortical thickening of the contiguous fibula. B, Pathologic fracture with exuberant callus in an ulna, which healed under antisyphilitic therapy. The lesion was at first considered to be an osteogenic sarcoma by some observers. The patient is known to have been well eight years later.

losing valuable time. It is interesting to note also that the rather large, circumscribed skeletal defects reflecting the early resorptive changes in Paget's disease may likewise prove confusing. Their appearance and significance in the calvarium are well recognized (so-called osteoporosis circumscripta cranii), but it is not generally appreciated that comparable defects may develop in other bones, e.g., the innominate bone or a tibia, as a forerunner of typical Paget transformation (Fig. A-16).

Continuing in the same vein, a solitary focus of fibrous dysplasia of bone may readily be mistaken for a benign neoplasm of one kind or another, if one is not altogether familiar with its roentgenographic and pathologic characteristics. Thus, it is not uncommon to find pertinent lesions in jaw bones, particularly, labeled as fibrous osteoma or ossifying fibroma, or lesions in large limb bones such as the femur or tibia interpreted as nonosteogenic fibroma. I am also aware of several instances in which a relatively large lesion of fibrous dysplasia in a limb bone, occupying a substantial part of the shaft, was overdiag-

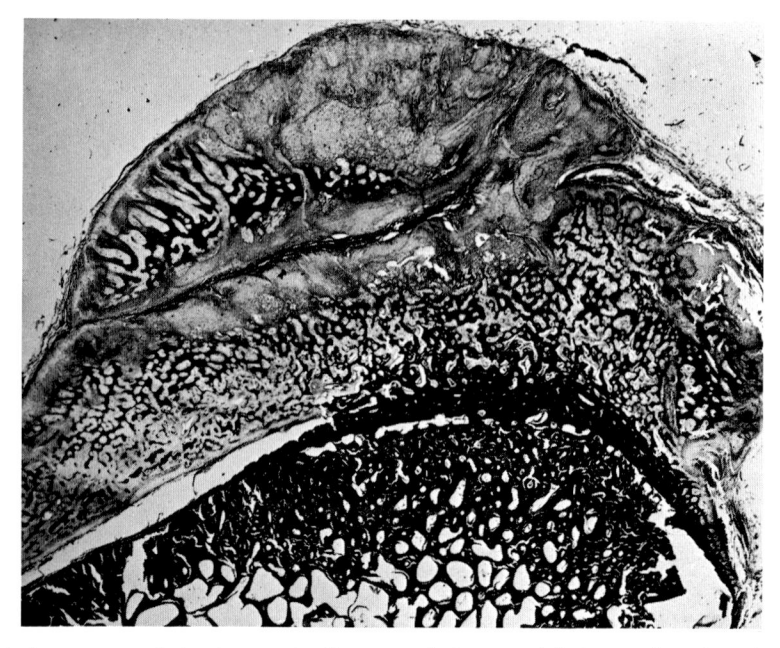

Fig. A-4. Low-power photomicrograph of a somewhat unusual instance of periosteal cartilaginous and osseous metaplasia leading to the formation of an exostotic tumor clinically and roentgenographically. The new bone formed by ossification of cartilage is layered over the original cortex (of a femur).

nosed as osteogenic sarcoma. When confronted with a solitary focus of fibrous dysplasia in a rib, a common location for it, radiologists seem prone to misinterpret such a lesion as a central cartilage tumor, despite its rather distinctive appearance (Fig. A-6, A).

In dealing with lesions held to represent osteogenic sarcoma, one must be particularly careful before resorting to ablation or radical resection to make certain that the condition does not represent some other, less serious lesion exhibiting active new bone formation for whatever reason.[2,24] That this problem in differentiation may at times constitute a formidable pitfall is evidenced by the fact that the five-year cures of osteogenic sarcoma, so-called, are undoubtedly padded by cases of periosteal ossification, myositis ossificans (in an active stage), ossifying hematoma, and exuberant fracture callus, among other conditions. I have personal knowledge of an appreciable number of such cases in which review of the pertinent roentgenograms and pathologic specimens indicated clearly that the lesions in question had been overdiagnosed, and that a surgical procedure far less drastic than amputation would have effected a clinical cure. It seems to be true, unfortunately, that pathologists not well versed in the subtleties of the diagnosis of skeletal lesions are sometimes stampeded into a diagnosis of osteogenic sarcoma by the observation of active osseous and cartilaginous metaplasia of connective tissue, even though the latter is situated outside of the bone and the background of the lesion as a whole is not that of an

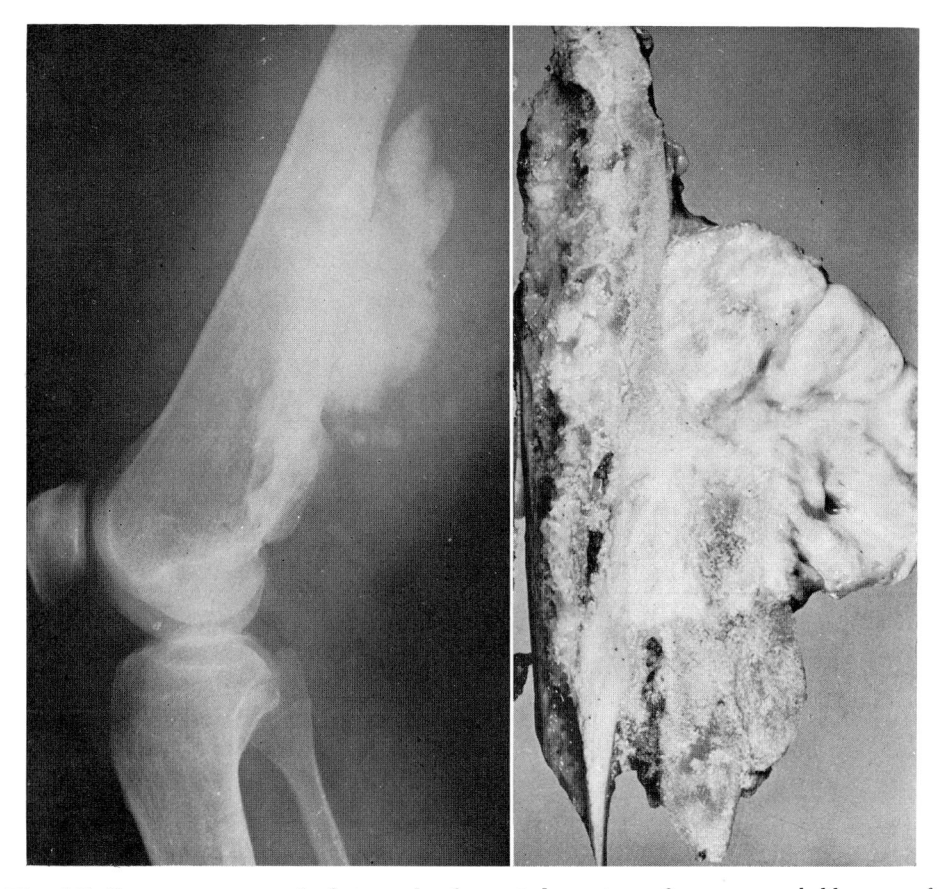

Fig. A-5. Roentgenogram and photograph of resected specimen from a remarkable case of metaplastic cartilage and bone formation within the connective tissue of the periosteum and/or the adjacent muscle tissue, simulating chondrosarcoma. A mass had been excised from the shaft of the femur thirty years previously; this mass reappeared nineteen years later and slowly progressed in size for about eleven years up to the time of resection. (Courtesy Dr. Lauren V. Ackerman, St. Louis, Mo.)

osteogenic sarcoma. It is important in this connection to stress once again that pertinent information in regard to the clinical history, the roentgen picture, and the surgeon's findings is essential in arriving at an intelligent opinion, self-evident though this may seem.

In such instances, one must be guided further by the principle that one must appraise a lesion in the light of its probable ultimate behavior rather than by its seemingly ominous cytologic appearance at the height of its activity. Stated more explicitly, localized foci of active osseous, and sometimes also cartilaginous, metaplasia of the connective tissue of muscle (so-called myositis ossificans) and of the periosteum tend with few exceptions to be self-limited rather than progressive. That is to say, they burn themselves out eventually, in the sense that in their end stage they come to be matured and reconstructed bony masses in-

390 Appendixes

capable of further significant growth. This appears to be true whether the lesion develops as a result of an injury (with or without associated hemorrhage) or whether it develops spontaneously due to causes unknown. Experienced orthopedic surgeons are well aware of this trend and of the desirability of waiting until the process of metaplastic ossification has fully subsided, rather than op-

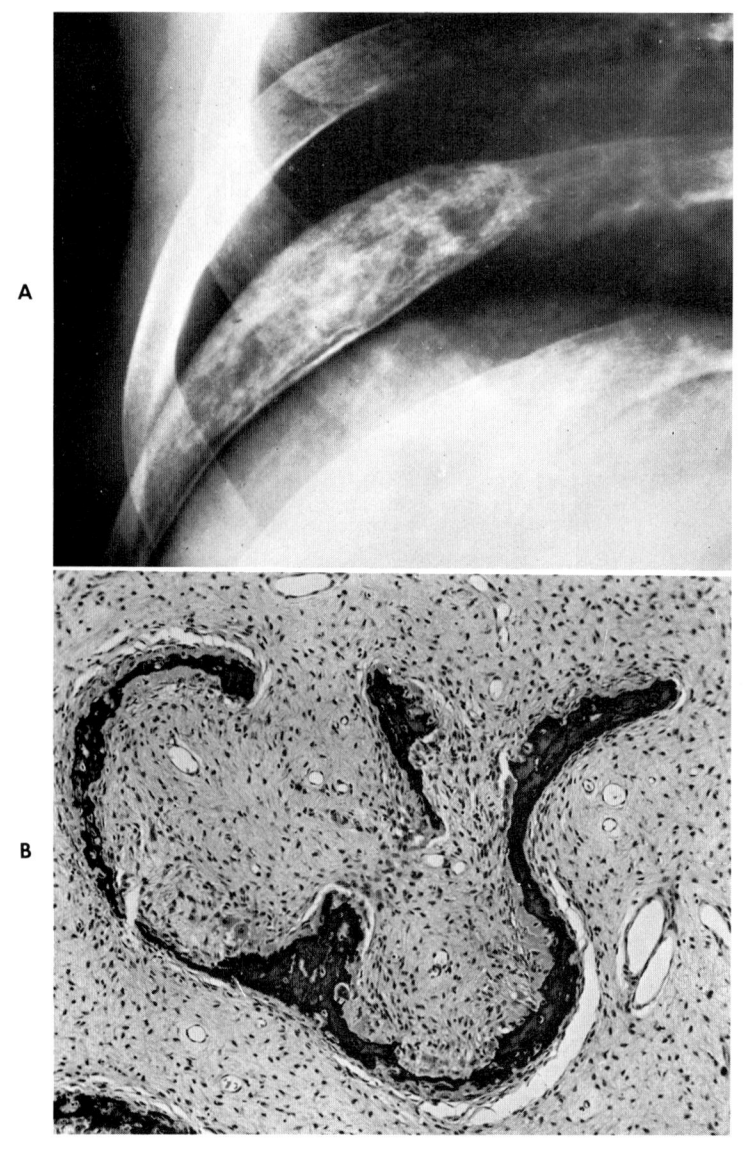

Fig. A-6. **A,** Roentgenogram of a fusiform, expanded, tumorlike lesion in a rib, which was resected and proved to be a focus of fibrous dysplasia. It was discovered in a routine chest film, and was apparently the only lesion the patient presented. **B,** Photomicrograph of a representative field from a comparable lesion of fibrous dysplasia. Note the delicate, spindly connective tissue stroma, in which curlicues of metaplastic bone have been deposited, mainly along the course of blood vessels.

erating prematurely at the risk of provoking renewed activity. One must take cognizance of the fact, however, that there are a few cases in the literature indicating that on rare occasions sarcoma may develop at a site of myositis ossificans[21] or of an ossifying hematoma[3] and lead to fatal pulmonary metastases. I have never observed such instances in my own experience and for that matter (quite aside from any consideration of myositis ossificans as a predisposing factor) I have encountered relatively few neoplasms that could be plausibly interpreted as extraskeletal osteogenic sarcoma, although neoplastic bone and cartilage may occasionally make their appearance as integral neoplastic components of malignant mesenchymal tumors of soft parts.

As noted, exuberant callus developing at a site of pathologic fracture due to whatever cause may sometimes be misinterpreted as an indication of a sclerosing osteogenic sarcoma. I have had occasion to review a case in which a pertinent lesion in an ulna, thought at first to represent a sarcoma, proved subsequently to be a gumma. Fortunately, the pathologist who interpreted the biopsy sections, though leaning in favor of osteogenic sarcoma, took so long to reach a definite decision that sufficient time elapsed for the lesion to heal under antisyphilitic therapy (Fig. A-3, *B*). Apropos of this case and others like it, experienced radiologists need scarcely be reminded that in dealing with equivocal skeletal lesions, as with equivocal lesions elsewhere, it is important to have the benefit of essential clinical data. In regard to the problem of pathologic interpretation, it may be helpful to emphasize again, as previously noted, that before a lesion can be interpreted as an osteogenic sarcoma, one must be certain that it is actually a sarcoma in the first place. In other words, however extensive or otherwise impressive the tendency to new bone formation may be, an essential prerequisite for the diagnosis of osteogenic sarcoma is the presence of a connective tissue stroma that is frankly sarcomatous. This is not intended to imply that the distinction is invariably a simple one to make (as noted in the case cited previously), and there are undoubtedly instances that call for nice judgment and mature experience.

The remainder of this discussion will be devoted to further consideration of a limited number of specific lesions of bone, which deserve special comment for one reason or another, namely, fibrous dysplasia of bone, the skeletal manifestations of histiocytosis X (eosinophilic granuloma, Schüller-Christian disease, and Letterer-Siwe disease), aneurysmal bone cyst, the skeletal changes in hyperparathyroidism, and monostotic Paget's disease.

Fibrous dysplasia of bone

My interest in fibrous dysplasia of bone dates back to 1938 when I described the distinctive skeletal pathologic changes and coined the name "polyostotic fibrous dysplasia" to designate them appropriately. Subsequently, the qualifying adjective "polyostotic" was dropped when it became evident that in many instances only a single bone is involved. The finding of associated skin pigmentation and of certain endocrine abnormalities, especially precocious sexual development in female patients, had previously been noted by Goldhamer and by Borak and Doll, among others, and emphasized particularly by McCune and Bruch, and by Albright and his associates. The latter group, especially, subsequently publicized these more dramatic cases in children presenting various extraskeletal abnormalities, as well as widespread severe skeletal alterations, and accomplished this so effectively that the changes described came to be designated as Albright's syndrome, although Albright himself subsequently recommended that the name fibrous dysplasia be generally adopted to apply to all pertinent cases of the disorder, irrespective of their severity.

In 1942 Jaffe and I[19] reviewed the entire subject on the basis of greater experience with it and expressed the view that the disease as a whole apparently represents a peculiar developmental anomaly in which the basic skeletal changes common to all cases may be supplemented, particularly in the more severe instances, by various extraskeletal aberrations; specifically, blotchy pigmentation of the skin, premature sexual development, premature skeletal growth and maturation, and hyperthyroidism, as well as cardiovascular and other developmental defects. The skeletal lesions apparently result from perverted activity of the bone-forming mesenchyme. Incidentally, Changus[4] has shown that the connective tissue cells differ from ordinary fibroblasts in that they are rich in alka-

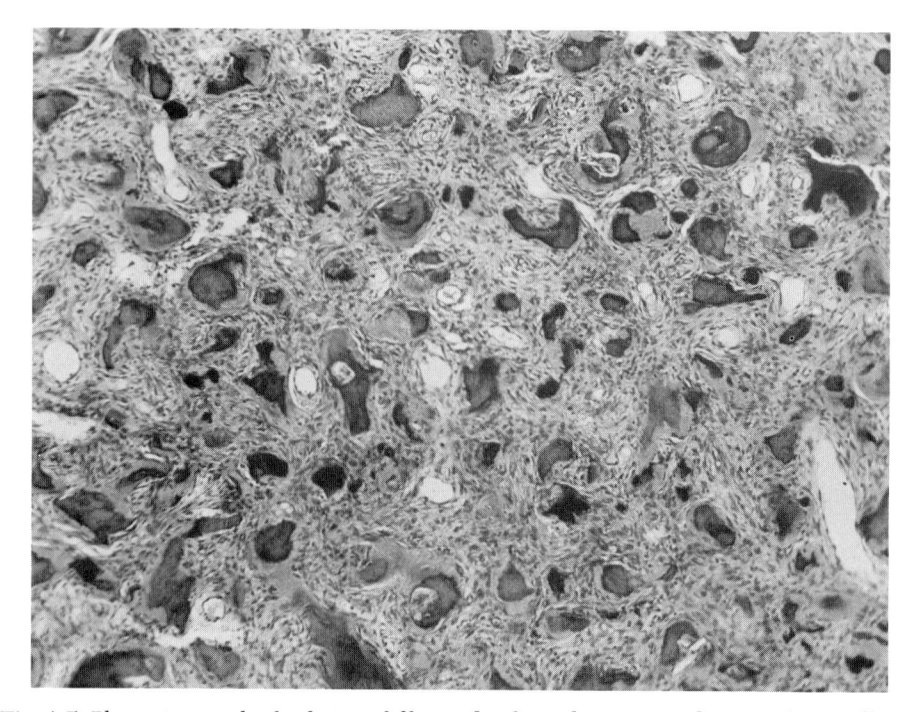

Fig. A-7. Photomicrograph of a lesion of fibrous dysplasia that presented as a rather small, circumscribed, lytic defect in a calvarium. This is a distinctive pattern frequently observed in lesions of fibrous dysplasia that develop within bones preformed in membrane (calvarium and jaw bones). ($\times 100$.)

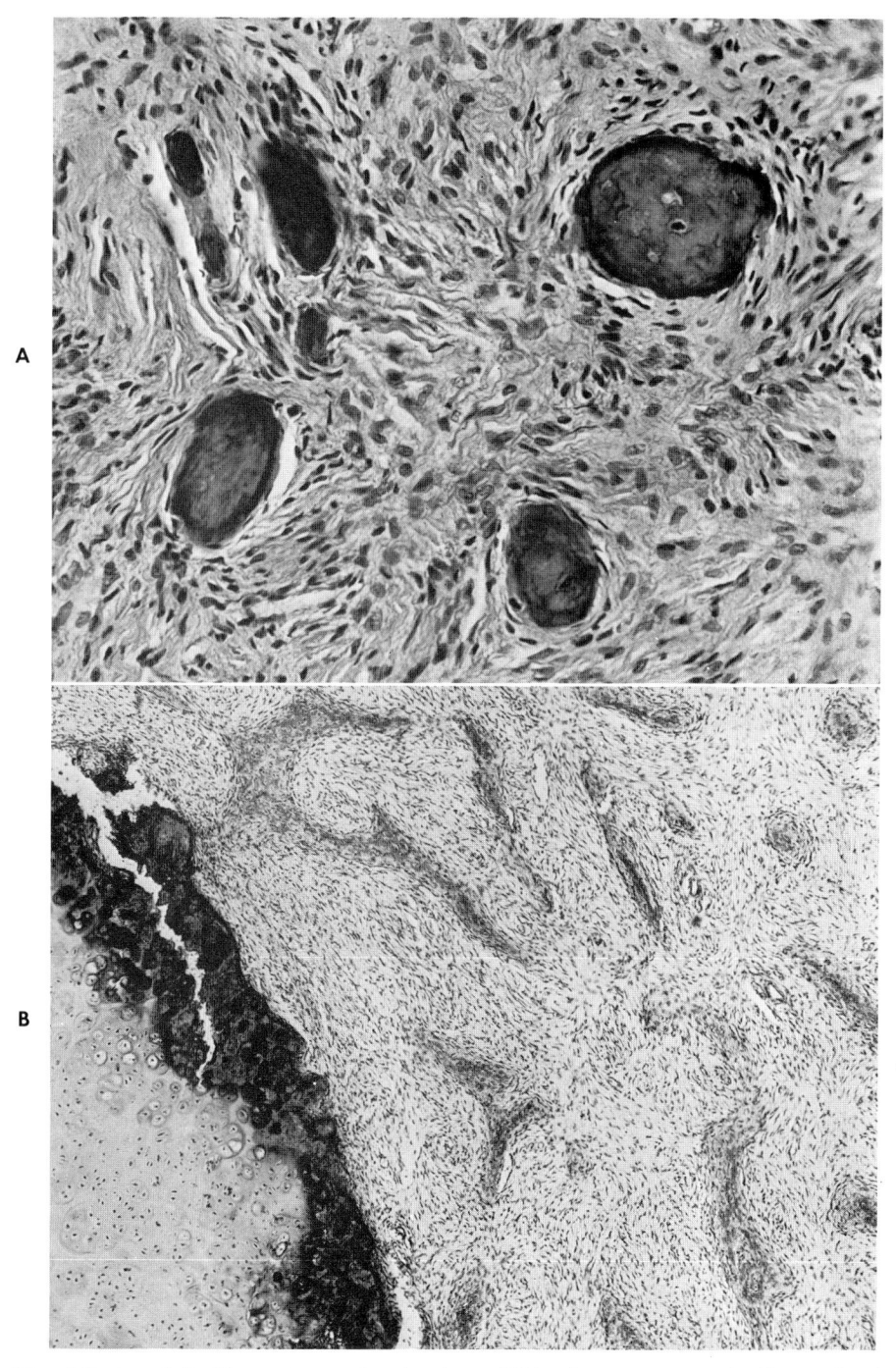

Some nonneoplastic lesions of bone that may be mistaken for tumors

Fig. A-8. A and **B**, Photomicrographs showing additional patterns seen in fibrous dysplasia. The lesion in **B** also shows an island of hyaline cartilage, heavily calcified around its periphery. **C**, Roentgenogram showing marked deformity and expansion of a femur affected by fibrous dysplasia. **D**, Roentgenogram showing widespread advanced changes of fibrous dysplasia in an adult. The initial (erroneous) impression was hyperparathyroidism, and the patient was operated for suspected parathyroid adenoma.

C

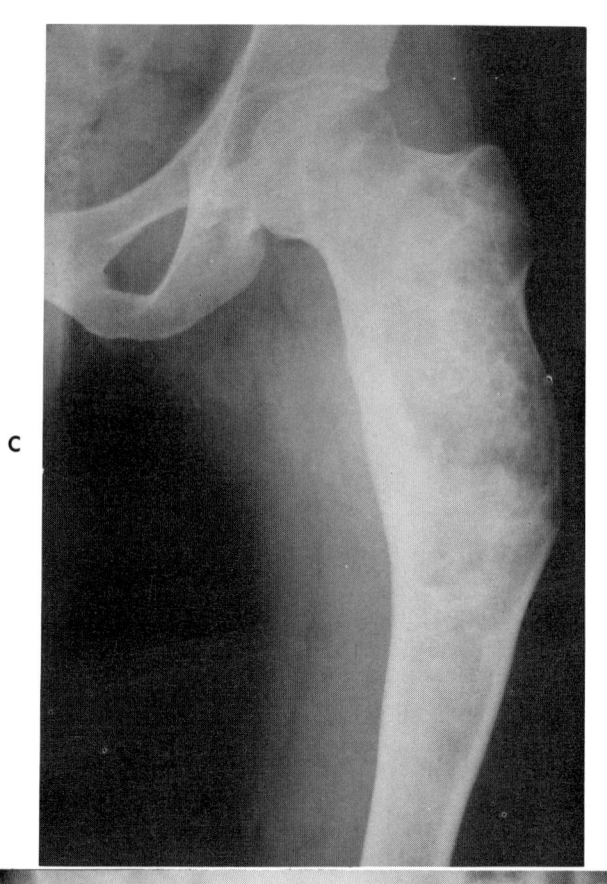

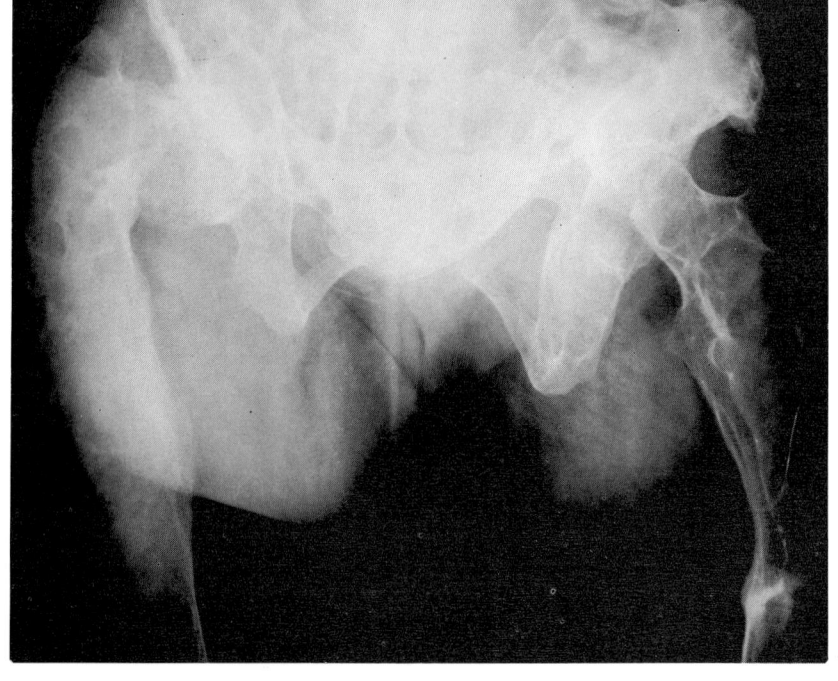

D

Fig. A-8, cont'd. For legend see p. 393.

line phosphatase. The affected bone areas may be expanded, bowed, and otherwise deformed (Fig. A-8, C) and are filled with a distinctive whitish, rubbery, and somewhat gritty fibrous tissue, which in occasional instances may also contain more or less prominent islands of hyaline cartilage. While occasional patients may exhibit the florid expression of the disorder in early childhood, many more show limited skeletal involvement, often predominantly unilateral or monomelic. The great majority (frequently adults) present only a single bone lesion, or a few at most, and by way of extraskeletal changes nothing more than perhaps an occasional patch of hyperpigmented skin. For valuable information on the natural history of fibrous dysplasia culled from a long-term follow-up study of some fifty cases, the reader is referred to the article (1962) by Harris, Dudley, and Barry.[7]

By way of differential diagnosis, it is worth noting that adult patients with fibrous dysplasia involving several or many bones are sometimes thought to have hyperparathyroidism and may even be subjected to a search for a parathyroid adenoma (Fig. A-8, D). I have knowledge of an appreciable number of such cases, and the literature contains reference to many more. Solitary foci of fibrous dysplasia, on the other hand, are not infrequently mistaken for tumors and, as such, treated more vigorously than is necessary (e.g., by block excision). Actually, their surgical removal is usually elective rather than mandatory. If such a lesion, however, is still expanding (in a jaw bone, for example), is painful or cosmetically deforming, or is prone to pathologic fracture, clinical cure can usually be accomplished by thorough curettement and packing with bone chips. On occasion, if the defect thus created is sufficiently large or so situated as to necessitate reinforcement of the affected area, one may resort to the use of an additional inlay strut. Irradiation of these bone lesions would seem to be contraindicated.

It is also pertinent here to consider briefly the question of malignant change in skeletal lesions of fibrous dysplasia. In recent years a veritable rash of case reports has amply confirmed the old observation of Coley and Stewart[5] that sarcomatous change may ensue in skeletal lesions of fibrous dysplasia, and these observations have been compiled by Schwartz and Alpert.[23] Malignant change may develop without prior irradiation, it may be observed in monostotic as well as polyostotic lesions, and it apparently occurs most often in bones of the craniofacial region and in large limb bones. It should be emphasized, however, that this complication is less common than it is in Paget's disease, and that its overall incidence appears to be of the order of a fraction of 1%.

Histiocytosis X (eosinophilic granuloma of bone, Schüller-Christian disease, and Letterer-Siwe disease)

In a review article[13] in 1953 under the above heading, I surveyed the accumulated evidence indicating that eosinophilic granuloma, Schüller-Christian disease, and Letterer-Siwe disease are all interrelated expressions of the same malady, for which the provisional designation of histiocytosis X was proposed for con-

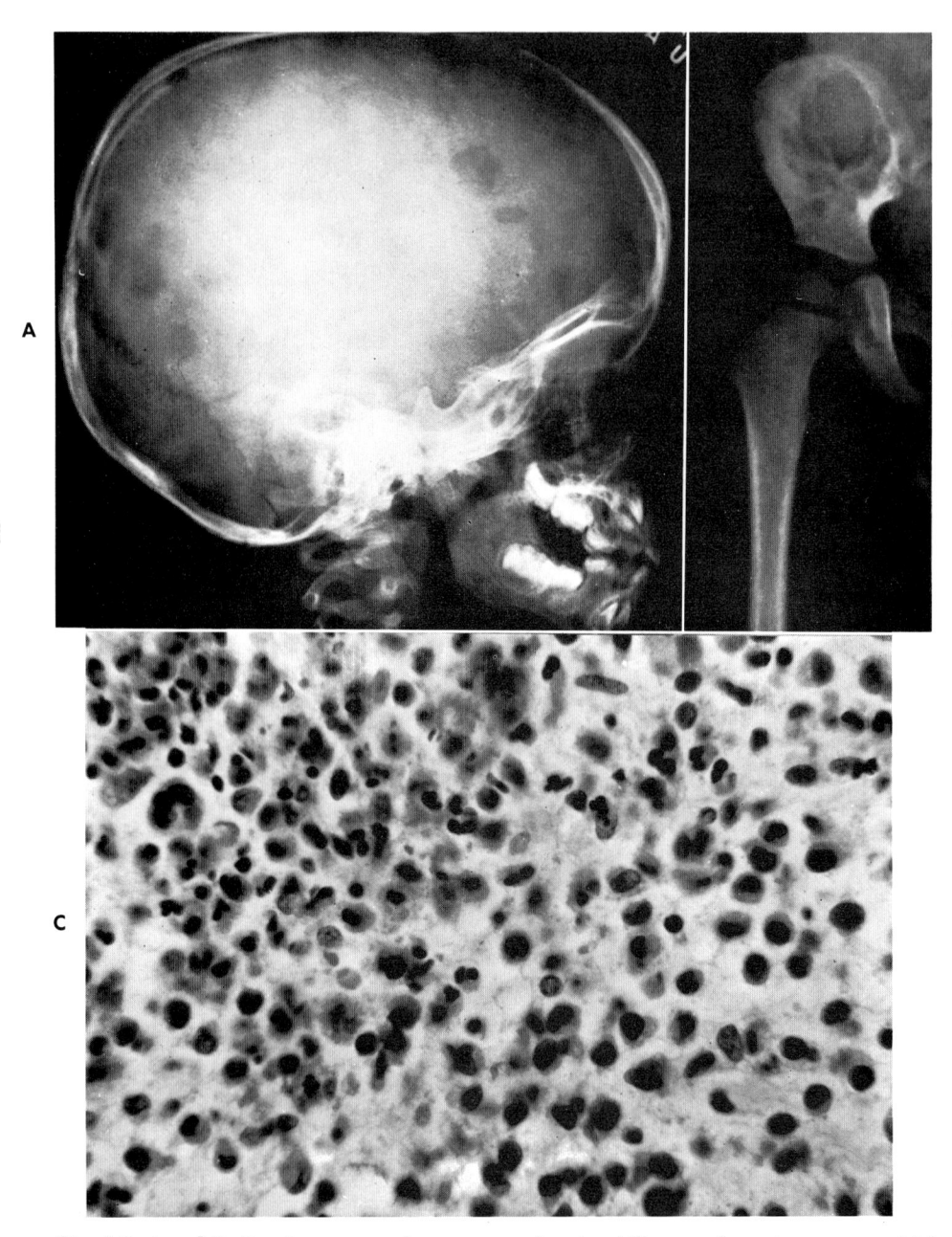

Fig. A-9. A and B, Roentgenograms from a case of eosinophilic granuloma in a young child, showing lytic, tumorlike defects in the calvarium and also in the wing of an iliac bone. C, Photomicrograph of a field from a lesion of eosinophilic granuloma showing (eosinophilic) leukocytes intermingled with histiocytes. (×400.)

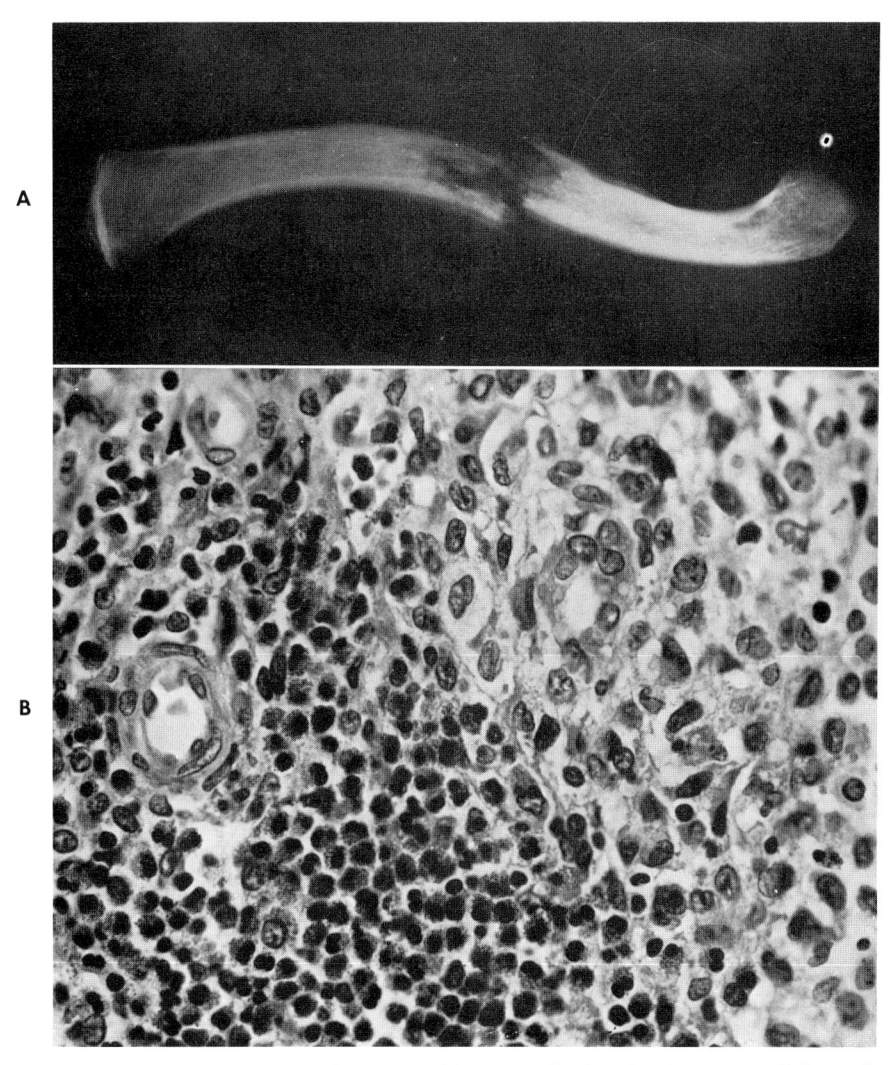

Some nonneoplastic lesions of bone that may be mistaken for tumors

Fig. A-10. **A,** Roentgenogram of a surgically removed clavicle showing pathologic fracture through a destructive tumorlike lesion, which proved to be an eosinophilic granuloma. Had the surgeon been aware of this possibility, conservative biopsy followed by roentgen therapy would have sufficed for cure. **B,** Photomicrograph of a lesion of eosinophilic granuloma. The leukocytes massed on the left are all eosinophils; the larger cells on the right are of histiocytic nature. (×450.)

398 Appendixes

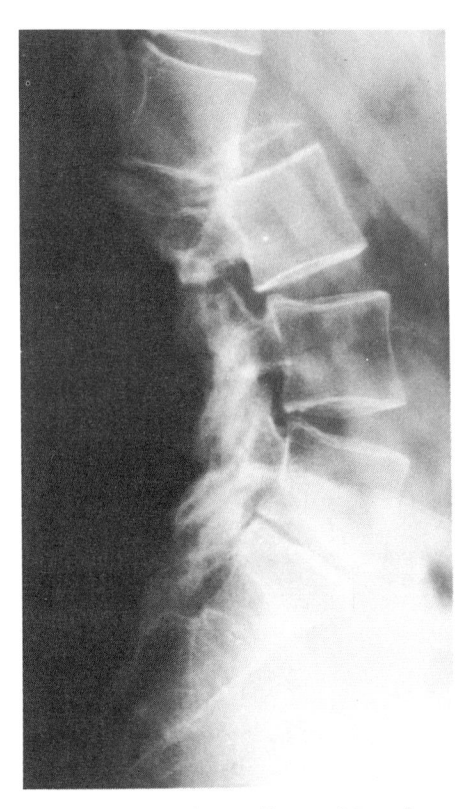

Fig. A-11. Roentgenogram showing complete collapse of L-2 due to a lesion of eosinophilic granuloma (biopsy), with remarkable luxation and angulation of the vertebral column proximal to it. (Courtesy Mr. Lloyd Griffith, Manchester, England.)

venient reference. The subject was again brought up to date in another paper[17] published in 1964. There are many features of the disease complex to suggest that it represents a reaction to some peculiar infection (possibly viral). A group of French investigators[1] in Paris have demonstrated cytoplasmic rod-shaped inclusion bodies in electron microscopic preparations from lesions of histiocytosis X (bone and lung). This observation has been confirmed by De Man,[6] but the significance of these bodies is still uncertain. According to this concept, the lesion of eosinophilic granuloma seems to represent the pathologic expression of early, rather rapidly developing reaction to the etiologic agent, and, as such, it may appear not only within bone, where its presence was first recognized, but also in other sites as well, notably in lymph nodes, the skin, the oral cavity (gingiva, palate, etc.), and the anogenital region, as well as in the lungs, the liver, kidneys, female genitalia, and possibly the cranial nerves and eye as well. It may be encountered not only as a skeletal lesion per se, in which case the prognosis is favorable, but also as a destructive skeletal focus developing in the clinical course of either the Letterer-Siwe or the Schüller-Christian syndrome. The latter apparently represent the acute (or subacute) and chronic forms, respectively, of the same systemic malady. Collaterally, the old idea stemming from Rowland and Thannhauser that so-called Schüller-Christian disease represents a disorder of lipid metabolism is no longer tenable.

Classification of histiocytosis X

Histiocytosis X, localized to bone (eosinophilic granuloma, solitary or multiple)
Histiocytosis X, disseminated, acute or subacute (Letterer-Siwe syndrome)
   With destructive skeletal lesions (esoinophilic granuloma)
   With transition to chronic phase (Schüller-Christian syndrome)
Histiocytosis, disseminated, chronic (Schüller-Christian syndrome)
   With destructive skeletal lesions (eosinophilic granuloma)
   With early extraskeletal lesions (indicate sites) resembling eosinophilic granuloma
   With acute or subacute exacerbation (Letterer-Siwe syndrome)
   With involvement predominantly of bones, lungs, pituitary, and/or brain, skin, mucous membranes (oral, anal, genital), liver, or lymph nodes, etc. (in varying combinations, as the case may be)

In regard to therapy and prognosis, we now know that the acute disseminated form of the disease (Letterer-Siwe) is not invariably fatal and that some infants and young children can be carried along for years into a more chronic phase (Schüller-Christian). Similarly, even in relatively serious, progressive cases of the chronic disseminated expression of the disease (Schüller-Christian) in adults, as well as children, presenting diabetes insipidus and/or extensive pulmonary infiltration as their major problem, it is often possible by alert and well-conceived clinical management to ward off a fatal outcome for some time and occasionally to induce a remission. Such management is concerned mainly with abatement of skeletal and extraskeletal foci through the use of adequate roentgen therapy, general supportive measures, prevention and control of potentially serious secondary infections by the judicious use of antibiotics, amelioration of diabetes insipidus by the use of Pitressin or irradiation, and the use of steroid (cortisone) therapy.

Aneurysmal bone cyst

The distinctive lesion we called aneurysmal bone cyst[9,11,12,16] represents a pathologic entity not uncommon that has gained general recognition,[20,25] although, as noted, individual instances of it are still mistaken by some for an unusual type of giant-cell tumor and even for osteogenic sarcoma. In a survey in 1957[16] I commented on observations gleaned from as many as fifty cases (encountered since 1948). The lesion develops in vertebrae and flat bones, as well as long bones. The affected site, whatever its location may be, is completely transformed and ultimately comes to resemble a peculiarly expanded, brownish, blood-filled sponge that, if untreated, may attain impressive size. The communicating pools of venous blood within this reservoir are bordered by connective tissue septa showing giant-cell reaction, especially within fields of blood extravasation, as well as more or less conspicuous reparative new bone formation, by way of attempted reconstruction. In regard to pathogenesis, I favor the view that the condition apparently results from some local circulatory disturbance, leading to

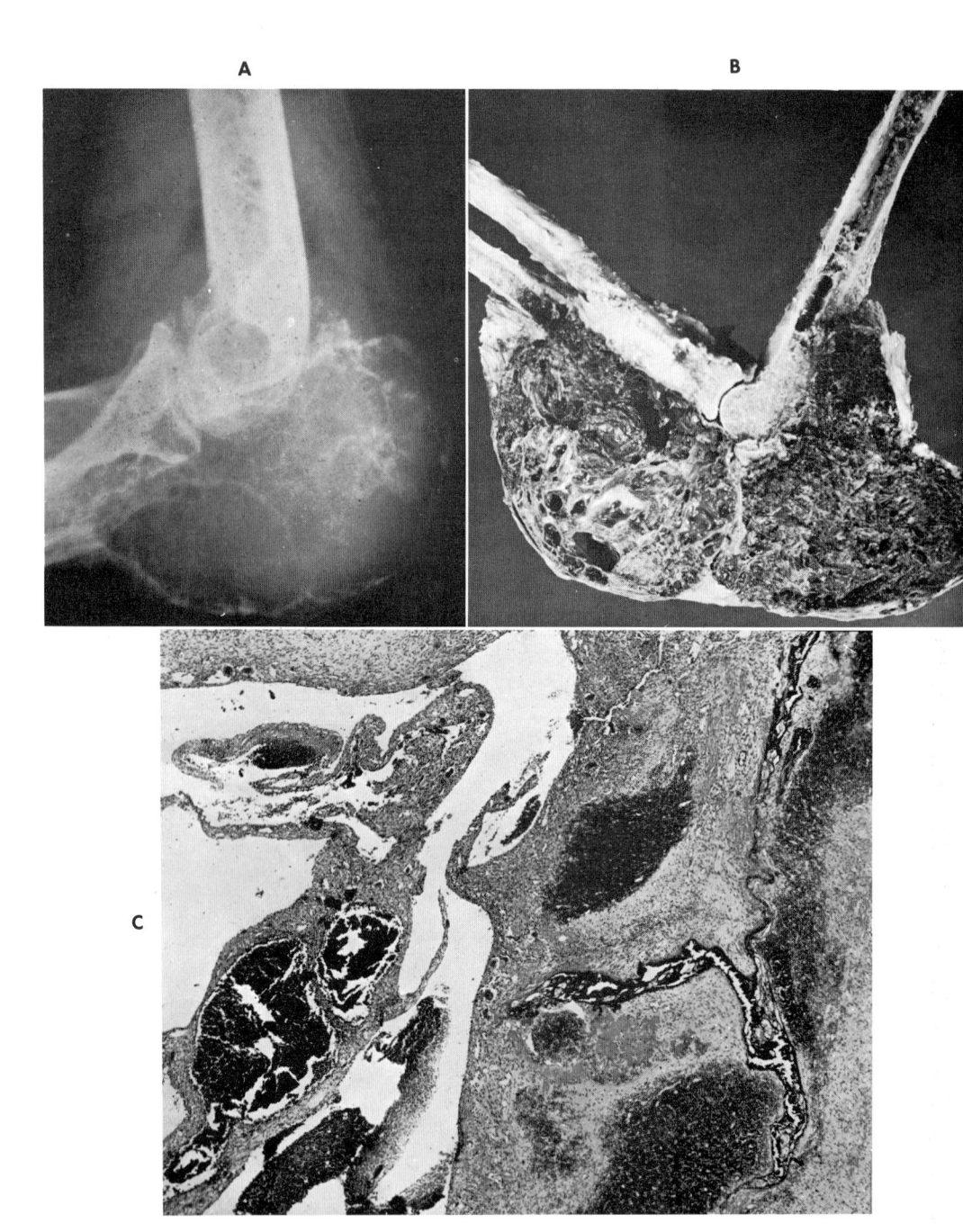

Fig. A-12. A, Roentgenogram of an aneurysmal bone cyst originating in and protruding from the upper end of an ulna. B, Photograph of the same lesion after it had progressed for another year. (Amputation was performed because useful reconstruction was no longer deemed feasible.) The lesion was spongelike in its architecture and composed of innumerable dilated blood-filled spaces lined by fibroosseous septa. C, Photomicrograph of a representative field of an aneurysmal bone cyst showing its essential pattern. Other fields may show more active osseous reconstruction or giant-cell reaction to hemorrhage.

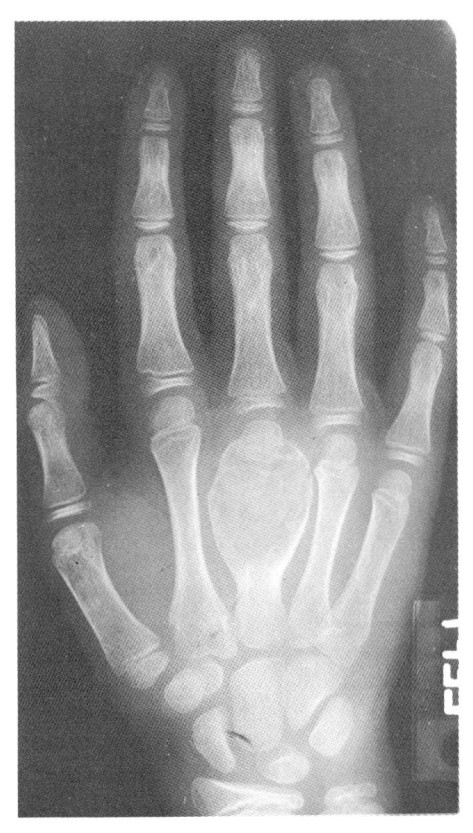

Fig. A-13. An aneurysmal bone cyst that has produced symmetrical expansion of the proximal shaft of a metacarpal bone.

markedly increased venous pressure and the development of a dilated and engorged vascular bed within the affected bone area. The anomalous circulation could conceivably result from intraosseous arteriovenous shunts.[18]

Aneurysmal bone cyst is not serious, if recognized and treated promptly, although it can have serious consequences if neglected (e.g., loss of a limb or spinal cord damage). It responds satisfactorily to thorough curettement and can be controlled also by roentgen therapy in moderate dosage. The latter is the treatment of choice in dealing with lesions in vertebral bodies or their neural arches, where an attempt at surgical extirpation might be hazardous.

Skeletal changes in hyperparathyroidism

In the modern era of early parathyroid surgery for suspected tumor, one seldom has the opportunity any longer to observe the devastating skeletal changes of "osteitis fibrosa cystica generalisata" of Recklinghausen. If one wishes to observe the curiously bent, broadened, extremely porotic and fractured bones reflecting the natural end stage of hyperparathyroidism, one must have recourse to museum specimens dating back forty years or more. Today, one is more likely

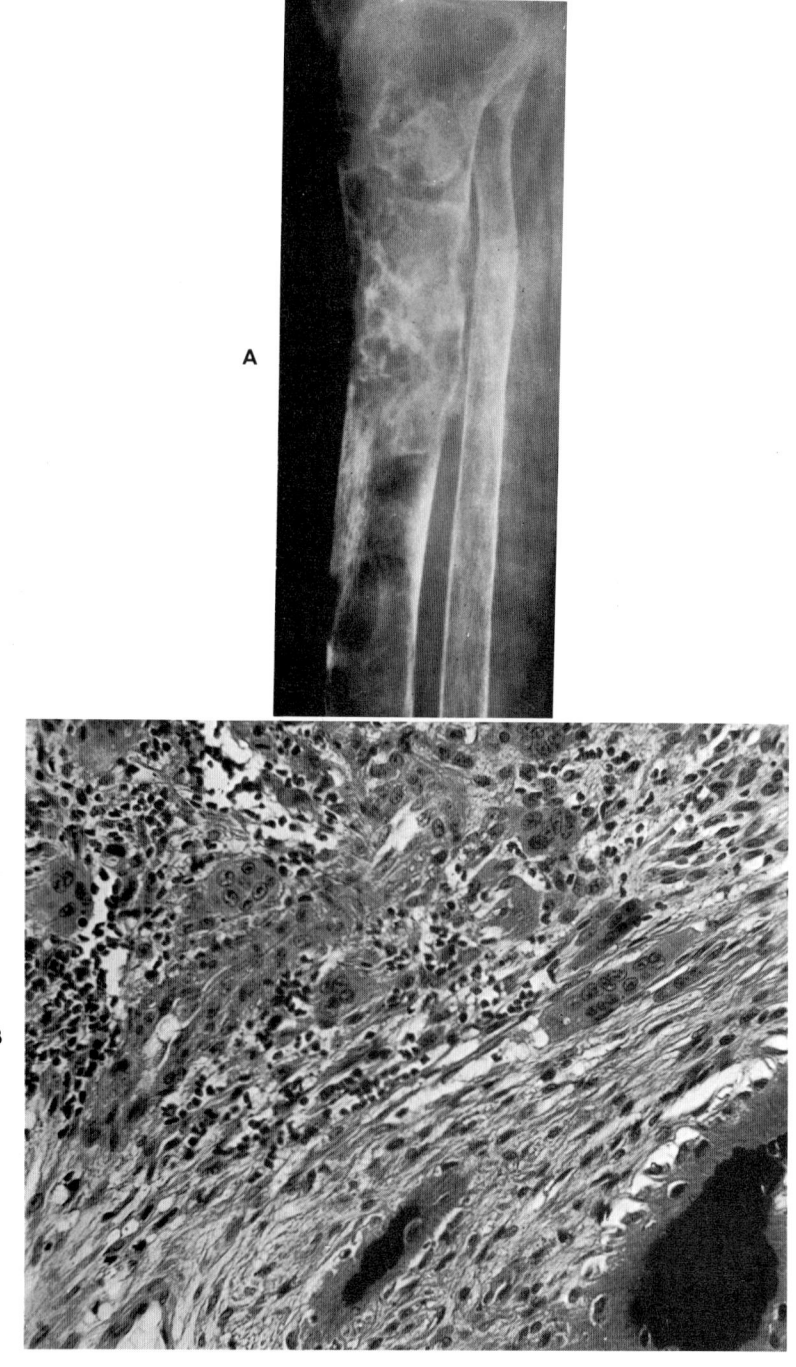

Fig. A-14. A, Roentgenogram of a tibia and fibula from a proved case of hyperparathyroidism with far-advanced skeletal changes. (The patient had also sustained a pathologic fracture of a femur, which failed to unite.) B, A representative field of a biopsy taken from the tibia showing extensive resorption and fibrous replacement of the bone, as well as conspicuous giant-cell reaction at a site of hemorrhage (so-called "brown tumor"). (×100.)

Some nonneoplastic lesions of bone that may be mistaken for tumors 403

to observe rather subtle roentgen evidences of skeletal resorption, such as cortical rarefaction and subperiosteal scalloping, requiring close scrutiny for their detection, and often even these are lacking. In other instances, it is true, the skeletal effects of hyperparathyroidism may be more pronounced and find expression in distinct cortical thinning of long bones, the presence of cystlike rarefactions (at sites of brown tumor, so-called) or perhaps pathologic fracture through a demineralized bone, going on to nonunion. In such cases, if one is aware of the possibility of hyperparathyroidism, confirmatory evidence of the diagnosis leading to surgical exploration will be readily furnished by such findings as granular mottling of the calvarium, resorptive changes in the phalanges, nephrocalcinosis and attendant renal damage, and significant serum chemical alterations, particularly persistent hypercalcemia and increased serum alkaline phosphatase activity, as well as significantly altered renal tubular reabsorption of phosphate.

If the observer is not alerted to the possibility of hyperparathyroidism by the history and the skeletal roentgen changes, he may be led to suspect carcinomatosis or multiple myeloma or perhaps senile or idiopathic osteoporosis. Also, it is not too unusual for localized rarefied defects resulting from hyperparathyroidism to be confused with giant-cell tumor, as previously noted, and occasionally with aneurysmal bone cyst.

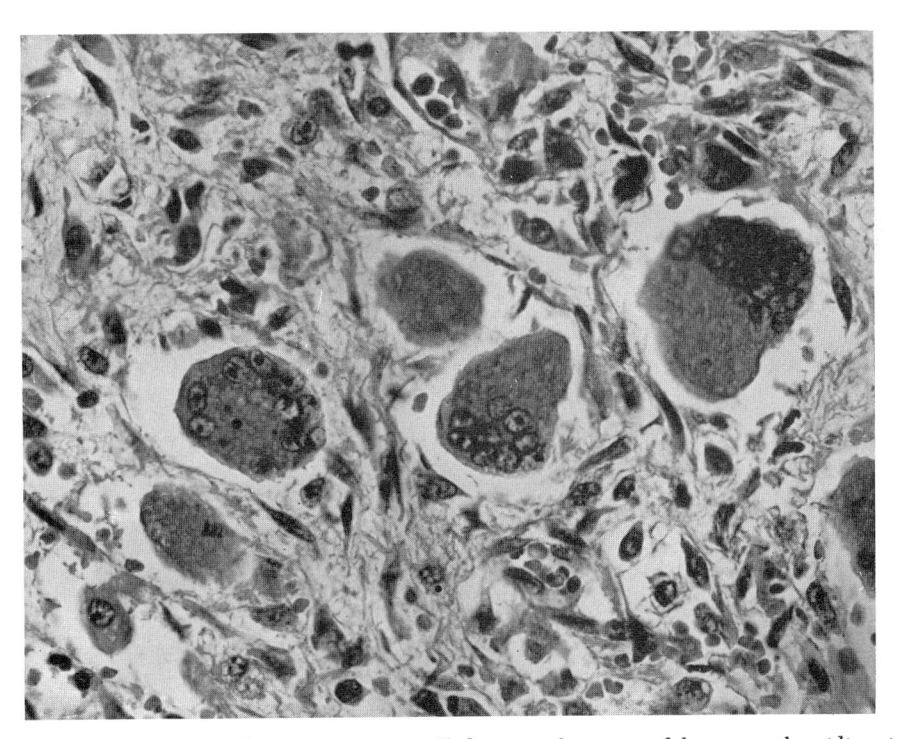

Fig. A-15. A field from a brown tumor, so-called, in another case of hyperparathyroidism intended to show that the large multinuclear cells are lodged within blood channels. This picture is quite different from that of genuine giant-cell tumor (see Figs. 12-10 and 12-11, taken at the same magnification). (×420.)

404   *Appendixes*

The treatment of primary hyperparathyroidism consists, of course, of surgical removal of the hyperfunctioning parathyroid tissue. In the great majority of instances, this will prove to be an adenoma of a single gland, although occasionally there may be two adenomas and, sometimes, hyperplasia of all four glands. The technical aspects of parathyroidectomy and the problems relating to postoperative care are beyond the scope of this discussion. It may be in order, however, to emphasize, as is now well known, that the surgeon must be prepared, if necessary, to search for an aberrant adenoma in the vicinity of the esophagus or in the superior mediastinum and to safeguard by appropriate means against renal suppression, as well as temporary postsurgical hypoparathyroidism manifested in tetany.

Paget's disease (monostotic)

This section will deal briefly with the recognition of relatively early monostotic lesions of Paget's disease, which still prove puzzling to many surgeons and radiologists. Just as foci of intense resorption and fibrous replacement of bone

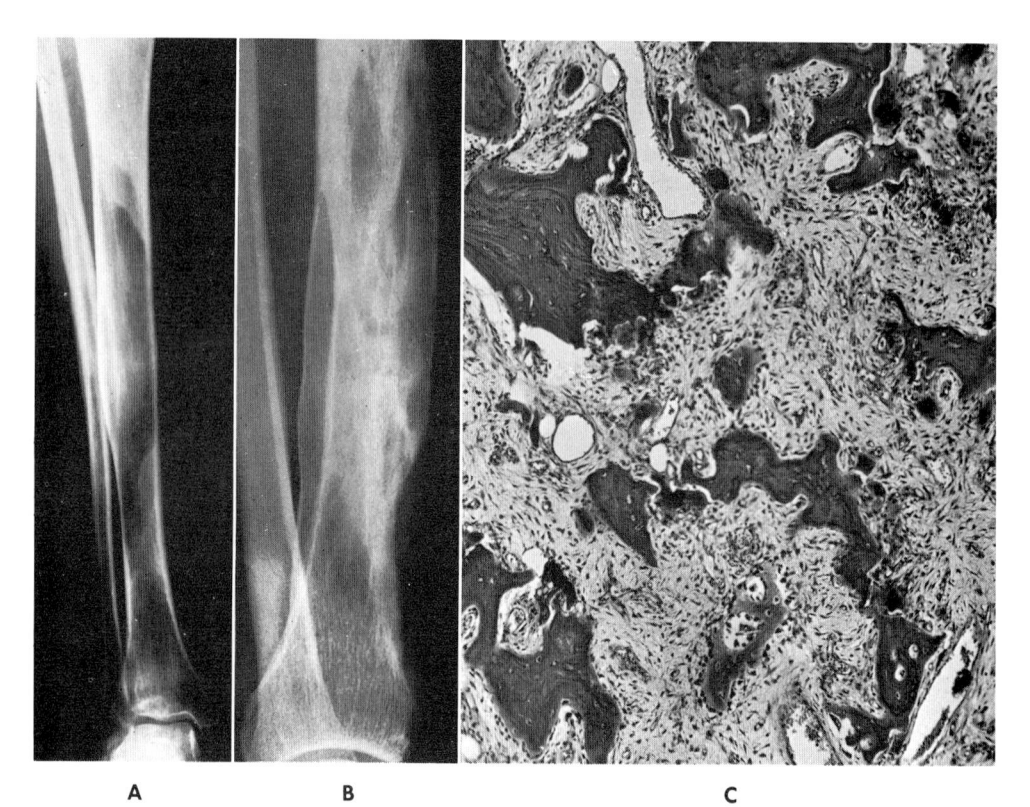

Fig. A-16. **A** and **B**, Roentgenograms of two instances of early monostotic Paget's disease involving the lower tibia. The lesion in each instance is still in a phase of active resorption and does not as yet show typical Paget transformation. **C**, Photomicrograph of a field from the biopsy of the lesion of Paget's disease illustrated in **B**. (×75.)

in hyperparathyroidism may be manifested roentgenographically in the appearance of localized defects sometimes mistaken for tumors (especially giant-cell tumor), so, too, the sizable circumscribed skeletal defects reflecting the early resorptive changes in Paget's disease may likewise prove confusing at times. Their appearance and significance in the calvarium are now well recognized (so-called osteoporosis circumscripta cranii). It seems not to be generally appreciated, however, that comparable defects may develop in other bones, e.g., an innominate bone, a tibia, or a humerus, as a forerunner of typical Paget transformation. When the tibia is involved, it is frequently the upper half of the shaft that is affected, although occasionally the lower end may display comparable changes (Fig. A-16, A and B). The rarefied defect often terminates sharply and is likely to be associated with some expansion of the shaft and thinning of its cortex, although there is not as yet any discernible coarse trabecular architecture. Altogether, if one is alert to the possibility, the roentgenographic picture of such lesions is sufficiently distinctive to suggest early monostotic Paget's disease (rather than a neoplasm or fibrous dysplasia), and even at this stage of its evolution, the microscopic changes observed in a biopsy specimen can be readily identified as those of Paget's disease (Fig. A-16, C). Treatment in such cases is concerned mainly with the relief of pain and discomfort and with reassuring the patient that the condition, if it remains localized, is not likely to have serious consequences.

The problem of sarcoma complicating Paget's disease is an important one, but this has already been discussed in the chapter on osteogenic sarcoma.

References

1. Basset, F., Nézelof, M. C., and Turiaf, M. J.: Présence en microscopie électronique de structures filamenteuses originales dans les lésions pulmonaires et osseuses de l'histiocytose x. Etat actuel de la question, Soc. Med. Hôp. Paris 117:413, 1966.
2. Brailsford, J. F.: Ossifying haematomata and other single lesions mistaken for sarcomata. The responsibility of biopsy, Brit. J. Radiol. 21:157, 1948.
3. Butler, F. E., and Wooley, I. M.: Osteogenic sarcoma arising from a calcified hematoma, Radiology 26:236, 1936.
4. Changus, G. W.: Osteoblastic hyperplasia of bone: histochemical appraisal of fibrous dysplasia of bone, Cancer 10:1157, 1957.
5. Coley, B. L., and Stewart, F. W.: Bone sarcoma in polyostotic fibrous dysplasia, Ann. Surg. 121:872, 1945.
6. De Man, J. C. H.: Rod-like tubular structures in the cytoplasm of histiocytes in "histiocytosis X," J. Path. Bact. 95:123, 1968.
7. Harris, W. H., Dudley, H. R., Jr., and Barry, R. J.: The natural history of fibrous dysplasia, J. Bone Joint Surg. 44-A:207, 1962.
8. Jaffe, H. L.: Aneurysmal bone cyst, Bull. Hosp. Joint Dis. 11:3, 1950.
9. Jaffe, H. L., and Lichtenstein, L.: Solitary unicameral bone cyst, with emphasis on the roentgen picture, the pathologic appearance and the pathogenesis, Arch. Surg. 44:1004, 1942.
10. Jaffe, H. L., and Lichtenstein, L.: Eosinophilic granuloma of bone. A condition affecting one, several or many bones, but apparently limited to the skeleton, and representing the mildest clinical expression of the peculiar inflammatory histiocytosis also underlying Letterer-Siwe disease and Schüller-Christian disease, Arch. Pathol. 37:99, 1944.
11. Lichtenstein, L.: Aneurysmal bone cyst. A pathological entity commonly mistaken for giant-cell tumor and occasionally for hemangioma and osteogenic sarcoma, Cancer 3:279, 1950.
12. Lichtenstein, L.: Aneurysmal bone cyst. Further observations, Cancer 6:1228, 1953.

13. Lichtenstein, L.: Histiocytosis X. Integration of eosinophilic granuloma of bone, "Letterer-Siwe disease" and "Schüller-Christian disease" as related manifestations of a single nosologic entity, A.M.A. Arch. Pathol. 56:84, 1953.
14. Lichtenstein, L.: Benign osteoblastoma. A category of osteoid- and bone-forming tumors other than classical osteoid-osteoma, which may be mistaken for giant-cell tumor or osteogenic sarcoma, Cancer 9:1044, 1956.
15. Lichtenstein, L.: Pathology: diseases of bone, N. Engl. J. Med. 255:427, 1956 (see Medical Progress).
16. Lichtenstein, L.: Aneurysmal bone cyst. Observations on 50 cases, J. Bone Joint Surg. 39-A:873, 1957.
17. Lichtenstein, L.: Histiocytosis X (eosinophilic granuloma of bone, Letterer-Siwe disease, and Schüller-Christian disease). Further observations of pathological and clinical importance, J. Bone Joint Surg. 46-A:76, 1964.
18. Lichtenstein, L.: Diseases of bone and joints, St. Louis 1970, The C. V. Mosby Co. (see pp. 180-183).
19. Lichtenstein, L., and Jaffe, H. L.: Fibrous dysplasia of bone. A condition affecting one, several or many bones, the graver cases of which may present abnormal pigmentation of skin, premature sexual development, hyperthyroidism or still other extraskeletal abnormalities, Arch. Pathol. 33:777, 1942.
20. Nobler, M. P., Higinbotham, N. L., and Phillips, R. F.: Cure for aneurysmal bone cyst: irradiation superior to surgery in analysis of 33 cases, Radiology 90:1185, 1968.
21. Pack, G. T., and Braund, R. R.: The development of sarcoma in myositis ossificans; report of 3 cases, J.A.M.A. 119:776, 1942.
22. Perkinson, N. B., and Higinbotham, N. L.: Osteogenic sarcoma arising in polyostotic fibrous dysplasia. Report of a case, Cancer 8:396, 1955.
23. Schwartz, D. T., and Alpert, M.: The malignant transformation of fibrous dysplasia, Am. J. Med. Sci. 247:350, 1964.
24. Shipley, A. M.: Ossifying hematoma and allied conditions, Arch. Surg. 41:516, 1940.
25. Tillman, B. P., Dahlin, D. C., Lipscomb, P. R., and Stewart, J. R.: Aneurysmal bone cyst: analysis of 95 cases, Mayo Clinic Proc. 43:478, 1968.

Appendix B

Tumors of synovial joints, bursae, and tendon sheaths

Although growths of joints, bursae, and tendon sheaths are, of course, not bone tumors, they do quite often develop in intimate association with contiguous bones and at times may erode and even extend into them. It was felt, therefore, that their comprehensive discussion in a chapter in the Appendix might enhance the usefulness of the book. This chapter includes the material presented in my survey in *Cancer*[43] in 1955, with some additions and minor changes to bring the subject up to date.

In view of their close pathologic relationship, it appears logical, as well as expedient, to consider the linings of synovial joints, bursae, and tendon sheaths as a single unit for the purpose of discussing tumors and tumorlike lesions. The deeper fibrous component of articular capsules and bursal walls, as well as the relatively inert tendons themselves, scarcely enter seriously into the problem of neoplastic proliferation, except insofar as one may note the rare occurrence of ordinary fibroblastic tumors and of the recently described malignant tumors of indeterminate nature that have been called clear-cell sarcomas of tendons and aponeuroses. The latter will be discussed further on.

In the old pertinent literature[24] one finds a number of lesions broadly classified as tumors that are not genuine neoplasms or whose pathologic interpretation is debatable. Thus, the common ganglion, developing as it does through myxoid degeneration and cystic softening of the connective tissue of a joint capsule or tendon sheath, constitutes a tumor only in the limited clinical sense of a swelling (Fig. B-1). Further, the condition of synovial, bursal, or tenosynovial osteochondromatosis may be convincingly interpreted as a self-limited metaplastic process rather than a genuine expression of neoplasia, as will be indicated presently. Continuing, the tumorlike lesions that have been called giant-cell tumor, xanthomatous giant-cell tumor, giant-cell myeloma, benign synovioma, and giant-cell synovioma (among other names) have long been a subject of controversial interpretation. My own view is that they may well represent peculiar hyperplastic, histiocytic granulomas of as yet undetermined etiology, rather than bona fide neoplasms. This concept is implied in the designation of pigmented villonodular synovitis, bursitis, and tenosynovitis,[33] as the case may be.

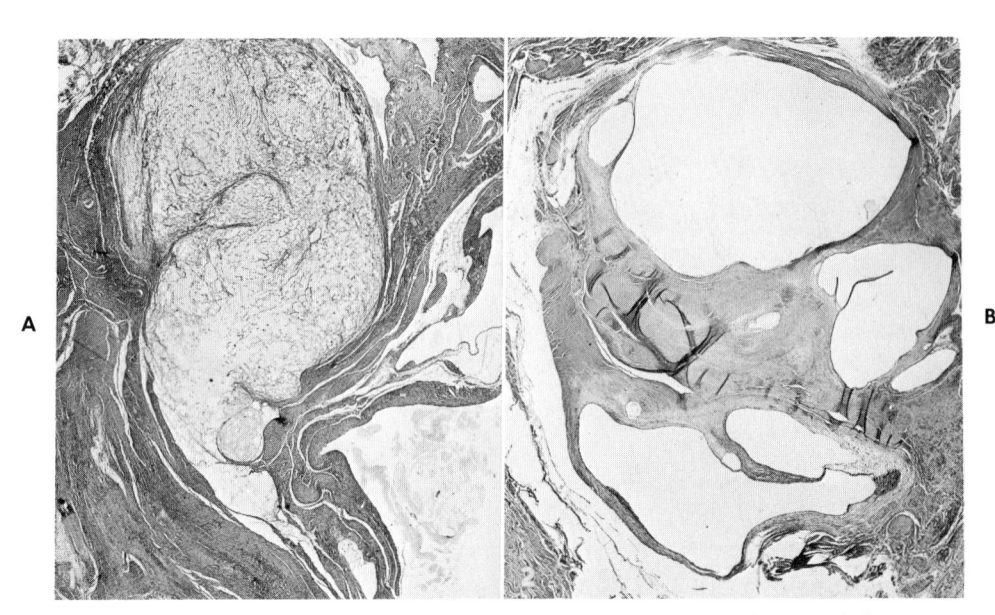

Fig. B-1. A, Ganglion formation through myxoid change and cystic softening of the connective tissue of a joint capsule. (×8.) B, Comparable multilocular cyst formation within the parameniscal connective tissue of a knee joint. (×9.) (From Lichtenstein, L.: Tumors of synovial joints, bursae, and tendon sheaths, Cancer 8:816, 1955.)

If one sets apart the conditions mentioned, there are actually relatively few undisputed tumors that are observed with any appreciable frequency. The benign tumors that are encountered occasionally on the lining surfaces of articular capsules and tendon sheaths are mainly of the nature of lipomas and hemangiomas, derived from the supporting fatty connective tissue and its blood vessels. Fibroma and chondroma also are listed in some old classifications,[9,36] but their occurrence, at least in the sense of genuine tumors of fibroblasts and chondrocytes respectively, seems questionable. In any event, if they do occur, they must be so rare as to constitute pathologic curiosities. As for primary malignant neoplasms, apart from a few unusual synovial chondrosarcomas,[26] the only one of practical importance is synovial sarcoma. This ominous neoplasm is being recognized with increasing frequency by pathologists, now that its specific cytologic features have been well defined, although the problem of effective treatment is still a formidable one. While the finding of such tumors as malignant hemangioendothelioma, liposarcoma, and fibrosarcoma, among others, is theoretically possible, actual recorded experience with them in the sites under consideration appears to be virtually nonexistent.

Cognizance should be taken here of the remarkable group of malignant tumors collected at the A.F.I.P. and reported by Enzinger[17] in 1965 under the provisional descriptive designation of *clear-cell sarcoma of tendons and aponeuroses*. Clinically, these peculiar neoplasms manifested notably slow but persistent growth, a strong tendency to repeated recurrence after attempts at surgical removal, and eventually, after several or many years, metastasis to regional lymph nodes, the lungs, and other viscera. More than half of them developed in the foot or ankle region, and a third in the tendinous tissues of the knee region. They were of limited size (averaging 4 cm. in greatest dimension), and in all of them firm attachment of the tumor to tendinous or aponeurotic structures was noted. Microscopically, they were composed of solid nests and fascicles of uniform cells with indistinct clear cytoplasm and round or ovoid nuclei with a prominent nucleolus. Enzinger was uncertain of the origin of these neoplasms, although he felt they differed in essential respects from synovial sarcoma and other tumors that he considered, including alveolar soft-part sarcoma.

I have seen only one instance (in the ankle region) and have little basis for any independent opinion, although it is difficult to understand how such cellular neoplasms could arise from the inert, collagenous connective tissue of the tendons and aponeuroses themselves. From a recent study of the ultrastructure of a tumor in point (patellar tendon), Kubo[41] inferred that "clear-cell sarcoma" may be a type of synovial sarcoma, but I think we must reserve judgment about this.

Tumorlike lesions of debatable pathologic nature

It seems appropriate here to consider further the nature of two specific lesions of uncertain pathogenesis, which may simulate tumors in the gross, if not in their microscopic, appearance. These have already been mentioned and are chondromatosis (or osteochondromatosis) of joints, bursae, and tendon sheaths and pigmented villonodular synovitis, bursitis, and tenosynovitis (so-called giant-cell tumor or giant-cell synovioma). This consideration is of practical importance as well as academic interest, having a bearing on appropriate treatment.

Osteochondromatosis

This condition is featured by the formation of numerous chondral and osseous bodies within the lining and sublining connective tissue of the affected structure. It is encountered far more often in joint capsules than in bursae or tendon sheaths, and the knee joint is its commonest site, although occasionally a hip, an elbow, a shoulder, or some other joint may be affected. When a knee joint is involved, for example, one may observe (on surgical exploration in the course of synovectomy) that the synovial lining of the joint proper, and perhaps of the suprapatellar pouch and posterior compartment as well, is studded by innumerable small, firm, flat or slightly raised, gray-yellow nodules. These have a tendency to become extruded so that the joint may contain numerous, sometimes hundreds, of free chrondal bodies. Whether or not these may be visualized roentgenographically depends upon whether they show sufficient calcification or osseous transformation to be radiopaque (Figs. B-2 and B-3).

On microscopic examination of the lining of an affected joint, one observes numerous foci of cartilaginous and/or osseous metaplasia in varying stages of development. The cartilage foci, as noted, may become calcified or converted to bone. At such sites there is initially focal nodular condensation of the con-

410 *Appendixes*

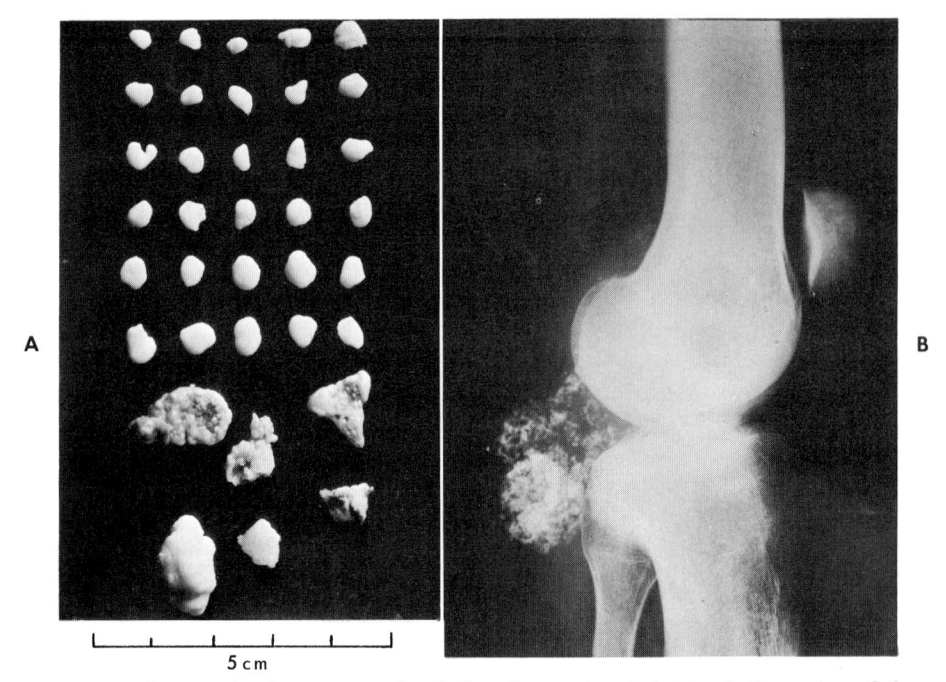

Fig. B-2. A, Photograph of numerous chondral and osteochondral joint bodies removed from an elbow in a case of osteochondromatosis. **B,** Roentgenogram of a lesion of osteochondromatosis of a popliteal bursa. Pictures such as this are sometimes misinterpreted as indicating the presence of chondrosarcoma. (From Lichtenstein, L.: Tumors of synovial joints, bursae, and tendon sheaths, Cancer **8:**816, 1955.)

nective-tissue cells, but the synovial lining elsewhere shows no characteristic alteration (Fig. B-4). Once the chondral or osseous bodies are formed, their growth potential appears to be distinctly limited. While the number of such bodies and conglomerate aggregates of them may be impressive at times, there appears to be no compelling reason to regard the process as neoplastic. Malignant change (to chondrosarcoma) has been reported,[49] but it is very unusual. Freund[22] and others have also expressed the view that the condition described represents a self-limited metaplastic process. In fact, spontaneous arrest and regression have been noted clinically by a number of observers,[22,51] which is scarcely the behavior one would expect of a neoplasm. I might add that in interpreting the synovial chondrosarcomas my colleagues and I have observed,[26] there was no reason to assume necessarily that these neoplasms had developed through malignant change in synovial chondromatosis.

Pigmented villonodular synovitis, bursitis, and tenosynovitis

This is the descriptive name Jaffe, Sutro, and I[33] devised in 1941 for a distinctive, yellow-brown, villous and/or nodular lesion encountered in joints and bursae, as well as in tendon sheaths. As indicated in the original paper, this lesion may take a number of forms, depending upon its site and whether it is localized or more diffuse, but it has the same essential character pathologically

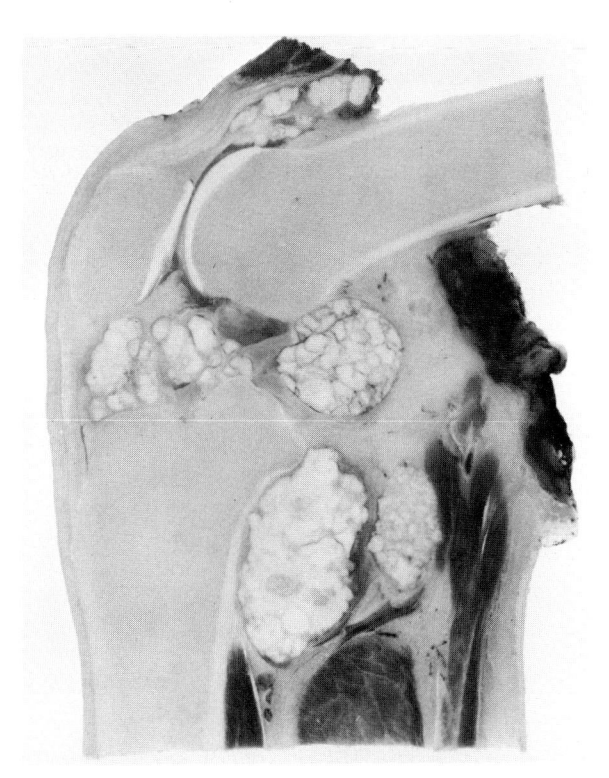

Fig. B-3. Sagittal section showing extensive synovial chondromatosis of a knee joint. The suprapatellar pouch and the bursae posteriorly are also involved. Such extensive involvement is unusual and may simulate chondrosarcoma. (From Goldman, R. L., and Lichtenstein, L.: Synovial chondrosarcoma, Cancer 17:1233, 1964.)

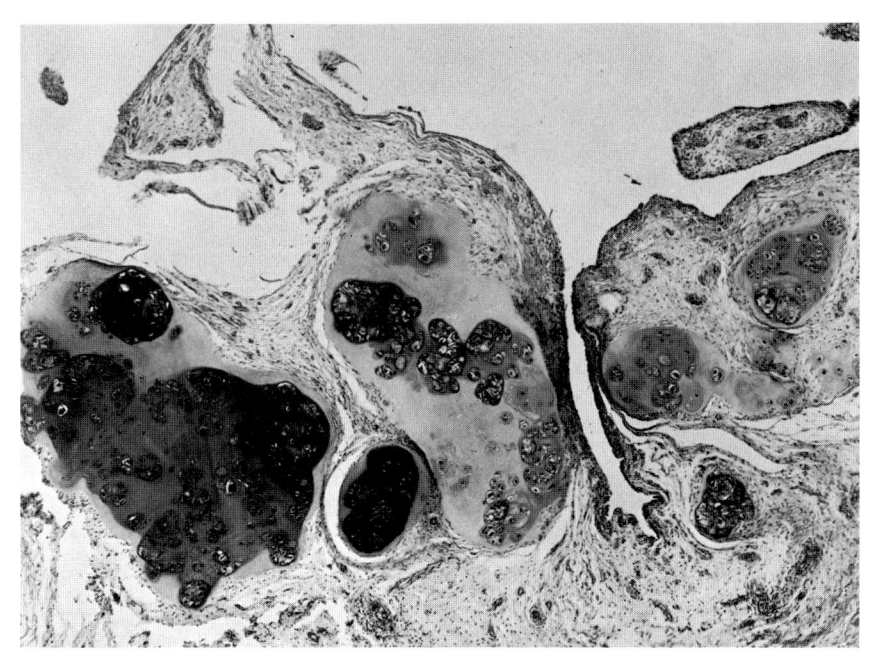

Fig. B-4. Synovial chondromatosis (knee joint). Some of the chondral bodies are calcified, but there was no osseous metaplasia in any of the sections examined. (×35.)

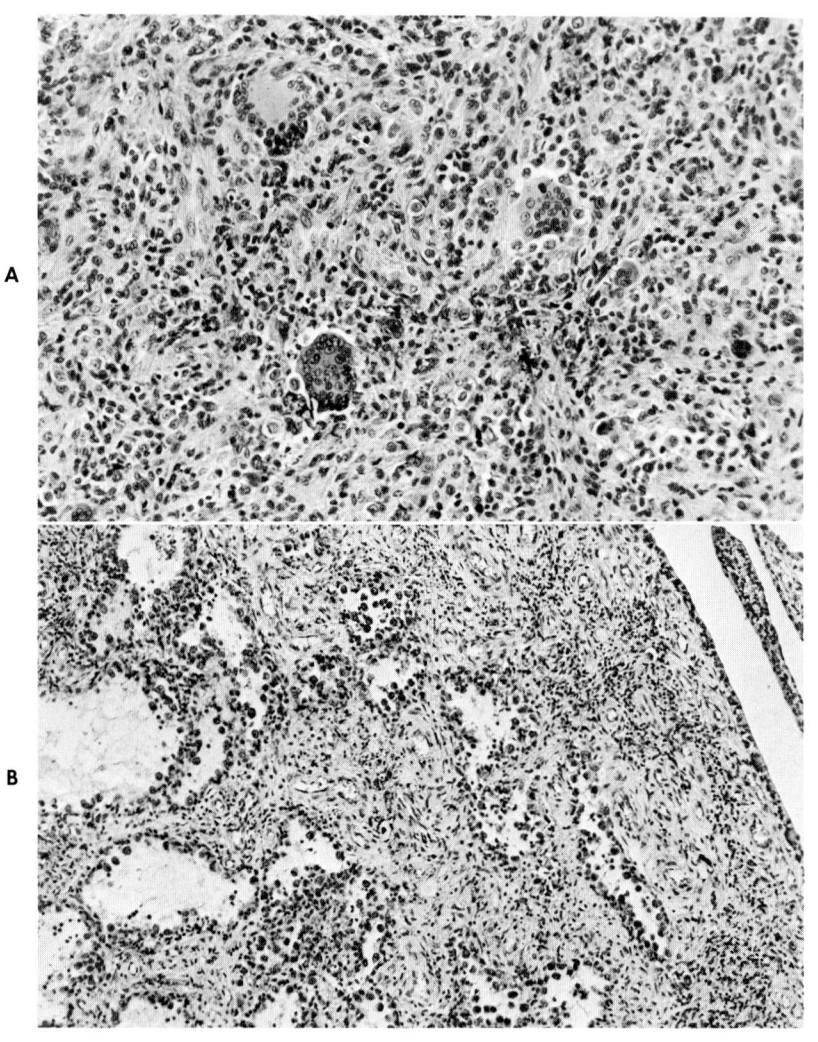

Fig. B-5. A, A field from a tendon sheath nodule of a finger (pigmented nodular tenosynovitis or giant-cell tumor, so-called), showing appreciable cellularity and the presence of occasional multinuclear cells. Many of the histiocytic stromal cells contained hemosiderin granules, nondiscernible at this magnification. (×100.) **B,** A field from a lesion of pigmented villonodular synovitis of a knee joint showing prominent synovial-lined spaces within the thickened synovial membrane. These apparently result from agglutination of villi and should not be misinterpreted as indicating the presence of synovial sarcoma. Other fields of this lesion showed appreciable collagenization, scattered multinuclear (giant) cells, and abundant hemosiderin deposition. (×125.) (From Lichtenstein, L.: Tumors of synovial joints, bursae, and tendon sheaths, Cancer **8:**816, 1955.)

in all these circumstances. Thus, it was pointed out that the diffuse villous or villonodular expression in joints (commonly, a knee joint) has its precise counterpart in bursae and its equivalent expression in tendon sheaths, although the latter is seen comparatively infrequently. The usual form of tendon sheath involvement is, of course, the familiar localized nodule (generally solitary, but occasionally multiple) previously designated as giant-cell tumor or myeloplaxoma by some and as xanthoma or xanthogranuloma by others (Fig. B-5, *A*). It was further demonstrated that this tendon sheath nodule is cytologically indistinguishable from the sessile or pedicled nodules observed in lesions of pigmented villonodular synovitis or bursitis. In an early stage of its evolution, it may likewise present a villonodular pattern, thus definitely linking it pathogenetically to the synovial and bursal equivalents of the condition.

For the sake of brevity, the complex cytologic details of the lesion in all these circumstances will not be reiterated here. Suffice it to state that, whatever its localization, the lesion in general is characterized in its early stages by appreciable vascularity and conspicuous hemosiderin deposition, as well as villous hypertrophy of the lining of the affected structure and agglutination of villi to form synovial-lined clefts. These eventually become incorporated in webbed, matted, or more solid areas (Fig. B-5, *B*). Concomitantly, one observes active proliferation of cells (occasionally in syncytial aggregates constituting giant cells) that appear to have a dual origin, being derived in part from synovial lining cells that have migrated downward and in part from the adventitial reticular cells of blood vessels. In any event, these prominent stromal cells, which may dominate the picture in an active lesion, soon manifest their tendency to function as macrophages through phagocytosis of hemosiderin, as well as lipid (usually cholesterol esters). Eventually, many lesions tend spontaneously to involute, in part or throughout, as a result of extensive fibrosis and collagenization. It seems altogether probable, incidentally, that roentgen-ray therapy accelerates this change. This evolutionary cycle may go on to substantial completion, as it commonly does in tendon sheath nodules of long standing, or may renew itself, as it does in the more exuberant lesions in the knee joint or in the popliteal space.

It is of practical importance to emphasize that at the height of proliferation of the histiocytic stromal cells, and especially before their phagocytic tendency becomes quite obvious, a casual observer unfamiliar with the lesion may gain the impression that it is a sarcoma. In fact, not a few pertinent cases in the old literature have been reported as such,[33] and undoubtedly many instances in the past have been treated by unnecessarily radical surgery. I have personal knowledge of several, seen in consultation, in which amputation of a lower limb had been seriously contemplated. In my own experience to date, I have not observed a single instance of pigmented villonodular synovitis, bursitis, or tenosynovitis in which malignant change ensued. Even the exuberant lesions in the knee joint that recurred after synovectomy were observed to clear up completely following roentgen-ray therapy in relatively small dosage,[23] which is scarcely the response one would expect if the lesion were a neoplasm.

This experience with the condition pointing to its benign character is apparently shared by De Santo and Wilson,[16] Jaffe and Selin,[34] Ackerman and del Regato,[1] and others. It should also be noted that Young and Hudacek[70] have reproduced some of the proliferative features of pigmented villonodular synovitis by inducing prolonged hemarthrosis in dogs under conditions of continued articular function, although the essential component of diffuse histiocytic proliferation was lacking. There has been some dissenting opinion, however, that warrants close scrutiny with a view to clarifying the situation. Thus, Bennett[4] has implied that there may well be transitions between the condition under discussion (which he prefers to regard as a neoplasm of specialized synovial lining cells) and malignant synovial tumors, and, collaterally, that some synovial sarcomas may develop through malignant change in originally benign growths. From his reported case material, however, one gathers that this interpretation is based largely upon inference rather than convincing follow-up observations. Continuing, Willis[67] agreed that the widespread, brown, seaweed-like synovial growths sometimes found filling a large joint (one expression of diffuse pigmented villonodular synovitis) are inflammatory and not neoplastic and that these frequently include small or large nodules closely resembling in structure the solitary "giant-cell growths." On the other hand, he feels that many of the solitary growths are neoplasms (benign synovioma) and attempts to explain this apparent contradiction by postulating that hyperplasia in these circumstances may at times pass insensibly into neoplasia.

Further, M. J. Stewart[59] and Wright[68] are unequivocally committed to the neoplastic view. The latter investigator, in particular, designates the condition under discussion as "benign giant-cell synovioma" and maintains that it may on occasion undergo malignant change and conversion to a special kind of synovial sarcoma, namely, the "well-differentiated, giant-cell type of malignant synovioma." In his paper on malignant synovioma, Wright includes two instances of this specific type (cases 43 and 44) situated in the knee and ankle regions, respectively, in which, after several unsuccessful attempts at local surgical extirpation, it was deemed necessary to amputate the affected lower extremity. It may be significant, however, that the duration of symptoms prior to radical surgery was as long as nine and fifteen years, respectively, and that both patients were well six years after amputation, despite the generally poor prognosis in cases of indubitable synovial sarcoma in which amputation is done as a late secondary procedure. Through the courtesy of Professors Willis and Stewart, I have had the opportunity of studying representative sections of one of these lesions, and my impression is that the diagnosis of sarcoma was based not upon cytologic evidence of frank malignancy (the picture was essentially that of pigmented villonodular synovitis) but rather upon the finding that the lesion had substantially encroached upon the surrounding muscle tissue. As a token of malignancy, this feature would be significant only if the lesion were an undisputed neoplasm, which brings us right back to the basic question in point.

The same problem in interpretation was highlighted by an unusual specimen that I have had occasion to examine. The patient in this instance was a 23-year-old man who, while in the service, had a biopsy of a lesion in a knee joint, which proved to be diffuse pigmented villonodular synovitis. The following year, because of persistence of pain and swelling of the affected knee, he received roentgen-ray therapy at a military hospital, the specific details of which are not available. Two years later, the knee joint was explored at our hospital because of a palpable, painful mass in the posterior knee region. At surgery, a firm, lobulated, fist-sized mass, situated beneath and slightly lateral to the head of the gastrocnemius muscle, was extirpated. Because the question of aggressiveness was raised by the examining pathologist, it was deemed desirable to obtain wider clearance by removing portions of the gastrocnemius and soleus muscles, the contiguous head of the fibula, the periosteum of the posterior tibia, and the posterior portion of the capsule of the knee. These structures, however, failed to show evidence of involvement. The mass measured 8.5 × 7.0 × 5.0 cm. in its greatest dimensions and weighed 160 grams; it was solid, firm, lobulated, and tan-brown in color and was invested by a thin connective tissue capsule, except on its raw undersurface. Here, in places, the lesion was encroaching upon muscle tissue by direct continuity. Thorough microscopic sampling of the mass showed pigmented nodular synovitis. The histiocytic stromal cells were of uniform appearance, contained abundant hemosiderin pigment, and presented only rare mitoses and no indication of nuclear atypism. It was felt that, although the lesion was encroaching upon muscle tissue by direct extension (not frank invasion), this in itself should not be construed as being indicative of a malignant or even of a neoplastic nature. Accordingly, the recommendation was made that radical surgery was not indicated and that prophylactic irradiation (in small to moderate dosage) of the bed of the extirpated lesion might be of value in forestalling possible local recurrence. This could not be instituted because of wound infection, but the patient presented no evidence of local recurrence over a three-year period of follow-up.

It should also be noted that on occasion, lesions of pigmented villonodular synovitis of the knee and also of the hip joint may erode contiguous articular bone ends and even extend through such apertures into the interior of one or more bones, producing roentgenographically discernible defects. I have observed material from several pertinent instances of hip joint involvement in which the proximal femur and acetabulum were penetrated and two of knee joint involvement in which the distal femur and upper tibia were implicated. A detailed account of six such cases, along with a summary of the pertinent literature, has been published by McMaster.[47] The recent observations of Schajowicz and Blumenfeld[56] indicate that such extension into one or more bones is actually a fairly common occurrence and should no longer occasion any surprise. These cases respond satisfactorily to conservative treatment, and the point is stressed that such direct extension into articular bone ends should not be construed as evidence of malignant change, disturbing as it may be to someone who observes it for the first time.

In the case of tendon sheath nodules of the nature of pigmented nodular tenosynovitis (so-called giant-cell tumor), it is well known that they also may induce pressure erosion of contiguous bones, especially phalanges of the fingers and toes (Fig. B-6), and occasionally even extend into such eroded bones. This complication has been discussed by Fletcher and Horn[21]; the point was stressed that such erosion is fairly common, if one looks for it, and should not be construed in itself as an indication of neoplastic aggressiveness. Incidentally, the interesting and rare tumor of a phalanx of a finger reported by Price and Valentine[54] as a "malignant giant-cell synovioma" seems clearly to have originated within bone and, however one chooses to interpret it, is not an instance of a malignant tendon sheath tumor.

Cognizance must be taken, however, of several case reports noting the rare occurrence of malignant change in tendon sheath growths having the pathologic character apparently of so-called giant-cell tumor. Thus, Kobak and Perlow[40] have reported an instance of "xanthomatous giant-cell tumor" thought to originate

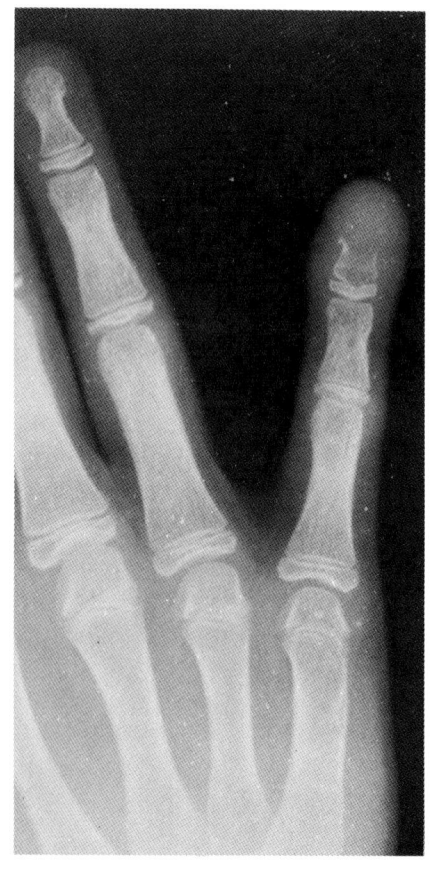

Fig. B-6. Roentgenogram showing partial destruction of a terminal phalanx of a finger by a tendon sheath node.

near the tendinous insertion of the triceps at the elbow, which recurred a number of times after local excision despite supplementary irradiation, also extended to the axillary lymph nodes, and within a year metastasized to the lungs and abdominal viscera. The authors point out that, while the cytologic picture "resembles closely a xanthomatous giant-cell tumor of tendon sheath origin," the stromal cells were obviously anaplastic and some of them presented atypical mitotic figures. Another pertinent case published by Decker and Owen[14] is that of a "giant cell tumor of tendon sheath" in the ankle region, apparently of fourteen years' duration prior to treatment, that recurred twice following surgical excision and, because of invasion and destruction of the tarsal bones, finally necessitated amputation of the leg, though too late to prevent metastases to the vertebral column and lung. In sections of the primary tumor, clues to the recognition of aggressiveness were increased cellularity in places, fusiform shape of the stromal cells, and an appreciable number of mitotic figures. To cite still another instructive case in point, I have had occasion to see material from a lesion of pigmented nodular tenosynovitis (in a second toe of a man of 74), which recurred twenty years or more after initial excision. The new mass was present for six months. The sections showed what I interpreted as incipient malignant change (inordinately cellular areas in which both stromal histiocytes and giant cells showed atypical hyperchromatic nuclei and mitotic figures), and accordingly, it was recommended that the affected toe be amputated. Experiences such as this are very unusual, however. The practical inference to be stressed is that, while tendon sheath nodes not infrequently recur locally after excision, it is only on rare occasions, apparently, that they undergo malignant change and hence require appropriate radical surgery without temporizing. On the other hand, it should be borne in mind that the overwhelming majority are innocuous and, if not neglected too long, may be effectively treated by conservative surgical excision.

Also noteworthy here is the recent report by Bliss and Reed[6] of some four frankly malignant tumors arising de novo from the tendon sheaths of the hand and wrist, under the title of "large cell sarcomas of tendon sheath." They stress the resemblance microscopically of their neoplasms to "benign giant cell tumors of tendon sheath" (pigmented nodular tenosynovitis in our terminology), although giant cells were scarce and the stromal cells were clearly malignant. These unusual neoplasms are apparently also rare, and I do not recall any in my own experience. They may conceivably represent the initially malignant, histiocytic counterpart of the common tendon sheath node. Several comparable case reports (in abstract form) have also been put on record by Gravanis[27] under the title, "malignant giant-cell tumors of tendon sheaths."

Benign tumors
Hemangioma

Reports of benign neoplasms composed of blood vessels, developing within the capsules of large joints, particularly the knee joint, have been well documented, although they are distinctly uncommon. The relatively few recorded instances have been of the nature of either circumscribed or more widespread cavernous hemangiomas. As a representative example of localized involvement of the knee joint, one may cite the case reported by Osgood[52] of an encapsulated, lobulated, reddish tumor mass that was attached by a pedicle to the infrapatellar fat pad. This growth measured 8 cm. in its greatest dimension and proved on pathologic examination to be a cavernous hemangioma. Its surgical extirpation was a simple task, and the patient, a 26-year-old woman who had complained of intermittent pain and disability for eight years, was completely relieved.

In other instances, virtually the entire joint capsule may be permeated by tortuous, engorged, thin-walled blood vessels, some of which may be of rather large caliber and prone to rupture, so that copious bleeding seriously interfaces with any attempt at surgical excision. For a comprehensive discussion of such diffuse hemangiomas of the knee joint, and particularly their clinical recognition and appropriate treatment, one may turn to the paper of Bennett and Cobey,[5] which presents a survey of twenty-nine cases, including five of their own. Cobey subsequently reported four additional pertinent cases. They pointed out that one may suspect the condition from the following findings: intermittent pain and swelling of the affected joint (often present since childhood and tending to be induced or aggravated by trauma), reduction in size of the swelling on elevation of the affected limb, and aspiration of blood from the affected joint. The presence of a hemangioma elsewhere is another helpful clue. With reference to treatment, Bennett and Cobey expressed the view that complete surgical excision is feasible only when dealing with relatively small or pedunculated hemangiomas of the capsule. For comparatively large or extensively ramifying hemangiomas, they favor roentgen-ray therapy because of its effectiveness, as well as the hazards of serious hemorrhage, impaired circulation, and infection attendant upon attempts at complete surgical removal. In one of their earlier cases, these complications led eventually to loss of a limb.

It may be noted in passing that other pertinent papers dealing with hemangiomas of articular capsules and their surrounding structures are those of Weaver[64] and of Sabrazès, Grailly, and Gineste.[55] A compilation of more recent references may be found in the case report by Stevens and his associates.[58]

As for hemangiomas of bursae, I have never encountered an unequivocal instance or found reference to one in the literature. A limited number of hemangiomas developing within and about tendon sheaths have been recorded, however. Thus, Burman and Milgram[8] collected some ten cases in the literature and reported six additional instances, the majority of which, however, involved one or another tendon and the peritendinous tissue rather than the tendon sheath primarily. The clinical picture in these cases was apparently too nondescript to permit any accurate impression prior to surgical exploration. It is worth noting also that in several instances disconcerting bleeding occurred during the course of attempted excision of the vascular tumor, suggesting that, as in dealing with ramifying hemangiomas of joints, it may be more expedient to resort to irradiation. The subject of hemangiomas of tendon sheath has also been discussed by Harkins,[29] Bate,[3] and Webster and Geschickter,[65] among others.

It may be mentioned here that several lymphangiomas apparently developing in tendons and their sheaths have been recorded—two by Huguenin and Oberling[30] and another by Faldini[18] that was apparently somewhat more cellular, being designated as a lymphangioendothelioma. From the meager data supplied in these reports, one can scarcely venture any helpful comment in regard to the clinical behavior of such tumors or their appropriate treatment.

Lipoma

Although it is conventional to list lipoma among the benign tumors affecting joints, its occurrence is distinctly unusual. One must be circumspect, moreover, about accepting casual mention of such observations at their face value, inasmuch as the subsynovial fat deposits may be rather thick normally, especially in a large joint such as the knee joint, and constitute synovial-covered pads or folds that bulge into the joint cavity. When a circumscribed protruding fatty mass shows distinct branching lobulation, there appears to be a sounder basis for accepting it as a neoplasm, and such growths are usually designated as arborescent lipomas. The relatively few recorded lipomas of one type or another have been encountered mainly in the knee and ankle joints.[24] An unusual instance of bilateral knee joint involvement has been reported by Arzimanoglu.[2]

The occurrence of fatty tumors in bursae has not been noted, to my knowledge. There are, however, several well-documented papers dealing with fatty growths held to represent lipomas of tendon sheaths. Thus Strauss,[61] in reporting a pertinent instance, collected some eighteen cases from the literature that he accepted as genuine lipomas of either simple or arborescent type. From these data, Strauss inferred that such growths develop slowly over a period of years, eventually causing some pain and disability, as well as obvious swelling and deformity of the affected part. He remarked further that their surgical excision may entail removal of the involved portion of the tendon sheath. Mason[46] also, in discussing comparable growths in the hand specifically, pointed out that the arborescent lipomas may take the form of numerous fatty villi developing along the course of the involved tendon sheath and that sometimes the tendon itself is thinned out or infiltrated by fat, so that partial resection of it is indicated. Among other pertinent references, those of Valdoni[63] and of White[66] may be cited. The latter, in describing a remarkable instance of arborescent lipoma developing along the course of tendon sheaths in the ankle region, observed that the shaggy fatty villi had spread not only over the parietal and visceral layers of the involved sheaths, but had also extended (after seven years or more) into the neighboring joints and penetrated the periosteum of the contiguous tarsal bones.

It may be noted here in passing that in some older papers[48] dealing ostensibly with tumors of tendon sheaths, one finds reference to lesions characterized by xanthomatous (cholesterol and cholesterol ester) deposits in tendons. These are obviously a manifestation of xanthoma tuberosum multiplex, an inbred disorder of cholesterol metabolism, and, as such, are not germane to a discussion of neoplasms.

Other benign tumors

When one considers critically the incidence of benign connective tissue tumors other than hemangioma and lipoma within joints, bursae, and tendon sheaths, one gets into rather dubious territory. As noted, both fibroma and chondroma are also listed in some review articles[9,35,36] dealing with tumors of tendon sheaths particularly, but unequivocal pathologic observations justifying their inclusion are singularly lacking. In this connection, one must be certain that what is interpreted as a fibroma does not actually represent a solitary lesion of pigmented nodular synovitis or tenosynovitis that has undergone involutional scarring or collagenization in the wake of substantial necrosis. In a general discussion of tumors of tendon sheaths, Jaffe[31] remarked that there are a few authentic cases of fibroma on record, but the pertinent references were not cited. With respect to the hand specifically, Mason[46] expressed the opinion that fibromas may take origin from tendons and their sheaths, as well as from joint capsules and intermuscular septa, although he qualified this statement to the effect that these are quite rare and that many so diagnosed were probably neuromas.

As for so-called chondromas, I adhere to the view of Freund[22] and Fisher[19] that the condition of synovial or bursal chondromatosis represents a self-limited metaplastic process. The same question of interpretation arises, of course, in connection with sessile or pedicled "chondromas" developing in tendon sheaths. One must also take cognizance here of the comparatively rare instances recorded by Buxton[9] and by Janik,[35] among others, in which a single cartilage growth of appreciable size was found attached to a tendon sheath, so that, in the course of surgical extirpation, resection of the sheath was deemed essential. Such cartilage growths appear actually to represent genuine neoplasms, but it is relevant to point out that, on occasion, sizable chondromas or chondrosarcomas may develop in the extraskeletal soft parts of extremities[60] without any relationship to tendon sheaths and that, by the same token, proximity does not necessarily establish a site of origin. Such subtleties, however, seem not to have been duly considered by the authors of the papers cited, and, from the sketchily recorded pathologic data, it is difficult to arrive at any independent judgment.

Malignant tumors

It is well known that malignant neoplasms of one type or another may extend into an articular capsule from a contiguous bone site. Thus, osteogenic sarcoma, chondrosarcoma, and reticulum-cell sarcoma developing in the lower end of a femur, for example, often spread eventually into the capsule of the knee joint at its attachment to the articular bone end. On the other hand, the only *primary* malignant tumor encountered with any degree of frequency in joints, as well as bursae and tendon sheaths, is the tumor that is appropriately designated as synovial sarcoma. As noted, the occurrence in these sites of other primary malignant tumors is so rare as to be of little practical moment. The remainder of this discussion will deal therefore with synovial sarcoma, emphasizing particularly current problems in diagnosis and treatment.

Synovial sarcoma

This is the designation that is preferred apparently by most investigators (synovial sarcomesothelioma, synovial sarcoendothelioma, malignant synovioma, and synovialoma are some of the other names employed). The cytologic hallmark of this tumor, whatever one chooses to call it, is the tendency of its primitive or mesenchymal spindle connective tissue cells to line spaces and ramifying clefts (presumably abortive joint spaces). Similarly in tissue-culture studies of a number of synovial sarcomas, Murray, Stout, and Pogogeff[50] observed that the tumor cells have the capacity to line slits or tubes and to secrete a mucinous substance, as well as to form strands of hyperchromatic fibrosarcoma-like cells supported by reticulin fibers. The over-all picture is somewhat reminiscent of that of a malignant mesothelioma in that there is a pseudoepithelial component within a dominant sarcomatous stroma. It seems logical, however, to maintain a sharp distinction between synovial sarcoma and mesothelioma, if only because the term "mesothelium" by anatomic definition is conventionally restricted to the layer of cells that lines the coelom or body cavity of the embryo and, subsequently, the serous membranes of the peritoneum, pleura, and pericardium.

Synovial sarcoma, though relatively uncommon as tumors of skeletal soft parts go, is not so rare as it is sometimes held to be. Thus, Bennett[4] was able to study fully thirty-two instances treated in military hospitals during the late war. Haagensen and Stout,[28] in a survey of the literature as of 1944, recorded as many as nine instances from their own files, and sizable groups of cases have been reported from other clinics. Similarly, I have had occasion to observe material from at least thirty cases seen in consultation within recent years.[44] A wealth of richly illustrated case material may be found in a fascicle by Goidanich and Battaglia.[25] For a discussion of synovial sarcoma in children particularly, the reader is referred to a paper by Crocker and Stout.[13] A generation ago, synovial sarcomas were often called "adenosarcomas" without full awareness apparently of their distinctive character, and it is altogether probable that even today some pathologists still fail to recognize instances of this neoplasm through unfamiliarity with its specific features. Although pertinent case reports, under whatever title, date back about sixty years, it is only in comparatively recent years that the serious clinical behavior of these tumors, the distinctive cytologic features leading to their identification, and the formidable problems entailed in their treatment have become subjects of common discussion. Among the papers in the American literature contributing materially to our understanding of synovial sarcomas have been those of Smith,[57] Knox,[39] De Santo, Tennant, and Rosahn,[15] Fisher,[20] Haagensen and Stout,[28] and Bennett.[4] The keen discussion by Knox[39] is particularly valuable for its pathologic insight, as well as its useful compilation and critical analysis of the older literature, as is also the article by Fisher.[20] Much valuable information was likewise elicited by Haagensen and Stout in a comprehensive survey of 104 cases, in which they attempted to analyze how the hitherto doleful results of treatment might be improved. Additional papers of value dealing with problems in therapy are those of Coley and Pierson,[12] Briggs,[7] Pack and Ariel,[53] and Tillotson, McDonald, and Janes,[62] among others.[45]

Clinical features
Age and sex incidence

Synovial sarcoma occurs in males more often than in females, but the differential is not great enough to be of much help in diagnosis. Also, it is observed most often in relatively young adults, although it is by no means unusual in adolescents or older adults and may, in fact, develop at almost any age.

Localization

With few exceptions, synovial sarcomas are encountered in the extremities, showing particular predilection for the lower extremity. The knee joint and the bursae in its vicinity account for a very considerable number. Thus, nearly half of the tumors surveyed by Haagensen and Stout developed in the knee region. The foot and ankle region is another relatively common site. In the upper extremity, the region of the hand and wrist constitutes a favorite site of origin, although occasional instances are observed in the elbow and shoulder regions. It seems to me that detailed statistical analysis that goes beyond these rough estimates suffers of necessity from the limitations of random sampling. Synovial sarcoma may sometimes be encountered in unusual sites, in the neck or in the sternoclavicular area, for example. It may be noted, also, that most synovial sarcomas do not arise in the synovial linings of joints, although a few undoubtedly do so and spread over the surface.

Nature and duration of clinical complaints

It has been observed repeatedly that synovial sarcomas tend to develop insidiously and that, rather paradoxically, despite their serious nature ultimately, several years may elapse before the patient is sufficiently concerned to seek surgical treatment. In the cases analyzed by Haagensen and Stout, for example, the mean duration of symptoms preoperatively was estimated at 2.6 years, while instances in which the patient was aware of a growth as long as four or five years are not at all uncommon. The presenting complaint is often that of a slowly enlarging swelling that is likely to be somewhat painful, especially on motion of the affected part. In some instances, a history of antecedent trauma may be elicited, but the significance of this appears rather doubtful. While these findings are likely to suggest the presence of a tumor, the possibility of synovial sarcoma specifically is usually not suspected at the outset. In the case of relatively deep-seated tumors in the knee region, particularly, the preoperative clinical impression may not be that of a neoplasm at all. The practical import of this in relation to surgical management is considered farther on.

Pathologic characteristics
Gross appearance

Synovial sarcoma often presents as a circumscribed tumor at the time of initial surgical exploration. Occasionally, it may already be widely infiltrating (e.g., in the sole of a foot) when first recognized. Also, when it develops within the synovial lining of a large joint such as the knee joint, as it sometimes does, it tends to spread diffusely over the articular capsule. The discrete growths are frequently comparatively small, measuring no more than 1 to 3 cm. in greatest dimension. The apparent encapsulation and limited size of such tumors are, of course, deceptive, and altogether their gross appearance is hardly calculated to convey an impression of potential seriousness. The neoplastic tissue, on section, may be grayish or more pink or yellow in color, and its consistency likewise varies, depending largely upon its mucin content and upon how fibrous its stroma happens to be. It should be noted also that some synovial sarcomas exhibit focal calcification and ossification (Fig. B-9), which may be roentgenographically discernible.[42] Another suggestive lead to their recognition is the presence commonly of small clefts or cystlike spaces within the tumor that contain viscid fluid. As indicated, however, the impression of synovial sarcoma is not often registered prior to microscopic examination, except perhaps as a shrewd surmise based largely upon the location of the tumor.

A synovial sarcoma that has been neglected or that has recurred after unsuccessful surgical treatment may become obviously aggressive. Specifically, it may invade the contiguous soft parts, extend into one or more of the adjacent bones, and eventually metastasize to the lungs and skeleton particularly. It is noteworthy, also, that the neoplasm exhibits a greater tendency to spread to regional lymph nodes than do most sarcomas of extremities[1,53] (a factor that must be taken into account in appropriate treatment).

Microscopic features

The distinctive features of synovial sarcomas and the variations in detail from case to case have been fully elaborated in a number of informative papers[4,28,37,62] and, for the sake of brevity, one may forego reiteration of detail. Suffice it to emphasize here that synovial sarcoma is characterized cytologically by the presence, in varying proportions, of two essential components: (1) a richly cellular, essentially spindle-cell stroma that frequently dominates the picture and that, in itself, is likely to create an impression of a primitive fibrosarcoma; and (2) random fields featuring peculiar clefts and/or glandlike structures lined by columnar or cuboidal cells, which may simulate epithelial lining cells (Figs. B-7 and B-8). As Haagensen and Stout have aptly remarked, the tumor is always composed of these two sharply contrasted tissue forms, one resembling fibrosarcoma, the other reproducing caricatures of synovial structures, and the two are

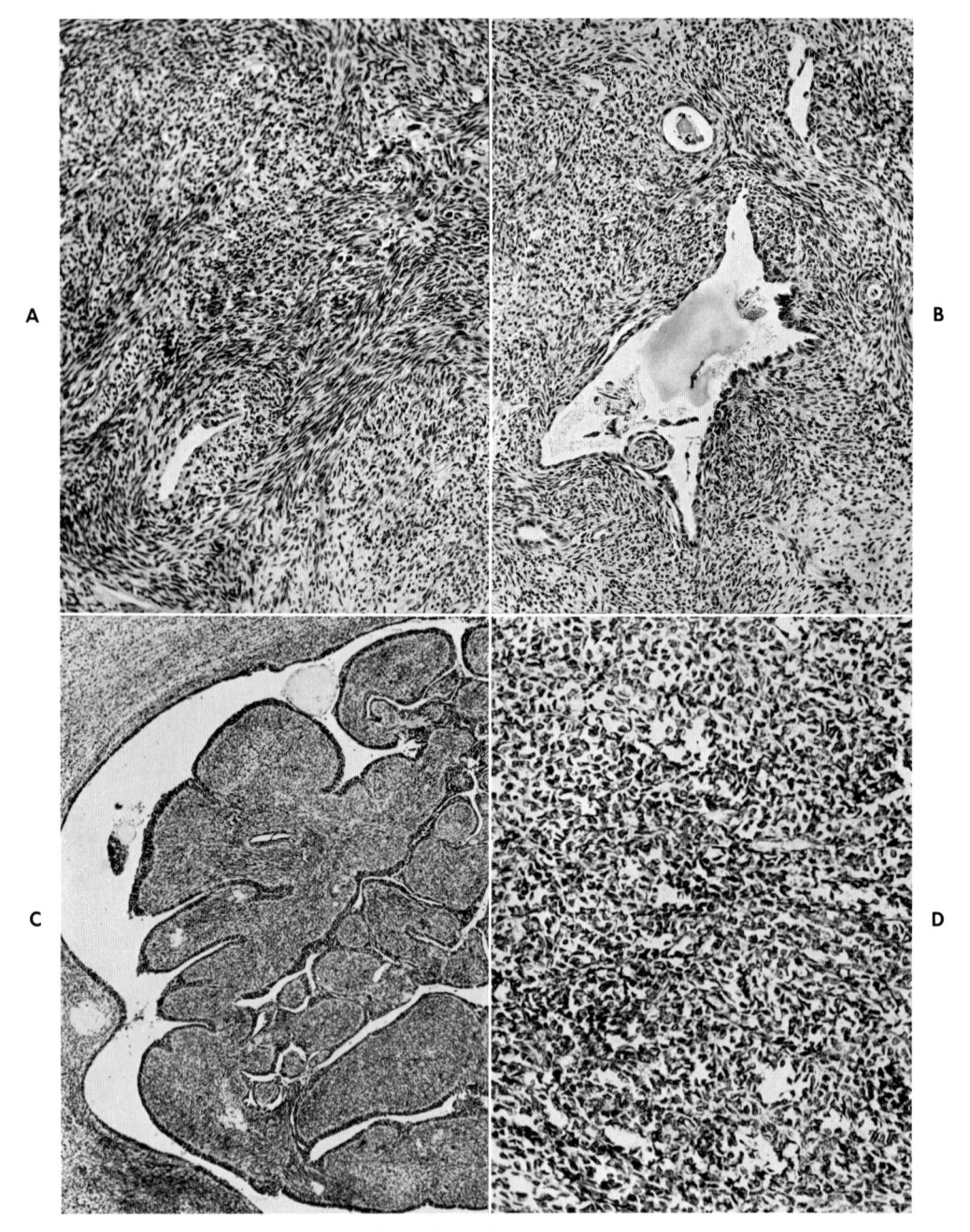

Fig. B-7. For legend see opposite page.

inextricably intermingled. When the specific synovial component is prominent, one can readily understand the old designation of adenosarcoma, and, by the same token, the diagnosis of synovial sarcoma should be fairly obvious to an observer familiar with the neoplasm (Fig. B-8). It is important to recognize, however, that fields showing telltale sinuous clefts and glandlike spaces may be so sparsely distributed as to require the examination of many tissue blocks for their detection. In such instances, an incisional biopsy specimen may well be inadequate for definitive diagnosis.

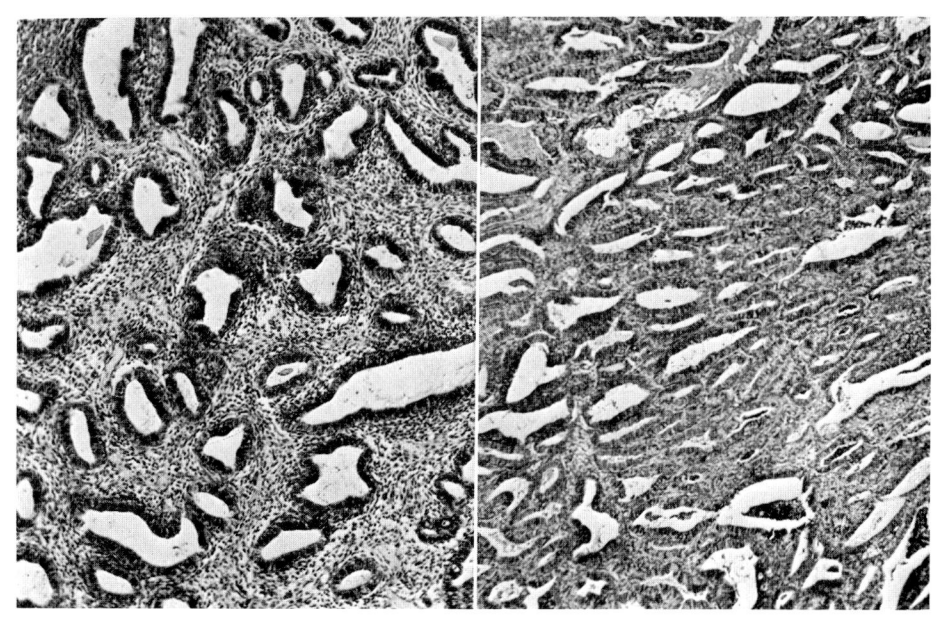

Fig. B-8. Selected fields of a synovial sarcoma situated in the ankle region of an 18-year-old boy, showing conspicuous pseudoglandular formation. Tumors such as this were formerly designated as adenosarcomas. At surgical exploration, this neoplasm was thought to be an organizing hematoma and, as such, was incised and curetted. (×84.) (From Lichtenstein, L.: Tumors of synovial joints, bursae, and tendon sheaths, Cancer 8:816, 1955.)

Fig. B-7. A, The cytologic pattern characterizing the major portion of a synovial sarcoma situated in the palm of a hand. From this picture alone of decussating bundles of spindle cells, one could venture an impression of sarcoma, though not necessarily of synovial sarcoma. (×110.) B, Another field of the tumor illustrated in A, showing the presence of smaller and larger spaces bordered by compacted tumor cells. The largest of these clefts also presents a telltale, whorled papillary tuft. Fields such as this are indicative of synovial sarcoma, but they were found only after many tissue blocks had been examined. (×110.) C, Still another random field of the synovial sarcoma of the hand illustrated in A and B, showing a comparatively large, invaginated tuft within a sinuous cleft. The tumor cells lining the spaces were compacted, flattened, and pseudoepithelial in appearance, as seen in higher magnification. (×80.) D, Cytologic pattern characterizing the major portion of another synovial sarcoma. (×190.) (From Lichtenstein, L.: Tumors of synovial joints, bursae, and tendon sheaths, Cancer 8:816, 1955.)

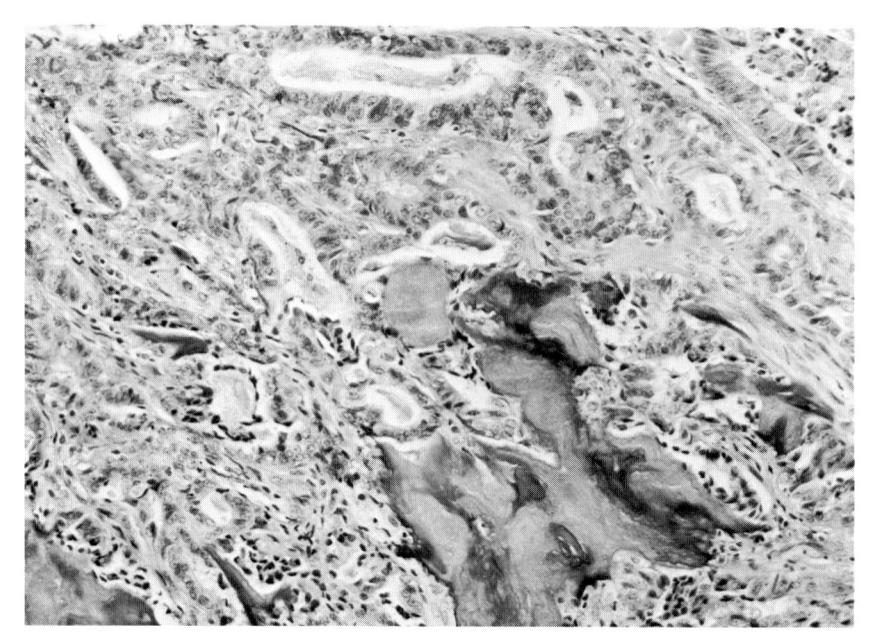

Fig. B-9. Photomicrograph of another synovial sarcoma showing pseudogland formation and extensive focal ossification (discernible roentgenographically.) (×160.)

Treatment and prognosis

As has been emphasized by many investigators, the results of treatment of synovial sarcoma to date have been discouraging on the whole, although it appears that some of the published cases were inadequately or injudiciously treated. Delay in recognition, lack of a concerted plan of attack, temporizing, and belated awareness of the seriousness of the tumor have all contributed to the picture of therapeutic failure. At present we are still striving for an effective approach to the situation. It must be frankly acknowledged, however, that the problem is inherently difficult, for we are dealing with a tumor whose behavior is treacherous and, in some respects, reminiscent of that of malignant melanoma. Despite the initial slow growth and circumscribed character of many synovial sarcomas, attempts at their surgical extirpation are followed in a high proportion of cases by local recurrence and extension and eventually by fatal dissemination, just as attempts to uproot an established bed of Oriental poppies may stimulate them to grow rampant through the garden like unrestrained weeds. Furthermore, synovial sarcoma may exhibit a dismaying persistence in spite of therapy and is capable of cropping up after a quiescent interval of as long as five or ten years or more, so that one hesitates to speak even of a ten-year cure. Still another handicap in planning a therapeutic program is the lack of substantial detailed information going beyond general impressions in regard to the precise manner and rate of spread of the neoplasm, whether by fascial planes, lymphatics, or venous channels.

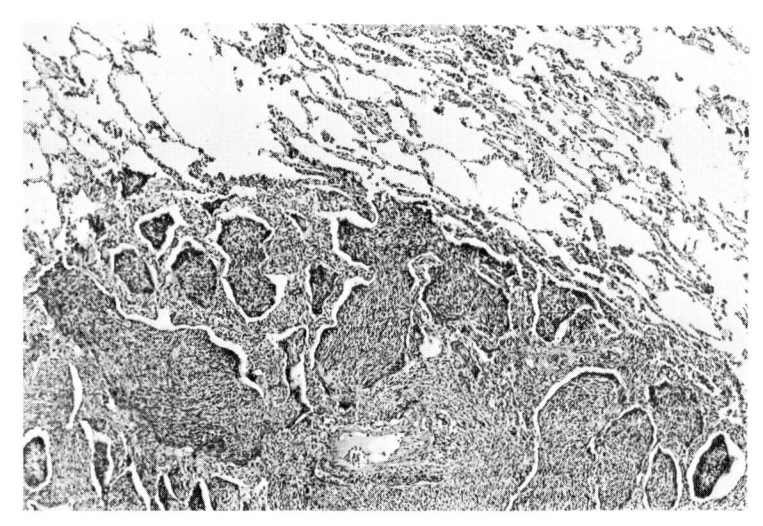

Fig. B-10. Photomicrograph of a metastatic focus of synovial sarcoma in the lung. The primary tumor developed in a leg, which had been amputated some months previously. Note that the neoplasm retains its distinctive architecture sufficiently well to permit ready recognition. (×48.)

It is small wonder, therefore, that the prevailing view in regard to prognosis, even under favorable auspices, is a somber one, brightened only by the consideration that the clinical course may be protracted over a period of several or many years. In fact, Haagensen and Stout were so pessimistic in their appraisal of the problem as to advocate immediate amputation as a routine procedure, even for synovial sarcomas that are relatively small and still circumscribed when first observed. Although fully recognizing the seriousness of the situation, I am inclined to regard this recommendation as a counsel of desperation, the necessity for which is far from proved at present. As a matter of fact, in a later paper (1959) on synovial sarcoma in children, Crocker and Stout[13] recommended a more conservative surgical approach. The remainder of this discussion will be devoted mainly to consideration of other, less drastic measures that appear to be well conceived in the light of experience to date and deserving of further clinical trial. Whether we shall have to be content ultimately with a survival rate perhaps no higher than 25%[53] because of the inherent nature of synovial sarcoma, or whether this can be increased under favorable auspices to a substantially higher estimate, can only be determined empirically. Somewhat encouraging is the review by Mackenzie[45] of some fifty-eight cases, in which the overall five-year survival rate was 51%.

It seems to be true, unfortunately, that the outcome in many instances is irrevocably prejudiced by the initial surgical approach to the presenting tumor (Fig. B-8), and, in this connection, the following suggestions may be advanced. In dealing with any tumor in the soft parts of the hand or foot or in the vicinity of the knee, elbow, and shoulder joints particularly, the possibility of synovial sarcoma should always be borne in mind, and it appears that even experienced surgeons may fail to anticipate this contingency. By the same token, in excising such tumors, one must scrupulously avoid crushing (with clamps or forceps), inadvertent incision, and especially blunt dissection. Needless to say, one should also strive for adequate clearance, and block excision would be advantageous, but this may not be feasible because of location. It was precisely because of the hazard of dissemination entailed in the injudicious removal of the primary growth that Haagensen and Stout advocated carefully performed incisional biopsy. While this recommendation may be well conceived theoretically, it seems to me to be unrealistic. For reasons already indicated, the likelihood is that section of a single sliver of tumor tissue selected at random would not provide an unequivocal diagnosis of synovial sarcoma, unless the pathologist were particularly fortunate as well as astute (Fig. B-7, *A*, *B*, and *C*).

The value of postoperative roentgen-ray irradiation of the tumor bed with a view to destroying any residual tumor nests that may be present at the periphery of the extirpated growth seems to be borne out clearly by our analysis[43] of the follow-up data available in the literature. While this view tends to controvert the much-repeated statement that roentgen-ray therapy for synovial sarcoma is of little avail, except perhaps for palliation, its validity is supported, on the other hand, by the clinical observations of Briggs[7] and of Pack and Ariel.[53] The time factor is important, however, and local irradiation should be started as soon as possible if it is to be effective. In view of the significantly high incidence of lymphatic extension, attention should also be directed promptly to the regional lymph nodes, both proximal and distal. Even if these are not palpably enlarged, the suggestion is ventured that prophylactic irradiation be employed for its possible benefit, and this should probably be pushed to the limit of skin tolerance. If enlarged regional lymph nodes are detected, surgical excision of the involved group may be preferred,[1] and, in this connection, one must consider the recommendation of Pack and Ariel[53] of dissection in continuity to encompass the intervening lymphatics, such as one might for extension of a malignant melanoma. In the face of a threat to the last effective barrier to uncontrollable dissemination, it would seem that one must accept the hazard of lymphedema of the affected extremity as a calculated risk.

The problem of coping with a tumor that recurs despite these therapeutic measures is formidable, though by no means hopeless. Needless to say, if it flourishes as a rapidly growing, frankly invasive neoplasm, one must have prompt recourse to amputation of the affected limb at an appropriate level, provided, of course, that the tumor has not already spread beyond bounds. In dealing with such aggressive tumors, the prognosis should be guarded, in spite of amputation. If, on the other hand, as in some observed cases, the recurrent growth is still discrete and relatively small, whether it be in the original surgical field or somewhat removed from it, one may resort again to meticulous excision, prompt supplementary roentgen-ray irradiation of the tumor bed, investigation of the regional lymph nodes if this has not already been done, and of course continued close follow-up. The question may be justifiably raised at this point of whether the patient is not placed in jeopardy by pursuing a conservative course for a recurrent malignant neoplasm. A recommendation of amputation under these circumstances would be justified, however, only if it offered a brighter prospect for cure, and thus far at least the recorded experience does not indicate convincingly that ablation of the affected limb is an attractive alternative.

In the event that a synovial sarcoma is already frankly invasive when first encountered, or if it is not amenable to surgical extirpation because of its bulk, because it is spread over a joint capsule, because it has already enveloped major vessels and nerves, or for whatever reason, one has no alternative but to resort to ablation of the affected part without undue delay (provided that there is no roentgen-ray evidence of metastasis). It seems worthwhile in such instances, if only to give the patient the benefit of every possible doubt, to supplement radical surgery with an attack on the regional lymph nodes, either by irradiation or surgical excision, whether or not these are obviously involved clinically.

In any event, in dealing with any particular instance, a note of distinct caution as to prognosis is in order, for synovial sarcomas, as indicated, have been known to metastasize after a latent period of as long as ten years or more.

References

1. Ackerman, L. V., and del Regato, J. A.: Cancer: diagnosis, treatment, and prognosis, St. Louis, 1971, The C. V. Mosby Co.
2. Arzimanoglu, A.: Bilateral arborescent lipoma of the knee, J. Bone Joint Surg. 39-A:976, 1957.
3. Bate, T. H.: Hemangioma of the tendon sheath, J. Bone Joint Surg. 36-A:104, 1954.
4. Bennett, G. A.: Malignant neoplasms originating in synovial tissues (synoviomata); a study of thirty-two specimens registered at the Army Institute of Pathology during the war-time period, 1941-1945, J. Bone Joint Surg. 29:259, 1947.
5. Bennett, G. E., and Cobey, M. C.: Hemangioma of joints; reports of five cases, Arch. Surg. 38:487, 1939.
6. Bliss, B. O., and Reed, R. J.: Large cell sarcomas of tendon sheath. Malignant giant cell tumors of tendon sheath, Am. J. Clin. Pathol. 49:776, 1968.
7. Briggs, C. D.: Malignant tumors of synovial origin, Ann. Surg. 115:413, 1942.
8. Burman, M. S., and Milgram, J. E.: Haemangiomas of tendon and tendon sheath, Surg. Gynecol. Obstet. 50:397, 1930.
9. Buxton, St. J. D.: Tumours of the tendon and tendon sheaths, Brit. J. Surg. 10:469, 1923.
10. Byers, P. D., Cotton, R. E., Deacon, O. W., Lowy, M., Newmau, P. H., Sissons, H. A., and Thomson, A. D.: The diagnosis and treatment of pigmented villonodular synovitis, J. Bone Joint Surg. 50-B: 290, 1968.
11. Cobey, M. C.: Hemangioma of joints, Arch. Surg. 46:465, 1943.
12. Coley, B. L., and Pierson, J. C.: Synovioma; report of fifteen cases with review of literature, Surgery 1:113, 1937.
13. Crocker, D. W., and Stout, A. P.: Synovial sarcoma in children, Cancer 12:1123, 1959.
14. Decker, J. P., and Owen, B. J.: An invasive giant-cell tumor of tendon sheath in the foot, Bull. Ayer. Clin. Lab. 4:43, 1954.
15. De Santo, D. A., Tennant, R., and Rosahn, P. D.: Synovial sarcomas in joints, bursae, and tendon sheaths; a clinical and pathological study of sixteen cases, Surg. Gynecol. Obstet. 72:951, 1941.
16. De Santo, D. A., and Wilson, P. D.: Xanthomatous tumors of joints, J. Bone Joint Surg. 21:531, 1939.
17. Enzinger, F. M.: Clear-cell sarcoma of tendons and aponeuroses. An analysis of 21 cases, Cancer 18:1163, 1965.
18. Faldini, G.: Linfo angio-endothelioma delle guaine tendinee, Chir. d. org. di movimento 12:417, 1928.
19. Fisher, A. G. T.: A study of loose bodies composed of cartilage or of cartilage and bone occurring in joints. With special reference to their pathology and etiology, Brit. J. Surg. 8:493, 1921.
20. Fisher, H. R.: Synovial sarcomesothelioma

(sarcoendothelioma), Am. J. Pathol. **18:** 529, 1942.
21. Fletcher, A. G., Jr., and Horn, R. C., Jr.: Giant cell tumors of tendon sheath origin; a consideration of bone involvement and report of two cases with extensive bone destruction, Ann. Surg. **133:**374, 1951.
22. Freund, E.: Chondromatosis of the joints, Arch. Surg. **34:**670, 1937.
23. Friedman, M., and Ginzler, A.: Xanthogranuloma of the knee joint; a report of two cases, Bull. Hosp. Joint Dis. **1:**17, 1940.
24. Geschickter, C. F., and Copeland, M. M.: Tumors of bone, ed. 3, Philadelphia, 1949, J. B. Lippincott Co., pp. 686, 706.
25. Goidanich, I. F., and Battaglia, L.: I Sarcomi Di Origiue Sinoviale, Chir. d. org. di movimento (Fasc. 5) **44:**235, 1957.
26. Goldman, R. L., and Lichtenstein, L.: Synovial chondrosarcoma, Cancer **17:**1233, 1964.
27. Gravanis, M. B.: Malignant giant-cell tumors of tendon sheath, Bull. Path. Am. Soc. Clin. Pathol., July, 1968, p. 130.
28. Haagensen, C. D., and Stout, A. P.: Synovial sarcoma, Ann. Surg. **120:**826, 1944.
29. Harkins, H. N.: Hemangioma of a tendon or tendon sheath; report of a case with a study of twenty-four cases from the literature, Arch. Surg. **34:**12, 1937.
30. Huguenin, R., and Oberling, C.: Lymphangiomes des tendons, Bull. cancer **20:**144, 1931.
31. Jaffe, H. L.: Tumors and tumorlike lesions. In Walters, W., editor: Lewis' Practice of surgery, vol. 3, Hagerstown, Md., 1954, W. F. Prior Co., Inc. (see chapter by Mayer, L., Surgery of tendons, pp. 98-100).
32. Jaffe, H. L., and Lichtenstein, L.: Synovial sarcoma (synovioma), Bull. Hosp. Joint Dis. **2:**3, 1941.
33. Jaffe, H. L., Lichtenstein, L., and Sutro, C. J.: Pigmented villonodular synovitis, bursitis and tenosynovitis; a discussion of the synovial and bursal equivalents of the tenosynovial lesion commonly denoted as xanthoma, xanthogranuloma, giant cell tumor or myeloplaxoma of the tendon sheath, with some consideration of this tendon sheath lesion itself, Arch. Pathol. **31:**731, 1941.
34. Jaffe, H. L., and Selin, G.: Tumors of bones and joints. In Ashford, M., editor: The musculoskeletal system: a symposium presented at the Twenty-Third Graduate Fortnight of the New York Academy of Medicine, October Ninth to Twentieth, 1950, New York, 1952, The Macmillan Co.
35. Janik, A.: Tumors of tendon sheaths, Ann. Surg. **85:**897, 1927.
36. King, E. S. J.: Concerning the pathology of tumours of tendon-sheaths, Brit. J. Surg. **18:**594, 1931.
37. King, E. S. J.: Tissue differentiation in malignant synovial tumors, J. Bone Joint Surg. **34-B:**97, 1952.
38. King, J. W., Spjut, H. J., Fechner, R. E., and Vanderpool, D. W.: Synovial chondrosarcoma of the knee joint, J. Bone Joint Surg. **49-A:**1389, 1967.
39. Knox, L. C.: Synovial sarcoma, Am. J. Cancer **28:**461, 1936.
40. Kobak, M. W., and Perlow, S.: Xanthomatous giant cell tumors arising in soft tissue; report of an instance of malignant growth, Arch. Surg. **59:**909, 1949.
41. Kubo, T.: Clear-cell sarcoma of patellar tendon studied by electron microscopy, Cancer **24:**948, 1969.
42. Lewis, R. W.: Roentgen recognition of synovioma, Am. J. Roentgenol. **44:**170, 1940.
43. Lichtenstein, L.: Tumors of synovial joints, bursae and tendon sheaths, Cancer **8:**816, 1955.
44. Lichtenstein, L.: Unreported data on file.
45. Mackenzie, D. H.: Synovial sarcoma. A review of 58 cases, Cancer **19:**169, 1966.
46. Mason, M. L.: Tumors of the hand, Surg. Gynecol. Obstet. **64:**129, 1937 (see Fig. 12 facing p. 129).
47. McMaster, P. E.: Pigmented villonodular synovitis with invasion of bone. Report of six cases, J. Bone Joint Surg. **42-A:**1170, 1960.
48. Morton, J. J.: Tumors of the tendon sheaths; their close biological relationship to tumors of the joints and bursae, Surg. Gynecol. Obstet. **59:**441, 1934.
49. Mullins, F., Berard, C. W., and Eisenberg, J. H.: Chondrosarcoma following synovial chondromatosis, Cancer **18:**1180, 1965.
50. Murray, M. R., Stout, A. P., and Pogogeff, I. A.: Synovial sarcoma and normal synovial tissue cultivated in vitro, Ann. Surg. **120:**843, 1944.
51. Mussey, R. D., Jr., and Henderson, M. S.: Osteochondromatosis, J. Bone Joint Surg. **31-A:**619, 1949.
52. Osgood, R. B.: Tuberculosis of the knee-joint. Angioma of the knee-joint, Surg. Clin. North Am. **1:**664, 1921 (see pp. 681-689).
53. Pack, G. T., and Ariel, I. M.: Synovial sar-

coma (malignant synovioma); a report of 60 cases, Surgery 28:1047, 1950.
54. Price, C. H. G., and Valentine, J. C.: Malignant giant-cell synovioma of phalanx, J. Clin. Pathol. 7:231, 1954.
55. Sabrazès, J., Grailly, R. De, and Gineste, G.: Les angiomes juxta-articulaires et articulaires. Deuxieme groupe. Les angiomes a la fois juxta-articulaires et articulaires, Gaz. hebd. d. sc. med. de Bordeaux 54:225, 1933.
56. Schajowicz, F., and Blumenfeld, I.: Pigmented villonodular synovitis of the wrist with penetration into bone, J. Bone Joint Surg. 50-B:312, 1968.
57. Smith, L. W.: Synoviomata, Am. J. Pathol. 3:355, 1927.
58. Stevens, J., Katz P. L., Archer, F. L., and McCarty, D. J.: Synovial hemangioma of the knee, Arthritis Rheum. 12:647, 1969.
59. Stewart, M. J.: Benign giant-cell synovioma and its relation to "xanthoma," J. Bone Joint Surg. 30-B:522, 1948.
60. Stout, A. P., and Verner, E. W.: Chondrosarcoma of the extraskeletal soft tissues, Cancer 6:581, 1953.
61. Strauss, A.: Lipoma of the tendon sheath; with report of a case and review of the literature, Surg. Gynecol. Obstet. 35:161, 1922.
62. Tillotson, J. F., McDonald, J. R., and Janes, J. M.: Synovial sarcomata, J. Bone Joint Surg. 33-A:459, 1951.
63. Valdoni, P.: Lipoma arborescente sistemico delle guaine tendinee delle mano e del piede, Chir. d. org. di movimento 15:509, 1931.
64. Weaver, J. B.: Hemangiomata of the lower extremities, with special reference to those of the knee-joint capsule and the phenomenon of spontaneous obliteration, J. Bone Joint Surg. 20:731, 1938.
65. Webster, G. V., and Geschickter, C. F.: Benign capillary hemangioma of digital flexor tendon sheath; case report, Ann. Surg. 122:444, 1945.
66. White, J. R.: Arborescent lipomata of tendon sheaths; a report of two cases, Surg. Gynecol. Obstet. 38:489, 1924.
67. Willis, R. A.: Pathology of tumours, ed. 2, St. Louis, 1953, The C. V. Mosby Co., pp. 694-696.
68. Wright, C. J. E.: Benign giant-cell synovioma; an investigation of 85 cases, Brit. J. Surg. 38:257, 1951.
69. Wright, C. J. E.: Malignant synovioma, J. Path. Bact. 64:585, 603, 1952.
70. Young, J. M., and Hudacek, A. G.: Experimental production of pigmented villonodular synovitis in dogs, Am. J. Pathol. 30:799, 811, 1954.

*Index**

A

Acid phosphatase (serum), 363
Adamantinoma, 14, **343-348**; *see also* Dermal inclusion tumors
   of jaw bone, 343
Adenocarcinoma, metastatic, 347
   microscopic pathology, *357*
Adrenal neuroblastoma, 267-268
Agnogenic myeloid metaplasia, 312
Albright's syndrome, 392
Albumin (serum), 291
Albuminuria, 294, 295
Alkaline phosphatase (serum), 219
   in metastatic carcinoma, 362
Alkeran, 305
Ameloblastoma, 343
Amyloidosis, 285, 296-298, *297*, 306
Aneurysmal bone cyst, 2, 63, 68, 138, 386, **399-401**
   gross pathology, *400, 401*
   location, 34
   malignant, 217
   microscopic pathology, *400*
   roentgenogram, *400*
Angioblastoma, 175, 343
Angioendothelioma, 175
Angiolipoblastoma, 332
Angiosarcoma, 14, 175
Anomaly, developmental, 9
Aponeurosis, clear-cell sarcoma of, 408-409
Azotemia, 295

B

Bence Jones proteinuria, 284, 289, 291-292, 296, 306
Benign tumors; *see* Tumors; specific diagnoses
Beryllium, 191
Biopsy, 1, 6; *see also* specific diagnoses
   desmoplastic reaction, 247
Bladder carcinoma, skeletal metastasis, 368
Bone abscess, chronic, roentgenogram, *271*

Bone aneurysm, malignant, 175
Bone cyst, 128, 386
   aneurysmal; *see* Aneurysmal bone cyst
   fibrosarcoma and, 250
   of humerus, 5
   location, 34
   roentgenogram, 5, *385*
   solitary unicameral, 34, 138
   subperiosteal, 372
Bone, new formation, 2
Breast carcinoma, 272
   castration in, 363
   7β, 17α-dimethyltestosterone, 365
   hormone therapy, 365
   hypercalcemia in, 362
   skeletal metastases, 355, *355-357*, 363
Bronchial carcinoma; *see* Lung carcinoma
Brown tumor, 135, 163, *403*
Bursae tumors, **407-431**
Bursitis, pigmented villonodular, 138, 407, **410, 413-417**

C

Calcium (serum), in metastatic carcinoma, 361
Callus, exuberant, 2, 391
Calusterone, 365
Calvarium
   hyperostoses of, 11
   metastatic carcinoma of, *353, 355, 356, 362, 364*
Carcinoma
   basal cell, 344
   colloid, of rectum, chondroma differentiation, 338
   direct extension, 352
   hematogenous dissemination, 352
   metastatic, 3, 5, 6, 13, **352-369**; *see also* specific primary and secondary sites
      aspiration biopsy in, 358-359
      autopsy findings, 354-355
      blood chemistry, 361-363
      calcium deposits, 361
      clinical findings, 352

---

*Page references to illustrations appear in italics. The more important references are in boldface.

Carcinoma—cont'd
  metastatic—cont'd
    Ewing's sarcoma differentiation, 257, 259, 262, 263, 270-272, 359
    hydroxyproline excretion, 354
    incidence, 352, 355
    location, 356, 358
    osteolytic versus osteoplastic, 359, *361*
    photoscanning in, 254
    plasma-cell myeloma differentiation, 359
    radiation therapy, 367
    roentgen appearance, 358-359
    roentgen survey, 352
    surgical eradication, 367
    therapy, 352, 367
Cartilage
  embryologic development, 71
  formation, 190
Cartilage tumors, 9-11, 29, 190
  benign, 35
  malignant changes, 192
Castration, serum acid phosphatase and, 363
Catecholamine excretion, 270
Chloroma, 313-314, *314*
Chondroblastic sarcoma, 71, **76-80**
  gross pathology, *78*
  location, 76
  low-grade, 10
  microscopic pathology, *77, 78, 80*
  multicentric, **80-82**, *81*
  roentgenogram, *76, 77, 79*
  surgery for, 76
Chondroblastoma, benign, 9-10, **45-56**, 70, 87, 138
  age incidence, 45, 55, 72
  atypical, 71-72, **82-84**, *83, 85*
  calcification in, 45, 48, 51, 55
  clinical complaints and features, 47-49
  differential diagnosis, 46-47
  evolutionary cycle, 51-53, *52*
  gross pathology, *46, 50*
  hemorrhagic extravasation, 51, 55
  location, 45-46, 55, 72
  malignant change, 7, 10, 54-55
  microscopic pathology, 51, *52, 53*
  multinuclear giant cells in, 51
  osseous transformation, 53
  pathology, 50-53
  prognosis, 53-55
  radiation therapy in, 54
  recurrence, 54
  roentgenogram, 45, *46-51*
  sex incidence, 45, 55, 72
  size, 47, 50
  surgery for, 53-54
  therapy, 53-55
Chondroid tumors, 10, **70-88**, *73, 81*
  age incidence, 74
  classification, 71
  location, 71, 72, 74
  malignant, 70, 71
  multicentric origin, 71, 75, 80-82, *81*
  poorly differentiated, 71, *73*, **74**

Chondroma, 420
  central, 29
  juxtacortical, 374
  periosteal, **372-375**, *373, 374*
    gross pathology, *374*
    microscopic pathology, *374*, 374, 375
    recurrence, 375
    roentgenogram, *373, 374*
    surgery for, 375
  surgery for, 339-340
Chondromyxoid fibroma, 10, 11, **57-69**, 70, 71, 72, 138
  age incidence, 58, 68
  atypical, **84, 86-87**, *87*
  clinical complaints and features, 58-62
  collagenization in, 66, 68
  differential diagnosis, 10, 57-58, 63, 66
  focal calcification, 72
  gross pathology, 57, *60*, 62-63
  hemorrhagic extravasation in, 66
  location, 34, 58-59, 68
  malignant change, 7, 10, 57, 67, 68
  microscopic pathology, 57, 63-67, *64, 65*, 84, 86
  multinuclear giant cells in, *65*, 66, 68
  prognosis, 67
  recurrence, 57, 67, 68
  reserve cells, 72
  roentgenograms, *58-62*, 68
    -pathology correlation, 62-63
  sex incidence, 58, 68
  size, 63
  surgery for, 67, 68
  treatment, 67, 68
Chondromyxoma, 35
Chondromyxosarcoma, 10
Chondro-osteosarcoma, 215
Chondrosarcoma, 36, 41, 46, 47, 54, 55, 57, 58, 66, 67, 68, 70, 84, 86, **190-214**, 384
  age incidence, 191, 193, 212
  beryllium compounds and, 191
  central, 9, 190, 191, 196, 198, *204*
    gross pathology, *207*
    history, 193-194
    microscopic pathology, *209, 210*
    postirradiation, 190
    pulmonary metastasis, 203-204
    roentgenogram, *202, 204-207, 210*
  chondroblastic, 71
  chordoma differentiation, 339
  clinical findings, 193-194, 196
  cure rate, 203
  differential diagnosis, 10
  Ewing's sarcoma differentiation, 262
  extension, 203-208
  juxtacortical, 378
  location, 29, 191, 193
  lymphatic spread, 208
  malignant change, 192
  mesenchymal, 71, **74-76**, *75*
  metastasis, 203-208
  microscopic pathology, 36, 192, 212-213
  in multiple exostosis, 27
  myxoid appearance, 10

Chondrosarcoma—cont'd
    osteogenic sarcoma differentiation, 191-192, 212, 215, 377, 378
    pathologic examination, 192
    periosteal, **377-378**, *378, 379*
    peripheral, 9, 17, 190, 191, 198-203, 212
        cartilage cap width in, 203
        gross pathology, *197, 199-201*
        history, 193
        microscopic pathology, *194, 197*
        in osteocartilaginous exostosis, 24, 25-28
        pathologic examination, 203
        recurrence, 202-203
        roentgenograms, *26, 27, 194, 197-202*
    pulmonary metastasis, 205, 208
    radiation therapy, 208
    radioactive sulfur therapy, 208, 211
    roentgenographic examination, 4, *37*, 143-144, 196
    sex incidence, 193
    surgery for, 190, 192, 202, 208, 211-212
    therapy, 2, 190, 192, 208, 211-212
    trauma and, 196
Chordoma, 14, **335-342**, *337-341*
    biopsy in, 336
    chondrosarcoma differentiation, 339
    clinical findings, 336
    colloid carcinoma of rectum differentiation, 338
    differential diagnosis, 338
    gross pathology, 336, *340, 341*
    location, 335
    metastasis in, 335-336
    microscopic pathology, 336, *337, 338*
    radiation therapy, 339, 341
    roentgenogram, 336, *337, 341*
    therapy, 339-340
"Clasmatocytoma," 317
Clinical management, **1-2**
Codman's tumor, 10
Consultation, 1-2
Cortical bone abscess, 89, 93, 101
Cortical defects, benign, 12, 122
Cyclophosphamide, 305
Cytoxan, 155, 305

D

Dermal inclusion tumors, 14, **343-348**
    differential diagnosis, 347
    gross pathology, 346, 347
    location, 343, 346
    metastasis, 344-345
    microscopic pathology, *346, 347*
    roentgenographic examination, *344-346*, 345-346
    surgery for, 347-348
    therapy, 347-348
    trauma in, 344, 345
Desmoid, periosteal, **371-372**, *371*
Desmoplastic fibroma, *130, 131*, 132
Desmoplastic reaction, 247
Diagnosis, 1-2, 5; *see also* specific diagnoses
Diaphyseal aclasis, 17
7β, 17α-dimethyltestosterone, 365
Dyschondroplasia, 42

E

Enchondroma, solitary, 9, **29-33**, *30*, 57, 62, 63, 68, 70, 180
    age incidence, 29, 43
    amitosis in, 35, 36, 43
    calcification in, 33-36, 43
    clinical features and history, 29-31, 43
    differential diagnosis, 34
    gross pathology, 34-35
    of humerus, 5
    location, 29, 42-43
    malignant change, 9, 36, 38, 43, 190, 193, 196, 198, 384
    microscopic pathology, *30*, 35
    ossification in, 33-36, 43
    pathology, 34-36
    preoperative irradiation, 38
    prognosis, 36, 38
    roentgenogram, 4, *30-34*, 43
    sex incidence, 29, 43
    surgery for, 36, 38, 43
    therapy, 36, 38, 43
    of vertebral column, 29
Enchondromatosis, skeletal, 9, **38-42**, *41, 42*, 190, 193, 198, *207*
    chondrosarcomatous changes, 41
    location, 40
    malignant change, 41
    microscopic pathology, *38, 209*
    multiple exostosis differentiation, 41-42
    with multiple hemangioma, 40, *42*
    roentgenogram, *39, 40, 207, 208*
Eosinophilic granuloma; *see* Histiocytosis X
Epiphyseal cartilage, anomalous, 53
Epithelioma, squamous cell, 347
Estrogen therapy, 365
    serum acid phosphatase and, 363
Ewing's sarcoma, 13, **256-276**
    age incidence, 259
    biopsy in, 256-257, 263, 264, 267
    blood examination in, 260
    chemotherapy for, 273, 275
    chondrosarcoma differentiation, 262
    clinical findings, 259-260
    differential diagnosis, 4, 256, 257, 259, 262
    eosinophilic granuloma differentiation, 263, 385-386
    fever in, 260
    glycogen content, 267
    gross pathology, *262, 263*, 264
    Hodgkin's disease differentiation, 272
    location, 259
    lymphosarcoma differentiation, 272
    malignant lymphoma differentiation, 257, 262, 263
    metastatic carcinoma differentiation, 257, 259, 262, 263, 270-272, 359
    metastatic neuroblastoma differentiation, 256, 257, *258*, 259, 263, 267-270
    microscopic pathology, 256-258, 264-267, *265, 266*
    multicentric origin, 13, 264, 273
    multiple myeloma differentiation, 257, 259

Ewing's sarcoma—cont'd
"onionpeel" effect, 261
osteogenic sarcoma differentiation, 262
osteolysis in, 262, 264
osteomyelitis differentiation, 2, *258, 269*, 385
pain in, 259-260
prognosis, 272-275
pulmonary metastasis, 256, *273*
radiation therapy, 190, 272-275
reticulin fibrils in, 267
reticulum-cell sarcoma differentiation, 256, 267, 317, 318, 323
roentgenogram, *3, 4*, 257, 261-264, *262, 263, 269, 273, 274*
metastatic bone lesions, 263-264
presenting bone lesion, 261-263
sex incidence, 259
skeletal involvement, differential diagnosis, 270-272
surgery for, 272, 274
therapy, 272-275
trauma in, 259
"Exostosis bursata," 24
Exostosis, hereditary multiple, 9, 17, *22*, 28, 190
chondrosarcoma and, 27
postirradiation, 25
roentgenogram, *23*
skeletal enchondromatosis differentiation, 41-42
Exostotic tumor, microscopic pathology, *388*

F

Fallout, radioactive, 232
Fat cells, tumor derivation, 14
Femur, metastatic carcinoma, roentgenogram, *360, 364*
Fibroblastoma, perineural, 188
Fibroma, 420
chondromyxoid; see Chondromyxoid fibroma
nonossifying, 121, 122, 133
nonosteogenic; see Nonosteogenic fibroma
ossifying, 115
Fibrosarcoma, 121, 132, 133, **244-255**
age incidence, 244
anaplastic, postirradiation, 162
biopsy, 247
bone cyst and, 250
central, 216
roentgen appearance, 4
therapy, 2
clinical complaints, 244, 246
differential diagnosis, 247
fibrous dysplasia and, 250
grading, 254
gross pathology, *246, 251, 253*
location, 244, 246
microscopic pathology, *245*, 249-251, 252-254
multicentric, 254
in osteocartilaginous exostosis, 26-27
osteogenic sarcoma differentiation, 216, 244
osteomyelitis and, 250
Paget's disease and, *248, 249*
parosteal, 244
periosteal, 370, 371, *376, 377*

Fibrosarcoma—cont'd
postirradiation, 248, *250*, 323, 386
prognosis, 254
radiation therapy, 254
roentgen diagnosis, 246
roentgenogram, 143-144, *245-248*
surgery for, 254
therapy, 254
Fibrous cortical defect, 121, 133, 137
Fibrous dysplasia, 11, 34, 63, 68, 128, **391-395**
benign osteoblastoma differentiation, 115
differential diagnosis, 387-388
fibrosarcoma and, 250
of humerus, 5
malignant change, 395
microscopic pathology, *390, 392, 393*
roentgenogram, *4, 390, 393*
Fibrous osteoma, 115
Fluoride, 305

G

Ganglion, 407, *408*
Ganglioneuroma, 13, 186, 270
Gastric carcinoma, skeletal metastasis, *359*
Gaucher's disease, *386*
Giant-cell reparative granuloma, 135, 138
Giant-cell tumorlike reaction, 135, *136*, 138
Giant-cell tumor (osteoclastoma), 12-13, 46, 56, 66, 68, 112, 119, 124, 128, **135-165**, *140*, 407, 413
age incidence, 138-139, 163
benign osteoblastoma differentiation, 115
benign, with pulmonary metastasis, 155
biopsy in, 158, 161
calcifying, 45, 55
cartilage-containing, 45
chondromatous, 66, 84, 137
clinical complaints and features, 138-143
definition, 137
differential diagnosis, 2, 4, 6, 135, 163, 386-387
enchondromatous, 72, 82, *83*
epiphyseal chondromatous, 45, 55
fibrosarcoma as, 248, 250
foam cells, 150
fracture in, 146
Grade I, *149*, 152, *153*, 155-156
Grade II, *140, 147, 149, 152, 153*, 156
Grade III, 151, 155, 156, 158
grading, 150-158, 163
gross pathology, 144-147, *145*
location, 34, 135, 139-142, 144
malignancy of, 151-153, *154*, 155, 156, 158
malignant change, 13
microscopic pathology, 137, 147-150, *149, 152-154*, 155
multinuclear cells, 135, 137, 148, 150, 163
in Paget's disease, 136, 141
prognosis, Grades I and II, 156
pulmonary metastasis, 136, 151, 155, *157*, 158
radiation and, 158, *161*
radiation therapy, 144, 146, 150, 161, 162
grading and, 155

Giant-cell tumor (osteoclastoma)—cont'd
  recurettement in, 162
  recurrence, 150-151, 153, 156, 162-163
  roentgenogram, 4, *136, 137, 139-143,* 144, *146, 148, 159-161*
  sex incidence, 138-139
  "soap bubble" appearance, 143
  surgery for, 144, 146, 150, 151, 158, 161, 162
  of tendon sheath, 416-417
  therapy, 12
    problems in, 158, 161-163
  variants, 9, 121, 135, 137-138, 163
"Giant osteoid osteoma," 12
Glomus; see Hemangiopericytoma
Granular-cell myoblastoma, malignant, 350
Granular-cell tumor, malignant, 250

H

Hemangioendothelioma, malignant, 14, **173-177**, 343
  incidence, 166
  microscopic pathology, 173, *174,* 175, *177, 178*
  multiple, 177
  radiation therapy, 177
  recurrent, 175
  roentgenogram, 175, *176,* 177, *178*
  surgery for, 177
  therapy, 177
Hemangioma, **166-173**, 175
  cavernous, 14
  incidence, 166
  of joints, **417-419**
  location, 166-168
  malignant change, 14, 175
  microscopic pathology, 168, *169,* 171, *174*
  multiple, with skeletal enchondromatosis, 40, 42
  plexiform, 14
  radiation therapy, 171, 177
  roentgenogram, 4, *167, 168,* 169, *170, 171, 172-173*
  "soap bubble" appearance, 172
  "sun ray" appearance, *168,* 171
  surgery for, 171
  therapy, 171
Hemangiomatosis, 166-167
Hemangiopericytoma (glomus), 14, **177-181**
  microscopic pathology, 178, 180, *181*
  pain in, 178, 180
  pulmonary metastasis, 180
  roentgenogram, 178, *180*
  surgery for, 178
Hematoma, ossifying, 2
Hematopoietic tissue, tumor derivation, 13
Hematopoietic tumors, skeletal manifestations, **311-329**
Histiocytosis X, 2, **395-399**
  classification, 399
  Ewing's sarcoma differentiation, 263, 385-386
  microscopic pathology, *396, 397*
  neuroblastoma differentiation, 386
  roentgenogram, *396-398*

Hodgkin's disease, 13, **323-328**
  biopsy in, 325
  Ewing's sarcoma differentiation, 272
  microscopic pathology, 327
  roentgen diagnosis, 324-325
  roentgenogram, *324-326*
Humerus, metastatic carcinoma, *353, 365, 366*
Hydroxyproline excretion, 354
Hypercalcemia, 289-291, 306
  microscopic pathology, *368*
  steroids in, 362
Hyperglobulinemia, 290-291
Hypernephroma, skeletal metastasis, *365, 366,* 367
Hyperostosis frontalis interna, 11
Hyperparathyroidism, 141, 386-387, 395, **401-404**
  brown tumors of, 135, 163
  microscopic pathology, *402, 403*
  plasma-cell myeloma differentiation, 289-290
  skeletal changes, roentgenogram, *402*
Hyperproteinemia, 289-291
Hyperuricemia, 292

I

Immunofluorescent antibody research, 238
Iodine, radioactive, 365

J

Joint, synovial; see Synovial joint tumors

K

Küntscher rod, 177

L

Leiomyosarcoma, 14, **349-350**
Letterer-Siwe disease, 395-399
Leukemia
  acute, 13, **312-314**
    myeloblastic, *314*
    "onionpeel" effect, 313
    roentgenogram, *313*
  chronic granulocytic, 311
  chronic lymphatic, roentgenogram, *315*
  chronic myeloid, 13, **311-312**, *312*
  plasma-cell, 280, 288-289, 306, 314
Lipoma, 14, **330-334**
  of joints, **419-420**
  parosteal, 375-376
  periosteal, 375-376
  roentgenogram, *331*
Lipomatosis, 330
Liposarcoma, 14, 15, **330-334**, *332, 333*
Lung carcinoma, 271-272
  hypercalcemia in, 361, *368*
  skeletal metastasis, 355
Lymphangioma, 14, 182, *182,* 419
Lymphangiomatosis, 167
Lymphoblastoma, follicular, 317

Lymphoma; *see also* specific diagnoses
  clasmatocytic, 318
  lymphoblastic, 13, 317
  lymphocytic, 13, 317
  malignant, 13
    Ewing's sarcoma differentiation, 257, 262, 263
    roentgenogram, *315*
Lymphosarcoma, 13, **315-317**
  Ewing's sarcoma differentiation, 272
  microscopic pathology, 315-316
  roentgenogram, *316,* 317

M

Maffucci's syndrome, 40, *42*
Malignant melanoma, skeletal metastasis, *353,* 355-356
Mandible, metastatic carcinoma, roentgenogram, *353*
Mastocytosis, 314
Medicolegal liability, 2
Melphalan, 305
Meningioma, 168
Mesenchymal chondrosarcoma; *see* Chondrosarcoma, mesenchymal
Mesenchymal connective tissue, tumor derivation, 13
Mesenchymoma, malignant, 15, 333, **350-351,** *351*
Mesothelioma, 421
Mesothorium, 231
Metaphyseal fibrous defect, 121
Monocytoma, 317, 318
Moore (metallic) prosthesis, 158
Multiple exostosis; *see* Exostosis, hereditary multiple
Multiple myeloma and apparently solitary myeloma, relationship of, 298-300, 306
Myelofibrosis, 311-312
Myeloma, 4, 144, 170
Myeloplaxoma, 413
Myositis ossificans, 2, *389,* 389-391
Myxoma, 10, 11, 35, 57, 66-67
Myxosarcoma, 10, 58, 66, 68, 86, 138

N

Needle biopsy, 1, 6; *see also* specific diagnoses
Nephritis, atypical, 294
Nerve tissue, tumor derivation, 13, **185-189**
Neurilemoma, 13, 185, 186-188, *187*
Neurinoma, 13, 186, 188
Neuroblastoma
  catecholamine excretion, 270
  eosinophilic granuloma differentiation, 386
  Ewing's sarcoma differentiation, 256, 257, *258,* 259, 263, 267-270
  metastasis, 13, 186
  microscopic pathology, *268,* 268-270
  roentgenogram, *258*
  with skeletal metastases, 267-270
Neurofibroma, 13, 185-186, *187*
  periosteal, **372**
  roentgenogram, 185, *186*

Neurofibromatosis, 185, 187, 188
  periosteal, **372**
Nitrogen mustard, 305
Nonchromaffin paraganglioma, malignant, 350
Nonneoplastic lesions, **384-406**
Nonosteoblastic connective tissue, tumor derivation, 12-13
Nonosteogenic fibroma, 12, **121-134,** 137
  age incidence, 125, 133
  clinical complaints and features, 125-128
  foam cells, 121, 124, 129, *130, 131*
  fracture and, 124-125, *125*
  gross pathology, 124, 128-129, 133
  hemosiderin in, 129, 131
  lipid in, 121, 129, *130,* 131
  location, 123, 125-126, 128, 133
  malignant change, 133
  in mass roentgenographic surveys, 122
  microscopic pathology, 12, 124, *129-131,* 129, 131, 132
  multinuclear giant cells in, 124, 129, *130, 131*
  multiple foci, 121, 124-125
  pathology, 128-132
  radiation therapy, 132-133
  roentgenogram, 4, *122-127,* 128, 133
  sex incidence, 125
  size, 128
  surgery for, 132, 133
  therapy, 132-133
Notochord
  embryology, 336
  tumor derivation, 14

O

Ollier's disease, 9, 40, 190, 198, *207-209; see also* Enchondromatosis, skeletal
Ossifying parosteal sarcoma, **240-242**
  biopsy in, 240
  pulmonary metastasis, 240
  recurrence, 250
  roentgenogram, *241*
  surgery for, 240
  therapy, 240
Osteoblastic connective tissue, tumor derivation, 11
Osteoblastoma, benign, 12, 99, **103-120**
  age incidence, 104, 119
  calcification in, 110, *114*
  clinical complaints and features, 104-110
  differential diagnosis, 112-115
  gross pathology, *109,* 110
  hemostasis in, 110
  location, 34, 104, 106
  malignant changes, 7, 12, 118-119
  microscopic pathology, 110, *111,* 112, *113, 114,* 119
  multicentric, 110, *114*
  multinuclear cells, 104
  pathology, 110-112
  prognosis, 117-118
  radiation therapy, 110, 117, 119
  roentgenogram, *105-109,* 110, 119
  sex incidence, 104

Osteoblastoma, benign—cont'd
  surgery for, 117, 119
  therapy, 117-118
Osteocartilaginous exostosis (osteochondroma), 9, 11, **17-28**
  age incidence, 17-18, 28
  bursae development, 24-25, *25*
  cartilage cap, *21, 22, 23, 24,* 25, 28
  cartilage resorption in, *20,* 23-24
  clinical complaints and features, 17-25
  fibrosarcoma in, 26-27
  gross pathology, *18,* 19, *21, 22*
  growth period, 23, 24, 28
  location, 17, 19, 28, 29
  malignant change, 190, 384
  marrow in, 23
  microscopic pathology, 23, *24*
  nerve compression in, 19
  pathology, 17, 19-25, 28
  peripheral chondrosarcoma and, 25-28, *26, 27*
  prognosis, 25
  roentgen examination in, 27
  roentgenogram, *19, 20,* 196
  sex incidence, 17-18
  size, 19, 21
  surgery for, 25, 27, 28
  therapy, 25-28
Osteochondroma; see Osteocartilaginous exostosis
Osteochondromatosis, 407, **409-410,** *410*
Osteochondrosarcoma, 215
Osteoclasts, 150
Osteogenic bone tumors, classification, 216
"Osteogenic disease," 9, 42
Osteogenic fibroma, 12, 103, 119
Osteogenic sarcoma, 12, 15, 46, 47, 103, 118, 119, **215-243,** *218,* 252, 386
  age incidence, 217
  benign osteoblastoma differentiation, 115
  biopsy in, 239
  blood chemistry, 219
  central (intramedullary), 233
  chondrosarcoma differentiation, 191-192, 212, 215, 377, 378
  clinical features, 217, 219
  cure rate, 204
  diagnostic criteria, 224
  differential diagnosis, 2, 4, 6, 9, 216-217, 237, 239, 388-389, 391
  Ewing's sarcoma differentiation, 262
  experimental production, 232
  familial incidence, 239
  fibrosarcoma differentiation, 216, 244
  gross pathology, *222-224*
  immunofluorescent antibody research, 238
  juxtacortical, 240, 380-382
  location, 219
  metastasis in, 228
  microscopic pathology, *223,* 224, *225-227,* 228
  multicentric foci, 230-233, *231, 232*
  myxoid fields, 10-11
  "onionpeel" effect, 217
  ossification in, 216, 220, 221
  in Paget's disease, 215, 217, 228-230, *229,* 233
  parosteal, 233, 240, 380-382

Osteogenic sarcoma—cont'd
  pathologic fracture in, 216, 219
  pathology, 220-221, 224, 228
  periosteal, *379,* 380-382, *381*
  postirradiation, 232-233
  prognosis, 233, 235, 237-239
  pulmonary metastasis, *227,* 228, *236,* 237, *238*
  radiation therapy, 239
  radium poisoning, 231-232
  recurrence, *234, 238,* 239
  roentgenogram, *3, 217, 218,* 219-220, *221, 234-236*
  sex incidence, 217
  surgery for, 233, 239
  telangiectatic, 217
  therapy, 233, 235, 237-239
  viral etiology, 238
Osteoid-osteoma, 11-12, **89-102,** 107, 110, 112, 114, 119
  age incidence, 90, 100
  clinical complaints, 90-91
  definition, 90
  diagnosis, 90-94
  etiology, 89, 97-98, 101
  evolution, 96-97
  giant, 98-99, 103-104, 114-115
  gross pathology, *92,* 94-95
  location, 90, 100
  microscopic pathology, 11, *94-97, 99*
  osteoblastic connective tissue derivation, 98, 100
  pain in, 90, 91, 100
  pathology, 94-99
  prognosis, 99-100
  radiation therapy, 100
  roentgen diagnosis, 92-94, 101
  roentgenogram, *91-98*
  size, 90, 100
  surgery for, 99-101
  treatment, 99-101
Osteoid tissue—forming tumor, 12, 103
Osteolytic phytosterols, 362
Osteoma, 11, 12
  gross pathology, *117*
  microscopic pathology, *116, 117*
  parosteal, 240
  roentgenogram, *116*
Osteomyelitis, 216
  Ewing's sarcoma differentiation, 2, 4, *269,* 385
  fibrosarcoma and, 250
  roentgenogram, *258*
  sclerosing nonsuppurative, 89, 94, 101
Osteoporosis circumscripta cranii, 387, 405
Osteosarcoma, 12, 118
Osteosclerosis, 311-312, *359, 361*
Overdiagnosis, 384-385

P

Paget's disease, 387
  calvarium in, 387, 405
  chondrosarcoma in, 190
  fibrosarcoma and, *248, 249*
  giant-cell tumor in, 136, 141

Paget's disease—cont'd
  monostotic, *404*, **404-405**
    osteogenic sarcoma in, 215, 217, 228-230, 233
    roentgenogram, *229*
Parosteal tumors, 376-377; *see also* specific diagnoses
Pathologic diagnosis, 2
Periosteal ossification, 2
Periosteum, bone tumors from, **370-383**; *see also* specific diagnoses
Phenylalanine mustard, 305
Phosphatase (serum)
  in metastatic carcinoma, 362
  in multiple myeloma, 290
Photoscanning, 354
Physaliphorous cells, 338
Phytosterols, osteolytic, 362
Plasma-cell leukemia, 280, 288-289, 306, 314
Plasma-cell myeloma (multiple myeloma), 13, **277-310**
  age incidence, 280, 307
  albuminuria in, 294-295
  amyloidosis and, 285, 296-298, *297*, 306
  ancestral cell, 278, 303-304
  atypical nephritis in, 294
  azotemia in, 295
  Bence Jones proteinuria in, 284, 289, 291-292, 296, 306
  biochemistry, 289-292
  biopsy in, 285, 289
  blood chemistry, 361
  calvarium in, 4, 5, 284, 286-287, 307
  cell maturation in, 302, 304, 306
  chemotherapy for, 305, 308
  clinical complaints and features, 280-284
  diagnosis, 284-285, 293, 306
  electrophoresis in, 277, 279, 306, 307
  Ewing's sarcoma differentiation, 257, 259
  extramedullary hemopoiesis, 294
  extraskeletal infiltration, 292-294
  genetic factor, 277
  gross pathology, 282
  as hematic neoplasm, 304
  hematology, 287-289, 306
  hypercalcemia in, 289-291, 306
  hyperglobulinemia in, 290-291
  hyperparathyroidism differentiation, 289-290
  hyperproteinemia in, 289-291
  immunoglobulin in, 277, 306
  incidence, 279
  laminectomy in, 305
  metastatic carcinoma differentiation, 359
  microscopic pathology, 279, 290, 301-304, *302*, *303*, 306-307
  pain in, 280, 281, 283
  pathologic examination, 301
  plasma-cell leukemia and, 288-289
  presenting skeletal lesions, 281, 283
  prognosis, 283-284, 307-308
  radiation therapy, 284, 305
  remission in, 284
  renal changes, 294-296, 306
  renal tubule proteinaceous casts in, *290*, 295-296

Plasma-cell myeloma (multiple myeloma)—cont'd
  roentgenogram, 4-5, *278*, *279*, *281*, *282*, *284*, *290*, 307
    skeletal alterations and, 285-287
  serum albumin in, 291
  serum phosphatase in, 290
  sex incidence, 280, 307
  solitary, *295*, 299
    relationship with multiple myeloma, 298-300, 306
  sternal puncture in, 285, *288*, *289*, 307
  subclassification, 279, 304
  therapy, 304-305, 308
  ultracentrifuge in, 277, 306
  uric acid in blood in, 292
  vertebral involvement, 286
Plasmacytoma, 301, 306
Prednisone, 305
Prognosis; *see also* specific diagnoses
  therapy and, 384
Prostatic carcinoma
  estrogen therapy, 365
  serum acid phosphatase in, 363
  serum alkaline phosphatase in, 362-363
  skeletal metastasis, 355, *358*, *362*, *363*
Pseudotumors, 370

R

Radioisotopes, in photoscanning, 354
Radiotherapy, 2, 6; *see also* specific diagnoses
  roentgen diagnosis and, 4
Radium poisoning, 231-232
Recklinghausen's neurofibromatosis, 185, 187, 188, 372
Renal carcinoma
  clear-cell, 175
  skeletal metastasis, 355, *365*, 367
Respiratory tract carcinoma, skeletal metastasis, gross pathology, *367*
Reticulomyeloma, 304
Reticulum-cell sarcoma, primary, 13, 316, **317-323**
  age incidence, 320
  biopsy in, 320
  clinical findings, 318
  Ewing's sarcoma differentiation, 256, 267, 317, 318, 323
  location, 320
  microscopic pathology, 317-318, *319*, *321*
  radiation therapy, 317, 320, *321*, *322*, 323
  roentgenogram, *318*, 320, *321*, *322*
  surgery for, 317, 320
  therapy, 2, 317, 320
Rhabdomyosarcoma, **350**
Rib, metastatic carcinoma, *357*, *361*
Roentgenograms; *see also* specific diagnoses
  "onionpeel" effect, 4
  perpendicular radiopaque striations, 3
  "soap bubble" effect, 4
  terminology, 5
  trabeculation, 5
  value of, 1, 2, **3-6**

Index

S

Sarcoma, 50, 58, 104
  alveolar soft-part, **350**
  angioblastic, 14
  chondroblastic; *see* Chondroblastic sarcoma
  clear-cell, 408-409
  differential diagnosis, 2, 413, 414
  giant-cell tumor and, 151, 156
  mesenchymal, 14
  neurogenic, 13, 188
  osteogenic; *see* Osteogenic sarcoma
  polymorphous cell, 317
  postirradiation, 2, 55, 133, 161-162, 341
  reticulum-cell; *see* Reticulum-cell sarcoma
  spindle-cell, 343
  synovial; *see* Synovial sarcoma
  telangiectatic, 175
Scapula, metastatic carcinoma, roentgenogram, *361*
Schüller-Christian disease, 395-399
Schwann cells, 13
Schwannoma, 13, 185, 186, 188-189, 372
Skeletal enchondromatosis; *see* Enchondromatosis, skeletal
Smooth muscle, tumor derivation, 14
Spine, metastatic carcinoma, *368*
Steroids, in hypercalcemia, 362
Subperiosteal fibrous cortical defect, 371
Surgery; *see also* specific diagnoses
  procedure of choice, 1
  radical, 2
  roentgen diagnosis and, 6
Sweat gland, adnexal skin tumor, 344
Sympathicoblastoma, 267
Symptomatology, 1
Synovial chondromatosis, 411
Synovial joint tumors, **407-431**
Synovial sarcoma, 343, 408, 414, **421-429**
  age incidence, 422
  clinical complaints and features, 422-423
  gross pathology, 423
  location, 422
  metastasis, microscopic pathology, *427*
  microscopic pathology, 421, 423-425, *424-426*
  prognosis, 426-429
  radiation therapy, 428

Synovial sarcoma—cont'd
  sex incidence, 422
  surgery for, 426-429
  therapy, 426-429
Synovioma, 414
Synovitis, pigmented villonodular, 138, 407, **410**, *412*, **413-417**
Syphilis, gumma, *387*, 391

T

Tendon, clear-cell sarcoma, 408-409
Tendon sheath tumor, **407-431**
Tenosynovitis, pigmented villonodular, 138, 407, **410**, *412*, **413-417**, *416*
Testis carcinoma, skeletal metastasis, 355
Therapy; *see also* specific diagnoses
  immediacy of, 2
  pathologic diagnosis and, 2
  prognosis and, 384
Thyroid carcinoma
  radioactive iodine in, 365
  skeletal metastasis, 355, 356, *364*
  thyroid extract in, 367
Tropical ulcer, 370
Tuberculosis, 3
Tumors, classification, **7-16**

U

Urticaria pigmentosa, 314

V

Vascular tissue, tumor derivation, 14
Vascular tumors in bone, **166-184**
Vertebra, metastatic carcinoma, *353*, *358*, 361, *361*
Viral oncogenesis, 238

W

Wilms' tumor, radiation therapy, 190

X

Xanthogranuloma, 121, *130*, 413
Xanthoma, 121, *130*, 131, 413